Handbook of
Family Violence

Handbook of
Family Violence

Edited by
VINCENT B. VAN HASSELT
University of California Irvine Medical Center
Orange, California

RANDALL L. MORRISON and
ALAN S. BELLACK
Medical College of Pennsylvania at EPPI
Philadelphia, Pennsylvania

and
MICHEL HERSEN
Western Psychiatric Institute and Clinic
Pittsburgh, Pennsylvania

Plenum Press • New York and London

Library of Congress Cataloging in Publication Data

Handbook of family violence.

Includes bibliographies and indexes.
1. Family violence — United States. I. Van Hasselt, Vincent B. [DNLM: 1. Family. 2.
Violence. HQ 809 H236]
HQ809.3.U5H35   1987   362.8′2   87-7204
ISBN 0-306-42648-X

© 1988 Plenum Press, New York
A Division of Plenum Publishing Corporation
233 Spring Street, New York, N.Y. 10013

Printed in the United States of America

To our parents

Contributors

Judith V. Becker
Sexual Behavior Clinic of the New York State Psychiatric Institute and Department of Clinical Psychology in Psychiatry of the College of Physicians and Surgeons, Columbia University, New York, New York

Alan S. Bellack
Department of Psychiatry, Medical College of Pennsylvania at the Eastern Pennsylvania Psychiatric Institute, Philadelphia, Pennsylvania

Carl A. Bersani
Department of Sociology, The University of Akron, Akron, Ohio

Connie L. Best
Department of Psychiatry and Behavioral Sciences, Medical University of South Carolina, Charleston, South Carolina

Angela Browne
Family Violence Laboratory, Horton Social Science Center, University of New Hampshire, Durham, New Hampshire

Huey-Tsyh Chen
Department of Sociology, The University of Akron, Akron, Ohio

Emily M. Coleman
Sex Offender Program, The Franklin County Mental Health Center, Franklin County, Massachusetts

Frank A. Elliott
Department of Neurology, Pennsylvania Hospital, University of Pennsylvania, Philadelphia, Pennsylvania

Anne Flitcraft
Department of Medicine, University of Connecticut, Farmington, Connecticut

Robert Geffner
Department of Psychology, University of Texas at Tyler, Tyler, Texas

Lisa Gleberman
Department of Psychology, University of Southern California, Los Angeles, California

Michel Hersen
Department of Psychiatry, Western Psychiatric Institute, University of Pittsburgh School of Medicine, Pittsburgh, Pennsylvania

Honore Hughes
Department of Psychology, University of Arkansas, Fayetteville, Arkansas

Theodore Jacob
Division of Child Development and Family Relations, University of Arizona, Tucson, Arizona

Kenneth E. Leonard
Research Institute on Alcoholism, Buffalo, New York

David Levinson
Operations Department, Human Relations Area Files, New Haven, Connecticut

Joseph S. Lucca
Department of Individual and Family Studies, Life and Health Sciences, University of Delaware, Newark, Delaware

Gayla Margolin
Department of Psychology, University of Southern California, Los Angeles, California

Susan V. McLeer
Department of Child Psychiatry, Medical College of Pennsylvania, Eastern Pennsylvania Psychiatric Institute, Philadelphia, Pennsylvania

Patricia L. Micklow
Judge, 96th District Court, Marquette County, Michigan

Randall L. Morrison
Department of Psychiatry, Medical College of Pennsylvania at the Eastern Pennsylvania Psychiatric Institute, Philadelphia, Pennsylvania

K. Daniel O'Leary
Department of Psychology, State University of New York, Stony Brook, New York

Mildred Daley Pagelow
Department of Sociology, California State University, Fullerton, California

Karl Pillemer
Family Research Laboratory, University of New Hampshire, Durham, New Hampshire

Alan Rosenbaum
Department of Psychiatry, University of Massachusetts Medical School, Worcester, Massachusetts

Andrea J. Sedlak
Westat Inc., Rockville, Maryland

Linda Gorin Sibner
Department of Psychology, University of Southern California, Los Angeles, California

Evan Stark
Department of Public Administration and Sociology, Rutgers University, Newark, New Jersey

Raymond H. Starr, Jr.
Department of Psychology, University of Maryland Baltimore County, Catonsville, Maryland

Suzanne K. Steinmetz
Department of Individual and Family Studies, Life and Health Sciences, University of Delaware, Newark, Delaware

J. Jill Suitor
Family Research Laboratory, University of New Hampshire, Durham, New Hampshire

Vincent B. Van Hasselt
Department of Psychiatry and Human Behavior, University of California Irvine Medical Center, Orange, California

David A. Wolfe
Department of Psychology, University of Western Ontario, London, Ontario, Canada

Vicky V. Wolfe
Department of Psychology, University of Western Ontario, London, Ontario, Canada

Preface

In the last decade there has been heightened clinical and investigative activity in the area of family violence. This, of course, is partly attributable to recent surveys showing a high incidence of family violence in the United States. For example, there are indications that nearly 30% of married women in this country are victims of physical abuse by spouses at some point in their marriage. Further, FBI statistics show that approximately 13% of all homicides are husband–wife killings. Moreover, it has been projected that such figures are likely to increase over the next several years.

Consistent with these trends, funding of family violence research by both federal and private agencies has increased. Indeed, federal agencies, such as the National Institute of Mental Health and the National Institute of Law Enforcement and Criminal Justice, have provided considerable support for work in this area. In addition, family violence, particularly wifebattering, child abuse, and sexual abuse of children has been the focus of media attention at the national level, and has generated intensive interest in both lay and professional publications. Moreover, there have been several recent governmental hearings and investigations regarding the prevalence of these problems.

Despite the fact that we still have much to learn about the victims and perpetrators of family violence, in recent years an increasingly large body of empirical data have been adduced about this issue. These data have appeared in disparate journals and books. That being the case, we and our editor at Plenum (Eliot Werner) felt that a *Handbook* now was warranted.

The *Handbook of Family Violence* is divided into four parts and includes 19 chapters. Part I (Introduction) consists of an overview of the field. In Part II (Theoretical Models) there are three chapters representing the psychoanalytic, social learning, and sociological perspectives. Part III (Forms of Family Violence) consists of eight chapters, ranging from the physical abuse of children, to marital rape, and to elder abuse. Chapters in this section present descriptions of the problems, epidemiological findings, assessment and treatment, case illustrations, current research status, ethical and legal issues, and future directions.

In Part IV (Special Issues) we have seven chapters: Violence among Intimates: An Epidemiological Review; Prevention of Wife Abuse; Neurological Factors; Alcohol, Alcoholism, and Family Violence; Domestic Abuse: The Pariah of the Legal System; Family Violence in Cross-Cultural Perspective; and Research Issues Concerning Family Violence.

Many people have contributed of their time and effort to bring this volume to fruition. First, we thank our gracious contributors for sharing their expertise with us. Second, we thank our technical assistants for their contributions: Mary Anne Frederick, Mary Jo Horgan, Florence Levito, Judith A. Kowalski, Jenifer McKelvy, Louise B. Moore, and Mary H. Newell. And finally, once again we thank our editor at Plenum, Eliot Werner, for agreeing about the timeliness of this project and for his willingness to tolerate the inevitable problems and delays.

Vincent B. Van Hasselt
Randall L. Morrison
Alan S. Bellack
Michel Hersen

Contents

III. FORMS OF FAMILY VIOLENCE

Handbook of
Family Violence

I
INTRODUCTION

1

Overview

VINCENT B. VAN HASSELT, RANDALL L. MORRISON,
ALAN S. BELLACK, and MICHEL HERSEN

PREVALENCE

The past decade has witnessed a dramatic increase in the scope and magnitude of clinical and investigative interest in family violence. Indeed, epidemiological, evaluation, and intervention efforts have encompassed a wide range of problems. Some of these include wife battering, physical and sexual abuse of children, incest, marital rape, and domestic homicide. More recently, elder or parent abuse and husband battering have been recognized as warranting attention as well. Heightened activity in this area is attributable to a number of factors. First, there is a growing awareness that violence in the home is a burgeoning public health problem. This has been evinced by research that has revealed alarmingly high prevalence rates of the various forms of violence and victimization. For example, epidemiological studies indicate that there were 929,310 documented cases of child abuse and neglect nationwide in 1982 (American Humane Association, 1984). This represents a 123% increase since 1976 and a 9% increase over 1981. With regard to spouse abuse, Steinmetz (1977a) estimated that out of the total married population of 47 million couples, 3.3 million wives and over a quarter of a million husbands are subjected to severe beatings from their spouses. Also, Federal Bureau of Investigation statistics show that as many as 13% of all homicides in the United States are husband–wife killings. And whereas husbands are responsible for substantially more violent acts, husbands and wives are relatively comparable in terms of committing domestic homicide (Gelles, 1972; Steinmetz, 1977b).

IMPACT

A second reason for the greater attention to family violence is the accumulation of clinical and research findings documenting the deleterious effects of this problem on its

---

VINCENT B. VAN HASSELT • Department of Psychiatry and Human Behavior, University of California Irvine Medical Center, Orange, CA 92668. **RANDALL L. MORRISON and ALAN S. BELLACK** • Department of Psychiatry, Medical College of Pennsylvania at the Eastern Pennsylvania Psychiatric Institute, Philadelphia, PA 19129. **MICHEL HERSEN** • Department of Psychiatry, Western Psychiatric Institute and Clinic, University of Pittsburgh School of Medicine, Pittsburgh, PA 15213.

3

victims. Illustrative of this point is a recent review by Browne and Finkelhor (1986) that examined initial and long-term effects of child sexual abuse. These investigators found a body of empirical data attesting to initial reactions of anxiety, depression, aggression, anger and hostility, and sexually inappropriate behavior in some portion of sexually abused children. Some consistent long-term difficulties were depression, self-destructive behavior, anxiety, and sexual maladjustment, to name a few. A similar overview of the clinical literature on consequences of physical abuse and neglect in children found consistent evidence of deficits in intellectual and academic functioning, as well as a variety of internalizing and externalizing disorders (e.g., depression, anxiety, aggressiveness, social withdrawal, conduct problems) in this population (Ammerman, Cassisi, Hersen, & Van Hasselt, 1986).

Numerous investigations also have clearly shown the physical and psychological toll exacted by wife battering. Many victims of this type of violence report such difficulties as somatic illness, depression (Gayford, 1975), suicide attempts, and drug or alcohol abuse (Stark, Flitcraft, & Frazier, 1983). The clinical literature is replete with descriptions of the severely damaging impact of other forms of family violence (e.g., incest, marital rape, elder abuse) on the physical, social, and emotional functioning of their victims.

SOCIAL AND LEGAL ACTIVISM

Another impetus for the expansion of direct services and the increased number of research endeavors in the area of family violence has been the widespread social and legal activism on behalf of the rights of victims. In particular. systematic lobbying and organizational activities by feminist groups and social welfare representatives have played a crucial role in heightening public and professional awareness of the extent and magnitude of family violence and in implementing steps to deal with the problem. For example, the plight of battered women was made known primarily as a result of actions by the women's movement, which also is responsible for the initial programs and service agencies (e.g., women's shelters and health centers, consciousness raising and support groups, women's law collectives, the National Organization for Women's Legal and Educational Defense Fund) for battered wives. An important study by Kalmuss and Straus (1983) has shown, in fact, that

> the level of feminist organization in a state is a significant determinant of the number of wife abuse services in that state. Moreover, the level of feminist organization is a more potent predictor of programs for battered women than is per capita income, political culture, individual feminist sentiment, or domestic violence legislation that allocates funds for services. (p. 372)

Kalmuss and Strauss (1983) also pointed out, however, that interest groups are unable to impact directly on policy and legislative initiatives: "Since they cannot pass legislation themselves, they must rely on lobbying, persuading, and pressuring policy makers" (p. 373). Fortunately, the tireless and concerted efforts of these groups have met with considerable success in achieving policy changes. By 1980, most states had enacted some form of domestic violence legislation. This included assignment of civil and/or criminal remedies for victims of family violence. For example, Act PC273D in California underscores the unacceptability of spouse abuse by making it a felony for an individual to hit and cause traumatic injury to his or her partner. Further, nearly half of the states in this country have passed laws that provide appropriations to domestic violence programs. Programs for the prevention and treatment of child abuse have been boosted substantially nationwide by the Child Abuse and Treatment Act. This bill has been beneficial in providing funding for research and demonstration projects designed to assess and remediate the problem. This piece of legislation also widens the traditional scope of child abuse programs by including victims involved in child pornography and infants with severe, life-threatening birth defects.

FUNDING AND DISSEMINATION

As part of the response to the large public outcry concerning the enormity and severity of family violence, increased state and federal funding of research and direct services has occurred in recent years. For example, the National Institute of Mental Health, National Institute of Law Enforcement and Criminal Justice, National Institute for Juvenile Justice and Delinquency Prevention, and the National Center on Child Abuse and Neglect are but a few of the federal agencies that have provided support for work in this area. This assistance has enabled investigators to garner information on the incidence of various forms of family violence, identify etiological factors, determine consequences, and develop prevention and treatment strategies for the various forms of violence in the home.

Further, dissemination of information and research findings to professionals and the general public has increased exponentially. Numerous governmental hearings and investigations on physical and sexual abuse of children and wife battering have been conducted over the past 5 years. In addition, dissemination of results of empirical studies has been carried out by professionals from a wide range of disciplines, including clinical and counseling psychology, sociology, psychology, psychiatry, public health, criminology, law, marital counseling, and social work. Most investigations are being published in the numerous professional journals (*Child Abuse and Neglect, Family Violence Bulletin, Journal of Family Violence, Journal of Interpersonal Violence, Violence and Victims, Victimology: An International Journal*) that have recently emerged as dissemination outlets specifically geared toward family violence research.

SCOPE OF THE HANDBOOK

Given the wide range of problems encompassed by family violence, coupled with the increased professional, public, and legislative attention it has received, we believe that the burgeoning information needed to be included under one cover in the form of a handbook. A sourcebook on family violence is, in our opinion, long overdue. In the present volume, we review the major developments in light of the theoretical perspectives, specific forms of family violence, and special issues relevant to the field. The book begins with chapters on each of the major theoretical orientations to family violence. Each of these chapters attempts to highlight the heuristic value of the different orientations for furthering both clinical and research endeavors. In Chapter 2, Susan McLeer provides a particularly thoughtful treatise regarding psychoanalytic perspectives on family violence. As many of our contributors elected to do in order to provide more detailed discussion, McLeer's chapter focuses on just one type of family violence: wife abuse. Applications of psychoanalytic theory to family violence have been the target of considerable criticism. McLeer's chapter helps the reader to understand controversial elements of the theory, and deals directly with some very difficult issues regarding the implications of the perspective.

In Chapter 3, K. Daniel O'Leary discusses social learning theory as it relates to family violence, and once again, devotes particular attention to spousal aggression. In Chapter 4, Carl Bersani and Huey-Tsyh Chen review sociological theories on family violence. As they demonstrate, "the sociological model" is more accurately a group of diverse sociological explanations for the phenomena of family violence. Here again, the issue of heuristic value receives particular consideration, as the authors conclude that theorizing and empirical research in family violence has been misaligned. One factor in this regard undoubtedly has been, as indicated earlier, the diversity of professions that have attempted to investigate the problem. Psychological, psychiatric, sociological, and legal perspectives have been emphasized in the literature on family violence. The research armamentarium, knowledge base, and interests of investigators from each of these camps have differed considerably. It is our hope that this book will serve to increase communication, understanding, and collaboration across clinicians and researchers from disparate orientations, and thus help to facilitate progress in the area. Alternatively, one must recognize that family violence is multiply determined. Any one theory can account for some, but not all, of the variance in the problem.

In Chapter 5, Gayla Margolin, Linda Gorin Sibner, and Lisa Gleberman review current knowledge on the topic of wife battering. The complexities of this literature are highlighted, beginning with a discussion of definitional issues. Assessment and treatment strategies are reviewed, including legal and education/community action alternatives to curtailing violence. (A more detailed account of prevention approaches is provided by Andrea Sedlak in Chapter 14.)

The next chapter (6), by Raymond Starr, provides an examination of similar issues as they apply to physical abuse of children. This chapter is, by design, limited to consideration of physical abuse. In many respects, the findings concerning physical abuse of children form the cornerstone of research and theory on family violence in general. More empirical data have been accrued on this problem than on any other form of family violence. Further, there are more reports available pertaining to treatment efficacy on this topic. Nevertheless, Starr's chapter concludes with a discussion of the many areas of uncertainty in the literature on child abuse, and the shortcomings of primary prevention efforts that have been carried out to date.

Physical abuse is but one type of violence that can occur within the home. Increasing attention recently has been focused on sexual violence and abuse within families. This problem takes three forms: child sexual abuse, incest, and marital rape. Perhaps as an outgrowth of the considerable clinical and investigative activity with physically abused children, child sexual abuse has received the most scrutiny. Child protection laws, which have resulted from widely publicized cases of child sexual abuses, also have brought child sexual abuse to the forefront. In Chapter 7, David Wolfe, Vicky Wolfe, and Connie Best discuss the impact of sexual abuse on child victims. Data regarding incidence and severity of child sexual abuse are presented. Common psychological sequelae in child victims are described, as are relevant assessment and treatment strategies.

Chapter 8, by Judith Becker and Emily Coleman, reviews the problem of incest. Here, characteristics of the perpetrators of intrafamily sexual abuse are described. Assessment measures for use with the offender are reviewed, and a cognitive-behavioral treatment package is outlined. Although intended specifically for use with perpetrators of incest, certain techniques that are covered may be appropriate for use with other sexual offenders, such as the husband who rapes his wife. However, as highlighted by Becker and Coleman, it is imperative to match the intervention strategy with the results of comprehensive assessment. This is necessary to provide an accurate focus on critical symptoms and/or dysfunctions exhibited by individuals in treatment for incestuous behavior.

In Chapter 9, Mildred Daley Pagelow reviews marital rape, which almost exclusively takes the form of wife rape. The complex issues surrounding marital exemptions in rape laws comprise a major portion of Pagelow's analysis. The role of economic pressures in keeping women in sexually abusive relationships is discussed. Other factors that may contribute to the incidence of marital rape also are offered, including the potential role of pornography. Issues in assessment and treatment of rape victims are considered, and comparisons and contrasts to the literature on nonmarital rape are provided.

Whereas child abuse and wife abuse have received the most clinical and investigative attention, and have been shown to be reaching epidemic proportions, other forms of abuse more recently have been reported to be occurring at disturbing rates. In Chapter 10, Suzanne Steinmetz and Joseph Lucca review the literature on husband battering. This problem frequently has been dismissed as inconsequential. However, the authors contend that husband abuse, like any form of violence within the family, is never insignificant. Although the imminent danger of any single attack against a husband by his wife may be minimal, the possibility of escalation, or counter-violence by the husband clearly exists.

A form of family violence that has been a topic of considerable media attention, but for which few empirical data are available, is elder abuse. The problem of battered elders is addressed in Chapter 11 by Karl Pillemer and J. Jill Suitor, who incorporate the gerontological literature on adult children–parent relationships and research on the quality of marital relationships in their analysis. These authors argue that beyond being a distinct phenomenon, elder abuse "can also be understood in part as an outgrowth of family conflict later in life."

In Chapter 12, Angela Browne reviews her findings on homicides committed by women involved in severely abusive relationships. Homicides between partners represent the most pernicious escalation of family violence. The FBI's Uniform Crime reports indicate that almost 20% of homicides occur within a family, and that about half of those involve a spouse killing his or her partner. Browne relates the occurrence of homicide by an abused woman to increasingly severe episodes of abuse within the context of that woman's perceptions of the potential danger and the survival alternatives available to her.

Epidemiological findings pertaining to domestic violence are reviewed in Chapter 13 by Evan Stark and Anne Flitcraft. The chapter examines the components and sequelae of domestic violence. In addition, it considers risk factors that could potentially be targeted for community interventions. Chapter 14 by Andrea Sedlak considers prevention issues in greater detail, and evaluates current knowledge regarding critical elements of primary, secondary, and tertiary prevention programs.

Although socioeconomic and cultural factors have been the focus of considerable study with regard to the etiology of family violence, neuropsychological and metabolic factors also have been implicated as possible causative variables. In Chapter 15, Frank Elliot provides a succinct overview of current data on these factors. Yet another disorder that may impact on the likelihood of family violence is alcoholism. Numerous investigators have cited alcohol use, or abuse, as a contributor to family violence. However, its precise role has yet to be determined. Kenneth Leonard and Theodore Jacob consider the multidimensional nature of alcoholism and alcohol use and their association with the similarly diverse problem of family violence in Chapter 16.

Family violence clearly is multifaceted, and multiply determined. Individual, familial, and societal-cultural variables must be taken into account in relation to both assessment and treatment. A highly relevant societal factor is the legal system. Treatment responses to family violence cannot be isolated from the backdrop of significant legal issues specific to this area. Indeed, offenders often are court referred for intervention. In Chapter 17, Patricia Micklow traces the history of the legal perspective on domestic violence and discusses current legislative initiatives enacted to deal with the problem. A number of critical legal issues are reviewed and future directions for legislative efforts are considered.

There has been much controversy surrounding the influence of cultural variables on the incidence and patterns of family violence. In Chapter 18, David Levinson examines cross-cultural data bearing on this issue, and presents findings from a study of 90 societies. Factors relating to family sexual types, (in)equality, and social organizations are described and their potential impact on family violence rates is discussed.

The book concludes with a chapter (19) on research issues, by Robert Geffner, Alan Rosenbaum, and Honore Hughes. Following an overview of conceptual and methodological issues in family violence research and treatment, these authors provide specific recommendations for future investigative strategies.

We trust that the information and recommendations presented throughout our handbook will stimulate additional clinical and research endeavors in this relatively new field of study. Further, we expect that the *Handbook of Family Violence* will be beneficial to practitioners, researchers, educators, legislators, public health officials, and students alike.

REFERENCES

American Humane Association. (1984). *Highlight of official child neglect and abuse reporting 1982.* Denver, CO: Author.

Ammerman, R. T., Cassisi, J. E., Hersen, M., & Van Hasselt, V. B. (1986). Consequences of physical abuse and neglect in children. *Clinical Psychology Review, 6,* 291–310.

Browne, A., & Finkelhor, D. (1986). Impact of child sexual abuse: A review of the research. *Psychological Bulletin, 99,* 66–77.

Gayford, J. J. (1975). Wife battering: A preliminary survey of 100 cases. *British Medical Journal, 1,* 194–197.

Gelles, R. J. (1972). *The violent home: A study of physical aggression between husbands and wives.* Beverly Hills, CA: Sage Publications.

Kalmuss, D. S., & Straus, M. A. (1983). Feminist, political, and economic determinants of wife abuse services. In D. Finkelhor, R. J. Gelles, G. T. Hotaling, & M. A. Straus (Eds.), *The dark side of families* (pp. 363–396). Beverly Hills, CA: Sage Publications.

Stark, E., Flitcraft, A., & Frazier, W. (1983). Medicine and patriarchal violence: The social construction of a "private" event. In V. Navaro (Ed.), *Women and health: the politics of sex in medicine* (Vol. 4, pp. 277–209). New York: Baywood.

Steinmetz, S. K. (1977a). *The cycle of violence: Assertive, aggressive and abusive family interaction.* New York: Praeger.

Steinmetz, S. K. (1977b). Wife beating, husband beating: A comparison of the use of physical violence between spouses to resolve marital fights. In M. Roy (Ed.), *Battered women: A psychosociological study of domestic violence* (pp. 63–71). New York: Van Nostrand Reinhold.

II
THEORETICAL MODELS

2

Psychoanalytic Perspectives on Family Violence

SUSAN V. McLEER

INTRODUCTION

"La Théorie, c'est bon, mais ça n'empêche pas d'exister."

Charcot, cited in Freud (1893)

On the occasion of the death of J. M. Charcot, Sigmund Freud wrote an essay eulogizing this great French neurologist (Freud, 1893). He reported that Charcot was heard to say that, "the greatest satisfaction man can experience is to see something new, that is, to recognize it as new." Charcot wondered how it happened that, in the practice of medicine, men could only see what they had already been taught to see. Throughout his life he remained open to new experiences; he acknowledged the need to order these experiences into a frame of reference, a theoretical formulation if you will, in order to enhance understanding and predictability. He valued theoretical medicine, but felt it was essential that one not be blinded by theoretical limitations. One day, when challenged by a group of students regarding the apparent conflict between a clinical innovation and the theoretical formulations of Young-Helmholtz, he replied, "La Théorie, c'est bon, mais ça n'empêche pas d'exister." And so it is, with Monsieur Charcot's words alive in our minds, that we dare approach phenomena as complex as family violence from a psychoanalytic perspective.

In the United States, violent crime occurs more frequently in the home than outside. Violence perpetrated amongst family members is more common than violence amongst strangers. (Borland, 1976; Dobash & Dobash, 1978; 1979; Freeman, 1979; Martin, 1976; Walker, 1979). Definitions of what constitutes violent behavior varies; reliable statistics are elusive. Three major types of clinical data are available for providing estimates regarding the prevalence of family violence in the United States. These include (a) national and state statistics of officially reported events; (b) interview data drawn from specifically identified subpopulation groups; and (c) studies utilizing random samplings of

SUSAN V. McLEER • Department of Child Psychiatry, Medical College of Pennsylvania, Eastern Pennsylvania Psychiatric Institute, Philadelphia, PA 19129.

11

the national population. Each of these techniques provides technical problems that investigators view as limiting. These specific limitations will be discussed as we present individual studies.

In this book, five major types of family violence have been identified: child physical abuse, child sexual abuse, spouse abuse, marital rape, and parent abuse. A brief review of the extent and severity of each of these forms of violence is in order.

Child Physical Abuse

Issues relating to definition immediately arise when discussing child physical abuse. For official reporting purposes, both instances of neglect and physical abuse, are frequently pooled together. Although this chapter will focus on violence, i.e., physical attacks on children, it should be noted that the majority of abuse cases do not involve battering, but neglect and/or emotional abuse.

> The so-called battered child syndrome is only the very final expression of child rejection. It is not necessary to beat or physically injure a child to abuse him, nor is physical abuse the sole or only form of rejection from the family unit that can be practiced. In battering, we are looking at the most extreme, and to society most violent, (but by no means the only) form of abuse. (Briggs, 1979, p. 4)

Whereas there is a spectrum of abusive behavior directed toward children, experts believe that there are distinct differences in the etiology, mode of transmission, perpetration, and clinical outcome of cases involving child neglect versus child physical abuse (Gil, 1970, Giovannoni & Becerra, 1979; Maden & Wrench, 1977; Steele & Pollack, 1974; Young, 1964). This distinction is important in developing policies and procedures for case identification and treatment programs. David Gil, in his nationwide survey of all reported cases of child physical abuse during 1967 and 1968, defined physical abuse as,

> the intentional, non-accidental use of physical force, or intentional and non-accidental acts of omission, on the part of a parent or other caretaker interacting with a child in his care, aimed at hurting, injuring, or destroying that child. (Gil, 1970)

In reviewing his data, he screened out 3,570 cases because they did not fit the criteria of intentional and nonaccidental acts. Approximately half of these cases were cases of child neglect. The physical abuse of one's child is not something that a parent is proud of, nor is it something that one readily admits to having done. Hence, case identification is difficult. With the advent of laws mandating the reporting of suspected abuse cases and with health professionals, teachers, and those professionals in areas providing human services maintaining a high index of suspicion for child abuse, reported cases have soared. Various national estimates ranging from 60,000 (Helfer & Kempe, 1968), 250,000 (Nagi, 1975), 500,000 (Light, 1974) to 1.5 million cases per year (Fontana, 1973; Gelles, 1979) have been offered by clinicians and researchers in the field. Again, these statistics are apt to include child physical abuse and neglect. The National Center on Child Abuse conservatively estimates that (a) one million children are abused or neglected each year; (b) 100,000 to 200,000 of these children are victims of physical abuse; (c) 60,000 to 100,000 are sexually abused, whereas the rest are neglected; (d) 2,000 children die each year because of abuse or neglect (cited in the *Child Abuse Prevention Handbook,* California Department of Justice, 1982).

The problem with statistics derived from officially reported cases is that the system for reporting results reflects a sampling bias based on socioeconomic factors. Likewise, not all cases are substantiated nor clearly defined with regard to whether physical abuse and/or neglect is present.

Straus, Gelles, and Steinmetz (1980) published the only major national study that did not rely on officially reported statistics. The research team interviewed 1,146 parents chosen by random sampling, throughout the United States. Each parent had at least one child living at home who was between the ages of 3 and 17. Violent episodes were categorized according to the Conflict Tactic Scale (CTS). (See Table 1.)

When a parent was asked about her/his behavior toward a randomly selected child in the family, 73% of the parents interviewed admitted to at least one occurence where some form of violence was used against the child. When the violent episode was limited to "severe violence" (kicked, bit, hit with fist, hit with something, beat up, threatened with knife and gun, used knife or gun), 3.6% of the parents interviewed gave a positive history. Gelles (1979), utilizing this data and extrapolating to the United States population of children between 3 and 17 years old, estimated that "between 1.4 million and 1.9 million children were vulnerable to physical injury from violence in 1975." Five major technical problems can be identified that affect the interpretation of Straus' data: (a) some of the questions asked of the families were open to interpretation, for example "beat up." (b) No questions were asked regarding children under the age of three. Nonetheless, we know that there are many abused children under three years of age. (c) Only one parent was interviewed regarding her/his behavior. Abuse could have been occuring in the other parent child dyad. (d) No single parent families were interviewed. These are families that often times have an even higher incidence of child physical abuse. (e) There was a refusal rate in the study; that is, 35% of the people refused to participate. This is not an insignificant subsample of the population. One could speculate that this subsample might well have a higher incidence of family violence than the study population.

In reviewing some of the studies on the prevalance of child physical abuse in the United States, we have examined some of the methodological problems inherent in the interpretation of the data. For the sake of brevity, the same discussion will not be elaborated in detail when examining estimates of other forms of family violence. Suffice it to say that all the data suffers from limitations imposed by sampling errors, inconsistencies in reporting events out of fear of public exposure, family disruption and legal ramifications, interpretation of interview questions, and varying definitions of what constitutes abuse.

Table 1. Conflict Tactic Scale

K. Throwing things at the spouse
L. Pushing, shoving, or grabbing
M. Slapping
N. Kicking, biting, or hitting with the fist
O. Hitting or trying to hit with something
P. Beating up
Q. Threatening with a knife of gun
R. Using a knife or gun

Note. From *Causes, Treatment, and Research Needs: Battered Women, Issues of Public Policy*, M. A. Straus, 1978. Washington, DC: U.S. Commission on Civil Rights.

Spouse Abuse

Returning to Straus's study of family violence (1978), one finds that of the 2,143 couples interviewed, 3.8% of the women had been the victims of violent physical attack (defined by the Conflict Tactic Scale, CTS, items N–R). Applying the 3.8% rate to the 47 million couples in the United States, one can extrapolate to 1.78 million wives being beaten by their husbands. The median frequency of such assaults were found to be 2.4 per year. A quick calculation shows that if one assumes an even distribution over time, (which one really cannot do, but in doing so one is provided with interesting comparison statistics), a woman is beaten every 7.4 seconds in the United States (McLeer, 1981). Straus's data additionally demonstrated a 4.6% incidence for violent physical attack (CTS N–R) perpetrated by women against men. The median frequency was 3.0 attacks. This data are misleading in that the question as to what percentage of violent acts by women were in response to blows initiated by husbands was not raised in the study. Furthermore, the strength differential of men and the fact that men are apt to use a more violent means of attack (Straus, 1978) results in a greater morbidity for women; it additionally has been demonstrated by other researchers that the intensity and frequency of violent attacks directed toward women within the marital dyad escalates in intensity and frequency over time. (Dobash & Dobash, 1979; Pagelow, 1981, Straus *et al.*, 1980). When violence escalates to the point of homicide, men and women are both at high risk. Of all murders, 25% occur in families; 50% of these are husband–wife killings. In these cases, husbands are the victims almost as often as wives: 48% versus 52% (Federal Bureau of Investigation, 1973). The data on homicides indicate that when a woman kills, it frequently is an act of self defense (Bende, 1980).

Parent Assault

The assault of elderly parents by adult children is a new area of investigation and good data are not available. Researchers believe underreporting of this form of family violence to be the worst yet. According to King (1983), ''Unlike children who are in regular contact with teachers, doctors, and other adults, infirmed elders are less likely to be noticed by those who might be alert to symptoms of abuse.''

King (1983) estimates that 500,000 elderly citizens are abused each year. The United States Committee on Aging, on the basis of actually reported cases, estimates a 4% incidence of parent abuse (United States Department of Health and Human Services, 1980). This estimate is consistent with the study of abuse of elderly citizens in the community done by Block & Sinnott (1979). If these estimates are correct, we could be talking about 900,000 to one million elderly citizens being the victims of physical abuse per year in the United States.

Sexual Abuse

Child sexual abuse and marital rape clearly constitute another expression of violence within the family system. Child sexual abuse is estimated at 80,000 to 250,000 occurrences per year (Sarafino, 1979). Seventy-five percent to 80% of the cases involve a parent or guardian (Nakashima & Zakus, 1979). Another way of looking at the same phenomena is with the data from Finkelhor's study (1981), where he estimates that 15% to 30% of all American women and 5% to 10% of all American men have been sexually victimized as children.

There is only one study that looks at a representative sample of women who were asked about rape and attempted rape within the marital dyad (Russell, 1982). Out of 644 women who had ever been married, 89 (14%) reported rape or attempted rape. This finding may be an underestimate because many women might not see a sexual encounter as rape but rather as a duty. Extrapolating to the United States population of 48 million married women, almost 8 million women are at risk for marital rape.

Family violence is a serious and common phenomenon. The morbidity is great, not only in terms of the physical injuries incurred, but also with regard to its contribution to emotional and social dysfunction. Those of us who work in the field and recognize the consequences of unremitting violence in the family, identify four overriding goals in the development of public health policies and procedures: (a) to protect the victim against further harm and/or death; (b) to interrupt the immediate cycle of violence; (c) to aid in the repair of damage and restoration of function for the victim and for the perpetrator of the violence; and (d) to prevent the perpetuation of violence in future generations.

In addressing the issue of a psychoanalytic perspective on family violence, one has to consider the domain attributed to psychoanalysis and psychoanalytic thought. Does a psychoanalytic perspective aid us in developing policies and procedures necessary to realizing our treatment goals? Has psychoanalysis aided us in identifying families at risk, in unraveling the complex phenomena contributing to the perpetuation of violence in the family, in developing rapid and effective treatment techniques that can be utilized by the vast numbers of people in need of help, and in developing methods for preventing the perpetuation of violence in future generations? What role has psychoanalytic thought played in the advancement of knowledge and application of that knowledge, by way of the skills possessed, by those who care for violent families?

In addition to examining the strengths and limitations of the application of psychoanalytic theory and technique to phenomena as complex as family violence, we will examine the child abuse literature, starting with the early classic papers that define the Battered Child Syndrome in 1967. This survey of the literature shall be used as a prototype for describing the developmental unfolding of knowledge, skills, and attitudes within the field. One of my hypotheses is that a literature develops according to a specific sequencing in the percentage of certain kinds of publications found during a specific period time. The hypothesized sequencing is as follows:

1. Descriptive, uncontrolled studies (D.U.C.) of the identified problem
2. Publication of uncontrolled interventions (I.U.C.) strategies
3. Publication of controlled empirical studies of both the identified problem (P.C.E.) and of interventions (I.C.); articles relating to controlled studies of the identified problem preceding the controlled intervention studies

Following the documentation of these specific developmental phases in literature, we will do a content analysis regarding the contribution of psychoanalytic theory and technique to the refinement of the knowledge, skills, and attitudes in the field of child abuse.

Professional experiences with child abuse, child sexual abuse, marital rape, and parent abuse have been more limited. The literature on spouse abuse emerged in the mid-1970s. Child sexual abuse came into prominence even later. Studies regarding marital rape and parent abuse are an even more recent phenomenon. Hence, the passage of time coupled with an analysis of the developmental sequencing of the literature regarding these other forms of family violence will be necessary in order to confirm the generalizability of the proposed model in the child abuse literature.

Psychoanalytic Tenets in the Family Violence Literature

In reviewing the past 18 years of the child abuse literature, the author utilized the psychological information service (PSYCINFO). An annotated printout was obtained covering the period from January, 1967 through May, 1985. The abstracts and, when necessary, the primary articles were reviewed by the author. Four categories of publications were identified:

1. DUC: descriptive, uncontrolled studies of parents and children in families where child abuse had been identified.
2. IUC: descriptions of interventions strategies not subjected to a controlled, research protocol.
3. PCE: empirical studies of parents and children in families where child abuse had been identified. In order to be placed in this category, studies had to have adequate control groups.
4. IC: controlled studies of interventions strategies.

Review articles were not placed in any of the listed categories, but were included in the total number of publications reviewed. The PSYCINFO search identified 1,223 references. For the purpose of this literature, analysis of the following categories were eliminated: institutional child abuse; child sexual abuse; animal studies and models; dissertations.

The author clearly acknowledges that institutional child abuse and child sexual abuse are serious forms of child abuse. However, both of these are forms of abuse that came into public and professional focus much later than ''The Battered Child'' of 1967. Hence, the development of literature in these two areas would most likely to out of synchrony with the child abuse literature and should be subjected to its own meta-analysis. In addition, animal studies and models are difficult to extrapolate to human behavior and so, were eliminated. Dissertations were not as readily available as publications, hence it was not possible to categorize the content of the dissertation without adding tremendously to the time and cost of the analysis. Therefore, dissertations were not counted in the total number of articles reviewed.

Eight hundred twenty articles were reviewed for the final analysis. It should be noted that this was not a sample of the child abuse literature, but was the entire population of interest; that is, literature in the PSYCINFO search. Thus, inferential statistics were not necessary in reporting the results of the analysis. The results of the study were reported as ratios and percentages of articles appearing in four discrete time periods: 1967–1969; 1970–1974; 1975–1979; and 1980–1985. Four hypotheses were stated prior to the initiation of the study:

Hypothesis 1 (H-1). Each stated time period will have a different pattern of distribution of articles in the four designated areas.

Hypothesis 2 (H-2). The period 1967–1974 will have the smallest percentage of articles utilizing controlled research protocols (PCE+IC). Conversely, 1967–1974 will have the largest percentage of articles that are descriptive and uncontrolled (DUC+IUC).

Hypothesis 3 (H-3). The period 1970–1979 will have the largest percentage of descriptions of uncontrolled treatments strategies (IUC).

Hypothesis 4 (H-4). The period 1980–1985 will have the largest percentage of articles documenting controlled studies of parents and children as well as intervention strategies (PCE+IC). Table 2 documents the results of the literature analysis of a total of 820 articles.

The four original hypotheses were confirmed by the data. Each time period has a different percent distribution of articles in the four categories (H-1). The time period 1967–1974 has 84 total articles, five of which are studies utilizing controlled research protocols (PCE+IC). This accounts for 6% of the articles. The period 1975–1979 has 19.1%, and 1980–1985 has 26.3% of the literature utilizing controlled research protocols. Conversely, 1967–1974 has 85.7% of the articles consisting of uncontrolled descriptions of parents, children, and intervention strategies. This compares to 63.5% in 1975–1979 and 52.9% in 1980–1985. This confirms Hypothesis 2. Hypothesis 3 stated that 1970–1979 would have the largest percentage of descriptions of uncontrolled treatment strategies. This is indeed true, with 44.4% versus 14.3% (1967–1969), 35% (1975–1979) and 30.7% (1980–1985). The period 1980–1985 has 26.3% of all articles utilizing a controlled research protocol. This compares with 9.5% (1967–1969), 4.8% (1970–1974) and 19.1% (1975–1979) and hence confirms H-4.

It might well be that the patterns found in the proliferation of literature on child abuse reflect the seriousness and urgency of the problem. If one examines the content of articles in the literature, it appears that the first five to seven years were concerned with the nature of child abuse (Bennie & Sclare, 1969; Fontana, 1968; Heffer & Kempe, 1968; Kempe, 1971; Laury & Meerloo, 1967a,b; Paulson & Blake, 1967; Polansky, DeSaiz, Wing, & Patton, 1968; Zalba, 1966, 1967). These articles announced that a serious problem existed, that the need for intervention was urgent, and that few resources were organized and available. In essence, the literature was a call for action. The Battered Child Syndrome was described in a clear manner in order that health professionals could identify children who were being battered. Early speculations regarding etiology were drawn from uncontrolled, select populations of abused children (Blumberg, 1974; Forrest, 1974; Freen, Gaines, & Sandground, 1974; Havens, 1972; Helfer & Kenipe, 1968; Laury & Meerloo, 1967; Lukianowicz, 1971; Schwartz, 1974; Silver, Dublin, & Lourie, 1969; Spinetta, 1978; Zalba, 1967). It was at this juncture that psychoanalytic thought had its major impact in developing theories regarding child abuse. Formulations regarding the individual psychopathology of parents, the subsequent psychological damage incurred by the abused child, and even speculations regarding the functioning of the family system, drew heavily on psychoanalytic theories regarding mechanisms of mental functioning and child development. These analytic hypotheses gained widespread recognition and accep-

Table 2. Distribution of Child Abuse Articles, 1967 to May, 1985

Category	1967–1969		1970–1974		1975–1979		1980–1985	
Total no. of articles	21		63		277		459	
	n	%	n	%	n	%	n	%
DUC	13	61.9%	28	44.4%	79	28.5%	102	22.2%
PCE	2	9.5%	3	4.8%	48	17.3%	85	18.5%
IUC	3	14.3%	28	44.4%	97	35.0%	141	30.7%
IC	0	0.0%	0	0.0%	5	1.8%	36	7.8%

tance as workers in the field desperately tried to understand and develop effective systems for intervention.

A failure in bonding between mother and child was cited as a significant element in precipitating child abuse (Ounsted, Oppenheimer, & Lindsey, 1974; Schwartz, 1974). Others spoke of the lack of family closeness or the rejecting attitude of the abusing parent toward the child (Smith, Hanson, & Noble, 1974). The projection, or transferring, of the abusing parent's negative characteristics onto the child was also noted as a major mechanism contributing to scapegoating (Green *et al.*, 1974). Another author suggested that the negativism toward the child was secondary to negative mental representations of the pregnancy and events around parturition (Asch & Rubin, 1974). A widespread opinion in the field that came to be accepted as dogma and was not subjected to empirical study until many years later was that abusing parents almost without exception were abused/neglected themselves; they had suffered early rejection and consequently had not developed the ability to love. Hence, as adults they were narcissistic, immature, and had poor ego control (Blumberg, 1974). It was recommended that treatment be aimed at improving the abused parent's self-image and ego strengths. A variation in the hypotheses regarding the developmental damage incurred by abusing parents was that they had been raised in the same style that they recreated in the pattern of rearing their own children (Steele & Pollock, 1974). These authors rejected the use of the adjectives *sadomasochistic, egocentric, narcissistic,* and *demanding,* all of which had been applied to abusive parents. They found these descriptions uniformly unhelpful and instead sought to identify consistent behavioral patterns that were unique for abusive parents. Abusive parents were noted to have high expectations of their children and demands for performance were found to be premature. Consequently, the child tended to be treated as if she or he were older than she or he really was. The parents too were viewed as having grown up in a home environment that placed individual demands on them as children. They were expected to be good, submissive, promptly obedient, and never in error (Steele & Pollock, 1974). Subsequently, the authors concluded, the parents felt unloved and unfulfilled. The expectations placed on them by their own parents were internalized. Consequently, they became self-critical and projected similar criticisms onto their own children. Other investigators, in describing parents who had grown up in abusive environments, noted that they utilized the defensive mechanism of identification with the aggressor as a means of coping with having been the recipients of their own parents' hostility (A. Freud, 1946, Laury & Meerloo, 1967). Because of this, the parental need for love and reassurance was considerable; not infrequently the parent would turn to her or his child for this "mothering." Hence, the phenomenon of role reversal (Morris & Gould, 1963), with the child being perceived as parent and not recognized as someone with her or his own needs.

Melnick and Harley (1969) utilized projective tests in studying some of the characteristics of abusive parents. Theirs was one of the first early studies to utilize control groups. Ten abusive and 10 control mothers were matched for age, social class, and education. Using the Thematic Apperception Test (TAT), the California Test of Personality (CTP), and the Family Concept Inventory (FCI), 18 personality variables were studied in order to explain hypotheses formulated in the child abuse literature. Abusive mothers scored high in TAT pathogenicity and dependency frustration; but scored lower on TAT need to give nurturance and the CTP self-esteem. Low scores were obtained on manifest rejection and family satisfaction in the FCI. These findings did not support hypotheses that abusive mothers were chronically hostile (Bennie & Sclare 1965; Calef, 1972) or overwhelmed by maternal responsibilities. However, they were not found to have normal personalities. Parents' lack of ability to empathize with their children seemed apparent. This, in conjunction with severely frustrated dependency needs, gave indirect support to the formulation of the history of emotional deprivation. In a definitive summary of the early literature (Spinetta & Rigler, 1972) noted that four summary conclusions could be drawn regarding the psychological characteristics of abusive parents.

1. The abusing parent was deprived as a child.
2. The abusing parent lacked accurate knowledge concerning child rearing.
3. The parents had characteristic defects that allow aggressive impulses to be expressed too freely.
4. Socioeconomic stresses were neither necessary nor sufficient causes of physical abuse.

Steele and Pollock (1974) elaborated on these findings in the literature and added their own observations from a sample of 60 families whom they intensively studied over a 5½-year period. These clinical investigators were aware that their sample was skewed, and that there was no control group. Their method of study was a conventional psychiatric evaluation, diagnosis, and therapeutic interview process designed to reach as deeply as possible into the patient's personality. Social work interviews and home visits supplemented the data. A primary finding in their study was that abusive mothers had what seemed to be a disruption of the maternal affectional system. This was seen to be secondary to the mother's own lack of mothering. Mothering was defined, according to Josselyn (1956), as the ability to show tenderness, gentleness, and empathy; to value a love object more than the self. The authors noted Benedek's description (1959) of how childhood memories upsurge when an adult becomes a parent, memories of what it was like to be a child and of how one was parented. Steele and Pollock emphasized that the initial disruption in the maternal affectional system grew out of that early phase of development providing the first primal identifications (Benedek, 1938, 1949, 1956, 1959). They hypothesized that the pleasure-giving mother is introjected as the primordial basis of the ego ideal and that the pain-producing mother becomes the *anlage* of the archaic, punitive superego (A. Freud, 1946; Spitz, 1958). That is, the abusive mother's own experience with her own parents, particularly mother, was filled with painful, non-satisfying experiences that resulted in accumulated memory traces that coalesced into a stable introject of a harsh, critical mother. This internalized maternal image becomes the core of the future abusive parent's superego, a superego characterized by excessive rules and expectations, hence resulting in the directing of excessive criticism and unrealistic expectations toward the next generation, the abusive parent's own children.

In addition, the authors postulated a basic defect in the confidence of abusive mothers, that is, that they lacked optimism regarding their own ability to maintain useful relationships with others and to expect consistency from others (Benedek, 1938; Erikson, 1950). Further along the developmental scale, Steele and Pollock noted that abusive parents also demonstrated a lack of identity consolidation (Erikson, 1956). The abusive parent seemed to have a loose collection of unintegrated, disparate concepts of the self. An opinion was offered that few of the parents in the Denver study had experienced a true, fully involved oedipal situation secondary to most of their conflicts and fixations being pregenital. Polanski *et al.* (1968) postulated a similar pregenital fixation. He noted that little behavior seemed to be regressive but instead indicative of massive early arrests and fixations of personality development. He stated that treatment would, hence, be arduous and long term in this population of people. However, it was noted by Steele and Pollock that abusive behavior toward older children, not infants, might well have a different dynamic and be caused by parental concerns over sexuality and competitiveness (Steele & Pollock, 1974; Zilboorg, 1932).

Martin, Beezeley, Conway, and Kempe (1974) reviewed the literature regarding the development of abused children. They noted that little had been written and that what was in print consisted of statements regarding the presence or absence of emotional disorders in these children. Little effort had been made to focus on specific areas of dysfunction. Speculations regarding abusive parents might well be extrapolated downward to the children. Here the parents were viewed as the recipients of abuse and neglect themselves and hence, representative of the end product. Martin and Beezley (1976) published an uncontrolled study of the personality characteristics of abused children ($N = 50$). The results of their study is noted in Table 3.

APPLICATIONS OF PSYCHOANALYTIC THEORY

What is clear in reviewing 18 years of child abuse literature is that the psychoanalytic formulations developed during the period 1967–1974 were viewed as having a high degree of credibility. Many of the psychiatrists in the field were analytically trained. Pediatricians working closely with their psychoanalytic colleagues also found psychoanalytic theory helpful in understanding the behavioral difficulties of their patients. Leaders in the child abuse fields, such as H. Martin, called for an extension of the work of such excellent analytic theorists as Anna Freud, Erik Erikson, and Margaret Mahler to understand the psychosocial development of a child raised in an abusive environment.

It is the contention of this author that there are some serious problems regarding the generalizability and validity of the application of psychoanalytic models of mental functioning to problems as complex as those involved in family violence. Furthermore, the widespread credibility of psychoanalytic formulations through the 1960s and mid-1970s resulted in the acceptance of inferential statements about metapsychological constructs as if they were equal to behavioral realities based on controlled clinical observations. Given that the empirical literature in the field of child abuse gained prominence only after 1975, one has to wonder if complacency with offered explanations and unrealistic expectations

Table 3. Characteristics of Abused Children

Characteristic	Percentage of children
1. Impaired capacity to enjoy life	66
2. Psychiatric symptoms, e.g., eneuresis, tantrums, hyperactivity, bizarre behavior	62
3. Low self-esteem	52
4. School learning problems	38
5. Withdrawal	24
6. Opposition	24
7. Hypervigilance	22
8. Compulsivity	20
9. Pseudo-mature behavior	20

Note. From "Personality of Abused Children," by H.P. Martin and P. Beezeley. In H.P. Martin and P. Beezeley (Eds.), *The Abused Child: A multidisciplinary Approach to Developmental Issues and Treatment*, 1976, Cambridge, MA: Ballingee Publishing Co. Reprinted by permission.

about psychoanalytic interventions resulted in a delay in delineating multicausal models for identifying families at risk, identifying specific areas of dysfunction in parents and children, and developing more effective and cost-efficient methods of minimizing and/or reversing dysfunction.

Two major theoretical issues are apparent when one considers the application of a psychoanalytic model of mental functioning to situations involving child abuse and other forms of family violence. First, the psychoanalytic situation is a relatively controlled situation in which intrapsychic phenomena are analyzed through the medium of the transference. It is assumed that mental mechanisms will be externalized and reflected in the transference and that these mechanisms will be relatively free from distortion or functional change secondary to external factors or biological assaults. For example, it would be inappropriate to analyze and draw conclusions regarding a person's psychic structure one day after a major flood has wiped out a person's home and killed three family members. Such an event would disrupt normal mental functioning. Likewise, a person who has acute bacterial meningitis or has an acute hypoglycemic episode would demonstrate a mode of mental functioning that differs considerably from that individual's norm. Let us put this phenomenon into the language of general systems theory. The patient who is not under biological assault nor overwhelmed by an external disaster and who meets the criteria for analyzability can enter into the psychoanalytic situation and analyze her or his psychological life, past and present, as if the system were a closed system. The patient's psyche in the midst of a flood or in the midst of a hypoglycemic episode is not functionally isolated and unaffected by other interfacing systems. Quite the contrary, we find ourselves dealing with an open system. A child, an adult, and an entire family enveloped in a violent abusive relationship likewise need to be understood as functioning according to the dynamic mechanisms that govern open rather than closed systems.

For those not versed in the language and theory of general systems, a brief review is indicated. A *system* is a real physical structure composed of interacting subelements that can be localized in space and time and that exhibit coherent characteristic functions or behavior over an extended period of time. Systems have specific properties that define function. A system itself may be a subelement of a larger system, or conversely, the subelements of a system may themselves be systems in interaction with superelements.

A system is more than the sum of its parts. Interactions among subelements endow a system with properties that its subelements, acting independently, do not have. A corollary is that the dysfunction of any element of the system effects the functional integrity of the whole.

Systems are located in space and time. There is a history and there is a future for any system. Each subelement has a developmental history that affects structural integrity. The larger system as a whole is likewise affected by the passage of time.

Systems are designed, or evolved, to perform characteristic functions, to achieve characteristic goals. Disruption in the systems' steady state will affect all the sub-systems, as self-regulation and return to the steady state is attempted.

Returning to the issue at hand, the psychoanalytic situation is by definition a relatively closed system (S. Freud, 1910, 1922, 1933; Jones, 1946; Rapaport & Gill, 1959; Stone, 1961). Psychoanalytic theory, specifically the psychoanalytic model of mental functioning with its developmental roots, is based on a verbal data base acquired within the confines of the psychoanalytic situation. The theory emerged and evolved when explanation was needed for apparent incongruities in behavioral observations (Arlow &

Brenner, 1964; S. Freud, 1895, 1900, 1901, 1905, 1915, 1923 [1922], 1923, 1926). Although inferences regarding mental functioning can be made outside of the psychoanalytic situation, it must be acknowledged that the generalizability of these inferences has a higher probability of being valid when the system approximates that one on which the model was based, mainly that of a relatively closed system. When the model is applied indiscriminately to situations involving family violence, we are on shakier ground in that we are now applying the model to an open system. Open systems behave differently than closed ones (Von Bertalanffy, 1968). Closed systems are simpler to analyze; causality is more apt to be understood by linear relationships and simple feedback loops. The technique, utilized by psychoanalysis, of isolating one subsystem as if it were a closed system in order to promote understanding of the subsystem and to develop functional models, is quite appropriate. This technique has been frequently utilized by scientists in their efforts to further understand the function of complex behavioral systems. Chemical reactions within complex metabolic pathways were first understood in isolation, as closed systems. Cardiac physiology was first understood in isolation from renal function. One simply must be cognizant of the differences in function of closed and open systems. Bowlby (1969) wrote

> Causality in the linear mechanistic sense . . . implies a strict determinism, causality involving feedback and organization in open systems does not. An open system that attains a steady state (as contrasted to a state of equilibrium in a closed system) may reach its characteristic final state from different initial states and in different ways.

This phenomenon Von Bertalanffy termed equifinality (1968).

The second major theoretical issue in applying a psychoanalytic model of mental functioning to situations involving child abuse and other forms of family violence is the tendency to confuse function with mechanism or cause (''Psychoanalysis, just like other fields, has used specific data, such as clinical examples, from which to form lower order inferences that in turn have been used to build more abstract generalizations'' [Rosenblatt & Thickstun, 1977].) Hence, one readily sees the importance of maintaining an accurate awareness of what kind of inference is being made from the data at hand (Klein, 1976; Meissner, 1981; Ricoeur, 1970; Waelder, 1962). The psychoanalytic model of mental functioning is, as we have previously stated, a model derived from the data base of verbal reports within the psychoanalytic situation and so, using Waelder's analysis (1962), is at the level of clinical interpretation. Applying this model to other clinical situations is one more step removed inferentially or, as Waelder noted, at the ''level of clinical generalization.'' We have discussed previously the criteria necessary for enhancing the validity of such generalizations. It is the author's contention that whereas descriptions of function are but one step removed from the data, constituting a small inferential leap, psychoanalytic theories, regarding developmental causality, or constructs, and the mechanism by which the intrapsychic system arrives at a particular structural or functional steady state, are further removed from the data base. Furthermore, the methodologies that are being utilized for the psychoanalytic formulations of developmental theories and models have serious technical difficulties relating to the reliability and validity of the instruments used for observation. In particular, I am referring to direct longitudinal observational studies of children. These technical considerations are even more confounded when one attempts to translate the manifest behavior of nonverbal children into a psychology of motivation (Gedo, 1982). Predictive statements regarding the developmental consequences of child abuse (mostly related to parents having been the recipients of abuse) found in the review of the psychoanalytic literature on child abuse not only violates the theoretical issue of applying rules affecting causality in closed systems to open systems, but also reflects an unacceptable inferential leap. One cannot move from function to mechanisms and causality so adroitly. These theoretical considerations are not inconsequential. The psychoanalytic perspective on the impact of child abuse on the future development of the child promotes a sense of therapeutic nihilism. This is not helpful to the development of creative research directed toward a more systematic untangling of the specific damages incurred secondary to abuse and the designing of effective and efficient therapeutic intervention techniques.

The final point on psychoanalytic perspectives of family violence is not theoretical but humanistic. As a psychoanalyst, I find myself in pain over what is happening in the field of psychoanalysis; in our institutes, in our journals, and in the field at large. Analysts, and collectively psychoanalysis, feel under tremendous attack. This chapter might well be perceived as but one more attack. It is and it is not. Under the intense bombardment of criticisms directed toward us, as analysts, we have become preoccupied with survival and warding off further attack. We fail to recognize the pervasiveness of psychoanalytic thought in our society. Our medical textbooks, our pediatric textbooks, our psychiatric textbooks all incorporate the psychoanalytic model of mental functioning and draw heavily on psychoanalytic perspectives in child development. In addition to the medical field, social work curricula and basic psychology courses all offer the psychoanalytic model as a model that has contributed significantly to understanding human behavior. Psychoanalysis still maintains a high degree of credibility among those on the front lines dealing with problems secondary to family violence. We have an obligation to be rigorous in our observations, our thinking, and the development of our hypotheses. We must help others recognize what aspects of our methodology and our theoretical models are directly applicable to clinical situations and which involve inferential leaps that are of questionable validity. The psychoanalytic perspectives on family violence has been helpful in the generation of hypotheses, However, our hypotheses have become much too familiar to the ear and are sometimes equated with proven truths. John Kenneth Galbraith has eloquently described this phenomenon of equating truth with familiarity and convenience.

> To a very large extent, of course, we associate truth with convenience—with what most closely accords with self-interest and individual well-being or promises best to avoid awkward efforts or unwelcomed dislocation of life . . . because familiarity is such an important test of acceptability, the acceptable ideas have great stability . . . I shall refer to these ideas henceforth as a conventional wisdom. Galbraith (1958)

Family violence is a horrible thing. To see a 2-year-old child with third degree burns from the waist down, to watch a one-year-old child die from an epidural hemorrhage or to see a 10-year-old who walks and talks like an 80-year-old stroke victim is an emotional experience that few forget. Psychoanalysts, directly and indirectly through their work with pediatricians and other mental health professionals, were on the front lines in mobilizing the entire country in effecting major social and legal changes necessary to protect children from serious battering. Psychoanalytic constructs were used for formulating hypotheses regarding family violence. Some of these were confirmed; some were not. We have been remiss in not recognizing that our words and theories have been imbued with a high degree of credibility. We have been too preoccupied with those who are attacking our profession. Consequently, we have behaved in a way that adds fuel to our critic's fire. We have been remiss in not maintaining a high degree of theoretical and technical rigor in the application of what we know from psychoanalytic situations to more complex phenomena in our society. Our explanations are received by many as familiar and comfortable and hence we have a false sense of security with regard to our understanding of family violence.

SUMMARY

In the data presented earlier in this chapter concerning the developmental sequencing of articles in the child abuse literature, the proliferation of empirical studies regarding the character of abusive parents and abused children, as well as controlled studies of specific therapeutic interventions was documented as beginning in the late 1970s and progressing through the early 1980s. These studies are most exciting and will be elaborated on in the subsequent chapters in this book. The psychoanalytic perspective was invaluable in the beginning and bogged down in the middle of our search for effective approaches on family violence. Multicausal models for the identification of families at risk, consistent with open systems analysis, have been developed (Ayoub, Jacewitz, Gold, & Milner, 1983; Conger, Burgess, & Barrett, 1979; Daniel, Hampton, & Newberger, 1983; Egeland, Breintenbucher, & Rosenberg, 1980, 1981; Gaines, Sandgrand, Green, & Power, 1978; Garabino & Sherman, 1980; Martin & Walters, 1982; McCabe, 1984; Milner, 1982; Milner, Gold, Ayoub, & Jacewitz, 1984; Pianta, 1984; Polansky, Cabral, Margura, & Phillips, 1983; Robertson & Milner, 1983; Sherrod, Attemeier, O'Connor, & Vietze, 1984; Starback, Krantzler, Forbes, & Barnes, 1984; Steinberg, Catalano, & Dooley, 1981). These models have been utilized to design questionnaires, easily filled out by families at high risk for battering. Empirical studies have demonstrated specific areas of psychological dysfunction in abused children (Allen & Oliver, 1982; Camras, Grow, & Ribordy, 1983; Egeland, Stroufe, & Erikson, 1983; Elmer, 1978; Friedrich, Einbender, & Loucke, 1983; Gaenbauer, 1982; George & Main, 1979; Giblin, Starr, & Agronan, 1984; Green, 1978; Halperin, 1983; Herzenberger, Potts, & Dillon, 1981; Hjorth & Harway, 1981; Hoffman-Plotkin & Twentyman, 1984; Jacobson & Straker, 1982; Kinard, 1980; Lewis, 1980; Oates & Peacock, 1984; Reidy, 1977; Schneider-Rosen & Cicchetti, 1984; Smetana, Kelley, & Twentyman, 1984; Wolfe & Mosk, 1983) and abusive parents (Anderson & Lauderdale, 1982; Barahal, Waterman, & Martin, 1981; Brunnguell, Crichton, & Egeland, 1981; Burgess & Conger, 1978; Butler & Crane, 1980; Crittenden, 1981; Crittenden & Bonvillian, 1984; Driscol, 1983; Egeland & Sroufe, 1981; Egeland & Vaughn, 1982; Frodi & Lamb, 1980; Frodi et al., 1978; Garabarino & Crouter, 1978; Garcia & Griffitt, 1978; Gaudin & Pollane, 1983; Hyman, 1977; Jones & McNeely, 1980; Justice & Duncan, 1976; Kevill & Kirkland, 1979; Kravitz & Driscoll, 1983; Larrence & Twentyman, 1983; Mash, Johnston, & Kovitz, 1983; Miller, 1984; Morgan, 1979; Nastasi & Hill, 1982; Newberger & Cook, 1983; O'Connor, et al. 1982; Passman & Mulhern, 1977; Paulson, Afifi, Thomason, & Chaleff, 1974; Paulson, Schwener, Afifi, & Bendel, 1977; Polansky, & Williams, 1978; Relich, Giblin, Starr, & Agronow, 1980; Rosen, 1979; Rosenberg & Reppucci, 1983; Salzinger, Kaplan, & Artenyeff, 1983; Spinetta, 1978; Twentyman & Plotkin, 1982; Wolfe, Fairbank, Kelly, & Bradlyn, 1983). Nonanalytic techniques have evolved that produce proven change in modes of mental functioning; hence, these techniques address multiple mechanisms for achieving desired end results in our patients (Barth, Blythe, Schinke, & Schilling, 1983; Egan, 1983; Ellis & Milner, 1981; Smith & Rackman, 1984; Wolfe & Sandler, 1981; Wolfe, Sandler, & Kaufman, 1981).

In summary, as I addressed the charge given to me prior to writing this chapter on psychoanalytic perspectives on family violence, Charcot's words still are loud and clear. The theory is good. It must not be a barrier to the realities of existence.

REFERENCES

Allen, R. E., & Oliver, J. M. (1982). The effects of child maltreatment on language development. *Child Abuse and Neglect 6*, 299–305.

Anderson, S. C., & Lauderdale, M. L. (1982). Characteristics of abusive parents: A look at self-esteem. *Child Abuse and Neglect, 6*, 285–293.

Asch, S. S., & Rubin, J. (1984). Post partum reactions: Some unrecognized variations. *American Journal of Psychiatry, 131*, 870–874.

Arlow, J., & Brenner, C. (1964). *Psychoanalytic concepts and structural theory*. New York: International Universities Press.

Ayoub, C., & Jacewitz, M. M., Gold, R. G., Milner, J. S. (1983). Assessment of a program's effectiveness in selecting individuals "at risk" for problems in parenting. *Journal of Clinical Psychology, 39*, 334–339.

Barahal, R. M., Waterman, J., & Martin, H. P. (1981). The social cognitive development of abused children. *Journal of Consulting and Clinical Psychology, 49*, 508–516.

Barth, R. P., Blythe, B. J., Schinke, S. P., & Schilling, R. F. (1983). Self-control training with maltreating parents. *Child Welfare, 62*, 313–324.

Bende, P. D. (1980). Prosecuting wives who use force in self defense: Investigative considerations. A report of the California Department of Justice, in *Peace Officer*, pp. 8–14.

Benedek, T. (1938). Adaptation to reality in early infancy. *Psycholoanalytic Quarterly, 7*, 200–215.

Benedek, T. (1949). The psychosomatic implications of the primary unit: Mother–child. *American Journal of Orthopsychiatry, 19*, 642–654.

Benedek, T. (1956). Psychobiological aspects of mothering. *American Journal of Orthopsychiatry, 26*, 272–278.

Benedek, T. (1959). Parenthood as a developmental phase. A contribution to the libido theory. *Journal of the American Psychoanalytic Association, 7*, 389–417.

Bennie, E. H., & Sclare, A. B. (1969). The battered child syndrome. *American Journal of Psychiatry, 125*, 975–979.

Block, M. R., & Sinnott, J. D. (1979). *The battered elder syndrome: An explanatory study*. Division of Human and Community Resources, College Park, Maryland: University of Maryland Press.

Blumberg, M. L. (1974). Psychopathology of the abusing parent. *American Journal of Psychotherapy, 28*, 21–29.

Borland, M. (1976). *Violence in the family*. Atlantic Highlands: Manchester University Press.

Bowlby, J. (1969). *Attachment and loss: Vol. I. Attachment*. New York: Basic Books.

Briggs, (1979). Overview. In Department of Health, Education, and Welfare (Ed.) *Child abuse and developmental disabilities: Essays*. Washington, DC: Government Printing Office. Publication No. (OHDS) 79-30226.

Brunnguell, D., Crichton, L., & Egeland, B. (1981). Maternal personality—Attitude in disturbances of child rearing. *American Journal of Orthopsychiatry, 51*, 680–691.

Burgess, R. L., & Conger, R. D. (1978). Family interaction in abusive, neglectful, and normal families. *Child Development, 49*, 1163–1173.

Butler, J. F., & Crane, D. R. (1980). Self-report schedules for use in assessing the marital adjustment of abusive and nonabusive parents. *American Journal of Family Therapy, 8*, 29–34.

Calef, V. (1972). The hostility of parents to children: Some notes on infertility, child abuse, and abortion. *International Journal of Psychoanalytic Psychotherapy, 1*, 76–96.

California Department of Justice. (1982). *The child abuse prevention handbook*. Sacramento, CA: Department of Justice.

Camras, L. A., Grow, J. G., & Ribordy, S. C. (1983). Recognition of emotional expression by abused children. *Journal of Clinical Child Psychology, 12*, 325–328.

Conger, R. D., Burgess, R. L., & Barrett, C. (1979). Child abuse related to life change and perceptions of illness: Some preliminary findings. *Family Coordinator, 28*, 73–78.

Crittenden, P. M. (1981). Abusing, neglecting, problematic, and adequate dyads: Differentiating by patterns of interaction. *Merrill-Palmer Quarterly, 27*, 201–218.

Crittenden. P. M., & Bonvillian, J. D. (1984). The relationship between maternal risk status and maternal sensitivity. *American Journal of Orthopsychiatry, 54*, 250–262.

Daniel, J. H., Hampton, R. L., Newberger, E. H. (1983). Child abuse and accidents in black families: A controlled comparative study. *American Journal of Orthopsychiatry, 53,* 645–653.

Dobash, R. E., & Dobash, R. P. (1978). Wives: The "appropriate" victims of marital violence. *Victimology, 2,* 426–442.

Dobash, R. E., & Dobash, R. P. (1979). *Violence against wives: A case against the patriarchy.* New York: Free Press.

Egan, K. J. (1983). Stress management and child management with abusive parents. *Journal of Clinical Psychology, 12,* 292–299.

Egeland, B. R., & Stroufe, L. A. Attachment and early maltreatment. *Child Development, 52,* 44–52.

Egeland, B., & Vaughn, B. (1982). Failure of "bond formation" as a cause of abuse, neglect and maltreatment. *Annual Progress on Child Psychiatry in Child Development, 1982,* 188–198.

Egeland, B. R., Breitenbucher, M., & Rosenberg, D. (1980). Prospective study of the significance of life stress in the etiology of child abuse. *Journal of Consulting and Clinical Psychology, 48,* 195–205.

Egeland, B. R., Breitenbucher, M., & Rosenberg, D. (1981). Prospective study of the significance of life stress in the etiology of child abuse. *Annual Progress in Child Psychiatry and Child Development, 1981,* 666–682.

Egeland, B., Stroufe, A., & Erikson, M. (1983). The developmental consequences of different patterns of maltreatment. *Child Abuse and Neglect, 7,* 459–469.

Ellis, R. H., & Milner, J. S. (1981). Child abuse and locus of control. *Psychological Reports, 48,* 507–510.

Elmer, E. (1978). Effects of early neglect and abuse on latency age children. *Journal of Pediatric Psychology, 3,* 14–19.

Erikson, E. (1950). *Childhood and society.* New York: W. W. Norton.

Erikson, E. (1956). The problem of ego identity. *Journal of the American Psychoanalytic Association, 4,* 56–121.

FBI uniform crime reports. (1973). Washington, DC: Government Printing Office.

Finkelhor, D. (1981). Sexual abuse: A sociological perspective. Paper presented at the National Conference for Family Violence Researchers. Durham, NH, 1981.

Fontana, V. J. (1968). Further reflections on maltreatment of children. *New York State Journal of Medicine, 68,* 2214–2215.

Fontana, V. J. (1973). *Somewhere a child is crying: Maltreatment–causes and prevention.* New York: MacMillan.

Forrest, T. (1974). The family dynamic of maternal violence. *Journal of the American Academy of Psychoanalysis, 2,* 215–230.

Freeman, M. (1979). *Violence in the home.* Westmead, England; Saxon House.

Freud, A. (1946). *The ego and the mechanisms of defense.* New York: International Universities Press.

Freud, S. (1959). Charcot. In E. Jones (Ed.), *Sigmund Freud Collected Papers* Vol. 1 (pp. 9–23). New York: Basic Books. (Originally published 1893).

Freud, S. (1955). Studies on hysteria. In J. Strachey (Ed.) *Standard Edition,* Vol. 2. London: Hogarth Press. (Originally published 1895).

Freud, S. (1953). The interpretation of dreams. In J. Strachey (Ed.) *Standard Edition,* Vol. 4, 5. London: Hogarth Press. (Originally published 1900).

Freud, S. (1960). The psychopathology of everyday life. In J. Strachey (Ed.) *Standard Edition,* Vol. 6. London: Hogarth Press. (Originally published 1901).

Freud, S. (1953). Three essays on sexuality. In J. Strachey (Ed.) *Standard Edition,* Vol. 7 (pp. 130–243). London: Hogarth Press. (Originally published 1905).

Freud, S. (1957). Five lectures on psychoanalysis. In J. Strachey (Ed.) *Standard Edition,* Vol. 11 (pp. 9–55). London: Hogarth Press. (Originally published 1910).

Freud, S. (1957). The unconscious. In J. Strachey (Ed.) *Standard Edition,* Vol. 14 (pp. 166–215). London: Hogarth Press. (Originally published 1915).

Freud, S. (1955). Beyond the pleasure principle. In J. Strachey (Ed.) *Standard Edition,* Vol. 18 (pp. 1–64). London: Hogarth Press. (Originally published 1920).

Freud, S. (1955). Two encyclopedia articles. In J. Strachey (Ed.) *Standard Edition,* Vol. 18 (pp. 235–254). London: Hogarth Press. (Originally published 1922/1923).

Freud, S. (1961). The ego and the id. In J. Strachey (Ed.) *Standard Edition,* Vol. 19 (pp. 1–59). London: Hogarth Press. (Originally published 1923).

Freud, S. (1959). Inhibitions, symptoms, and anxiety. In J. Strachey (Ed.) *Standard Edition* Vol. 20 (pp. 75–172). London: Hogarth Press. (Originally published 1926).

Freud, S. (1964). New introductory lectures on psychoanalysis. In J. Strachey (Ed.) *Standard Edition*, Vol. 22 (pp. 1–182). London: Hogarth Press. (Originally published 1933).

Friedrich, W. N., Einbender, A. J., & Leucke, W. J. (1983). Cognitive and behavioral characteristics of physically abused children. *Journal of Consulting and Clinical Psychology, 51*, 313–314.

Frodi, A. M., & Lamb, M. E. (1980). Child abusers' responses to infant smiles and cries. *Child Development, 51*, 238–241.

Frodi, A., Lamb, M. E., Leavitt, L. A., Donovan, R. L., Neff, C., & Sherry, D. (1978). Fathers' and mothers' responses to the faces and cries of normal and premature infants. *Developmental Psychology, 14*, 490–498.

Gaenbauer, T. J. (1982). Regulation of emotional expression in infants from two contrasting caretaking environments. *Journal of the American Academy of Child Psychiatry, 21*, 163–170.

Gaines, R., Sandgrund, A., Green, A. H., & Power, E. (1978). Etiological factors in child maltreatment: A multivariate study of abusing, neglecting, and normal mothers. *Journal of Abnormal Psychology, 87*, 531–540.

Galbraith, J. K. (1958). *The affluent society*. New York: The New American Library.

Garbarino, J., & Crouter, A. (1978). Defining the community context for parent–child relations: The correlates of child maltreatment. *Child Development, 49*, 604–616.

Garbarino, J., & Sherman, D. (1980). High-risk neighborhoods and high-risk families: The human ecology of child maltreatment. *Child Development, 51*, 188–198.

Garcia, L. T., & Griffitt, W. (1978). Authoritarianism-situation interactions in the determination of punitiveness: Engaging authoritian ideology. *Journal of Research and Personality, 12*, 469–479.

Gaudin, J. M., & Pollane, L. (1983). Social networks, stress and child abuse. *Children in Youth Services Review, 5*, 91–102.

Gedo, J. E. (1982). On black bile and other humors. *Psychoanalytic Inquiry, 2*, 181–191.

Gelles, R. J. (1979). *Family violence*. Beverly Hills, CA: Sage.

George, C., & Main, M. (1979). Social interactions of young abused children; Approach, avoidance, and aggression. *Child Development, 50*, 306–318.

Giblin, P. T., Starr, R. H., & Agronun, S. J. (1984). Affective behavior of abused and control children: Comparisons of parent–child interactions and the influence of home environment variables. *Journal of Genetic Psychology, 144*, 69–82.

Gil, D. G., (1970). *Violence against children*. Cambridge, MA: Harvard University Press.

Giovannoni, J., & Becenna, R. (1979). *Defining child abuse*. New York: The Free Press.

Green, A. H., (1978). Self destructive behavior in battered children. *American Journal of Psychiatry, 135*, 579–582.

Green, A. H., Gaines, R. W., & Sandground, A. (1974). Child abuse: Pathological syndrome of family interaction. American Journal of Psychiatry, 131, 882–886.

Halperin, S. M. (1983). Family perceptions of abused children and their siblings. *Child Abuse and Neglect, 7*, 107–115.

Havens, L. L. (1972). Youth, violence and the nature of family life. *Psychiatric Annals, 2*, 18–29.

Helfer, R. E., & Kempe, C. H. (1968). *The Battered Child*. Chicago, IL: University of Chicago Press.

Herzberger, S. D., Potts, D. A., Dillon, M. (1981). Abusive and nonabusive parental treatment from the child's perspective. *Journal of Consulting and Clinical Psychology, 49*, 81–90.

Hjorth, C. W., & Harway, M. (1981). The body-image of physically abused and normal adolescents. *Journal of Clinical Psychology, 37*, 863–866.

Hoffman-Plotkin, D., & Twentyman, C. T. (1984). A multimodal assessment of behavioral and cognitive deficits in abused and neglected preschoolers. *Child Development, 55*, 794–802.

Hyman, C. A. (1977). A report on the psychological test results of battering parents. *British Journal of Social and Clinical Psychology, 16*, 221–224.

Jacobson, R. S., & Straker, G. (1982). Peer group interaction of physically abused children. *Child Abuse and Neglect, 6*, 321–327.

Jones, E. (1946). A valedictory address. *International Journal of Psychoanalysis, 27*, 7–12.

Jones, J. M., & McNeely, R. L. (1980). Mothers who neglect: Differentiating features in their daily lives and implications for practice. *Corrective and Social Psychiatry and Journal of Behavioral Technology, 26*, 135–143.

Josselyn, I. (1956). Cultural forces, motherliness and fatherliness. *American Journal of Orthopsychiatry, 26*, 264–271.

Justice, D., & Duncan, D. F. (1976). Life crisis as a precursor to child abuse. *Public Health Reports, 91*, 110–115.

Kempe, C. H., (1971). Pediatric implications of the battered baby syndrome. *Archives of Diseases in Childhood, 46,* 28–37.

Kevill, F., & Kirkland, J. (1979). Infant crying and learned helplessness. *Journal of Biological Psychology, 21,* 3–7.

Kinard, E. M. (1980). Emotional development in physically abused children. *American Journal of Orthopsychiatry, 50,* 686–696.

King, N. (1983). Exploitations and abuse of older family members: An overview of the problem. *Responses, 6,* 1–2, 13–15.

Klein, G. S. (1976). *Psychoanalytic theory: An exploration of essentials.* New York: International Universities Press.

Kravitz, R. I., & Driscoll, J. M. (1983). Expectations for childhood development among child-abusing and nonabusing parents. *American Journal of Orthopsychiatry, 53,* 336–344.

Larrence, D. T., & Twentyman, C. T. (1983). Maternal attributions and child abuse. *Journal of Abnormal Psychology, 92,* 449–457.

Laury, G. V., & Meerloo, J. A. (1967a). Mental cruelty and child abuse. *Psychiatric Quarterly Supplement, 41,* 203–254.

Laury, G. V., & Meerloo, J. A. (1967b). Subtle types of mental cruelty to children. *Child and Family, 6,* 28–34.

Lewis, M. (1980). Peer interaction and maltreated children: Social network and epigenetic models. *Infant Mental Health Journal, 1,* 224–231.

Light, R. J. (1974). Abused and neglected children in America: A study of alternative policies. *Harvard Educational Review, 43,* 356–398.

Lukianowicz, N. (1971). Battered children. *Psychiatria Clinica, 4,* 257–280.

Maden, M. F., & Wrench, D. F. (1977). Significant findings in child abuse research. *Victimology, 2,* 196–224.

Martin, D. (1976). *Battered wives.* San Francisco: Glide.

Martin, H. P., & Beezeley, P. (1976). Personality of abused children. In H. P. Martin (Ed.), *The abused child: A multidisciplinary approach to developmental issues and treatment* (pp. 105–111). Cambridge, MA: Ballinger.

Martin, H., Beezeley, P., Conway, E., & Kempe, C. H. (1974). The development of abused children. I. A Review of the Literature. *Advances in Pediatrics, 21,* 25–44.

Martin, M. J., & Walters, J. (1982). Familial correlates of selected types of child abuse and neglect. *Journal of Marriage and the Family, 44,* 267–276.

Mash, E. J., Johnston, C., & Kovitz, K. (1983). A comparison of the mother–child interactions of physically abused and nonabused children during play and task situations. *Journal of Clinical Child Psychology, 12,* 337–346.

Meissner, W. W. (1981). Metapsychology—Who needs it? *Journal of the American Psychoanalytic Association, 29,* 921–938.

Melnick, B., & Hurley, J. R. (1969). Distinctive personality attributes of child abusing mothers. *Journal of Consulting and Clinical Psychology, 33,* 746–749.

Miller, S. H. (1984). The relationship between adolescent childbearing and child maltreatment. *Child Welfare, 63,* 553–557.

Milner, J. S. (1982). Development of a Lie Scale for the Child Abuse Potential Inventory. *Psychological Reports, 50,* 871–874.

Milner, J. S., & Wimberly, R. C. (1979). An inventory for the identification of child abuse. *Journal of Clinical Psychology, 35,* 95–100.

Milner, J. S., & Wimberly, R. C. (1980). Predictive and explanation of child abuse. *Journal of Clinical Psychology, 36,* 875–884.

Milner, J. S., Gold, R. G., Ayoub, C., & Jacewitz, M. M. (1984). Predictive validity of the child abuse potential inventory. *Journal of Consulting Psychology, 52,* 879–884.

Morgan, S. (1979). Psychoeducational profile of emotionally disturbed abused children. *Journal of Clinical Child Psychology, 8,* 3–6.

Morris, M. G., & Gould, R. W. (1968). Role reversal: A concept dealing with neglected/battered child syndrome. In *The neglected/battered child syndrome* (pp. 29–49). New York: Child Welfare League of America.

McCabe, V. (1984). Abstract perceptual information for age level: A risk factor for maltreatment. Child Development, 55, 267–276.

McLeer, S. V. (1981). Spouse abuse. In G. P. Sholevar (Ed.), *The handbook of marriage and marital therapy.* New York: Spectrum.

Nagi, R. (1975). Child abuse and neglect programs: A national overview. *Children Today, 4,* 13–17.

Nakashima, I., & Zakus, G. (1979). Incestuous families. *Pediatric Annals, 8,* 29–30, 32–33, 36–37, 40–42.

Nastasi, B. K., & Hill, S. D. (1982). Interactions between abusing mothers and their children in 2 situations. *Bulletin of the Psychonomic Society, 20,* 79–81.

Newberger, C. M., & Cook, S. J. (1983). Parental awareness in child abuse: Cognitive-developmental analysis of urban and rural samples. *American Journal of Orthopsychiatry, 53,* 512–524.

Oates, K., & Peacock, A. (1984). Intellectual development of battered children. *Journal of Developmental Disabilities, 10,* 27–29.

O'Connor, S., Vietze, P., Sherrod, K., Sandler, H., Gerrity, S., & Altemeier, W. (1982). Mother–infant interaction and child development after rooming-in: Comparison of high-risk and low-risk mothers. *Prevention in Human Services, 1,* 25–43.

Ounsted, C., Oppenheimer, R., & Lindsey, J. (1974). Aspects of bonding failure: The psychopathology and psychotherapeutic treatment of families of battered children. *Developmental Medicine and Child Neurology, 16,* 447–456.

Pagelow, M. D. (1981). *Women and battering victims and their experiences.* Beverly Hills, CA: Sage.

Passman, R. H., & Mulhern, R. K. (1977). Maternal punitiveness as affected by situational stress: An experimental analogue of child abuse. *Journal of Abnormal Psychology, 86,* 565–569.

Paulson, M. J., Afifi, A. A., Thomason, M. L., & Chaleff, A. (1974). The MMPI: A descriptive measure of psychopathology in abusive parents. *Journal of Clinical Psychology, 30,* 387–390.

Paulson, M. J., & Blake, P. R. (1967). The abused, battered and maltreated child: A review. *Trauma, 9,* 1–3.

Paulson, M. J., Schwener, G. T., Afifi, A. A., & Bendel, R. B. Parent Attitude Research Instrument, (PARI): Clinical vs. statistical inferences in understanding abusive mothers. *Journal of Clinical Psychology, 33,* 848–854.

Perry, M. A., Wells, E. A., & Doran, L. D. (1983). Parent characteristics in abusing and nonabusing families. *Journal of Clinical Child Psychology, 12,* 329–336.

Pianta, B. (1984). Antecedents of child abuse: Single and multiple factor models. *School Psychology International, 5,* 151–160.

Polansky, N., Cabral, R. J., Magura, S., & Phillips, M. H. Competitive norms for the childhood level of living scale. *Journal of Social Service Research, 6,* 45–55.

Polansky, N. A., & Williams, D. P. (1978). Class orientations to child neglect. *Social Work, 23,* 397–401.

Polansky, N. A., DeSaix, C., Wing, M. C., Patton, J. D. (1968). Child neglect in a rural community. *Social Casework, 49,* 467–474.

Rapaport, D., & Gill, M. M. (1959). The points of view and assumptions of metapsychology. In M. M. Gill (Ed.), The *Collected Papers of David Rapaport* (pp. 795–811). New York: Basic Books.

Reidy, T. J. (1977). The aggressive characteristics of abused and neglected children. *Journal of Clinical Psychology, 33,* 1140–1145.

Relich, R., Giblin, P. T., Starr, R. H., Agronow, S. J. (1980). Motor and social behavior in abused and control children: Observations of parent–child interactions. *Journal of Psychology, 106,* 193–204.

Ricoeur, P. (1970). *Freud and philosophy.* New Haven, CT: Yale University Press.

Robertson, K. R., & Milner, J. S. (1983). Construct validity of the child abuse potential inventory. *Journal of Clinical Psychology, 39,* 426–429.

Rosen, B. (1979). Interpersonal values amongst child-abusive women. *Psychological Reports, 45,* 819–822.

Rosenberg, M. S., & Reppucci, N. D. (1983). Abusive mothers: Perceptions of their own and their children's behavior. *Journal of Consulting and Clinical Psychology, 51,* 674–682.

Rosenblatt, A. D., & Thickstun, J. T. (1977). *Modern psychoanalytic concepts in a general psychology.* New York: International Universities Press.

Russell, D. (1982). *Rape in marriage.* New York: MacMillan.

Salzinger, S., Kaplan, S., & Artenyeff, C. (1982). Mothers' personal social networks and child maltreatment. *Journal of Abnormal Psychology, 92,* 68–76.

Sarafino, E. P. (1979). An estimate of a nationwide incident of sexual offenses against children. *Child Welfare, 58,* 127–34.

Schneider-Rosen, K., & Cicchetti, D. (1984). The relationship between affect and cognition in maltreated infants: Quality of attachment in the development of visual self-recognition. *Child Development, 55,* 648–658.

Schwartz, B. K. (1974). Easing the adaptation to parenthood. *Journal of Family Counseling, 2,* 32–39.

Sherrod, K. B., Altemeier, W. A., O'Connor, S., & Vietze, P. M. (1984). Early prediction of child maltreatment. *Early Child Development in Care, 13,* 335–350.

Silver, L. B., Dublin, C. C., & Lourie, R. S. (1969). Does violence breed violence? Contributions from a study of child abuse syndrome. *American Journal of Psychiatry, 126,* 404–407.

Simons, B., & Downs, E. F. (1968). Medical reporting of child abuse: Patterns, problems and accomplishments. *New York State Journal of Medicine, 68,* 2324–2330.

Smetana, J. G., Kelly, M., & Twentyman, C. T. (1984). Abused, neglected, and maltreated children's concepts of moral and social convention transgressions. *Child Development, 55,* 277–287.

Smith, J. E., & Rachman, S. J. (1984). Nonaccidential injury to children: II. A controlled evaluation of a behavioral management programme. *Behavior Research and Therapy, 22,* 349–366.

Smith, S. M., Hanson, R., & Noble, S. (1974). Interpersonal relationships in child rearing practices in 214 families of battered children. *British Journal of Psychiatry, 125,* 568–582.

Spinetta, J. J. (1978). Parental personality factors in child abuse. *Journal of Consulting and Clinical Psychology, 46,* 1409–1414.

Spinetta, J. J., & Rigler, D. (1972). The child-abusing parent: A psychological review. *Psychological Bulletin, 77,* 296–304.

Spitz, R. (1958). On the genesis of superego components. *Psychoanalytic Study of the Child, 13,* 375–403.

Starbuck, G. W., Krantzler, N., Forbes, K., & Barnes, V. (1984). Child abuse and neglect in Oahu, Hawaii: Description and analysis of 4 proported risk factors. *Journal of Developmental and Behavioral Pediatrics, 5,* 55–59.

Steele, B. F., & Pollock, C. B. (1974). A psychiatric study of parents who abuse infants and small children. In R. E. Helfer & C. N. Kempe (Eds.), *The battered child* (pp. 89–133). Chicago, IL: University of Chicago Press.

Steinberg, L. D., Catalano, R., & Dooley, D. (1981). Economic antecedents of child abuse and neglect. *Child Development, 52,* 975–985.

Stone, L. (1961). *The psychoanalytic situation.* New York: International Universities Press.

Straus, M. A. (1978). Causes, treatment, and research needs: Battered women: Issues of public policy. Washington, DC: Consultation: U.S. Commission on Civil Rights. January 30–31, 1978.

Straus, M. A., Gelles, R., & Steinmetz, S. (1980). *Behind closed doors: Violence in the American family.* New York: Doubleday.

Twentyman, C. T., & Plotkin, R. C. (1982). Unrealistic expectations of parents who maltreat their children. An educational deficit that pertains to child development. *Journal of Clinical Psychology, 38,* 497–503.

U.S. Department of Health and Human Services. (1980). *Elder abuse.* Washington, DC: Government Printing Office. DHHS. Publication No. (OHDS). 81-20152.

Von Bertalanffy, L. (1968). *General systems theory.* New York: George Braziller.

Waelder, R. (1962). Psychoanalysis, scientific method and philosophy. *Journal of the American Psychoanalytic Association, 10,* 617–637.

Walker, L. E. (1979). *The battered woman.* New York: Harper.

Wolfe, D. A., & Sandler, J. (1981). Training abusive parents in affective child management. *Behavior Modification, 5,* 320–335.

Wolfe, D. A., & Mosk, M. D. (1983). Behavioral comparisons of children from abusive and distressed families. *Journal of Consulting and Clinical Psychology, 51,* 702–708.

Wolfe, D. A., Sandler, J., & Kaufman, K. (1981). A competency-based parent training program for child abusers. *Journal of Consulting Clinical Psychology, 49,* 633–640.

Wolfe, D. A., Fairbank, J. A., Kelly, J. A., & Bradlyn, A. S. (1983). Child abusive parents' physiological responses to stressful and nonstressful behavior in children. *Behavioral Assessment, 5,* 363–371.

Young, L. (1964). *Wednesday's children: A study of child neglect and abuse.* New York: McGraw-Hill.

Zalba, S. R. (1966). The abused child: A survey of the problem. *Social Work, 11,* 3–16.

Zalba, S. R. (1967). The abused child: II. A typology for classification in treatment. *Social Work, 12,* 70–79.

Zilboorg, G. (1932). Sidelights on parent–child antagonism. *American Journal of Orthopsychiatry, 2,* 35–43.

3

Physical Aggression between Spouses

A Social Learning Theory Perspective

K. DANIEL O'LEARY

Before a theoretical analysis of spousal aggression is presented, it is imperative that one first understands the theory that supports the analysis. There are numerous theoretical accounts of aggression as reflected in Geen and Donnerstein's (1983) book, *Aggression: Theoretical and Empirical Reviews*. In addition, Gelles and Straus (1979) inventoried 15 theories that they felt were relevant to the understanding of violence between family members. The theories ranged from psychopathology or intrapsychic models to macrosociological models. Further, Gelles and Straus (1979) attempted to provide an integrated theoretical account of violence between family members. However, as Gelles (1983) later noted, the attempt to integrate resulted in a model that was "long on heuristic value and equally long and complex to examine," (p. 156). Consequently, Gelles moved from a model that attempted to integrate a plethora of concepts to a "more middle-range theory and set of theoretical propositions." He turned to exchange theory as a means of explaining family violence, a model that has been quite valuable in both sociological and social psychological research.

In this chapter, an attempt will be made to apply social learning theory (Bandura, 1969, 1977) to family violence and in particular to spousal aggression. Social learning theory is first and foremost a cognitive theory, one that more than any other cognitive theory has been placed in a social context. I am in total agreement with Gelles that theoretical accounts of aggression must now be middle-ground theories that attempt to explain some but not all of the phenomena of aggression. Aggression in general is probably one of the most frequently researched topics in psychology—particularly during the 1960s and 1970s. Indeed, a host of variables have been found to relate to aggression, varying from brain abnormalities (Mark, Sweet, & Erwin, 1975) to sugar ingestion (Prinz, Roberts, & Hartman, 1980) to police intervention policies (Sherman & Berke,

K. DANIEL O'LEARY • Psychology Department, State University of New York, Stony Brook, NY 11794–2500. Preparation of this chapter was supported in part by NIMH Grant MH35340.

1984). However, as Gelles (1983) stated, it is impossible to relate adequately all these accounts of aggression to family aggression. Instead, it seems most efficacious to select empirically verifiable variables presumed to be most relevant to spouse abuse. In this chapter, the following topics will be covered: major psychological conceptualizations of aggression, social learning theory, and criteria for evaluating theories. Next, the major portion of this chapter will be devoted to a theoretical account of spousal aggression. Included in this account will be violence in the family of origin, stress, aggression as a personality style, alcohol abuse, and relationship dissatisfaction. Finally, an evaluation of a social learning account of spousal aggression will be presented as will the generalizability of the spousal aggression model to child abuse.

In psychology, the early major theoretical accounts of aggression had to do with instinctual impulses (Freud, 1933; Lorenz, 1966), heritability and the XYY chromosome abnormality (Jacobs, Brunton, & Melville, 1965), and aggressive drives (Dollard, Doob, Miller, Mowrer, & Sears, 1939; Fesbach, 1964). The theoretical accounts based largely on instinctual or drive theory perspective have been found to be lacking in a number of ways. Most importantly, the instinctual accounts of aggression are often so general that they are not easily subject to empirical verification or refutation. The XYY abnormality accounts for a very small amount of aggressive behavior in a very minor portion of the population. The aggressive drive theories assume that frustration arouses an aggressive drive that can only be reduced through some form of aggressive behavior. In this frustration-aggression model, frustration is a necessary and sufficient condition for aggression. It is known that aggression does not always follow frustration and that many of the complexities of aggressive behavior are best explained by social variables.

WHAT IS SOCIAL LEARNING?

Social learning theory was given rudimentary form by Albert Bandura in 1969 in his book, *Principles of Behavior Modification,* and it was given more complete form in 1977 in his book, *Social Learning Theory*. Prior to Bandura's expositions, the two other major behavioral accounts of human behavior emphasized one dimension of psychological functioning to the relative neglect of others. For example, Skinner (1938, 1953) focused on the role of reinforcement of behavior; he placed almost sole emphasis on observable behavior, and he encouraged research aimed at predicting and controlling behavior. The Skinnerian emphasis came to be known as operant conditioning because of the central role of observable behavior and the manner in which behavior operates or interacts with the environment. In 1958, Wolpe published *Psychotherapy by Reciprocal Inhibition,* in which several treatment procedures were set forth based on principles of classical conditioning developed by Pavlov. More central in Wolpe's book was a procedure called systematic desensitization, an anxiety-reduction procedure, which became one of the best known and widely used behavior therapy procedures with adults. The pioneering work of Wolpe and Lazarus (Lazarus, 1971) was central in the establishment of modern behavior therapy practices with adults. However, the exposition of social learning theory by Bandura was the first major theoretical exposition of learning theory that incorporated three major regulatory systems of behavior: operant conditioning, classical conditioning, and cognitive mediational processes. In 1969, Bandura used cognitive mediational processes to integrate operant, classical, and vicarious learning. In 1979, and especially in 1986, Bandura used cognitive processes, namely, vicarious, self-regulatory, and self-reflective processes in the acquisition of knowledge. In turn, he changed the name of his exposition to social cognitive theory. Previous learning theorists, such as Tolman (1932, 1959), had given cognitive processes a central role in the determination of behavior, but no theorist had given a comprehensive account of the three regulatory systems prior to Bandura. An example of the integration of the three regulatory processes is given in the following statement:

> At this (cognitive) level stimulus inputs are coded and organized; tentative hypotheses about the principles governing the occurrence of rewards and punishments are developed and tested on the basis of differential consequences accompanying the corresponding actions; and, once established, implicit rules and strategies serve to guide appropriate performances in specified situations. Symbolically generated affective arousal and covert self-reinforcing operations may also figure prominently in the regulation of overt responsiveness. (Bandura, 1969, p. 63)

Bandura did not discount the role of differential reinforcement in molding behavior; instead he emphasized that the consequences of behavior do more than reward and punish behavior. Three functions of the response consequences were noted: informing, motivating, and reinforcing. In terms of the informational function, people observe the effects of their behavior and they form hypotheses about which behaviors are most appropriate in varied situations. This information then serves as a guide for future action. The motivational function of response consequences, according to Bandura, serves to create expectations that certain actions will have benefits and others will not. By imagining certain outcomes of our behavior, we can "convert future consequences into current motivators of behavior" (1977, p. 18). As Bandura noted, we do not wait until our house has burned down to purchase fire insurance. Instead, we engage in foresightful behavior. The reinforcing function of the consequences of our social behavior appear to occur when we are aware of the behaviors that are being rewarded. For most behavior, especially social behavior, reinforcing consequences are relatively ineffective unless the subject is aware of the reinforcement contingency. Given this fact, Bandura argues that the notion of response strengthening is at best a metaphor because response strengthening resulting from the consequences of our behavior was heretofore viewed as an automatic phenomenon. Instead, the consequences of our behavior play a key role in the regulation of previously acquired behavior, although Bandura believes that such consequences are inefficient ways of learning new behavior.

Learning through modeling is the method by which most human behavior is learned according to social learning theory. We observe others and from these observations, we form ideas of how new behaviors are performed. In turn, these coded observations serve as guides for further actions. Bandura's theories were probably most influential in this area of modeling, in that he explicated the processes that govern observational learning. More specifically, he elaborated four processes that influence whether one will engage in previously modeled behavior: attentional processes, retentional processes, motor reproduction processes, and motivational processes. In brief, it is held that people do not learn much by observation of others unless they attend to them and unless they remember what they observed. If we both attend to and remember what we observed, we also have to be able to perform the behaviors we saw, heard about, or read about. Of course, we need not be able to perform exactly the behaviors in question, such as when we observe someone serve in tennis, kick a soccer ball, or engage in a dance routine. As Bandura (1977) noted,

> In most everyday learning, people usually achieve a close approximation of the new behavior by modeling, and they refine it through self-corrective adjustments on the basis of informative feedback from performance and from focused demonstrations of segments that have been only partially learned. (p. 28)

Finally, we will engage in modeled behavior if the modeled behavior results in outcomes that are positive. There is an important difference in the acquisition (learning) of a behavior and the performance of a behavior; we may learn how to do things through modeling that we might never do because the modeled behavior had such disastrous consequences for the individual or because we perceive that engaging in such behavior would have disastrous consequences for us. In summary, we will engage in modeled behavior if we attend to the modeled event, if we can encode that event in our memories, if we can physically perform the specific behavior or some approximation thereof, and if we believe that engaging in such behavior will have positive consequences for us.

A social learning theory analysis recognizes the role of antecedent determinants of behavior. In contrast to some learning theory analyses, the social learning analysis indicates that stimuli influence the likelihood of particular behaviors through their predictive function, and not because of some automatic association of events and behavior. As Bandura (1977) emphasized, "Contingent experiences create expectations rather than stimulus–response connections" (p. 59). In 1986, he stated:

> Contrary to claims that behavior is controlled by its immediate consequences, behavior is related to its outcomes at the level of aggregate consequences, rather than immediate effects. . . People process and synthesize contextual and outcome information from sequences of events over long intervals about what behavior is needed to produce given outcomes. (p. 13)

We learn to avoid situations because we predict that we will have aversive experiences if we encounter those situations. Once established, avoidant behavior is hard to eliminate because the avoidance does not allow the individual to ascertain that negative events may no longer occur. Consistent with this view that the pairing of experiences renders stimuli predictive of response consequences is the evidence demonstrating that when a neutral event consistently occurs prior to provoked assault between animals, the predictive event alone produces fighting. Furthermore, we do not have to experience events directly in order to develop emotional reactions to them. We learn by observing that positive or negative events occur. Finally, in a process often called classical conditioning, there is a pairing of neutral stimuli with unconditioned responses. However, for almost all social behaviors, the process is not automatic; humans do not learn from repeated paired experiences unless they recognize that events are correlated.

Of special importance is the ability of humans to arouse emotions in themselves by imagining varied experiences. We can frighten ourselves by thinking about various frightening experiences—whether we ever personally experienced the events or not. It is extremely common for depressed clients to report that they imagined certain negative events (e.g., doing poorly on the job, wife with male friend, or child getting ill) and then to feel "down." Some sexual offenders report becoming very sexually aroused by imagining certain erotic scenes and then acting on these images.

Behavior Change Processes. In contrast to some theorists, Bandura placed key emphasis on the utility of psychological methods in changing psychological functioning. As he stated, "The value of a theory is ultimately judged by the power of the procedures it generates to effect psychological changes" (1977, p. 4). In changing anxious and avoidant behavior, the most effective means of producing psychological change have been performance based. That is, in order to help individuals overcome fears we have to get them to behave differently. However, the explanation of the behavior change process has been largely cognitive in social learning theory. According to Bandura (1977), psychological changes, regardless of the method used to achieve them, occur because of altered expectations of personal efficacy. An efficacy expectation is the conviction that one can successfully execute the behavior required to produce certain outcomes. An outcome expectation refers to an individual's estimate that a given behavior will produce certain outcomes. (p. 79)

As you might guess, a client or patient may believe that a given behavior would produce certain outcomes but doubt whether he could perform the behavior in question. People's beliefs in their ability to perform important behaviors (efficacy expectations) determine whether they will engage in those behaviors. The stronger our efficacy expectations, the greater the efforts we will make in trying to overcome obstacles. Therapeutic efforts to alter efficacy expectations may focus on changing our accomplishments by providing us with vicarious experiences in which we see others perform anxiety-provoking behavior without adverse consequences, by verbally persuading us that we can perform certain behaviors, and by reducing emotional arousal that often debilitates performance.

Reciprocal Determinism. According to the social learning perspective, human behavior is a function of continual reciprocal interaction between personal, behavioral, and environmental determinants. Of special importance is the premise that we can influence our own behavior and our environment. We can be considered partially free in that we can influence future conditions by our own behaviors. Although our courses of action are themselves determined, we exert some influence over the factors that govern our choices. As Bandura so aptly argued, "Because of the capacity for reciprocal influence, people are at least partial architects of their own destinies" (1977, p. 206).

Bandura's theory uses many practical examples of daily life, and his depictions are replete with social examples. As such, his theory is a social learning theory. He emphasizes the influence of people on people. Bandura's theory is the most popular theory of human behavior. It gained such popularity because it incorporated many of the traditional theories of learning, such as operant and classical conditioning, but gave the findings usually associated with those theories a distinctive cognitive flavor. In some clinical settings, Bandura has had a very strong influence. His concept of efficacy expectations has received more attention than almost any concept in adult clinical research in the past decade. According to two psychologists, Hilgard and Bower (1975), "In broad outline, social learning theory provides the best integrative summary of what modern learning theory has to contribute to practical problems" (p. 605).

As was apparent in my presentation of Bandura's social learning theory, the theory is clearly a cognitive theory. Previous learning theories, such as classical conditioning and operant conditioning, were depicted as operating in an automatic fashion through the pairing of various events. Bandura's social learning theory, in contrast, has a consistent cognitive theme in that almost any learning of a social nature occurs because it provides an individual with information, and the common denominator of any change process is the alteration of efficacy expectations. The decided emphasis on cognitive factors by Bandura is reflected in his 1986 book, *Social Foundations of Thought and Action: A Social and Cognitive Theory*. In order to provide a framework for an evaluation of a social learning theory approach to spousal aggression, it is first necessary to enumerate certain criteria for a good theory.

Criteria for Evaluating Theories

Many researchers describe their theory of a particular phenomenon. However, many so-called theories do not even meet minimal criteria for theories. The best method for building theories is still a matter of considerable debate (Sjoberg & Nett, 1968), but there is some consensus about characteristics of a good theory. According to Hergenhahn (1982), theories should have the following characteristics:

1. A theory synthesizes a number of observations.
2. A good theory is heuristic, that is, generates new research.
3. A good theory must generate hypotheses that can be empirically verified. If such hypotheses are confirmed, the theory gains strength; if not, the theory is weakened and must be revised or abandoned.
4. A theory is a tool and as such cannot be right or wrong; it is either useful or not useful.
5. Theories are chosen in accordance with the law of parsimony: of two equally effective theories, the simpler of the two must be chosen.
6. Theories contain abstractions, such as numbers or words, which contain the formal aspects of the theory.
7. All theories are attempts to explain empirical events and they must, therefore, start with empirical observations. (p. 21)

After reviewing a social learning approach to spousal aggression, we will return to these criteria to assess how well extensions of a social learning theory account for spousal aggression.

Theoretical Analysis of Spousal Aggression

Why is Spousal Aggression a Special Case of Aggression? Before turning to an elaboration of a social learning analysis of spousal aggression, it is important to know why an analysis of spousal aggression should be different from any general theory of aggression. Straus (1977) appropriately noted that family aggression and spousal aggression are different from many other acts of aggression. Among these differences are the following:

1. Spousal aggression occurs within a social group, the family, which is different from other small groups. Statuses and roles in the family are assigned on the basis of age and sex rather than interest and competence as is the case in most social groups.

2. There are conflicting normative expectations within a family about violence, but there is a long-standing implied right or obligation to use force on family members by husbands.

3. Commitment to family makes it difficult to leave the situation if violence occurs. Legal, moral, financial, and affective commitments make it especially hard for individuals to leave families even though violence has occurred.

4. Emotional involvements characterize most families, and it appears that this high emotional involvement may in fact be a partial cause of some of the violence in the family.

5. Until very recently, physical violence in the home was seen as a private matter, and, as such, was not the subject of much research and legal attention.

6. The family is a highly stressful unit because of the inherently unstable nature of the group.

This author agrees that commitment, emotional involvement, sanctions of family violence, and the private nature of the family make the occurrence of physical aggression in the family different from aggression in other social units, such as the workplace, school or college, or military. The last characteristic noted by Straus (1977), the stressful nature of the family, appears to be debatable as a unique aspect of social units. That is, for some individuals, family life may be an excellent source of solace and support, not stress.

Prevalence of Spousal Aggression. Now that we have some notion of the special characteristics of family violence that differentiate it from other types of physical aggression, let us turn to a brief summary of some important facts about spousal aggression. At a minimum, approximately 30% of American wives are the victims of some act of physical aggression by their husbands (Straus, Gelles, & Steinmetz, 1980). Based on our own research, it appears that at least half of all United States citizens, male and female, will be the recipient of at least one act of physical aggression by their partner at some point in their marriage (O'Leary et al., 1986). Furthermore, approximately 10% to 15% of the women in the United States will be victims of repeated and serious physical aggression from their partners (Straus et al., 1980). We found that women in beginning marriages engage in physical aggression against their husbands more frequently than husbands physically aggress against their wives, and we also found that women in beginning marriages engage in physical aggression against their husbands that is not reciprocated. However, we believe that the impact of men's physical aggression on women is usually more deleterious than women's physical aggression toward men. Further, in the extreme form of spousal aggression, that is, murder, of all female murder victims in 1985, 30% were killed by husbands or boyfriends. In contrast, 6% of all male murder victims were killed by wives or girl friends (U. S. Dept. of Justice, 1985).

Clinical Accounts of Spousal Aggression. Several clinical descriptions of spousal aggression can provide a framework for studying the phenomenon. Walker (1979) described the cycle of violence, and her clinical portrayal has been influential in aiding therapists to understand how the cycle can be broken. Walker depicted three phases of violence: a tension-building phase, an acute-violence phase, and a repentance phase. In the tension-building phase, the aggressor engages in minor threats and other verbally aggressive acts; the victim tries to cope by accepting blame or by verbal counterattacks. During the acute-violence phase, physically aggressive acts occur that are often marked by uncontrollable rage. The victim may attempt to fight back at first, but soon the victim learns that passivity is the best method of getting the violence to stop. According to Walker, this phase lasts from 2 to 24 hours. Following the acute-violence phase comes the repentance phase in which the batterer attempts to win his partner's forgiveness by solicitation, favors, and discussion.

Another clinical description of spousal violence is provided by Deschner (1984), who depicted seven stages of violence which incorporate Walker's three phase notions and Patterson's coercion model. The seven stages of violence as described by Deschner (1984) are as follows:

1. Mutual dependency. Two very needy individuals form a conjugal relationship with the hopes that all their needs will be met by their partner. Many promises are exchanged and passionate feelings are generated. A very exciting but isolated relationship forms. The battered woman often feels that her husband is like a child who must be taken care of.

2. Noxious Event. Some seemingly minor event, such as the wife not being home when the husband arrives, may be perceived as very negative.

3. Coercions Exchanged. The abuser-to-be makes attempts to stop what he views as the undesired behavior by means of threats and verbal denunciations. A spiraling of negative interchanges occurs.

4. "Last Straw" Decision. The climax occurs when the potential abuser decides the situation is intolerable. According to Deschner, this decision is critical. If it is never made, violence can be avoided. However, the history of verbal attacks and the cultural

values about what is appropriate and what is not appropriate influence the speed by which climax is reached.

5. Primitive Rage. Rages occur in response to the previous judgment. Possessions in the house and perhaps walls or doors may be destroyed. The batterer kicks, bites, or chokes the victim.

6. Reinforcement for Battering. According to Deschner, nearly all battered women agree that unless they are physically stronger than their spouses, the best way of coping with a fury of rage is to become submissive. Struggling and or counterattack are not productive and in fact will escalate the violence. Inadvertently, the victim is reinforcing the partner's aggression. As Deschner further notes, if the victim is not too badly injured, the victim may even further reward the batterer by "making placating gestures, such as taking all the blame on herself or trying harder to please him by providing food, housework, or sex." These placating gestures may even further serve to reinforce the batterer.

7. Repentance Phase. The batterer may swear that such an incident will never occur again. He may apologize to the victim and may even act affectionately. Finally, the batterer may even abdicate the position won by the violent coercion.

A Social Learning Theory Account of Spousal Aggression. The social learning account of spousal aggression to be presented here is a model that is currently being tested in our longitudinal study of spousal aggression, in which we are following couples from premarriage to 36 months after marriage. The model incorporates five major factors that predict spousal aggression:

1. Violence in the family of origin
2. Aggression as a personality style
3. Stress
4. Alcohol use and abuse
5. Relationship dissatisfaction

The depiction of the manner in which these variables interact in a fashion leading to spousal aggression is depicted in Figure 1, and a set of postulates associated with this model are presented in Table 1.

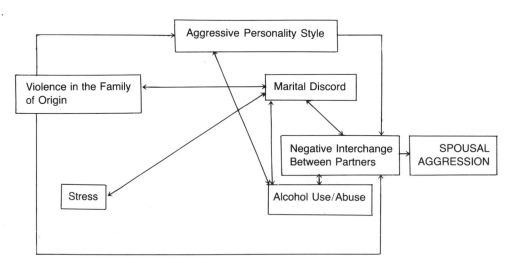

Figure 1. A social learning model of spousal aggression.

Violence in the Family of Origin

1. *Observation of parental aggression.* Parents who are physically aggressive with one another serve as models for generalized aggressive behavior and for spouse-specific aggression. If one observes a parent use physical aggression in a functional manner, (i.e., it leads to a desired effect such as making the partner cease an action or making the partner engage in some activity) one's own likelihood of using physical aggression should increase. Many individuals who hit their partner did not observe their parents hitting, and many individuals who did see their parents engage in physical aggression do not later hit their spouse. Prior observation of physical aggression is not a prerequisite for physical aggression against one's spouse; it is a condition that increases the probability that an individual will engage in spousal aggression. Finally, observation of physical aggression between parents does not operate in a direct fashion to produce spousal aggression. Many other factors intervene between the observation of parental aggression and the occasion for spousal aggression.

2. *Being beaten as a child.* Almost all parents of preschoolers report that they use physical punishment to discipline their children. However, when parents hit a child frequently or beat a child for engaging in undesired behavior, they inadvertently serve as a model for immature coping behavior. That is, the parent who beats a child indicates that one way to deal with frustration is to lash out physically against another. One sometimes even hears a parent apologize to a child after harshly hitting him or her claiming, "I just lost control." This parent will thus serve as an aggressive model for a child who will learn to be aggressive with others outside the home, and who may later excuse himself or herself for engaging in aggressive behavior by the "loss of control" rationale. Beating children may serve to increase their anxiety and hostility. Finally, being beaten as a child may lower self-esteem, which is known to correlate with spousal aggression.

Aggressive Personality Style

1. *Aggressive-impulsive personality style.* Individuals who have conduct problems as children and adolescents would most likely exhibit aggressive-impulsive personality styles as adults, because such patterns are relatively stable in general and particularly so for those in the upper ranges of such personality styles. When we measure aggressive personality styles of adults, we are often assessing anger (e.g., "Sometimes I feel like smashing things; Stupidity makes me angry; I rarely (often) get angry either at myself or at other people"). However, it is necessary to assess anger, for without anger physical aggression would not occur, and elevated anger scores would make physical aggression more probable.

2. *History of physical fighting.* One can assume that individuals with a long history of physical fighting were intermittently successful in such fights. These outcomes in elementary, junior and senior high school serve to reinforce aggressive behavior in general, and they should make the occurrence of spousal aggression more likely. Although it would be assumed that same-sex physical fighting should be more likely than opposite sex fighting, even frequent same sex fighting would make spousal aggression more probable than if such fighting did not occur. More critically, however, one would predict that spousal aggression would be more probable if an individual engaged in dating aggression against an opposite sex partner than if there were only a history of physical aggression against a same sex partner.

Stress

Stress is a background variable that makes physical aggression more likely if other variables such as observation of parental aggression and history of fighting are present. Stress *per se* is not sufficient to produce aggression. Many individuals when stressed will become depressed and socially isolated; others will become angry and physically aggressive given certain predisposing factors. Males and females react to certain stressful events differently, and it is necessary to assess coping with stress and the types of stressors that have the most negative impacts separately for men and women. Stress serves as an arousal or triggering mechanism such that at some level stress will make the individual more likely to respond in one of his or her less desirable but somewhat stylistic manner.

Alcohol

Alcohol depresses cortical control and makes aggression more probable. When taken in excess, alcohol will make spousal aggression more likely even when the predisposing factors to spousal aggression like observation

(Cont.)

of parental aggression and physical history of hitting are not present. Alcohol will make spousal aggression more likely in both men and women.

Marital (Relationship) Discord

Without discordant marital interaction at some recent time, no physical aggression will occur. In young couples, general marital discord need not be present, but in older couples, general discord will be one of the major predictors of spousal aggression. In almost all couples, however, a negative interchange between the partners occurs before spousal aggression.

From our own research, as well as the research of others, we know that demographic variables, such as age, education, and income are significantly related to spousal violence. In fact, Straus *et al.* (1980) catalogued 20 characteristics that have been found to be related to spouse abuse. However, multivariate analyses are notably absent from the spouse abuse research, and, as a consequence, the unique portions of variance associated with spouse abuse by particular variables is unclear. For example, I know of no published account of spouse abuse that indicates whether the critical unique variance in demographic variables associated with such abuse is explainable by age, income, education, or some combination thereof. At this point, we can only point to correlates of spouse abuse. Because so many factors have been associated with spouse abuse, the analysis presented here will use only those psychological factors presumed to have the greatest relevance to spousal aggression. A more elaborate model of spousal aggression was presented by O'Leary and Arias (1987a), that incorporates contextual variables (i.e., individual characteristics, couple characteristics, and societal characteristics); situational variables (i.e., precipitating events and appraisal of the precipitating event); and outcome variables (i.e., conflict resolution method chosen, consequences of resolution method chosen, and appraisal of consequences of resolution method chosen). This model (see Fig. 2) is reasonably comprehensive, but we do not have measures of all of these variables to include in a

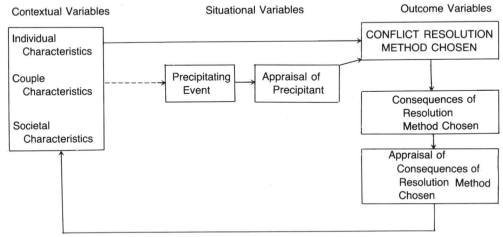

Figure 2. Theoretical model of the etiology of spouse abuse: → represents strong, causal relationship; ⟶ Represents weaker, causal relationship. Taken from O'Leary and Arias (1987b), Prevalence, correlates and development of Spouse Abuse. Chapter to appear in R. DeV. Peters and R. J. McMahon (Eds.), *Marriage and families: Behavioral treatments and processes.* Copyright 1987 by Brunner/Mazel, New York. Reprinted by permission.

single multivariate analysis. However, the more elaborate model does consider certain cognitive and reinforcement variables that are central to any full social learning analysis. We are currently conducting longitudinal research on our model, that is designed to assess the relative power of the different variables in predicting spouse abuse. In cross-sectional research and in some longitudinal research during the next 5 years, we will also expect to test certain hypotheses regarding cognitive and reinforcement factors as they relate to spousal aggression. In brief, our basic model under present examination is presented, because we have measures of all variables described to allow us to test empirically the efficacy of this model in predicting spousal aggression. As we develop the cognitive and reinforcement measures to allow us to examine empirically more complex models of spousal aggression, we will test more expansive models, such as the one presented by O'Leary & Arias (1987b).

VIOLENCE IN THE FAMILY OF ORIGIN

It has become a well-accepted fact that a disproportionate number of individuals who engage in physical aggression against their partners come from homes in which they saw their parents hit one another (Straus *et al.*, 1980). In fact, although a large number of factors have received attention in the etiology of spousal aggression, the intergenerational transmission of marital violence has received more attention than almost any other correlate of spouse abuse (cf. Arias, 1984; Steinmetz, 1977). The theoretical rationale for the intergenerational transmission of marital violence is derived from social learning theory. More specifically, modeling or observational learning has been used as a mechanism to explain why certain individuals acquire physical aggression as an appropriate response to a spouse.

Arias (1984) reviewed the role of observational learning as it pertains to spousal violence, and noted that modeling has three types of effects on the observer: (a) the acquisition of new responses or patterns of behavior; (b) the inhibition/disinhibition of previously learned behaviors and (c) response facilitation (Bandura, 1977). Acquisition of new responses refers to the learning and performance of a novel response (for the observer) in a new situation similar to the response displayed by the model in similar situations. Inhibition or disinhibition of previously learned behaviors refers to a decrease or an increase, respectively, in the probability that the observer will perform a response already existing in his or her repertoire of responses as a function of the observed punishing or rewarding consequences of the model's behavior. Response facilitation refers to an increase in the probability of occurrence of a response already existing in the observer's repertoire as a function of observing the model engaging in a similar response. The difference in response facilitation and response disinhibition is the social desirability of the modeled behavior: response facilitation refers to an increase in a socially desirable behavior; response disinhibition refers to an increase in the probability of a socially undesirable behavior.

In her application of social learning theory to conjugal violence, Arias (1984) indicated that, of the three effects just noted, the transmission of violence across generations is likely caused by disinhibition of previously learned behavior. She used Bandura's claim that modeling is generally more successful in producing disinhibitory effects than in producing facilitation effects to support her point that the transmission of conjugal violence across generations is likely a response disinhibition effect. More specifically, the disinhibition effect is more likely to occur because the socially undesirable behavior is usually positively reinforcing for the actor. In turn, the durability of the modeling effect is determined in large part by the reinforcement contingencies for engaging in the modeled behavior. With regard to conjugal violence, especially male to female violence, the negative consequences for engaging in physical aggression are often delayed (deterioration of the marital relationship, separation, and divorce). As such, the punishing consequences of a male engaging in conjugal violence are probably not strong enough to result in a suppression of the behavior.

In their book, *Social Learning and Personality Development,* Bandura and Walters (1963) indicated that similarity of sex and age of the model to the observer were important factors influencing the modeling effect. However, similarity of probable consequences was held to be more important than similarity of sex and age. Nonetheless, all other things being equal, one would predict that similarity of sex of the model to the observer would be predictive of whether an observer will engage in the modeled behavior. That is, males who observed their fathers hit their mothers would be more likely to hit their wives than if they saw their mothers hit their fathers.

Research on intergenerational transmission of aggression has focused on whether men who observed their fathers hit their mothers or those who observed their mothers hit their fathers, are more likely to engage in physical aggression against their partners than those who did not. Research on this issue has also focused on the topic of whether women who observed their fathers hit their mothers are more likely to approve of physical aggression against a wife and whether they themselves are more likely to be physically attacked by their husbands than women who did not observe their fathers hit their mothers. Most research has focused on father to mother aggression because such aggression is more likely to come to the attention of legal authorities and mental health professionals than mother to father aggression.

Observation of Spousal Violence and Attitudes Toward Aggression. As predicted by social learning theory, Ulbrich and Huber (1981) found in a stratified cluster sample of approximately 1,100 women and 900 men, that for men, exposure to fathers hitting mothers was associated with approval of a husband hitting his wife. For women, exposure to fathers hitting mothers was not predictive of their approval of a husband hitting his wife. Interestingly, however, exposure to mothers hitting fathers was predictive of a woman's approval of a husband hitting his wife. Unfortunately, Ulbrich and Huber did not assess the approval of wife to husband hitting, and it is not possible to conclude from their research that exposure to a same-sex model is predictive of approval of physical aggression by a husband or wife regardless of the victim's gender.

Exposure to Parental Violence and Spousal Aggression. A number of studies have indicated that there is an association between observation of fathers hitting mothers and subsequent spousal violence. This finding is most consistent for men; the findings regarding the effects of observation of parental violence on females is not consistent.

Pagelow (1981) obtained data on approximately 350 battered women who were staying in shelters. These women provided information about their own and their husbands' families concerning the origin of aggression. Forty-three percent of the battered women reported that they saw or heard their fathers hitting their mothers whereas 70% of the men were reported to have heard or seen their fathers hitting their mothers. Of course, the data are potentially biased in that the women were reporting on violence in their husbands' families. Further, all of these subjects were from shelters, which limits the generalizability of the results. Finally, there was no nonviolent control group matched for socioeconomic status.

Rosenbaum and O'Leary (1981) obtained data from 32 couples in which the husbands had physically aggressed against their wives, 20 discordant couples in which physical aggression was not a major presenting problem, and 20 maritally satisfied couples. For women, there was no association between exposure to marital violence and being a victim of subsequent spousal violence. For men, there was a significant association between exposure to marital violence and being a member of the physically abusive group. Although this finding was useful in that it was the first in which the reports of abusive men were obtained directly, it did not look at the direct association between observation of marital violence and subsequent spousal violence. Instead, it looked at exposure to marital violence and group membership, that is, whether one was in an abusive or nonabusive group. However, a subsequent study by O'Leary and Curley (1986), using an identical methodology to Rosenbaum and O'Leary (1981), did look at the association between exposure to parental violence and subsequent spousal violence for men. For women, again, there was no association between exposure to parental violence and being a victim of spousal violence.

Straus *et al.* (1980), in their representative sampling research with over 900 men and 1,100 women, found a significant association between witnessing parental violence and physically aggressing against a spouse for men and women. Further, they also looked at same-sex modeling effects of interparental violence. They did not predict same-sex modeling effects, and they did not report statistical analyses of their data on this topic. However, they reported that 13% of their sample observed father to mother aggression and 8.5% observed mother to father aggression. Apparently, boys who observed violence by the father were not affected more than daughters who observed violence by the mother. In brief, there did not seem to be a sex-specific modeling effect, but there did seem to be a general modeling effect.

Kalmuss (1984), in a reanalysis of the Straus *et al.* (1980) data with severely abused individuals, again did not find a sex-specific modeling effect. Sixteen percent of the respondents reported witnessing parental violence, and there were no differences in the rates reported by men and women. Whereas the probability of engaging in severe aggression was approximately 1% for the total sample, the probability of engaging in severe aggression was 8% of the individual, either male or female, had observed interparental violence.

Arias (1984), in a study of 369 young couples about to be married, found that exposure to interparental violence was associated with aggressive attitudinal and personality styles. However, exposure to interparental aggression was significantly associated with aggression against a current mate for males but not for females. On the other hand, exposure to interparental violence was associated with physical aggression against other people for women but not for men. Stepwise logistic regression analyses showed that the effect of interparental violence on women's extrafamilial physical aggression was mediated by aggressive predispositions. With these analyses, she inferred that observation of violence has a direct modeling effect for men but an indirect effect for women (See Figs. 3 and 4, from O'Leary & Arias, 1987b). These results should be replicated by others before great stock is placed in them for theory building. However, if these results were to be replicated, they point to the need to have different theoretical models of spousal aggression for men and women.

It is important to note here that the amount of variance accounted for by observation of father hitting mother or mother hitting father is quite small in some samples. For example, in our own research with 393 couples, observation of either parent hitting the other is significantly associated with partner aggression, but it accounted for less than 4%

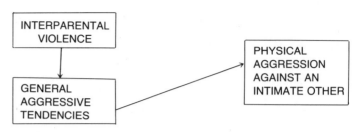

Figure 3. Model of women's premarital physical aggression most supported by the resulting empirical relationships.

of the variance in spousal aggression. Many individuals who see their parents hit each other do not engage in spousal aggression. Such results lead us to emphasize strongly the need for multiple predictors of spouse abuse (Tyree, Malone, & O'Leary, 1987).

Being the target of very harsh discipline or beatings by parents has also been shown to correlate with spouse abuse (Rosenbaum & O'Leary, 1981; Straus *et al.*, 1980). Although this variable has received less attention in the prediction of spouse abuse than has the observation of physical aggression between parents, we found it to be approximately equal to observation of parental fighting in predicting spousal aggression (Rosenbaum & O'Leary, 1981). We believe that more attention should be paid to the type of discipline one receives as a child in models of spousal aggression. Straus *et al.* (1980) presented some very interesting data regarding the role of physical punishment received as a child and later spouse abuse. Of special interest was their finding that the link between being hit as a teenager and hitting a marriage partner was not as strong for women as it was for men.

In sum, modeling accounts of spousal aggression indicate that there is clearly an effect of observing parental violence on both men and women. One study using multivariate analyses indicates that the effect of observing parental violence appears to have a more direct influence on men than women. More specifically, whereas observing violence is associated with a higher rate of spousal aggression for both men and women, this effect seems to be a direct one for the men whereas it operates through an aggressive personality style for women. The role of harsh physical discipline that one receives as a child has received less attention by most investigators than observation of spousal aggression but it is clearly a factor to place in any model of spouse abuse, and it should receive more attention in the future.

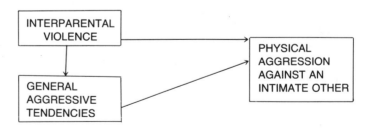

Figure 4. Model of men's premarital physical aggression most supported by the resulting empirical relationships.

Stress does not have the same effects on all people. In fact, some persons seek out environments that would seem stressful to most individuals. For example, some individuals choose to play tennis in very hot weather whereas others would find such activity unbearable. Some love to dance in discotheques where the decibel level is over 100 and the lights flash incessantly; others report they get vertigo in these environments. Simply stated, certain environmental factors, such as extreme heat and noise *per se,* often have no effect on aggression. As Mueller (1983) argued, the presence of an environmental stressor is not sufficient for the occurrence of aggressive behavior. He presented a theoretical model that suggests characteristics of situations that differentiate aggression-inducing environments from those that have little or no effect. First, he pointed out that many environmental stressors are arousing, and this arousal serves as a generalized drive for behavior. In addition, drive serves its greatest motivating effects on the predominant response mode. If the individual is predisposed to act in an aggressive manner, the environmental stressor should make aggression more likely. Second, environmental stressors can produce stimulus overload, in which the individual becomes overwhelmed and unable to process information effectively. Third, stressors can interfere with ongoing behavior and engender feelings of loss of control. Fourth, according to Mueller, stressors can make one annoyed, irritable, and uncomfortable; as he further comments, the fact that negative affect can increase aggression is both intuitively obvious and empirically demonstrated (e.g., Berkowitz, 1969). Finally, each of these four factors, arousal, stimulus overload, interference with ongoing behavior, and feelings of annoyance, can interact to influence aggression. Following the presentation of this model, research was presented to Mueller to show that heat, noise, personal space invasions, and crowding, especially for men, make the probability of aggression higher. There is almost no research on the effects of these variables on spousal violence, but Michael and Zumpe (1986) found that violence by men toward women increases in the summer and that the increases were independent of opportunity for contact between perpetrator and victim. Interestingly, in concordance with the social learning orientation of this chapter, it is clear that in experimental studies of environmental stressors, cognitive variables moderate the influence of aggression. One would expect the same result to hold with spousal violence. As predictability and perceived control over environmental events is greater, spousal violence should be less frequent.

Stress seems to be associated with marital violence, and this finding has been replicated by a number of investigators (e.g., Barling & MacEwen, 1986; Neidig & Friedman, 1984; O'Leary, Arias, Barling, & Rosenbaum, 1985; Straus, 1980). Straus concluded that it is not stress *per se* that is the cause of marital violence. Violence is but one of many responses to stress. One may leave the situation, become depressed or anxious, develop physical symptomology, or drink heavily. In his research, most people who experienced a high level of stress did not engage in spousal aggression. He argued that stress is a mediating variable that may occur in combination with other variables to make violence more likely. For example, if a male reported low stress levels and his father hit his mother, the probability of his assaulting his spouse was 5%; however, if a male reported high stress levels and his father hit his mother, the probability of his assaulting his partner was 17%.

In the military there are certain types of stressors that predispose men to engage in spousal aggression. For example, there is a very clear chain of command in the military with a firm hierarchical, authoritarian model. This model works well in the military but if it is used within the family it may create extreme controversy. For example, a link between stress and child abuse was found by Shwed and Straus (1979) in the Air Force. They found that the prevalence of child abuse was higher in the Air Force than in the civilian sector, and contrary to patterns in the civilian sector, fathers tended to be more abusive than mothers. Stress-related factors that predisposed men to child abuse were low rank, geographical isolation, and a job description associated with violence.

Within the Marine Corps, Neidig (1985) found that the longer a man was a drill instructor, the more likely he was to engage in spousal aggression. More specifically, 28% of husbands who had been drill instructors less than one year engaged in spousal violence. In contrast, 42% of the drill instructors who had been in the billet more than one year engaged in spousal violence. As Neidig stated,

> the linear relationship between length of time on the drill field and increasing conflict and declining marital satisfaction suggests strongly that marital conflict and dissatisfaction can be accurately understood as an occupational hazard for this billet. (p. 4)

The fact that there is partial self-selection of drill instructors might lead some to conclude that personality style of the drill instructors was the critical variable. However, length of time as a drill instructor suggests that the training and job play a significant role in the instigation of aggression, and these factors operate over and above personality styles.

In a sample of young civilian couples, O'Leary, Arias, Rosenbaum, and Barling (1985) found that stress was significantly related to spousal aggression for men and women. Similarly, Makepeace (1983), using an undergraduate population, also found that stressful events predicted physical aggression with one's partner for men and women. Finally, Riggs (1986), using an undergraduate population, also found that physical aggression with one's dating partner was predicted by stress levels for men and not for women.

Based on a social learning analysis, one would expect that heightened levels of emotional arousal would have a number of negative consequences. It also appears that heightened levels of arousal for which individuals have no explanation generally become labeled and felt as anger in hostile contexts and as euphoria in positive contexts. As Bandura (1986) noted, given people's strong propensity to interpret events, it is unlikely that they will experience arousal for long without producing an explanation for it. From this perspective, stress and the often concomitant anxiety or anger are the products of two separate factors, heightened visceral arousal and cognitive self-labeling of the arousal as anxiety or anger. In this vein, the stress management literature has led therapists to help spouse abusers to identify stress symptoms, to identify stressors contributing to their symptoms, and to help these individuals to learn coping skills to deal with the stressors they encounter. For example, Novaco (1978) showed in a laboratory provocation situation that subjects who learned relaxation, especially when coupled with cognitive coping instructions, were able to demonstrate increased self-control over anger as evidenced by self-report measures and by physiological indexes.

In summary, there is common agreement that environmental stressors do not cause spousal aggression *per se*. Instead, they enhance the likelihood that aggression will be more likely, given other factors such as an aggressive personality style. Because of the moderating effects of cognitive variables on stressful events, it is necessary to have more sophisticated testing of stress factors. In an investigation of the effects of life stressors, MacEwen and Barling (in press) showed that for women stress predicted marital aggression one year later after controlling for age, education, and initial level of marital aggression.

It has long been known that aggression is one of the most stable characteristics of human behavior. In fact, with the exception of intelligence, no other behavior of humans is more stable. For example, the test–retest correlation of the Iowa Test of Basic Skills (a group intelligence test), is .89 for a 3-year interval for children in Grades 3 and 6 (Cronbach, 1977). The test–retest correlation of ratings of aggression for children assessed at Grades 3 and 6 was .63 (Olweus, 1979). More data on the stability of aggression and intelligence have been obtained on children than adults, but Olweus (1979) summarized the data on aggression and intelligence, with intervals from 2 to 18 years for aggression and with intervals up to 5 years for intelligence. Essentially, the stability coefficients for intelligence are in the range of .80 to .90, whereas stability coefficients for aggression are in the range of .50 to .80 (coefficients corrected for attenuation).

Our own data on spousal aggression, with 393 couples assessed at premarriage, 6 months, and 18 months after marriage indicate remarkable stability for spousal aggression (O'Leary et al., 1986). More specifically, the data on the stability of physical aggression between partners as measured by the Conflicts Tactics Scale (CTS) using Pearson correlations, on continuous CTS data, were as follows for men:

- premarriage to 6 months   .66
- 6 months to 18 months   .78
- premarriage to 18 months   .49

For women the data were the following:

- premarriage to 6 months   .63
- 6 months to 18 months   .76
- premarriage to 18 months   .57

Given these stability figures, one wonders how well aggressive personality styles predict partner aggression. Arias (1984), using the Jackson Personality Research Form, found that high aggression scores were significantly associated with physical aggression against a partner for men and women. Furthermore, using logistic regression analyses with 369 couples about to be married, she found that controlling for the observation of interparental violence, there was a significant association between aggressive personality styles (high aggression scores on the Jackson PRF) and partner aggression for men and women. However, as noted earlier in this chapter, when one controlled for aggressive personality styles, the observation of interparental violence was significantly associated with partner aggression only for men. For women, the influence of observing parental aggression was moderated by aggressive personality styles. Alternatively stated, observation of parental aggression was only predictive of spousal aggression if the women had adopted an aggressive personality style.

Multivariate analyses of the reports of physical aggression in junior and senior high school and in postsecondary school have proven especially useful in predicting partner aggression. In preliminary analyses of 369 women 18 months after marriage, Tyree, Malone, and O'Leary (1987) found a canonical correlation of .61 between reports of physical aggression with others (parents, friends, and acquaintances) and spousal aggression. For 369 men, the canonical correlation between reports of physical aggressing against others and spousal aggression was .45. These correlations are among the highest one sees in the literature on aggressive personality styles and other measures of aggression, and we are anxious to see if these findings replicate in our longitudinal sample at a later point in the marriages. Of special interest was the finding that physical aggression seems to be a more generalized behavioral characteristic for women than men. That is, based on correlational analyses of spousal aggression and general aggression, women's aggression was more predictable across situations. These data as well as others presented earlier lead us to believe that within a few years a sophisticated theoretical analysis of spousal aggression will probably posit different causal variables in predicting spousal aggression for men and women.

Use of personality variables as predictor and outcome variables in behavioral research lost favor in the 1960s and 1970s, but there appears to be a resurgence of interest in personality variables by some behavioral researchers who are attempting to use standardized self or other ratings of stylistic factors in process and outcome research (cf. O'Leary & Wilson, 1987). In the spouse abuse area differences of opinion have been so great regarding DSM-III diagnoses for use with aggressors and victims of spouse abuse that there is a move by the Council of Representatives of the American Psychological Association to create a Diagnostic and Statistical Manual separate from the American Psychiatric Association or one that is based on decision making with more equal representation by psychologists and psychiatrists than exists at present (Landers, 1986). One of the major issues leading to rancor among psychologists and psychiatrists has been the possible use of the diagnostic label masochistic personality disorder for battered women. Although it is not a major subject of discussion, one might also raise the issue of the applicability of the DSM-III diagnosis Disorders of Impulse Control to men or women who frequently physically aggress against their partner. The criterion for Intermittent Explosive Disorder and Isolated Explosive Disorders—absence of signs of generalized impulsivity or aggressiveness—does not fit with the clinical picture of many men who physically abuse their spouses, their children, and even sometimes their pets. The category Atypical Personality Disorder has absolutely no diagnostic criteria other than "Disorders for Impulse Control that cannot be classified elsewhere" (American Psychiatric Association, p. 298, 1980). The diagnostic category should receive attention in any revision of DSM-III because of the relevance to spousal aggression. Whereas some individuals who physically aggress against their spouses evidence generalized aggressive tendencies, others do not.

Alcohol Use

Alcoholism or alcohol use is one of the most frequently discussed topics related to spousal aggression. Unfortunately, the reported incidence of alcohol use during physically aggressive interchanges varies greatly. As Rosenbaum and O'Leary (1981) noted, rates vary between 21% (Bard & Zacker, 1974) and 95% (Roy, 1977). More common estimates of alcohol use and spousal aggression range from about 40% to 60% (e.g., Fotjik, 1977, 67%; Gayford, 1975, 44%; Gelles, 1972, 48%). Consistent with the highly varying use of figures are professional judgments about the role of alcohol in spousal violence. For example, Bard and Zacker (1974) suggest that alcohol may be associated with reduced levels of violence and may in fact have a calming effect, reducing the possibility of violence in a family quarrel. Although alcohol is indeed a depressant, it also functions to reduce inhibitions and increase the probability of unacceptable behaviors. Congruent with a cognitive or social learning perspective, alcohol serves as an expectancy effect in that many individuals believe that they will be less controlled when they imbibe alcohol. This fact has been repeatedly shown in the area of sexual arousal when subjects are given actual alcohol or nonalcoholic drink mixtures (O'Leary & Wilson, 1987). Further, subjects with a history of light drinking also excuse spousal violence more when the aggressor has been ingesting alcohol than when the aggressor has not had any alcohol (Jouriles & Collins, 1986).

Rosenbaum and O'Leary (1981) found that alcohol use was significantly associated with spousal aggression. They found that 40% of the abusive husbands were clearly alcoholic by the most conservative standards, according to the Michigan Alcoholism Screening Test. In contrast, only 5% of the control group of satisfactorily married husbands matched for socioeconomic status were alcoholic. This latter figure is similar to the national rate of alcoholism of 5% according to the Third Special Report to the United States Congress on Alcohol and Health from the Secretary of HEW (NIAAA, IFS no. 53, November 30, 1978). A second control group, a group of maritally distressed husbands who did not present at a marital clinic for problems of spouse abuse, had an alcoholism rate of 20%, suggesting that marital discord and alcohol use may serve a complex interactive role.

In a study with 393 couples about to be married, O'Leary, Arias, Rosenbaum, and Barling (1985) used the Short Michigan Alcoholism Screening Test and found that alcohol use was significantly associated with physical aggression against a partner for men and women. Further, when those individuals in this sample who scored clearly in the alcoholic range on the Short Michigan Alcoholism Screening Test were analyzed, it was found that they were more likely to be physically aggressive with their partner than individuals who did not drink heavily.

Stuart and Leonard (1983) presented evidence for a model that emphasizes the interactive effects of alcohol and contextual cues in the drinking situation. The results indicate that given the presence of instigative cues, a moderate dose of alcohol increases the probability that an aggressive response will occur. According to Stuart and Leonard, the empirical evidence does not support a simple expectancy effect. They disavow the assumption that the act of drinking rather than intoxication is responsible for the acting-out behavior. Of special interest in their chapter on general aggression was their emphasis on the fact that many intoxicated subjects behave nonaggressively when they compete under nonthreatening conditions. They therefore argue against a purely pharmacological disinhibition model that posits that alcohol releases primitive, repressed aggressive impulses by weakening cortical control or a censorship system. In a recent substantive review of the effects of alcohol on aggression, Chritchlow (1986) concluded that whereas the alcohol–crime link was popularized in the 19th century and has continued to be popular, it also must be recognized that this link may be more sociocultural than pharmacological.

Relationship (Marital) Dissatisfaction

When I was working with couples who presented with problems of physical abuse, I believed that marital discord was a key causal factor in predicting spouse abuse. More specifically, in the Rosenbaum and O'Leary (1981) research, marital discord was the most significant correlate of spouse abuse. Rosenbaum (1980) used discriminant analyses to assess the most important factors that differentiated abusive from nonabusive couples. When wife data were considered separately, and when wife and husband data were considered together, the most important variable in discriminating the abusive from nonabusive groups was marital satisfaction. Marital satisfaction was far more important than witnessing parental violence, being a victim of beatings as a child, having conservative attitudes toward women, alcohol use, and general assertiveness. These results seemed so strong and seemed to make such sense clinically that Rosenbaum (1980) proposed a model of spousal violence in which marital discord was the key link in the causal chain leading to physical aggression.

Our view of the role of relationship dissatisfaction changed, however, when we began examining factors associated with partner aggression in young couples. In our sample of 393 couples about to be married, we found that 42% of the women and 33% of the men reported that they had engaged in at least one act of physical aggression against their partner in the past year. In addition, at 6 and 18 months after marriage, females also reported more aggression against their partners (37% vs. 27% and 33% vs. 26% respectively). As there are a number of plausible reasons why an individual might underreport acts of physical aggression against his or her partner, prevalence estimates were also calculated using self-reports of either the aggressor or the victim. Across these three assessment periods, the prevalence rates were approximately 10% higher when using this either/or index. All of these prevalence rates of partner aggression are at least twice as high as in any previous reports of married individuals, and in fact, they are higher than we obtain in our marital therapy clinic at the State University of New York at Stony Brook. When we looked at the relationship satisfaction scores of couples prior to marriage who were physically aggressive and those that were not physically aggressive, we did find significant differences between the two groups (O'Leary *et al.*, 1985). However, the scores of the two groups on a modified version of the Locke-Wallace Marital Adjustment Test indicated that the mean scores of the physically aggressive subjects were all above 100. Therefore, we had to reconceptualize our view of the causal factors in spouse abuse because individuals who engaged in physical aggression against their partner and even those who reported being victims of physical aggression had mean relationship satisfaction scores that were above 100, the usually accepted cutoff for relationship dissatisfaction (Jouriles & O'Leary, 1986). More specifically, if an individual receives a score of 100 or greater on this measure, he or she indicates that the couple has few disagreements on many important issues (sex, finances, philosophy of life), and that he or she is quite satisfied with the marital relationship. Thus we certainly conclude that marital dissatisfaction is not a necessary condition for spousal aggression.

In interviews with our subjects, it is clear that some form of disagreement takes place that in one way or another precedes any physical aggression. In that sense, some relationship dissatisfaction is critical in the development of aggression against one's partner. However, as evident from the material presented in the previous paragraph, the dissatisfaction with the relationship in these cases is not pervasive. Furthermore, there are many couples who report some physical aggression against their partner as well as very high relationship satisfaction scores. In sum, it appears that a very negative interaction with a partner is a key link in the etiology of aggression but that these negative interactions do not need to be pervasive. Partners do not simply come home and hit their partner without some negative interaction. They may come home in an angry mood, but something in the partner interaction must also go awry for spousal aggression to occur.

Consistent with the approach presented here, we have argued elsewhere that when some event occurs that could trigger an angry reaction in some individuals (e.g., partner comes home one hour late), it is the individual's appraisal of the event that will determine whether it is seen as especially negative or not (O'Leary & Arias, 1987b). As mentioned earlier, Deschner (1984), in her seven-stage model of partner aggression, indicates that some noxious event occurs in the chain of events leading to physical abuse. This noxious event is something perceived as unpleasant by the victim to be. Several days after the partner aggression, the event may seem very trivial to even the aggressor. Deschner

(1984) further points to another stage in the abuse process, "Coercions Exchanged," a stage in which the abuser-to-be makes an attempt to stop the unpleasant behavior by means of threats or denunciations. The crucial stage, however, according to Deschner is the "Last Straw Decision" phase when the potential abuser decides that the situation is intolerable. As she noted, if this decision is never reached, the violence is avoided.

With couples who have been married for many years and who have been discordant for a significant portion of those years, it is likely that the appraisal of an event will be negatively colored by the marital discord (Schacter & O'Leary, 1985). In addition, it also appears that some individuals get very easily aroused by events that leave others minimally affected. The appraisal of events as negative and the subsequent negative interchanges are crucial in the development of partner aggression.

AN EVALUATION OF SOCIAL LEARNING THEORY

Using the criteria of theories discussed earlier in the chapter, let us now evaluate how well social learning principles can be applied to spousal aggression.

Social learning theory has been one of the basic theories that has driven some specific hypotheses regarding the etiology of marital violence. More specifically, the modeling of violence has been one of the most frequently tested assumptions in this area. It has proven fruitful in that the modeling hypotheses have received repeated empirical support.

Social learning theory is based on cognitive theory and it spawns hypotheses regarding the influence of various social events on human behavior. With the exception of assessing attitudes toward violence, there have been very few research investigations that have used variables that flow directly from the cognitive elements of social learning theory. It is in this context, however, that social learning theory has its greatest potential. Personal efficacy as a theoretical construct has proven useful in many clinical arenas, and it could well prove useful in other areas, such as marital interventions and in understanding the etiology of aggression. The model of spousal aggression presented in this chapter contains several important gaps in terms of social learning theory as presented by Bandura in 1977, and it lacks a focus on reinforcement that has been a cornerstone of behavior theories since Skinner. Although Bandura moved to a decidedly cognitive view of reinforcement in his 1986 book, *Social Foundations of Thought and Action: A Social and Cognitive Theory,* some emphasis on reinforcement is necessary in a social learning model of spousal aggression.

Whether social learning theory or more restricted models of spousal aggression prove most useful in the near future remains to be seen. As noted early in this chapter, I believe that the more restrictive models of spousal aggression will prove most useful in a heuristic sense in the next decade. However, I also believe that social learning theory provides a very fruitful rubric for conceptualizing aggression in general and in particular spousal aggression. As indicated in the title of this chapter, we are not testing the validity of social learning theory in general. Instead, we are evaluating the effects of a social learning perspective in interpreting spousal aggression data.

With regard to the criteria of a good theory, the social learning model does allow one to synthesize a number of observations, and it does point the way to new research as evidenced by the cognitive research issues just discussed. Certain hypotheses are generated from the social learning theory approach, such as the roles of modeling and its parameters, cognitive strategies and their parameters, and reinforcement and its parameters. The social learning approach to spousal aggression has proven useful in that it attempts to explain events with some clear grounding to empirical observations, and some accounts of partner aggression have been able to explain approximately 50% of the variance in the physical aggression of males toward females (e.g., Riggs, 1986). When one considers the law of parsimony and applications of social learning theory to spousal aggression, social learning theory may be wanting. Social learning theory has become expansive, and does not generally consider only one or two factors as they predict behavior. Contributions of experimental, social, and clinical psychology all have found their way into social learning theory, and issues of affect, behavior, and cognition all come under a modern day social learning theory. Perhaps the cognitive direction in which Bandura moved in 1986 will provide a synthesis of the information and principles contained in what we have come to regard as a social learning theory approach to clinical problems (O'Leary & Wilson, 1987). At present, however, it appears that a social learning approach to spousal aggression is not an especially parsimonious approach to spousal aggression. However, I believe that aggression, and spousal aggression in particular, is a multidetermined phenomenon that will require complex models for prediction and understanding.

We now need models that allow us to conceptualize many data sources and many empirical relations. One model has been presented to aid in the conceptualization of spousal aggression. Within the next year, we will have evaluated this model with our sample of 400 young couples in a 3-year longitudinal study. Most importantly, we need to examine the strengths of relationships among the variables and to ascertain the percentage of overall variance and the percentage of unique variance accounted for by the variables under question (cf. Broderick & O'Leary, 1986). Most of the excellent research in the area of spouse abuse has come from sociologists who have conducted large sample research (cf. Straus *et al.*, 1980). This research has highlighted many of the risk factors, particularly of a demographic and social nature, that are associated with spouse abuse. What is not known from this research, however, is the relative contribution of the variables of interest and the unique variance associated with these variables.

Whether the same theoretical model presented earlier would apply equally well in predicting child abuse remains to be seen. Some integration of a model of spousal aggression (abuse) and child abuse could readily occur because history of family violence, aggressive personality style, stress, alcohol use, and marital discord relate to spouse abuse and to child abuse. However, a full child abuse model would have to include variables different from a spouse abuse model, such as parenting skills and temperament and behavior of the child. In addition, because child abuse often exists in single parent homes, it is necessary to consider predictors of child abuse outside a marital relationship. However, in keeping with the notion of developing middle-ground theories, we already have data which begin to allow us to argue for separate models of spousal aggression for men and women, and we certainly believe sophisticated child abuse and spouse abuse models will differ.

ACKNOWLEDGMENTS

Special thanks go to Julian Barling, Chris Murphy, and Evelyn Sandeen for their editorial suggestions.

REFERENCES

American Psychiatric Assocation. (1980). *Diagnostic and Statistical Manual of Mental Disorders* (3rd ed.). Washington, DC: Author.

Arias, I. (1984). *A social learning theory explication of the intergenerational transmission of physical aggression in intimate heterosexual relationships.* Unpublished doctoral dissertation. State University of New York, Stony Brook, NY.

Bandura, A. (1969). *Principles of behavior modification.* New York: Holt, Rinehart, & Winston.

Bandura, A. (1977). *Social learning theory.* Englewood Cliffs, NJ: Prentice-Hall.

Bandura, A. (1986). *Social foundations of thought and action: A social and cognitive theory.* Englewood Cliffs, NJ: Prentice-Hall.

Bandura, A., & Walters, R. H. (1963). *Social learning and personality development.* New York: Holt, Rinehart & Winston.

Bard, M., & Zacker, J. (1974). Assaultiveness and alcohol use in family disputes. *Criminology, 12,* 283–292.

Barling, J., & Rosenbaum, A. (1986). Work stressors and wife abuse. *Journal of Applied Psychology, 71,* 346–348.

Berkowitz, L. (1969). The contagion of violence: An S-R mediational analysis of some effects of observed aggression. In W. J. Arnold & M. M. Page (Eds.), *Nebraska symposium on motivation* (pp. 95–135). Lincoln, NE: University of Nebraska Press.

Broderick, J. E., & O'Leary, K. D. (1986). Contributions of affect, attitude, and behavior to marital satisfaction. *Journal of Consulting and Clinical Psychology, 54,* 514–517.

Chritchlow, B. (1986). The powers of John Barleycorn: Beliefs about the effects of alcohol on social behavior. *American Psychologist, 41*(7), 751–764.

Cronbach, L. J. (1977). *Educational psychology* (3rd ed.). New York: Harcourt Brace Jovanovich.

Deschner, J. P. (1984). *The hitting habit: Anger control for battering couples.* New York: The Free Press.

Dollard, J., Doob, L. W., Miller, N. E., Mowrer, O. H., & Sears, R. R. (1939). *Frustration and aggression.* New Haven, CT: Yale University Press.

Fesbach, S. (1964). The function of aggression and the regulation of aggressive drive. *Psychological Review, 103,* 119–131.

Fotjik, K. M. (1977). *Wife-beating.* Ann Arbor-Washtenaw County NOW Wife Assault Task Force, 1917 Washtenaw Avenue, Ann Arbor, Michigan 48124.

Freud, S. (1933). *New introductory lectures on psycho-analysis.* New York: Morton.

Gayford, J. J. (1975). Wife battering: A preliminary survey of 100 cases. *British Medical Journal,* 195–197.

Geen, R. G., & Donnerstein, E. I. (1983). *Aggression: Theoretical and empirical reviews.* New York: Academic Press.

Gelles, R. (1972). *The violent home: A study of physical aggression between husbands and wives.* Beverly Hills, CA: Sage.

Gelles, R. J. (1983). An exchange/social control theory. In D. Finkelhor, R. J. Gelles, G. T. Hotaling, & M. A. Straus (Eds.), *The dark side of families: Current family violence research* (pp. 151–165). Beverly Hills, CA: Sage.

Gelles, R. J., & Straus, M. A. (1979). Determinants of violence in the family: Toward a theoretical integration. In W. R. Burr, R. Hill, F. I. Nye, & I. L. Reiss (Eds.), *Contemporary theories about the family* (pp. 549–581). New York: Free Press.

Hergenhahn, B. R. (1982). *An introduction to theories of learning.* Englewood Cliffs, NJ: Prentice-Hall.

Hilgard, E. R., & Bower, G. H. (1975). *Theories of learning* (4th ed.). Englewood Cliffs, NJ: Prentice-Hall.

Jacobs, P. A., Brunton, M., & Melville, M. M. (1965). Aggressive behavior, mental sub-normality and the XYY male. *Nature, 208,* 1351–1352.

Jouriles, E. N., & Collins, R. L. (1986). *Women's attitudes concerning the justification of relationship aggression: Effects of alcohol consumption by the assailant and the subjects' drinking experience.* Unpublished manuscript. State University of New York, Stony Brook, NY.

Jouriles, E. N., & O'Leary, K. D. (1986). *Short marital adjustment test: Psychometric properties and cutting scores.* Unpublished manuscript. State University of New York, Stony Brook, NY.

Kalmuss, D. (1984). The intergenerational transmission of marital aggression. *Journal of Marriage and the Family, 46,* 11–19.

Landers, S. (1986, November). DSM by APA? *Monitor.* American Psychological Association. Washington, DC. p. 7.

Lazarus, A. A. (1971). *Behavior therapy and beyond.* New York: McGraw-Hill.

Lorenz, K. (1966). *On aggression.* New York: Harcourt Brace Jovanovich.

MacEwen K. E., & Barling, J. (in press). *Multiple stressors, violence in the family of origin, and marital aggression.* A longitudinal study. *Journal of Family Violence*

Mark, V. H., Sweet, W., & Erwin, F. (1975). Deep temporal lobe stimulation and destructive lesions in episodically violent temporal lobe epileptics. In W. S. Fields & W. S. Sweet (Eds.), *Neural bases of violence and aggression.* (pp. 379–400). St. Louis, MO: Warren Green.

Makepeace, J. M. (1983). Life events, stress and courtship violence. *Family Relations, 30,* 97–102.

Michael, R. P., & Zumpe, D. (1986). An annual pattern in the battering of women. *American Journal of Psychiatry, 143,* 637–640.

Mueller, C. W. (1983). Environmental stressors and aggressive behavior. In R. G. Geen & E. I. Donnerstein (Eds.), *Aggression: Theoretical and empirical reviews* (pp. 51–76). New York: Academic Press.

National Institute on Alcohol Abuse and Alcoholism (NIAAA) (Nov., 1978) *Third special report to U.S. Congress on alcohol and health* (HEW, IFS No. 53). Washington, DC: U.S. Government Printing Office.

Neidig, P. H. (1985). Domestic violence in the military. Part II: The impact of high levels of work-related stress on family functioning. *Military Family, 5*(4), 3–5.

Neidig, P. H., & Friedman, D. H. (1984). *Spouse abuse: A treatment program for couples.* Champaign, IL: Research Press.

Novaco, R. W. (1978). Anger and coping with stress: Cognitive behavioral interventions (pp. 135–173). In J. P. Foreyt & D. P. Rathesen (Eds.), *Cognitive behavior therapy: Research and applications.* New York: Plenum Press.

O'Leary, K. D., & Arias, I. (1987a). Marital assessment in clinical practice. In K. D. O'Leary (Ed.), *Assessment of marital discord.* Hillsdale, NJ: Erlbaum.

O'Leary, K. D., & Arias, I. (1987b). Prevalence, correlates, and development of spouse abuse. In R. deV. Peters & R. J. McMahon (Eds.), *Marriage and families: Behavioral treatments and processes.* New York: Brunner/Mazel.

O'Leary, K. D., & Curley, A. D. (1986). Assertion and family violence: Correlates of spouse abuse. *Journal of Marital and Family Therapy, 12*(3), 281–290.

O'Leary, K. D., & Wilson, G. T. (1987). *Behavior therapy: Application and outcome.* Englewood Cliffs, NJ: Prentice-Hall.

O'Leary, K. D., Arias, I., Rosenbaum, A., & Barling, J. (1985). *Premarital physical aggression.* Unpublished manuscript. State University of New York, Stony Brook, NY.

O'Leary, K. D., Barling, J., Arias, I., Rosenbaum, A., Malone, J. & Tyree, A. (1986). *Prevalence and stability of spousal aggression.* Manuscript submitted for publication.

Olweus, D. (1979). *Aggression in the schools: Bullies and whipping boys.* New York: Halstead Press, Wiley.

Pagelow, M. D. (1981). Factors affecting women's decisions to leave violent relationships. *Journal of Family Issues, 2,* 391–414.

Prinz, R. J., Roberts, W. R., & Hartman, E. (1980). Dietary correlates of hyperactive behavior in children. *Journal of Consulting and Clinical Psychology, 48,* 760–769.

Riggs, D. S. (1986). *Conflict resolution in dating couples: A multiple predictor approach.* Unpublished manuscript. State University of New York, Stony Brook, NY.

Rosenbaum, A. (1980). *Wife abuse: Characteristics of the participants and etiological considerations.* Unpublished doctoral dissertation. State University of New York, Stony Brook, NY.

Rosenbaum, A., & O'Leary, K. D. (1981). Marital violence: Characteristics of abusive couples. *Journal of Consulting and Clinical Psychology, 49,* 63–71.

Roy, M. (1977). *Battered women: A psychosociological study of domestic violence.* New York: Van Nostrand Reinhold.

Schacter, J., & O'Leary, K. D. (1985). Affective intent and impact in marital communication. *The American Journal of Family Therapy, 13*(4), 17–23.

Shwed, J. A., & Straus, M. A. (1979). *The military environment and child abuse.* Unpublished manuscript. University of New Hampshire.

Sherman, L. W., & Berke, R. A. (1984). Deterrent effects of arrest on domestic violence. *American Sociological Review, 49* (2), 261–271.

Sjoberg, G., & Nett, R. (1968). *A methodology for social research.* New York: Harper & Row, Publishers.

Skinner, B. F. (1938). *The behavior of organisms: An experimental analysis.* Englewood Cliffs, NJ: Prentice-Hall.

Skinner, B. F. (1953). *Science and human behavior.* New York: Macmillan.

Steinmetz, S. K. (1977). *The cycle of violence.* New York: Praeger.

Straus, M. A. (1977). A sociological perspective on the prevention and treatment of wife beating. In M. Roy (Ed.), *Battered women: A psychosociological study of domestic violence* (pp. 194–238). New York: Van Nostrand Reinhold.

Straus, M. A. (1980). *Social stress and marital violence in a national sample of American families.* Symposium on Forensic Psychology and Psychiatry, New York Academy of Sciences. Annals of the New York Academy of Sciences.

Straus, M. A., Gelles, R. J., & Steinmetz, S. K. (1980). *Behind closed doors: Violence in the American Family.* New York: Anchor Books.

Stuart, P. T., & Leonard, K. E. (1983). Alcohol and human physical aggression. In R. G. Geen & E. I. Donnerstein (Eds.), *Aggression: Theoretical and empirical reviews* (pp. 77–102). New York: Academic Press.

Tolman, E. C. (1932). *Purposive behavior in animals and men.* New York: Naiburg.

Tolman, E. C. (1959). Principles of purposive behavior. In S. Koch (Ed.), *Psychology: A study of a science.* (Vol. 2, pp. 92–157). New York: McGraw-Hill.

Tyree, A., Malone, J., & O'Leary, K. D. (1987). *Physical aggression with others as a predictor of spousal violence.* Unpublished manuscript. State University of New York, Stony Brook, NY.

Ulbrich, P., & Huber, J. (1981). Observing parental violence: Distribution and effects. *Journal of Marriage and the Family, 43,* 623–631.

U.S. Department of Justice. (1985). *Uniform Crime Reports.* Washington, DC: U.S. Government Printing Office.

Walker, L. (1979). *The battered woman.* New York: Harper & Row.

Wolpe, J. (1958). *Psychotherapy by reciprocal inhibition.* Stanford, CA: Stanford University Press.

4

Sociological Perspectives in Family Violence

CARL A. BERSANI AND HUEY-TSYH CHEN

INTRODUCTION

It is common knowledge that not many years ago the problem of family violence was virtually ignored. It has not been that many years since a diversity of disciplines began to offer explanations for our "newly discovered" phenomena. Our popular literature now calls what was previously ignored "private" violence, as contrasted to the more visible public violence to which our theorists and researchers in sociology have always directed their efforts. Although sociologists are late arrivals in the study of family violence, a cursory view of this literature indicates that some sociological perspectives are now being included in the attempt to understand more fully the phenomena of violence in the family. (See Star, 1980, and Straus, 1974, for assessments as to why the late entry of sociology.)

Usually, when sociologists enter a new field, their initial efforts are to critique definitions; assess the nature and extent of the problem; identify the major social factors associated with the problem; challenge previous research on methodological grounds; and question the limitations of theories dominating the field. As sociologists entered the study of family violence, they repeated this pattern. For a discussion of specifics of this pattern in family violence, as well as additional citations, see Gelles (1983, 1985).

As to theory, sociologists apply a very diverse set of perspectives in their investigation of a very wide range of social problems. Implicit in this diversity is the view that the kinds of questions needed to understand fully a problem are more likely to appear if several levels of social reality are recognized as contributing sources. Thus, sociological perspectives embrace the microscopic as well as macroscopic levels of analysis, and recognize that each type of theory is really introducing a set of questions among many which could be examined.

One portion of the model's continuum deals with interpersonal relations and social groups. The other portion concentrates on aspects of the social structure, society, culture, and intersocietal comparisons (Ritzer, 1986). Sociologists are interested in a variety of

CARL A. BERSANI and HUEY-TSYH CHEN • Department of Sociology, The University of Akron, Akron, OH 44325.

social relations. The never ending process of socialization is an important foundation for this level of analysis. Some possibilities from the array of possible interpersonal relations are more suitable in inducing and maintaining violence in the family setting than others. Social groups as parties to family violence are another level of interest to sociologists. Family and nonfamily groups are characterized by patterns of interaction, by group and individual identities, and by norms meant to guide group and individual behavior. It also becomes necessary to grasp the history of relational and interactional processes of families because a part of our understanding of how family violence evolves and is sustained will come from this type of analysis.

However, interpersonal relations could themselves reflect the consequences of macrophenomena such as social structure and culture. Therefore, we must also include macroscopic levels of analysis from our sociological model. At this level of analysis, sociologists are interested in such phenomena as social and cultural structures within societies and contrasts between societies. A social structure is identifiable by a predictable design in interrelationships, separate in part from the individuals composing the structure. Illustrations of structures may range from such an abstraction as the economy to the federal government, stratification, and the family. Culture—be it societal or subcultural—refers to the sharing among segments of the population of such things as beliefs, norms, and value goals.

In terms of structural factors, for example, Gelles and Cornell (1985) developed the following list of 11 unique characteristics, the variance of which contributes either to a supportive and warm family climate or a violence-prone environment: amount of time together, range of activities/interests, intensity of involvement, impinging activities, right to influence, age and sex differences, involuntary membership/ascribed roles, insulation/privacy, inequality, extensive knowledge of social biographies, and change/stress/ instability.

In terms of culture, many writers (Gelles, 1979; Pagelow, 1984; Straus, Gelles, & Steinmetz, 1980) charge that the background for family violence in our society is a cultural-normative system that promotes, stimulates, and rewards male aggressiveness. Pagelow (1980) discusses this cultural approval of violence theme in her discussions of toys, sports, media, role models, and the like.

It should be evident that the sociological model is broad in coverage. However, our review of sociological explanations for the family violence phenomena in this chapter will not exhaust all possible perspectives. We will restrict our analysis to those sociological perspectives that have caught the attention of family violence scholars.

THE ISSUE OF FAMILY VIOLENCE THEORY

There exist a considerable number of theoretical works and empirical studies from the field of criminology that offer contributions to understanding violent behavior as well as nonviolent behavior. Bahr (1979) summarizes and applies the major theoretical contributions and empirical findings from criminology to family structure and interaction. It is not totally clear why this body of literature has generally been ignored by students of family violence.

One apparent reason that family scholars do not turn to the field of criminology is that theorists and researchers in the field of family violence do not consider family violence as equivalent to criminal violence. With the exception of homicide against a relative, police and court practices also indicate a similar position. It is commonly recognized that much of what would be called aggravated assaults in other circumstances become domestic disturbances or comparably minor offenses if they occur in domestic situations.

This directs attention to the question of whether it is necessary to theorize about family violence as a special case. This question, in turn, also raises the issue of the relevancy of theory development by specialists who focus on one type of family violence: child abuse, incest, elder abuse, wife battering, sexual abuse, and so forth.

Gelles (1985) and Gelles and Straus (1979) have argued for a body of theory and explanation directed at the global category of family violence. Although violence *per se* is not unique, they maintain that the acts of violence occurring between family members are special enough to justify separate analysis.

Gelles and Straus (1979) offered a very extensive and convincing discussion as to why special family violence theorizing is appropriate. Our brief review will not do justice to their explanation. Nevertheless, we can focus on a few central points. They stress that certain variables (i.e., intimacy, privacy) are much more evident in the family than outside it. Not only are certain variables much more visible but the uniqueness of the interrelationship (i.e., amount of time spent together, age and sex differences) in family settings tends to set families apart from other social groups. In addition, critical variables can be readily discovered and observed in family settings.

Finkelhor (1983) and Pagelow's (1984) review of the literature recognize that absolute commitment to specialization in family studies does create factionalizing tendencies that do not benefit theory and research. It is possible that emerging rivalries for scarce resources in the family violence social movement will enhance confusion, rather than enlighten money givers. By examining the commonalities and the differences between types of family violence (offenders and victims), theory and research can be enriched.

Beyond social factors identified by Gelles and Cornell (1985), one commonality among types of family violence is what Pagelow (1984) called power differentials, and Finkelhor (1983) abuse of power. Another commonality is the spectrum of effects on family violence victims: weakened self-esteem, shame, and helplessness (Finkelhor, 1983; Pagelow, 1984). Finkelhor (1983) also pointed out more than one form of abuse often occurs in the same situation. Pagelow (1984) made a careful distinction between power differentials (i.e., victims are powerless relative to abusers), and power/powerlessness. This latter commonality refers to the abuser's sense of powerlessness. Abusers feel unable to gain sufficient control within their family in any other way, or are not able to gain control of the larger social environment, and take it out on their families.

A great deal of our theories and research do, indeed, focus on one form of family violence and may assume more differentiation than does exist. At this stage, however, this specialization makes good sense because there are features of victim types and situations that differ (Bandura, 1973; Dobash & Dobash, 1976).

Nevertheless, for the sake of uncovering common theoretical connections, Finkelhor (1983) and Pagelow (1984) have stressed that these endeavors must also strive to uncover commonalities among forms of family violence. Russell's (1984) book dealing with sexual exploitation is illustrative of the search for common causal connections of seemingly incompatible forms of sexual exploitation: rape, child sexual abuse, and sexual harassment in the workplace. The leading sociologists in this field, Straus, Gelles, and Steinmetz (Breines & Gordon, 1983) stress in a number of their works the similarities in patterns and causes for violence against children and against spouses particularly. In their own words:

> As the historical data show, and as the statistics [1975 national probability sample of families] we review in the following section bear out, the problem is one of family violence. Fathers and mothers hitting children, children hitting one another, and spouses physically battling each other are all part of the same topic—violence in the American family. (Straus, Gelles, & Steinmetz, 1980, pp. 12–13)

Accordingly, the purpose of our review is to explore these theories that stress this latter approach. This review will include three microlevel perspectives: resource, exchange/control, and symbolic interaction, and five macrolevel perspectives: subculture of violence, conflict, patriarchal, ecological, and general systems.

One final point concerns interpretation of the writings we include in this chapter. In explaining and interpreting these works and also striving for brevity and clarity, we have resisted the temptation—to the best of our ability—of interpreting in ways the authors themselves may never have expressed. On the other hand, because we anticipate some readers will not have a background in sociology, we introduce the theoretical roots of many of the theories included in this chapter.

RESOURCE THEORY

One of the central concepts in sociological theory has traditionally been power. Founding fathers of sociology, such as Karl Marx (1964) and Max Weber (1956), for example, regarded social classes as outcomes of differentials in power that determine who gets how much of scarce resources, such as wealth and privileges. The best known discussion of power in family relations has been done by Blood and Wolfe (1960). They perceive a close relationship between power and resources in a family. Power is viewed by them as the potential ability of one member to influence the behavior of another, whereas a resource is anything one member makes available to help others satisfy needs or goals. Blood and Wolfe indicate that the balance of power in a family will favor the spouse who contributes the greater resources. The spouse with the greater number of resources tends to have power over his or her partner. They argue (1960, p. 29) that "the balance of power in particular families and in whole categories of families is determined by the comparative resourcefulness of the two partners and by the life circumstances within which they live."

Whenever husbands exercise excessive power in American society, Blood and Wolfe believe, it is not because their wives subscribe to patriarchal belief systems, but because husbands can contribute more resources to the marriage. Husbands win power by virtue of their own skills and accomplishments in comparison with their wives. This argument has been labeled resource theory (e.g., Allen & Straus, 1977). The same name has been subsequently used for Goode's (1971) efforts to apply the concept of power in explaining family violence.

The major theoretical effort in this area has been made by Goode (1971). According to Goode, the family, like all other social systems, is a power system. However, Goode felt the term *power* covers a grab bag of phenomena and he prefers to use the term *force* as a substitute and the term *overt force* or *violence* for the actual exercise of physical force.

Within a family, Goode argues, force is supported by external social structures.

Family patterns are expressed in laws, such as parental rights and obligations, laws of custody, and property rights, and are backed up by the police and the courts. Force is important in stabilizing a family structure. If no force existed, the structural strength of a family would be undermined.

In addition, the legitimacy of force is consolidated by socialization. People are socialized not only to know that force is real and strong, but also to believe it is right and desirable. We use force and its threat in order to socialize our children, and in doing so we also teach them that force is useful.

Based on such observations, Goode proposed a famous proposition regarding the relationships among force, other resources, and violence:

> the greater the other resources an individual can command, the more force he can muster, but the less he will actually display or use force in an orderly manner. (p. 628)

Goode observed that all of the following resources affect a family member's power: success, prestige, and position outside the family; age; gifts; job and services; political authority; intelligence and relevant knowledge; friendship, love, and attraction; and so on. Because different social classes and ethnic groups have different levels of access to alternative resources that would help them to redress their balance of exchange with family members, and also different alternative sources of pleasure and contentment, different levels of family violence can be expected. Lower-class people, who have fewer resources than the rest of society, often experience greater frustration and bitterness. Their problems are expressed in an imbalance of transactions within the family and difficulty in balancing the flow of gifts, loyalty, and affection. As a consequence, members of the lower strata may be more inclined to resort to family violence than other parts of society. Empirical research on the resource theory has produced inconsistent findings. For example, Allen and Straus's (1980) study provided some evidence that the more resources people have the less likely they are to commit family violence. However, Stark and McEvoy (1970) showed the opposite.

Goode (1971) mentioned that normative structure may influence the degree that a spouse uses violence as an ultimate resource to induce the other spouse to perform some behavior when the other spouse lacks other resources, such as money or prestige. Rodman (1972) provided some evidence that the use of violence as an ultimate resource in a family is, in fact, contingent on the cultural context. He demonstrated that this pattern of violence appears only in a society that is weak or ambiguous in legitimizing the exercise of power. In the United States, norms regarding the distribution of marital power are ambiguous because equalitarian norms have not completely replaced the traditional patriarchal norms of families and the high incidence of family violence in this country may result partly from this ambiguity.

When traditional normative expectations undergo rapid changes, as they are now, members of the family may use violence in order to maintain superiority over other family members who have traditionally inferior roles. As a result, the changing expectations of women and their demands of equality may actually increase violence against them. This suggests that status inconsistency theory is another way to conceptualize the relationship between power and violence (e.g., Kelly & Chambliss, 1966; Lenski, 1954). Status inconsistency applies to a person who has high rank in one status hierarchy (i.e., education) and low rank in another (e.g., income). The theory argues that status inconsistency creates a dilemma when such a person interacts with others. The individual tends to evaluate himself or herself according to the higher status hierarchy, whereas the others tend to evaluate the person in terms of the lower. The inconsistency will result in stress or dissatisfaction, which, in turn, will lead to the development of antisocial attitudes and behavior, such as political radicalism, to remove the inconsistency.

In family situations, males may be traditionally regarded as having a higher ascribed status, such as father or husband, but their achieved status in areas such as education and income, or occupation, may fail to measure up with the ascribed status. O'Brien (1971) suggested that this inconsistency may result in family violence when the husband feels threatened in his traditional status by a more educated or skillful wife and resorts to physical violence to maintain dominance. The studies by O'Brien (1971) and Gelles (1976) showed some support for this theory, in that families with high status inconsistency have more violent incidents than families with low status inconsistency. Husbands who fail to perform adequately in their traditional role as income provider, or who are lower than their wives in education, occupation, job skills, and so on, are more likely to use violence.

EXCHANGE/SOCIAL CONTROL THEORY

The exchange/social control theory proposed by Gelles (1983) to explain family violence is drawn largely from exchange theory, and to a lesser degree from social control theory. It will be useful to review briefly both of these theories before discussing Gelles.

According to exchange theorists (e.g., Blau, 1964; Homans, 1961, 1974), the fundamental assumption of exchange theory is that persons engage in behavior either to earn rewards or to escape punishment. Homans' exchange theory mainly focuses on social interactions within a dyad and relies on a set of general propositions deriving from behavioral psychology and from classical economics. Examples of his propositions are as follows (Homans, 1974). The success proposition states that: "For all actions taken by persons, the more often a particular action of a person is rewarded the more likely the person is to perform that action" (1974, p. 16). The value proposition states that: "The more valuable to a person is the result of his action, the more likely he is to perform the action" (1974, p. 25). And the rule of distributive justice holds that, "A man in an exchange relation will expect that the rewards of each man be proportional to his costs—the greater the rewards, the greater the costs—and that the net rewards, or profits, of each man be proportional to his investments—the greater the investments, the greater the profit" (Homans, 1961, p. 75).

Blau (1964) basically accepts Homans' theory, but Blau goes further and turns his attentions to larger social structures. Blau considers that although the desire for rewards is what initially attracts individuals into the social interaction, the seeds for the emergence of social structure are also being sown. For example, social differentiation can emerge from the initial social interaction. In a group situation, differences in status and power begin to develop because different members make different contributions to the group. Blau indicates that not all social transactions are symmetrical and based on equal social change; that is, members do not always receive rewards in proportion to their investments. Symmetrical exchange gives way to coercive power, in which the low-ranking members receive fewer returns. Blau moves from Homans' microsociological phenomenon of exchange to the macrosociological concern of power.

Social control theory is frequently used to explain juvenile delinquency. Social control theory assumes that committing crime is part of human nature (e.g., Nettler, 1978;

Vold & Bernard, 1985). In other words, people will commit crime if left alone without nurturing. Accordingly, an essential question in social control theory is why most people do not commit crimes. The answer to this question is that most people have adequate control mechanisms. Crimes occur when the controlling forces, which ordinarily restrain people from committing crimes, either become weak or were not strong to begin with. Therefore, situations where people commit crimes are regarded as resulting from the weakness of controlling forces that should have restrained them from doing so. There are a variety of control theories and only two frequently mentioned ones are reviewed here. Reckless (1973) proposed a containment theory and argued that criminality is caused by failure of inner containment and outer containment. Inner containment consists of self-control, good self-concept, ego strength, superego, goal-directedness, etc., whereas outer containment consists of effective family living and support groups, and includes such factors as consistent moral front, reasonable norms and expectations, cohesion, etc.

Whereas Reckless provides a general framework for control theory, Hirschi (1969) attempted to devise a set of testable hypotheses. Hirschi considered that persons who are closely bonded to social groups, such as their families, school, and peers, would be less likely to commit delinquent acts. He suggested that four basic elements bond individuals into society: attachment, commitment, involvement, and beliefs. *Attachment,* or sensitivity toward and concern for the opinions of others, is the most important element necessary for internalization of values and norms. *Commitment* is the rational investment of time and energy one has in conventional society that is risked by engaging in deviant behavior. *Involvement* describes the constriction of possibilities for delinquent activities. Finally, *belief* refers to the acceptance of the moral validity of conventional rules.

Drawing from exchange theory and social control theory, Gelles (1983) proposed an exchange/social control model of family violence. According to Gelles, this model is what Robert Merton (1967) called a middle-range theory, consisting of a set of testable propositions, which Gelles believes is more suitable and valuable than other family violence theories.

Gelles accepts the basic assumption of exchange theory that human interaction is guided by the pursuit of reward and avoidance of punishment and costs. Following Homans (1961, 1974) and Blau (1964), he also believes an individual who provides a reward to another thereby places him or her in debt, so that the second individual must furnish benefits to the first in return. The interaction will continue if rewards come equally to both parties, but if not, it will be broken off. However, Gelles argues, unlike regular social interactions, intrafamilial relations cannot be broken off easily. As a consequence, when family members perceive injustice in a daily interaction, they become angry and resentful, and conflict and even violence result. On the other hand, Gelles also accepts the thesis of social control theory that individuals must have control mechanisms to prevent them from committing crimes.

Attempting to apply these two theoretical traditions to family violence, Gelles says that according to the general principle of exchange theory, we should expect that people will use violence in the family if the costs of being violent do not outweigh the rewards. And, from social control theory, we can expect that family violence occurs in the absence of social controls that would bond people to the social order and negatively sanction family members from acts of violence. Accordingly, Gelles derives the following general proposition of family violence: ''People hit and abuse other family members because they can'' (1983 p. 157).

This general proposition is further expanded into the following propositions:

(1) Family members are more likely to use violence in the home when they expect that the costs of being violent are less than the rewards.

(2) The absence of effective social controls over family relations decreases the costs of family members being violent toward one another.

(3) Certain social and family structures serve to reduce social control in family relations, and therefore reduce the costs and/or increase the rewards of being violent. (p. 158)

Gelles also claims that three major factors in social and family structure reduce external social control of the home and increase the rewards of being violent: inequality, privacy, and the image of the "real man." The normative power structure in society in general and in the family in particular promotes sexual and generational inequality. This inequality weakens social controls and reduces the costs of being violent for those with sexual and generational advantages. Husbands are usually bigger than their wives and children, have higher status positions, and earn more money. Because of this, they can use violence without fear of being struck back hard enough to be injured and do not fear economic or social sanctions against them in return.

The private nature of the family makes neighbors more reluctant to report that they overhear incidents of family violence because they fear intervening in another person's home. Similarly, judges, prosecutors, and policemen are also reluctant to intervene in family violence because court intervention may result in divorce or separation in order to protect a woman, or removal of a child from a home in order to protect the child. Courts usually wish to avoid putting the legal system in the position of breaking up a family to protect individual members.

Finally, being labeled as a child beater or a wife beater may not necessarily imply the loss of social status. Some subcultures, in fact, consider aggressive sexual and violent behavior as proof that someone is a real man. Rather than risk status loss, the violent family members may actually have a status gain. Even in situations where violence is a status loss, the violent individuals can employ accepted vocabularies or motives to explain their untoward behavior. For example, violent fathers or mothers might explain their actions by saying they were drunk or lost control.

SYMBOLIC INTERACTION PERSPECTIVE

Symbolic interaction is one of the most important perspectives in contemporary sociology. Because of its importance we will discuss it briefly, despite the fact that conceptual aspects of this approach have not been incorporated as part of a theory of family violence or by theorists addressing the question of an integrated theory (Gelles & Straus, 1979).

The core of this perspective is *self* as an ever emerging social product derived from participation in a process of social interactions. The self is not a set of established traits as some psychological theories affirm (Davis, 1980). This view stresses that a fluidity is given to social existence by the processes by which individuals designate, define, and interpret behavior. Individuals give behaviors meaning. Symbolic interaction has the capacity to correct inadequacies of sociological theorizing because it can offer researchers a framework and measuring instruments to analyze microprocesses within macrosocial events (Turner, 1986). (For a systematic summary of symbolic interaction theory see Rose, 1962. Rose offers a detailed set of assumptions and propositions.)

Interactional theorizing in general, and symbolic interaction in particular, demonstrate considerable diversity (Turner, 1986). Nevertheless, Stryker (1967) highlighted several indications of researchable questions that can be helpful in the study of family violence through the use of symbolic interaction.

The first concerns differential commitment to family identities. What accounts for differentials? This approach considers how males, for example, view themselves; how congruent these views are with the definitions of significant others; and what "cross-pleasures" exist from others in the individual's total social world (Stryker, 1967).

A second question for research deals with the consequences of differential commitment to family identities. Stryker (1967) feels that diverse family behaviors, one of which is family violence, are influenced by the degree of commitment to familial identities—the extent to which a person is motivated to carry out a role. A third question for research concerns an examination of the effects of identities—based on diverse spheres of activity—on each other, and on the behavior within one sphere versus another.

Stryker (1967) raised a fourth research question about the relationship of crisis to identity. Multiphased crises threaten identity because identity depends on the stability of interactions between others and self. He notes that the ease of identity alteration in crisis situations has not been found to be functional because it may induce other problems in relationships.

The fifth area for research deals with role taking. In role taking, anticipations of how others will respond may not always be accurate. Furthermore, when a couple moves through stages in the marriage, may not role taking differ in its consequences as role relationships change (Stryker, 1967)?

One basic premise of symbolic interaction is worth examining as a final research question. Symbolic interactionists have argued that the meaning held by individuals about things and words has been largely ignored by sociologists and psychologists in their search for determinants of behavior. For symbolic interactionists, the central research concept is the study of how to account for behavior (Vold, 1986). Therefore, conditions, whether psychological or sociological, should be evaluated according to the meaning those conditions have for the individual.

Gelles and Straus (1979) suggested that a symbolic interaction view of family violence would explore the different meanings of violence people hold (how they develop, persist, and are modified), and the consequences of such meanings in situational settings. To them this perspective would address such things as the process that is involved in the "construction of violence," and the dynamics of the situation.

In terms of identity, the dynamics of the situation, and the construction of violence, Hepburn's (1973) theoretical paper is illustrative of such processes. Hepburn calls attention to the dominance of harmony in the interaction between friends and within families supposedly embedded in a subculture of violence. This raises the question of how routine interactions, on occasion, result in violent behavior.

Hepburn (1973) stated that public identities are acquired and maintained through interaction with others. But in enduring dyadic relationships self–other identities are taken for granted, for they are stable and established unless, or until, they are questioned and threatened. For the purpose of our review we will concentrate on dyadic relationships. In dyadic or family relationships, relational rules or norms are created to reaffirm social identities and avoid assaults on identities and self-esteem.

Assaults (negative evaluations) on an identity may produce a violent response by the person whose role and status expectations have been violated. Although violations of the relational rules may be deliberate or accidental, what is crucial is the meaning the offended person attributes to the offender's intention (Hepburn, 1973).

A violent response is also influenced by the accountability and the claiming behavior one expects from others. These can increase the potential for violence. Self–other identities indicate the agreed upon manner in which the parties are available to each other and might reveal extensive/intensive knowledge of social biographies held by each. If this is the case, the offending person may be held accountable—that person knows better. The other element that adds to the potential for violence is claiming behavior. Prior interactions of participants in an existing relationship reflect an established pattern for claiming behavior. If one person violates or completely rejects aspects of the claiming pattern, conflict in the form of violence may be enhanced (Hepburn, 1973). One or more of the previously described variables offers threats to a person's social identity. Hepburn (1973) discussed the conditions under which three "tactics of threat-reduction" will be utilized: avoidance, acceptance, and retaliation.

However, Hepburn's theoretical paper not only includes the microlevel of analysis, but also embraces at least five independent structural factors that he views as critical in triggering physical violence: subculture of violence, previous experience, intoxicants, the presence of an audience, and closing of alternatives—the cost of failure in retaliation.

Symbolic interaction does not include all the variables helpful in accounting for violent family behavior. But it does call our attention to some variables in need of intensive attention that so far have been largely neglected. Ultimately, in our move toward an integrated theory, the final result will be incomplete unless it is enriched by a set of ideas—of which we have mentioned only a few—contained in the symbolic interactionist perspective.

SUBCULTURE OF VIOLENCE THESIS

The subculture of violence thesis is an influential statement on the sociology of violence, more a cultural than a social-structure explanation (Wolfgang & Ferracuti, 1967, 1982). Wolfgang and Ferracuti's position, deduced from a number of studies on criminal violence and child-rearing studies, is that coexisting within the main culture there are subcultural orientations toward violence, especially among certain ethnic groups and among certain lower-income groups. Although *subculture* is not precisely defined, it is a patterned way of life similar in some ways to the dominant culture but different in other ways.

What this thesis suggests, then, is simply that among the cluster of values that make up, for example, the range of modern American life-styles, there exists a differential orientation to violence reflected in the cultural differences in values, beliefs, and norms regarding the appropriate conditions for violent behavior. In some situations a violent response is a subcultural response—it is normative in that subculture. What that subculture values may be learned definitions of toughness, the worth of human life, the character of masculinity, the meaning of honor and deference. Some normative rules may dictate violent responses for even trivial remarks. These norms have a life of their own. Regardless of the depth of belief in the norms, failure to act in a certain way in a specific circumstance may result in ridicule rather than in social rewards and respect (Wolfgang & Ferracuti, 1982). On the other hand, these authors state, not all participants partake of the subculture's values nor convert them into action. According to Wolfgang and Ferracuti, violence proneness will differ among participants in a subculture, because it is also dependent on psychological factors held by individuals in the subculture. Wolfgang and Ferracuti (1967) state:

> The development of favorable attitudes toward, and the use of, violence in this subculture involve learned behavior and a process of differential learning, association, or identification. (p. 324)

Although the Wolfgang and Ferracuti thesis is not concerned as to how such subcultures originate, they do embrace differential association and social learning theories as part of their thesis. For them, such theories provide a theoretical bridge between an individual's violent behavior and his commitment to a subcultural value. In effect, normative violent responses are learned and transmitted. The underpinnings for this, according to Wolfgang and Ferracuti, begin with the family because the family is our initial and major source for socialization. For some, relationships among family members not only nurture violent responses but are a central reinforcing element in socialization to violence.

The patterned way of life described by the Wolfgang and Ferracuti thesis is usually located in a specific geographical location. But they also stress that a subculture may also be widely distributed spatially.

This is possible because each family lives in its own social world or is embedded within its own social network. Its social network is not necessarily a clone of one evident in the family next door or of any other family of the same class. The others within each social network tolerate and reinforce values and norms about male dominance, deference, and the like. In some networks, this socialization taps aspects of psychogenic traits of some males in molding of attitudes that lead to striving for positive reinforcement of those highly desirable and valued qualities that men should possess. However, during their early and continuous socialization, these males have not been deeply inculated with sophisticated alternatives for resolving pressures, threats, and grievances. The dilemma of unresolved threats to male dominance and deference invites reactions, one being violence.

We assume a number of men experience a wide variety of threats and assaults to their self-esteem, many of which cannot be dealt with on a case-by-case basis. For some such men the most accessible target for aggression, and the most frequent source of challenges to self-esteem, may well be the intimate relationship within the family. Official homicide and assault data suggest this. Studies describing the ''marriage license as a hitting license'' (Pagelow, 1984) suggest that the family is a cradle for violence.

Portions of the thesis receive some limited support. Other findings suggest that violence among groupings of blacks and within the South are better explained by structural factors, such as economic inequality (Vold, 1986). Curtis (1975a,b) has expanded the thesis to include social structure variables, thus expanding the subculture of violence thesis to include the impact of social condition variables on behavior.

Wolfgang and Ferracuti do not apply their thesis to violence within upper-status groups. However, the Milwaukee study (Bowker, 1983) appears to have extended the thesis to apply to all socioeconomic groups. Bowker offered a theoretical interpretation based on empirical findings that he had not anticipated. The essence of the theory is that some male peer subcultures justify wife beating and violence against other family members. Bowker reported that the data strongly suggest that to the extent a battering husband is integrated into these subcultures, the more severely he is likely to beat his wife.

Specifically, Bowker's (1983) findings led him to the following theoretical interpretation. Battering males have been socialized with standards of gratification that demand complete domination over wives and children. Bowker recognizes the patriarchal ideas existing in our society. He also acknowledges that many of the batterers have been in families where they and their mothers were dominated by their fathers. However, Bowker states that the fullest development of these standards, reinforcing the use of violence in family settings, occur in those men who are heavily submersed participants in social relationships with male peers who are constantly supporting and reinforcing these standards of gratification through dominance. He views this phenomena as constituting a subculture of violence consisting of males in supportive social relationships. Associates of the subculture socialize each other by defining situations calling for violence, by inculcating each other about beliefs, values, and norms concerning male dominance as well by their main focus: making certain wives are kept in line. For such subcultural participants the centers for socialization and support are the workplace, informal involvement in sports activities, socializing in bars, and the like.

Recall that the Wolfgang and Ferracuti subculture of violence thesis is not explicitly meant to account for upper-status violence. It is of interest that according to the Milwaukee findings, the subculture of violence thesis is not confined to a single social class, geographical area, occupational grouping, race, or religion. It appears in all environments. Such findings call for a reassessment of the class, ethnic, and geographical emphasis that Wolfgang and Ferracuti place on their version of the subculture of violence.

The primary intent of the Wolfgang and Ferracuti subculture of violence thesis (1967) is to call attention to a normative system shaping the conditions under which violence is a normal outcome. In spite of this, they have been criticized for not addressing the question of how such values and norms, as cultural patterns, originated in the first place.

Building on White's (1975) concept of a culture as a system, and the explanation by Wolfgang and Ferracuti (1967) of how the subculture relates to the larger society, Carroll (1980) addressed the question by proposing a cultural-consistency theory. This theory allowed him to derive hypotheses for future empirical research.

His theory is based on the premise that cultural values can either increase or keep down the amount of violence in the family in certain ethnic groups. To Carroll, cultural consistency is meant to call attention to cultural patterns that are an integrated system of ideas and beliefs being shared by members of a subculture. These ideas and beliefs guide behavior in all areas of life. These ideas and beliefs may not deal with violence directly, but they either do or do not set conditions for violent responses.

He uses two ethnic groups as illustrations in applying his cultural consistency theory: Mexican-American families and Jewish-American families. The Mexican-American families are thought to have higher levels of family violence. Carroll (1980) proposed that this is caused by the main values of the subculture. For this ethnic group family violence is thought to be a result of the great importance placed on such values as severe male dominance, strict discipline, and the general recognition that other family members are under the control (submission) of the father. Subcultural transmission is assured through social learning and the desire to sustain the status males hold in the subculture. Thus, the boy becomes an adult and treats his family members in much the same way his father did. Carroll (1980) noted the recent changes in the formal normative structure of Mexican-American families as such families assimilate and views such changes as possibly increasing family violence.

Carroll (1980) noted that Jewish-American families through history have been known for having low rates of family violence. In applying his cultural-consistency theory of family violence to Jewish-American families, Carroll cited a number of sources that identify the pursuit of knowledge as a central value in the Jewish-American subculture. This value suggests a norm of intellectuality or rationality. Carroll argued that other norms coexist with intellectuality, such as articulateness, argumentativeness, and parent–child bargaining. Accordingly, the climate of conflict is part of a stable family life. The distinction in such norms is that they are primarily used as legitimate means for family problem solving and these norms do not encourage physical responses.

Drawing from various sources, Carroll views families in this subculture as being in perpetual conflict. But the aggression is channeled into verbal expression rather than physical aggression. Sarcasm, screaming, ridicule, interruptions, and contradictions expressed by family members might well be the basis for family violence within some groupings. But it is argued that for this ethnic group such behaviors are an interwoven part of the normal pattern of everyday social interaction. This particular type of conflict style among members appears to indicate a degree of equalitarianism within families that allow a mode of conversational interaction that may reduce frustration and stress. (See a discussion in Coser, 1956, in regard to how social conflict can be functional for a group. Also note how cultural-consistency theory does answer some of the theoretical problems and disappointing findings of "catharsis" theory in Straus, Gelles, & Steinmetz, 1980.)

Brisson's (1981) research suggests the possibility that two types of men are involved in domestic violence. The first type is generally violent outside as well as within their intimate relationships. Ideally, this type best reflects the subculture of violence thesis. The second type is violent in "relationship-specific" situations. That is, violence occurs only with intimate partners. Ongoing research by the authors (Bersani & Chen, 1985) of this chapter partially addresses the question of the subculture of violence thesis.

Our study group consists of males convicted of domestic violence. We are in the process of collecting court data for the 4-year period prior to the court conviction for domestic violence. Data to be collected at a later time will trace these domestic violators as victims of crime. The data we are now collecting include demographic characteristics and charges of prior as well as subsequent domestic violence, other violence, property offenses, and all other offenses. Our research should provide a limited test of the major theme that certain categories best reflect the Wolfgang and Ferracuti thesis. In other words, we will attempt to identify Brisson's first type. If our data provide support for Brisson's (1981) insight, the ramifications for treatment models will be far reaching.

CONFLICT PERSPECTIVE

The conflict perspective has a view of society that is radically different from a traditional functionalist position. Functional theorists hold the social order constant and recognize the vital functions deviance plays in it. Ideally, deviance identifies problem areas within the social order, thereby alerting the institutional structure.

Although sociologists have been critical of this approach, no one functionalist likely supported all the attributes that have been associated with its name (Poloma, 1979). Despite efforts by Merton and others (Poloma, 1979), the main thrust of this perspective does not serve us well for the purpose of understanding family violence. It leaves individuals abstractly occupying status roles, and a social system achieving its consensus equilibrium (when all other means fail) by the coercion of the state (Davis, 1980). It provides limited insight into the sources or consequences of family violence. Nor does it deal with conflicting aspects of the normative structure itself as a contributing factor.

With a conflict perspective of violence, conflict could be viewed as one of the elements involved in social interactional processes within dyads and groups characterized by positions of dominance and submission (Steinmetz, 1978). However, the conflict perspective involves at least two distinct interpretations, drawn from two 19th-century sources, Simmel and Marx. The Marxist version (adopted and modified by Dahrendorf) views intense conflict as the pervasive feature of society itself, and also of social change (Davis, 1980). Bipolar opposition of interests is the essence of a capitalist society, therefore conflict is an inevitable feature of social process and social change. The literature in family violence generally ignores this version. (For a discussion of how this version is integrated with the works of other theorists see Collins, 1975.)

Family violence theorizing reflects Simmel's version of conflict. This version views conflict as one of the universal forms of social interaction. Coser and other value-conflict proponents reflect Simmel's notion of conflict as simply one of the processes of social interaction. Coser's observation that imbalances, tensions, and conflicts of interest occur among interrelated parts of a social system, and essentially constitute normal systems adaptation is consistent with this version (Davis, 1980). Criminological studies and theorizing in family violence reflect this version.

Coser's version of conflict still remains one of the most comprehensive available to us. Among the phenomena covered by his propositions are the causes, violence, duration, and functions of conflict (Turner, 1986). Coser's usefulness in our understanding of family violence is centered on his discussions of internal violence as a mechanism for conflict resolution. Our subsequent discussion will introduce some of his thinking on this topic.

Coser (1967) does not view conflict as reflecting a difference in interest as much as he views conflict as a method of advancing one's self-interests. He (1967) cited Dahrendorf's observation to the effect that organized conflict groups use less violent means than those that lack organization. It is difficult to visualize members of families as logically organized for conflict and conflict resolution. In his volume *The Functions of Social Conflict,* Coser (1956) stated that when group members are deeply involved with one another, a very high degree of their energies are likely mobilized by conflicts, and that these conflicts can be very intense in character.

As an extreme illustration, Coser, in his 1967 volume, discussed the social circumstances in the ghetto setting where failure of conflict resolution may lead to a violent response. Although characteristic of that setting, the process is also applicable to middle-class and working-class settings. The central feature is a restricted role-set. This means the male is involved with relatively few persons in relatively unsegmented relationships. Accordingly, the lack of the social support that would come from a broadly based social system foundation, through involvement in a variety of groups, is a form of deprivation.

On the other hand, it is recognized that multiple conflict opportunities do exist for others who do have broad base, complex role-sets, and who do have segmented types of relationships. However, they would generally not be very intense because they frequently involve only a segment of the personality, a single issue, and do not polarize the individuals on all issues (Coser, 1967).

But what of the individual isolated from social participation and lacking asssociational ties other than his intimate role-set? The chances are a good deal higher that conflicts, if they happen, may not only occur on a number of issues, but the conflict will reflect higher degrees of both intensity and violence (Coser, 1956).

Family violence theorists have incorporated aspects of this general framework and have added to it in their own works. For example, Sprey (1969, 1974) views the family system as a process of continuous confrontation among its members. Harmony is viewed as problematical rather than normal. Family confrontations occur between individuals with conflicting interests in what can be viewed as their common circumstances and violence is an option for advancing the interest of one member when other means of accommodation fail or are not utilized. For Sprey this is a real possibility because he does not view the family as resulting from some kind of preconceived consensus. In stressing this thought he cites Irving Horowitz's statement of why families come into existence: "the contradictory yet interrelated needs, and designs of men" (1967, p. 268).

Sprey's (1974) discussion of a most central question concerning reciprocity between individuals builds on Simmel's discussion of the stranger. What does it mean when one considers that the nature of family living brings family members closer to each other? To Sprey this means that moving apart can be a necessary outcome. So the intimacy of family life creates not only intense awareness of the uniqueness of other members, but confrontation as well. To the extent that the "stranger" in others is rejected, and one member attempts to possess others totally, then reciprocity ceases to be an effective means of conflict resolution.

The analysis by Gelles and Straus (1979) of work by Straus and Steinmetz (1974) and of Steinmetz and Straus (1974), identified a number of similarities between their perspective and the perspective proposed by Sprey. For these theorists, as for Sprey, violence in the family is a powerful option for achieving one's self-interests and a likely outcome of confrontations when other means are ineffective. Steinmetz (1977, 1978), in particular, distinctly stresses Weber's concepts of authority and of power in family systems. In research by Steinmetz (1977), it appears that the most conflict-ridden families are those in which an individual claims the superordinate position of authority, but lacks the power to have that authority obeyed. She cites a member of sources and illustrations that convey the incongruency between authority and power. One such illustration—hardly uncommon— is the possibility of violence when a parent of a teenager still retains the legal authority to control, but the relationship does not provide the power to carry it out. In similar fashion, Steinmetz (1978) applied the same incongruency to wife battering.

In the discussion of the impact and function of conflict in group structures, Coser (1957) followed the lead provided by Simmel by raising two central questions. Coser says: Can we assume in a stable relationship between a married couple that the absence of conflict must be associated with an absence of hostile feelings? Also, can one not assume strength in a marital relationship, instead of a weakness, if hostile feelings are present and marital conflicts occur? Essentially, what this means is that partners are not reluctant to verbalize hostile expressions. In our subsequent discussion we shall deal with these major points expressed by Coser, as well as his position of the role of negotiation and reasoning in situations of conflict.

Findings from the 1975 national probability sample reported by Straus, Gelles, and Steinmetz (1980) have a bearing on the positive functional aspects of conflict theory proposed by Coser (1967) and the violence-avoiding strategy proposed by catharsis theory (Bach & Weyden, 1968).

Coser's position is that violence is an unlikely option if spouses also make use of negotiation and reasoning in situations of conflict. Straus *et al.* (1980) report findings that are in direct opposition to Coser's position. Those couples highest in conflict and highest in use of reasoning as a means of conflict resolution were the most violent couples. In the opposite end of the continuum are couples reporting never or rarely using negotiation or no occasions for conflict. This category had a very low rate of violence, indeed! These latter findings as well may not also fit the conflict prediction (Straus *et al.*, 1980), because Coser predicts that repressing frustration and aggression eventually erupts into violence.

One of the postulates of Bach's catharsis theory (''creative'' aggression) is that ventilating aggression verbally is a means of recognizing the differences among interacting parties. For Coser (1957) hostile expressions may strengthen the relationship, and therefore minimize physical violence. Other previous studies report relationships in the reverse direction. Findings reported by Straus *et al.* (1980) found an extremely dominant reverse pattern as well. Those in the national survey reported very clearly that the more violent responding couples made the greater use of ventilation.

It is apparent that Coser's reasoning as a strategy for conflict resolution, and catharsis theory's postulate that ventilating aggression verbally is a means for conflict resolution do not receive empirical support as presently formulated.

On the other hand, Carroll (1980), who built on White's (1975) concept of a culture as a system and the ways in which a subculture relates to the larger society (Wolfgang & Ferracuti, 1967), offered a cultural-consistency theory. As indicated elsewhere, he argued that an integrated system of certain ideas and beliefs guiding subcultures—although not directly dealing with norms directing violence—may or may not set the conditions for violent responses. For one of his subcultures it appears that one can argue that the very low rates of violence among Jewish-Americans may be related to both Coser's reasoning strategy for conflict resolution and also what is identified in Bach's catharsis theory as ventilating.

It is apparent that neither reasoning nor ventilating *per se* is the ''magic bullet.'' Such strategies for conflict resolution cannot make sense in a vacuum.

Theoretically, what is needed is not only an enhanced understanding of intrafamily processes, but also the placement of that family within the context of the totality of values and beliefs with which they identify and that may set the conditions for violence. Conflict theorists have not yet reformulated elements of the general theory by taking into account some of the problems and inconsistencies discussed earlier.

PATRIARCHAL PERSPECTIVE

When one searches for an underlying foundation providing support for the claim that structural inequality exists among family members, patriarchy comes to mind. Curtis (1986) cited a number of sources that differ in their definition of patriarchy. He argued against a standard definition for this theoretical concept. His view is that the concept is a generalization about social relations that calls for sociological explication. Although patriarchal writers refer to power (legitimate as well as crude), Curtis (1986) considers that sociologically the most important source of power, and the one that underlies patriarchy, is authority. Authority gives one person, rather than another, the right to make decisions that may impact on all members of the group. (For a detailed discussion of power versus authority, and family power structures, see the article by Curtis, 1986.) To Curtis, the study of the family reveals many aspects of patriarchy, because a patriarchal system's chief institution is the family. Gelles (1983) accepted the notion that structural gender inequality can be part of a causal model, but rejected the notion that a theory of sexism (prejudice) can account for family violence.

Writers of this perspective subscribe to a sociocultural model for explanation. Nevertheless, this perspective is distinct from other perspectives. It is considered by Gelles (1983) as one of the most macrolevel approaches to explaining wife abuse. This view holds that other perspectives theorize and research domestic violence within a limited focus, or, in effect, attempt to explain a pervasive problem away by attributing it to individual pathological qualities or assuming malfunctional family interaction.

For this perspective, the core principle in accounting for pervasive spouse violence is that the traditional family reflects an arrangement of domination by males. The social structure supports gender inequality, and this inequality is rooted in the history and in the traditions of Western societies. Marriage is viewed as the central element of a patriarchal society (Yllo, 1983). When one considers the similarity in physical pain and injury, legal reluctance to process family violence as criminal violence would be viewed by this perspective as evidence of the influence of patriarchal norms. The recent emergence of informal structure versus formal structures for assisting victims would also be viewed as confirmation that society's concern for those victimized by this system of male domination is not as intense as it is for those in other adverse circumstances.

Among the early writers explicating this perspective was Martin (1976) in her book *Battered Wives,* and her discussion of theories and related findings makes it worth reading. Violence within the family for Martin is more than merely private interaction among family members, it is a complex problem whose roots lie in our historical traditions: our attitudes toward women, toward marriage, and the services of criminal and civil law, as well as our social service agencies. In short: "The economic and social structure of our present society depend upon the degradation, subjugation, and exploitation of women" (Martin, 1976, p. xv).

Because traditional role activities are changing, Martin (1976) feels that both sexes are experiencing difficulty in living up to traditional expectations; therefore resentment and blame are now more freely expressed concerning expectations that traditional roles be fulfilled. Interestingly, preliminary analysis of the 1985 national representative sample of American families suggested to Straus (1986) that family violence has decreased compared to findings collected during 1975, that were also based on a national representative sample of American families (Gelles & Straus, 1979; Straus *et al.,* 1980).

The volume best known for building a strong case for this perspective as well as reflecting a similarity to Martin's theme, is Dobash and Dobash's (1979) *Violence against Wives.* The Dobashes' view is that the cause of violence against wives and others who are powerless in the family stems from the subordinate positions they occupy in relation to men. The power differentials are especially confronted, maintained, and reinforced within the intimate relationships of a patriarchal family system. The Dobashes identified two central features for the foundation of patriarchy. The first is the manner in which social relationships routinely reinforce the dominating and controlling position of men. The second feature is the sanctification of a system of social relationships from which violence between men and women may result. The very underpinnings of such relations are sustained by an ideology embedded in our system of institutions, including our religious, political, and economic systems (Dobash & Dobash, 1979). Their documentation of this difficult-to-test perspective is impressive. Through an extensive use of data from around the world and by interviewing victims, they trace its roots in history and its persistence in our time.

Socialization processes are a key element in making superordinate-subordinate relationships appear not only acceptable but natural to both sexes (Dobash & Dobash, 1979). For those who are successfully socialized, radical challenges to inequities seem to be outside the predictable order of things. Such challenges are seen as unnatural. Social learning exposures teach that the natural and legitimate statuses for females are marriage and motherhood. All outside activities and responsibilities to family members are in some ways restricted by this reality. Subordination is a cultural legacy of the patriarchal family. Dobash and Dobash (1979) note that social and legal changes in the status of women, in marriage, and in regard to wife beating do occur, so that patriarchy in an absolute sense cannot exist. Nevertheless, they note that these changes have not significantly affected patriarchal ideals, nor greatly modified the hierarchical nature of family organization.

Although their studies do not explore other forms of intrafamily violence, they do recognize that other family members are also subject to violent encounters. They would expect some social, historical, and interpersonal distinctions, but they would also expect similarities. Thus, for the Dobashes (1979) the underpinnings for other forms of intra-family violence are similar to those for the wife. These sources are unequal status, authority, and power. The Breines and Gordon (1983) paper reflects this position. Their argument is that the social contexts of intrafamily violence not only include gender, but also have generational inequalities at the core. (For an insightful assessment [by advocates of this perspective] of the diverse scholarly research dealing with several forms of family violence proposed by various theoretical orientations, the Breines and Gordon, 1983, paper is required reading.)

Finally, such sources as caring and legal agencies are analyzed. Dobash and Dobash (1979) review in detail many of the practices and policies of these agencies, and evaluate their implications for either the reduction or continuation of family violence, as well as the general tolerance level for wife beating. The implications that can be derived from those policies and practices are, for the Dobashes, not always clear. Often policies and practices within an agency are contradictory. At any rate their analysis is an impressive display of how victims are exposed to the ''social reconstruction'' of reality.

In like fashion Stark, Flitcraft, and Frazier (1979) document how intervention and referrals to an emergency medical center function to ''socially construct'' battering victims. The thrust of this process is the introduction of strategies that make victims feel personally responsible. However, Stark et al. (1979) charge that medical providers are influenced by patriarchal logic (structural inequality) that goes beyond merely perpetuating sexism. Their theory and evidence lead them to conclude that broader social forces are involved when females do resist and challenge their status in society. These theorists assume that wife battering is increasing, and consider that the supposed increase is not solely due to the declining power of the patriarchal family, but, more importantly, to the introduction of more females into the labor force. This threatens the survival of the capitalist social order because of the loss of control over women's labor power. In short, their broadbase theory accounts for family violence as due to the continued erosion of family, political, and economic domination by males.

Their view, thus, is that the medical emergency staff are mere representatives of male-bonded networks of our capitalist social order attempting to slow the process of change in social relationships (Stark et al., 1979). This analysis by Stark et al. radically differs from that of the Dobashes. The Dobashes recognize the contributions of society, but they also focus on how males within intrafamily settings utilize violence to maintain their power.

Some writers (Gelles, 1983; Gelles & Cornell, 1985) have criticized the Dobashes' theory for being a single-factor (patriarchy) attempt to explain violence against women in family settings. On the other hand, Pagelow (1984) also recognized that the major focus of the theory is the patriarchal orientation of American society, but feels that the theory is strengthened because it borrows from social learning theory and also from conflict theory.

It is of considerable interest that leading sociologists of family violence include selected elements stemming from this perspective (Martin, and the Dobashes in particular) in their own theoretical orientation and research. Space does not allow specification of such connections, but works by Straus *et al.* (1980), and Straus (1980) are illustrative. Nor is Bowker's (1983) theory and research unrelated to the patriarchal perspective. Although Bowker argues for a male peer subculture of violence, he does place family violence within a framework of patriarchal family dominance.

One can casually state that traces of patriarchy are detected in the works of certain other theorists. But it is quite clear that the patriarchy perspective is under attack. Some of the alleged criticisms directed against this perspective have already been mentioned. Nevertheless, a few brief remarks are necessary.

The works of Martin (1976) and Dobash and Dobash (1979) have used historical and case-study research designs in linking spouse battering, primarily, to a patriarchal system. In the Straus, Gelles, and Steinmetz (1980) tradition, however, power differentials are theorized and examined within family settings, essentially as if exploration of the nature of patriarchy is not relevant. The Dobashes (1979) appear to view such an approach as a "sacred" dependence on data gathering that places limits on the development of theory. This single methodological approach would not lead to an understanding of the role played by our historically structured institutions (Empey, 1985). We interpret these remarks to mean that better understanding of particular intrapersonal power struggles within families would not necessarily lead to understanding of the societal sources that sustain and assure the continued production of intrafamily violence.

Yllo (1983) expressed this view. For him interpersonal power family researchers assume that societal equalitarian norms have replaced patriarchal norms and, therefore, the latter norms have no empirical importance. They do not recognize that the legitimization of male behavior in families comes first and foremost from the larger social structure. The status of patriarchal norms in society in any period of time is, therefore, always a relevant research question.

As to the patriarchal perspective, Pagelow (1984), as previously noted, feels this perspective has borrowed from social learning theory and conflict theory. Nevertheless, the criticism offered by Washburne (1983) is valid. Proponents of this perspective are noted for limiting their theoretical discussion of family violence to spouse violence without incorporating abuses against children. The Dobashes (1979) do identify the connection of other forms of family violence relationship to social, historical, and interpersonal forces. However, even they do not intensely explore the nature of these relationships. Nor do they explore the commonalities and dissimilarities among forms of family violence despite their recognition that such forms stem, in part, from similar social forces.

As regards to methodology, the patriarchal perspective's stress on the qualitative approach produces works rich in detail, but weak in generalizability (Yllo, 1983). Of course there is no research method that does not have its limitations: areas where information is lost, information is not sought, or where information is in the hands of subjective integration and interpretation.

Each of these approaches must first explore the full range of questions that their theory has the potential to address. In turn, the question each perspective raises can be dealt with more completely by the utilization of a wider range of research designs than have thus far been evident (Saunders, 1986; Yllo, 1983). At this stage, a theory is often associated with a specific research method, instead of collaboration among researchers using a range of research designs. To the point, Yllo (1983) for one demonstrates how patriarchal social context can be subject to examination by using a quantitative methodology.

ECOLOGICAL PERSPECTIVE

Some psychologists (e.g., Bronfenbrenner, 1977, 1979) believe, like sociologists, that human behavior can best be understood by taking into account aspects of the environment beyond the immediate situation containing the individual. However, because of discipline differences, these psychologists prefer to label their work as the ecological perspective and tend to draw references mainly from psychological literature. Following this tradition, Garbarino (1977) and Belsky (1980) have attempted to develop an ecological perspective to explain child maltreatment. Generally speaking, both of them accept Bronfenbrenner's (1977, 1979) approach: that a person's environment can be understood as a series of settings, each nested within the next broader level, from the microenvironment of the family to the macroenvironment of society.

The early medical perspective regarded child abuse as qualitatively deviant from normal caregiver–child relationships. However, Garbarino (1977) shares the same views as sociologists and attempted to place the phenomenon of child abuse into an ecological perspective that emphasizes the ''social context'' of the abuse. In rejecting the idea of ''pure content-free'' child abuse, Garbarino believes that child abuse is related to what normal caregivers do with children, and to what the society and its institutions as a whole consider normal childrearing behavior. He sets out, therefore, to identify sufficient and necessary conditions under which child abuse can occur. To him, in order for any particular sufficient condition to cause a specific effect, all relevant necessary conditions must be met. In other words, if one or more required necessary conditions is absent, the sufficient condition will have little effect. In child abuse cases, there are many child abuse prone families, but obviously not every abuse prone family ends up with actual child abuse. Clearly, there are many families with sufficient conditions for child abuse but, in order to help them, it is vital to understand the necessary conditions that might move them from potential to actual abusers.

The greatest emphasis in the study of sufficient conditions for child maltreatment (both abuse and neglect) has been placed on role malfunction, that is, incompetence in the role of caregiver. Role malfunction is influenced by three major factions: role reversal, clarity of expectations, and minimal normative change. Maltreating parents often appear to have had little experience or opportunity to rehearse the role of caregiver, and do not know what to expect. Some of them have unrealistic expectations of children, even expecting the children to help meet their needs. They may also refuse to reorder their priorities to give the children's needs an appropriate place.

Another aspect of role malfunction is that these maltreating parents tend to have lives out of control. Abusive parents often perceive themselves as incompetent in facing stress or dealing with various problems. Finally, role malfunctions can also result from unsuccessful coping with unplanned or unwanted children, chronic transience, unpredictable or undependable income sources, and unsatisfactory transition to and mastery of key roles (e.g., caregiver, worker).

In terms of necessary conditions for child abuse, Garbarino identifies two major ecological factors. The first is that there must be cultural justification for the use of force against children. Children, in such a culture, may be defined as the property of caregivers and caregivers are authorized to use physical force against them. Garbarino argues that American society fulfills this necessary condition.

The second necessary condition for child abuse is the family's isolation from potent support systems, either family, neighborhood, or community. A social support system can serve as an important buffer in stressful situations, such as marriage difficulties, unemployment, unwanted pregnancy, crowded housing conditions, and special children (e.g., premature, retarded, etc.). Without social support, there is more stress, and therefore greater chance of abuse. Social isolation creates a context that permits child maltreatment.

Gelles (1983) believes that Garbarino's perspective, so far, is one of the few well-developed causal models and is surprised that it has not been applied to other forms of family violence. What is of more interest is that as far as we are aware, no empirical research adequately examines this model even with child abuse.

Belsky (1980) also attempted to use the ecological perspective to develop a general conceptual framework in which different research on child maltreatment can be integrated. Unlike Gabarino, Belsky's work has focused on classifying ecological variables to guide future empirical research.

Belsky's conceptual framework draws heavily on Tiorbergen's (1951) concern for the need to consider ontogenic development and also especially on Bronfenbrenner's (1977, 1979) ecological framework of human development (microsystem, exosystem, and macrosystem).

Using the ideas of Tiorbergen and Bronfenbenner, Belsky argues there are four levels of ecological analysis that are useful in the understanding of child abuse and neglect: ontogenic development, the microsystem, the exosystem, and the macrosystem.

Ontogenic Development. Ontogenic development refers to the history that individual parents who abuse their children bring with them to the family and the parenting role. An examination of the childhood histories of abusive parents is essential in this stage.

A consistent finding in past research is that the abusive parents were themselves abused when they were children. However, Belsky argues that because many parents who were mistreated in childhood do not mistreat their children, it is doubtful that a parent's experience as a child is sufficient, by itself, to account for abusive or neglectful behavior as an adult. Perhaps parents' developmental histories play a role in the abuse and neglect process by predisposing them, as adults, to become abusers. This childhood abuse may interact with additional personal, social-situational, and cultural factors to create an abuse cycle. The study of Conger, Burgess, and Barrett (1979), for example, provided some support of this argument. They found that childhood rearing is associated with later child maltreatment only when parents are subject to rapid life changes.

In addition to childhood exposure to violence and aggression, a few clinical studies (e.g., Elder, 1977) suggest that the absence of experience in caring for children may play an important role in the abuse and neglect process. However, Belsky argues that these clinical studies have to be interpreted cautiously, for there can be little doubt that many parents are lacking in child care experience but do not mistreat their children. Again, Belsky suggests a more systematic study of the relationship between prior experience in child care and subsequent caregiving competence, especially with respect to how it interacts with other ecological factors.

The Microsystem. The microsystem concerns the family setting, that is, the immediate context in which child maltreatment takes place. The traditional studies of child abuse in the family have focused on the parents. However, there is growing awareness that the abused children are, at least potentially, contributors to their own maltreatment. A disproportionate number of mistreated children were born prematurely, reveal a lack of social responsiveness, or are retarded or handicapped.

However, Belsky stresses that within the microsystem of the family child maltreatment must be considered an interactive process; although children may play a role in their own abuse or neglect, they cannot cause it by themselves. The work by Burgess and Conger (1978) in examining patterns of family interaction in abusive and nonabusive households clarified this process. They showed that in certified abusive and neglectful families there was less interaction between family members than there was in matched control families, and that mothers from maltreating families displayed 40% less positive interaction (e.g., affectionate and supportive behavior) and 60% more negative behavior (i.e., threats and complaints) than control mothers. Most intriguing is that children from abusive households displayed almost 50% more negative behavior than their counterparts from control families.

Following Bronfenbrenner (1979), Belsky argues that the major assumption underlying the ecological perspective is that the causes of child abuse are ecologically nested within one another. Therefore, a full understanding of the child's contribution to his or her own maltreatment in the abuse process can be achieved only by examining other aspects of the microsystem of the family. Because the parent–child syndrome (the crucible of child abuse) is nested within the spousal relationship, what happens between husbands and wives has implications for what happens between parents and their children. For example, the child abusive households are frequently found to have a high degree of marital conflict and discord. Similarly, the success of the married couple's transition to parenthood and the availability of economic and human resources may also relate to the abuse and neglect process.

The Exosystem. The exosystem represents the formal and informal structure (e.g., work situation, neighborhood, social networks) that do not themselves contain the developing person but impinge on or encompass the immediate settings in which that person is found and thereby influence, delimit, or even determine what goes on within them.

A frequently mentioned variable that links this system to child abuse is unemployment. Job loss is usually associated with frustration, stress (i.e., lack of monetary resources), and increased parent–child contact (resulting from the unemployed parent's spending more time at home), which in turn affects child maltreatment. Similarly, other work-setting-related variables, such as job satisfaction, alienation, and so forth, are also found as causative agents in the abuse process.

In addition, formal and informal social supports also relate to child abuse. It has been repeatedly found that child-abusing families are isolated from formal and informal support systems that can provide emotional and material assistance (including child-care service).

The Macrosystem. The macrosystem contains the cultural values and belief systems that foster the abuse or neglect of children through the influence they exert on ontogenic development and the micro- and exosystems.

The United States has higher levels of violence in comparison to other Western nations. Belsky argues that the societal willingness to tolerate violence sets the stage for the occurrence of family violence. More specifically, there is a general acceptance, if not sanctioning, of physical punishment as a means of controlling children's behavior. Not only is such punishment practiced with extraordinary frequency in this country, but it is also explicitly condoned by authorities or experts such as educators, police officers, judges, etc. The problem may be reinforced by the belief that children are property to be handled as parents choose.

Accordingly, despite the fact that advances are being made in the fight for children's rights, it is doubtful that maltreatment can be eliminated so long as parents rear their offspring in a society in which violence is tolerated, corporal punishment is condoned as a child rearing technique, and parenthood itself is construed in terms of ownership. Finally, Belsky points out that what happens in the micro- and exosystems on child abuse and neglect is invariably influenced by the macrosystem of child maltreatment.

GENERAL SYSTEMS THEORY

Some sociologists feel that traditional sociological theories, when applied to family violence, result in formulations that are static in nature and narrow in analytical power. Straus (1973) and Giles-Sims (1983) have turned to general systems theory (e.g., Buckley, 1967) in hopes of developing a more comprehensive and dynamic framework for explaining family violence. Before discussing Straus and Giles-Sims' works, it is important to have a basic idea of what general systems theory is.

The general systems theory attempts to provide a multidisciplinary overview of all scientific efforts and a unified set of concepts that can be used to generate hypotheses applicable in many fields. Boulding (1956) argued the general systems theory is the ''skeleton of science'' that aims to provide a framework for systematically structuring particular disciplines and particular subject matters in an orderly and coherent body of knowledge. Throughout the history of sociology, some theorists have used the idea of systems. For example, Spencer (1910) viewed society as an organization, similar to many biological organizations in a number of ways, such as growth, differentiation, and mutual dependence of parts, etc. Modern sociological theorists, such as Parsons (1951), rely heavily on general systems theory. Parsons (1968, p. 458) considers that the term *system* may apply ''both to a complex of interdependencies between parts, components, and processes that involve discernible regularities of relationship, and to a similar type of interdependency between such a complex and its surrounding environment.'' Buckley (1967) also made important contributions by systematically elaborating the systems approach. Buckley saw general systems theory as an attempt to examine how relationships are brought about, organized, and maintained. He hopes that it can consolidate the avalanche of many unrelated findings and provide an insightful framework for interpreting their output.

As a theory, the general systems theory combines several key concepts or constructs which must be understood to understand the larger theory (e.g., Berrien, 1968). Only a few of these key concepts are briefly discussed in the following.

A system acquires inputs from its environment, and these inputs are transformed by throughput into outputs that are subsequently returned to the environment. The event of input—throughput—output is cyclical. The following key concepts may help to understand how a system operates:

System Boundary. Each system has a boundary which separates it from its environment.

Open and Closed Systems. A system is considered open if it exchanges information, energy, or materials with its environment. A closed system can survive without interacting with its environment. Totally open or totally closed systems are rare. Usually, a social system is relatively open or relatively closed.

Positive and Negative Feedback. Negative feedback is a message that output has reached some predetermined maximum level and should be cut off or reduced. Positive feedback means that the output is less than some maximum, and the system should allow more input. Feedback enables a system to regulate itself, and thus enhances its probability of survival.

Morphostasis (or Homeostasis) and Morphogenesis. Morphostasis or homeostasis refers to a tendency toward stability. This state is maintained by negative feedback. Morphogenesis, however, is the system-enhancing behavior that allows for innovation and change.

Goal. A system is goal oriented. The interrelated parts guide the joint behavior of a system in accordance with its purpose.

In general, the basic tenet of the general systems theory is that the whole is more than the sum of the parts. Instead of breaking down a system into smaller parts for study, we will have greater insights if we look into the interaction between the subunits.

The general systems theory may have profound implications for theorizing about family violence. Its emphasis on the holistic view, the interchange between environment and family, the element of morphostatis versus morphogenesis, the impacts of positive and negative feedback, etc., may provide rich ideas for future development toward understanding family violence. However, the fertile ground of general systems theory is only tentative ground. An understanding of family violence cannot be achieved by these abstract concepts alone. A set of comprehensive prepositions and hypotheses may be generated, but their validity and relevance to family violence must be verified. With this in mind, we can proceed to the discussion of the efforts of Straus (1973) and Giles-Sims (1983).

Straus (1973) attempted to apply a general systems theory approach to explain family violence. Following the general systems theory tradition, he argued that family violence is a product of the system rather than of individual pathology. Feedback, which is essential for the operation of family as a system, generates stability or conflicts, such as violence. Positive feedback from violent acts produces an upward spiral of violence, and negative feedback serves to maintain the level of violence within tolerable limits.

According to Straus (1973), the general systems theory must go beyond analysis of the relationships among antecedent variables (e.g., social structure), precipitating variables (e.g., stress and frustration), and consequent variables (e.g., violence). It must include at least three crucial elements: (a) alternative courses of action or causal flow; (b) the feedback mechanisms that enable the system to made adjustments; and (c) system goals. That is, the feedback must be cybernetic feedback that controls the operation of the system in relation to its goals.

Straus uses eight propositions taken from Scheff (1966) to illustrate how the general systems theory relates to family violence. These eight propositions are as follows:

1. Violence between family members has many causes and roots. Normative structures, personality traits, frustrations and conflicts are only some.
2. Much more family violence occurs than is ever reported.
3. Most violence is either denied or considered normal.
4. Stereotyped family violence imagery is learned in early childhood from parents, siblings, and other children.
5. The family violence stereotypes are continually reaffirmed for adults and children through ordinary social interaction and the mass media.
6. Violent acts by violent persons may generate positive feedback, that is, these acts may produce the desired results.
7. Use of violence, when contrary to family norms, creates additional conflict over the original violence.

8. Persons who are labeled as violent may be encouraged to play out a violent role, either to live up to the expectations of others or to fulfill their own self-concept of being violent or dangerous.

Straus argued that these propositions represent the idea that violence is a system product. Violence in the family is increased through positive feedback, such as (a) labeling; (b) creation of secondary conflict over the use of violence; (c) reinforcement of the violent acts through successful use of such violence; and (d) the development of role expectations and self-concepts, such as being tough or violent.

The problem is that these propositions can be more or less developed from existing knowledge without general systems theory. Straus must be aware of this limitation. Moreover, he claims that the propositional format is incapable of including all the diverse elements in mind at once and does not make explicit the cybernetic and morphogenetic processes that are at the heart of systems analysis (p. 116). In order to overcome the problem, Straus introduces a computer flow chart that includes numerous steps of numerous causes, processes, and consequences of family violence. The flow chart is so tedious and complicated that it loses one of the essential characteristics of a theory or model: it is not parsimonious. Neither is it clear how Straus's general systems theory, in its present form, is useful in generating other testable propositions or models.

The book entitled *Wife-Beating: A Systems Theory Approach,* written by Giles-Sims (1983), is supposed to go further in systematically elaborating Straus's work on the general systems theory. It turns out, however, that Giles-Sims' intention is to use the ideas and concepts of general systems theory to raise various questions for investigation. Various interesting questions are raised and examined in her work, but there is no major theoretical breakthrough in family violence. However, many useful hints are provided about how to conceptualize and investigate the various processes and consequences of family violence. Her major contribution is Chapter 8, where she identified six temporal sequences which lead to wife battering.

Stage 1. The Establishment of the Family System. In this stage of any family, the groundwork is laid for ongoing patterns of interaction, boundaries are established, and system-governing rules evolve. Three systems questions are related to this stage. First, how is the new family system effected by patterns in other systems? At the beginning of any relationship, each person already has norms, values, and responses. A person's history of conflict and violent experiences provides clues to patterns of conflict and violence in subsequent relationships. For example, persons with violent childhood experiences are more likely to be physically violent to a child and/or to a spouse than those without such experiences.

Second, how did the commitment that established the boundaries of the system evolve over time? According to Giles-Sim's data, some women increase their commitment to a man even when he has a history of violence. Women tend to dismiss this or be sympathetic to it. However, according to the systems perspective, this pattern of dismissal or sympathy means that the women did not focus on past violence as a warning signal. They overlooked possible warning signals, even when the man had hit them before they married or started living together.

The pattern of a woman's commitment to a man results from social structure, parents, relatives, friends, etc. The role of single parent or divorced women is heavily stigmatized in American society, and therefore many women feel under pressure to become more committed in a relationship, even to the point of marriage. However, from a systems perspective, the increasing commitment represents a positive feedback loop that encourages violence in the future.

Third, have rules already been established concerning the use of violence, and the distribution of power? One important area of marriage expectations that may affect conflict processes is the relative power of males and females. For example, a man may use violence as a response to a woman's attempt to break off the relationship. Histories of violence in other systems of either the man or the woman, or sometimes both, determine the response to violence in the new system. In addition, male–female power is one of the most important forces determining the pattern of violence. If a man feels that he should or must have power in the relationship, he may use violence to enforce that power. If a woman accepts that a man should have that power, she may accept his violence.

Stage 2. The First Incidence of Violence. This stage focuses on the question: How did what happened between the couple at the time of the first violent incident affect the possibility of future incidents? According to the systems perspective, the feedback will give the answer to this question. If the violent person's goals (expressive and/or instrumental) are satisfied, positive feedback occurs, and the possibility of future violence is enhanced. Almost all the women in Giles-Sims' sample were willing to forgive and/or forget after the first incident. This lack of response also represents positive feedback to the violence.

Stage 3. Stabilization of the Violence. At this stage the question is: How much violence can develop within this system before negative feedback forces a halt? How does an interactional system develop when the members of the system are in conflict over goals? Systems theory predicts that behavior that receives positive feedback will escalate and tend to become an established part of the system. Each act of violence, therefore, is grounds for further conflict. As an example, violence creates a feud between families. After a while each forgets where it really started and become concerned only with getting revenge for the past acts of the other party. Some abused wives did fight back, but many did not. When women give in, their response represents positive feedback to violence, and it soon becomes an established pattern. When corrective responses do not keep violence within acceptable ranges, it will lead to a change in the basic rules of the system, a morphogenesis. For example, after a certain amount of escalation has occurred, corrective action within the system does not work. The battered woman must turn to outsiders, such as relatives, friends, police, or formal social control agencies for help. If these actions receive positive feedback, the process of escalation may be revised. Otherwise, the pattern of violence will be further strengthened.

Stage 4. The Choice Point. The question here is: When do patterns of wife battering become intolerable? Are there criteria for intolerability other than amount of violence?

The change-precipitating incident is not necessarily either the most violent or the most recent. The incident that stands out in the minds of women who come to shelters seeking help as most important and most critical in their decisions often occurred a few weeks to several months or even a few years previously.

These battered women described three important factors in their decisions: (a) fear the children would be hurt, (b) resentment at husbands who let the children see their mother being beaten, and (c) exposure of the violent pattern to people outside the family.

Stage 5. Leaving the System. This stage includes the following questions: Can the boundaries of the system shift and if so, how? How does one member of the system leave, and possibly become a member of another system? How does the battering member of the system respond? It was found that many of the women in shelters had been close to another person for at least a few months, indicating that women in those cases sought and found alternate sources of feedback from outside the family system in the period between the critical incident and the time they came to the shelter. The battered women and their confidants formed a relationship that crossed the boundaries of the original system. This bridging relationship was important for these women, because the family system had been their total involvement for so long that they required a new support system to act as a bridge between the original family system and the larger social system.

As the boundaries of the system opened, women became more aware of new opportunities and sources of information, such as public educational programs, media coverage, or word of mouth, and conflict developments between the original family system and the new emerging one. The outcome depends on the strength and different goals within the two systems and within the individual woman.

Stage 6. Resolution or More of the Same. Three questions relate to this stage: After the stay at the shelter, will the original family system be restructured so that future violence will not be encouraged? If women choose not to return to that system, can they establish new and satisfying systems to replace it? How likely is it that women who return to the original system will return to the same pattern, and that violence will recur?

Twenty-four percent of the women in Giles-Sims' sample were reinterviewed 6 months after they came to the shelter. Of those reinterviewed, 58% had returned to the man, at least temporarily, after leaving the shelter. Forty two percent were married to and/or living with the man at the time of the second interview.

Of all the follow-up couples, 56% reported at least one incident of violence in that interim period. Women who returned and never left reported the highest percentage of violent incidents, more than women who returned and left or those who never went back. Returning to a relationship that has an established pattern of violence is, in some cases, the same as continuing to comply with it. If the system has not been changed, the return represents positive feedback to established patterns.

EPILOGUE: WHERE WE ARE AND WHERE WE ARE GOING

During the 1970s, sociologists challenged the narrow vision of the psychiatric or medical model that explained family violence by personality disorders. Contrary to common beliefs that the family is a loving and happy social unit, sociologists have shown that family violence is a widespread phenomenon, influenced by many social forces.

Family violence is now recognized as a pervasive social problem, and issues of incidences, definitions, and the like are being addressed. In order to develop a comprehensive understanding of family violence, sociologists and other social scientists must now develop a systematic body of theories amenable to empirical verification.

The theories and perspectives reviewed in this chapter indicate that sociologists and social scientists are addressing this problem. Developing a comprehensive and useful perspective requires ongoing empirical verification (qualitative and quantitative) directly tied to a theory or model. Empirical testing can provide enlightening information that refines or expands aspects of a theory or model. Unfortunately—so far—theorizing and empirical research in family violence has not been a cooperative activity. Only a small number of studies have directly attempted to test formally theories or perspectives, such as the resource theory or the patriarchal perspective, and the research designs of such studies are often not sufficiently vigorous or sophisticated to address validity issues (Campbell &

Stanley, 1963) such as internal validity (Does the research rule out confounding sources?), or external validity (Are the research findings generalizable?).

The discrepancy between theory and research in family violence may be attributed to theorists who are eager to argue for specific theories instead of carefully developing them so that they can be subject to research verification. This discrepancy may be also due to empirical researchers who are occupied in compiling empirical data without careful prior thought to theory considerations. For example, patriarchal theorists and researchers should offer insight as to how one longitudinally or cross-sectionally measures and observes variations in patriarchal systems. Nor have general systems theorists provided, thus far, any new insights that can be empirically verified. We conclude with the thought that in future scientific studies of family violence more emphasis should be placed on systematically refining and integrating theory and research.

References

Allen, C. M., & Straus, M. A. (1977). Resources, power, and husband-wife violence. In M. A. Straus & G. T. Hotaling (Eds.), *The social courses of husband–wife violence* (pp. 188–208). Minneapolis, MN: University of Minnesota Press.

Bach, G. R., & Wyden, P. (1968). *The intimate enemy.* New York: Avon Books.

Bahr, S. J. (1979). Family determinants and effects on deviance. In W. R. Bur, R. Hill, R. I. Nye, & I. L. Reiss (Eds.), *Contemporary theories about the family* (pp. 615–643). New York: The Free Press.

Bandura, A. (1973). *Aggression: A social learning analysis.* Englewood Cliffs, NJ: Prentice-Hall.

Belsky, J. (1980). Child maltreatment: An ecological integration. *American Psychologist, 35,* 320–335.

Berrien, F. (1968). *General and social systems.* New Brunswick, NJ: Rutgers University Press.

Bersani, C. A., & Chen, H. T. (October, 1985). *A format for treatment and comparison outcomes: Court ordered treatment of "spouse" abusers versus other court sanctions.* Paper presented at the Midwest Criminal Justice Meetings, Chicago, IL.

Blau, P. M. (1964). *Exchange and power in social life.* New York: Wiley.

Blood, R. O., & Wolfe, D. M. (1960). *Husband and wives: The dynamics of married living.* Glencoe, IL: Free Press.

Boulding, K. E. (1956). General systems theory—The skeleton of science. *Management Science, 2,* 197–209.

Bowker, L. H. (1983). *Beating wife-beating.* Lexington, MA: D. C. Heath.

Breines, W., & Gordon, L. (1983). The new scholarship on family violence. *Signs: Journal of Women and Culture and Society, 8* (31), 490–531.

Brisson, N. J. (1981). Battering husbands: A survey of abusive men. *Victimology: An International Journal, 6,* 338–344.

Bronfenbrenner, U. (1977). Toward an experimental ecology of human development. *American Psychologist, 32,* 513–531.

Bronfenbrenner, U. (1979). *The ecology of human development.* Cambridge, MA: Harvard University Press.

Buckley, W. (1967). *Sociology and modern systems theory.* Englewood Cliffs, NJ: Prentice-Hall.

Burgess, K., and Conger, R. (1978). Family interaction in abusive, neglectful and normal families. *Child Development, 49,* 1163–1173.

Campbell, D. T., & Stanley, J. C. (1963). *Experimental and quasi-experimental designs for research.* Chicago, IL: Rand McNally.

Carroll, J. C. (1980). A cultural-consistency theory of family violence in Mexican-American and Jewish-ethnic groups. In M. A. Straus & G. T. Hotaling (Eds.), *The social causes of husband-wife violence* (pp. 68–81). Minneapolis, MN: University of Minnesota Press.

Collins, R. (1975). *Conflict sociology.* New York: Academic Press.

Conger, R., Burgess, R., & Barrett, C. (1979). Child abuse related to life changes and perceptions of illness: Some preliminary findings. *Family Coordinator, 28,* 73–78.

Coser, L. A. (1956). *The functions of social conflict.* New York: The Free Press.

Coser, L. A. (1967). *Continuities in the study of social conflict.* New York: The Free Press.

Curtis, L. A. (1975a). *Criminal violence: National patterns and behavior.* Lexington, MA: D. C. Heath.

Curtis, L. A. (1975b). *Violence, race, and culture.* Lexington, MA: D. C. Heath.

Curtis, R. F. (1986). Household and family in theory on inequality. *American Sociological Review, 51,* 168–183.

Davis, N. J. (1980). *Sociological constructions of deviance.* Dubuque, IA: Brown.

Dobash, R. E., & Dobash, R. P. (August, 1976). *Love, honour and obey: Institutional ideologies and the struggle for battered women.* Paper presented at the annual meeting of the Society for the Study of Social Problems, New York.

Dobash, R. E., & Dobash, R. P. (1979). *Violence against wives.* New York: The Free Press.

Elder, G. (1977). Family history and life course. *Journal of Family History 2,* 279–304.

Empey, L. T. (1985). The family and delinquency. *Today's delinquent, 4,* 5–46.

Finkelhor, D. (1983). Common features of family abuse. In D. Finkelhor, R. J. Gelles, G. T. Hotaling, & M. A. Straus (Eds.), *The dark side of families* (pp. 17–28). Beverly Hills, CA: Sage.

Garbarino, J. (1977). The human ecology of child maltreatment: A conceptual model for research. *Journal of Marriage and the Family, 39,* 721–735.

Gelles, R. J. (1976). *The violent home: A study of physical aggression between husbands and wives.* Beverly Hills, CA: Sage.

Gelles, R. J. (1985). Family violence. In Turner, R. H. & J. F. Short (Eds.), *Annual Review of Sociology* (Vol 11, pp. 347–367). Palo Alto, CA: Annual Reviews.

Gelles, R. J. (1983). Violence in the family: A review of research in the seventies. In D. H. Olson & B. C. Miller (Eds.), *Family studies review yearbook, Vol. 1,* No. 1 (pp. 873–885). Beverly Hills, CA: Sage.

Gelles, R. J. (1983). An exchange/social theory. In D. Finkelhor, R. J. Gelles, G. T. Hotaling, & M. A. Straus (Eds.), *The dark side of families: Current family violence research* (pp. 151–165). Beverly Hills, CA: Sage.

Gelles, R. J., & Straus, M. A. (1979). Determinants of violence in the family: Toward a theoretical integration. In W. R. Bur, R. Hill, R. I. Nye, & I. L. Reiss (Eds.), *Contemporary theories about the family-research-based theories* (Vol. 1, pp. 549–581). New York: The Free Press.

Gelles, R. J., & Straus, M. A. (1979). Violence in the American family. *Journal of Social Issues, 35,* 15–39.

Gelles, R. J., & Cornell, C. P. (1985). *Intimate violence in families.* Beverly Hills, CA: Sage.

Giles-Sims, J. (1983). *Wife-beating: A systems theory approach.* New York: Guilford Press.

Goode, W. J. (1971). Force and violence in the family. *Journal of Marriage and Family, 33,* 624–636.

Hepburn, J. R. (1973). Violent behavior in interpersonal relationships. *The Sociological Quarterly, 14,* 419–429.

Hirschi, T. (1969). *Causes of delinquency.* Berkeley, CA: University of California Press.

Homans, G. C. (1961). *Social behavior: Its elementary forms.* New York: Harcourt, Brace, Jovanovich.

Homans, G. C. (1974). *Social behavior in its elementary forms.* (2nd ed.), *New York: Harcourt, Brace, Jovanovich.*

Horowitz, I. L. (1967). Consensus, conflict and co-operation. In N. J. Demerath III & R. A. Peterson (Eds.), *System, change and conflict* (p. 268). New York: Free Press.

Kelly, K. D., & Chambliss, W. J. (1966). Status consistency and political attitudes. *American Sociological Review, 31,* 375–382.

Lenski, G. E. (1954). Status crystallization: As a non-vertical dimension of social status. *American Sociological Review, 19,* 405–413.

Martin, D. (1976). *Battered wives.* San Francisco: Glide.

Marx, K. (1964). *Selected writings in sociology and social philosophy.* T. B. Bottomore & M. Rubel (Eds.) New York: McGraw-Hill.

Merton, R. K. 1967. *On theoretical sociology.* New York: The Free Press.

Nettler, G. (1978). *Explaining crime* (2nd ed.). New York: McGraw Hill.

O'Brien, J. E. (1971). Violence in divorce prone families. *Journal of Marriage and the Family, 30,* 692–698.

Pagelow, M. D. (1984). *Family violence.* New York: Praeger.

Parsons, T. (1951). *The social system.* Glencoe, IL: Free Press.

Parsons, T. (1968). Systems analysis social systems. *International encyclopedia of the social sciences* (Vol. 15).

Poloma, M. M. (1979). *Contemporary sociological theory.* New York: Macmillan.

Reckless, W. C. (1973). The crime problem (5th ed.). New York: Appleton-Century-Croft.

Ritzer, G. (1986). *Social problems.* New York: Random House.

Rodman, H. (1972). Marital power and the theory of resources in cultural context. *Journal of Comparative Family Studies, 3,* 50–59.

Rose, A. M. (1962). A systematic summary of symbolic interaction theory. In A. M. Rose (Ed.), *Human behavior and social processes* (pp. 3–19). Boston, MA: Houghton Mifflin.

Russell, D. E. H. (1984). *Sexual exploitation: Rape, child sexual abuse, and workplace harassment*. Beverly Hills, CA: Sage.

Saunders, D. G. (1986). When battered women use violence: Husband-abuse or self-defense? *Victims and Violence, 1,* 47–56.

Scheff, T. J. (1966). *Being mentally ill*. Chicago, IL: Aldine.

Spencer, H. (1910). *The principles of sociology*. New York: Appleton.

Sprey, J. (1969). The family as a system in conflict. *Journal of Marriage and the Family, 31,* 699–706.

Sprey, J. (1974). On management of conflict in families. In S. K. Steinmetz & M. A. Straus (Eds.), *Violence in the family* (pp. 110–119). New York: Harper & Row.

Star, B. (1980). Patterns of family violence. *Social Casework, 61,* 339–346.

Stark, R., & McEvoy, I. J. (1970). Middle-class violence. *Psychology Today,* vol. 4, 52–54.

Stark, E., Flitcraft, A., & Frazier, W. (1979). Medicine and patriarchal violence: The social construction of a ''private'' event. *International Journal of Health Services, 9(3);* 461–493.

Steinmetz, S. K. (1977). *The cycle of violence*. New York: Praeger Publishers.

Steinmetz, S. K. (1978). Violence between family members. *Marriage and Family Review, 1,* 1–16.

Steinmetz, S. K., & Straus, M. A. (Eds.). (1974). *Violence in the family*. New York: Harper & Row.

Straus, M. A. (1973). A general systems theory approach to a theory of violence between family members. *Social Science Information, 12,* 105.

Straus, M. A. (1974). Forward. In R. G. Gelles, *In the violent home: A study of physical aggression between husbands and wives* (pp. 13–17). Beverly Hills, CA: Sage.

Straus, M. A. (1976). Cultural and social organizational influences on violence between family members. In R. Prince & D. Barrid (Eds.), *Configurations: Biological and cultural factors in sexuality and family life.* Lexington, MA: D. C. Heath.

Straus, M. A. (1980). Sexual inequality and wife beating. In M. A. Straus & G. T. Hotaling (Eds.), *The social causes of husband-wife violence* (pp. 86–93). Minneapolis, MN: University of Minnesota Press.

Straus, M. A. (October, 1986). *Family violence*. Paper presented at the Family Violence Seminar sponsored by NEOUCOM (Northeastern Ohio Universities College of Medicine).

Straus, M. A., & Steinmetz, S. K. (1974). Violence research, violence control, and the good society. In S. K. Steinmetz & M. A. Straus (Eds.), *Violence in the family* (pp. 321–324). New York: Dodd, Mead.

Straus, M. A., Gelles, R. J., & Steinmetz, S. K. (1980). *Behind closed doors*. Garden City, New York: Anchor Books.

Stryker, S. (1967). Symbolic interaction as an approach to family research. In J. G. Manis & B. N. Meltzer (Eds.), *Symbolic interaction* (pp. 371–383). Boston, MA: Allyn & Bacon.

Tiorbergen, N. (1951). *The study of instinct*. London: Oxford University Press.

Turner, J. H. (1986). *The structure of sociological theory*. Chicago, IL: Dorsey Press.

Vold, G. B. (1986). *Theoretical criminology*. New York: Oxford University Press.

Vold, G. B., & Bernard, T. J. (1985). *Theoretical criminology* (3rd ed.). New York: Oxford University Press.

Washburne, C. K. (1983). A feminist analysis of child abuse and neglect. In D. Finkelhor, R. Gelles, G. T. Hotaling, & M. A. Straus (Eds.), *The dark side of families* (pp. 289–292). Beverly Hills, CA: Sage.

Weber, M. (1956). *From Max Weber: Essays in sociology*. H. H. Gerth & C. Wright Mills (Trans. and Ed.). New York: Oxford University Press.

White, L. A. (1975). *The concept of cultural systems*. New York: Columbia University Press.

Wolfgang, M. E., & Ferracuti, F. (1967). *The subculture of violence*. Beverly Hills, CA:

Wolfgang, M. E., & Ferracuti, F. (1982). *The subculture of violence* (2nd ed.). Beverly Hills, CA: Sage.

Yllo, K. (1983). Using a feminist approach in quantitative research. In D. Finkelhor, R. Gelles, G. T. Hotaling, & M. A. Straus (Eds.), *The dark side of families* (pp. 277–288). Beverly Hills, CA: Sage.

III

FORMS OF FAMILY VIOLENCE

5

Wife Battering

GAYLA MARGOLIN, LINDA GORIN SIBNER, and LISA GLEBERMAN

Of all forms of family violence, wife battering ranks second, following child abuse, in terms of the attention it now receives in public, professional, and scientific communities. This attention has been painstakingly slow to develop. It has come about only through the untiring efforts of concerned individuals, primarily feminists, who were on the front lines of providing direct services to battered women. Efforts to make known the enormity and severity of this problem have borne the following results: the number of shelters in the United States has grown from two in 1974, to 200 in 1978, to an estimated 780 today (Bowker & Maurer, 1985). On February 2, 1985, the House of Representatives passed the Family Violence Prevention and Services Amendment, which appropriated $65 million over a 3-year period to assist states in preventing violence within families and in the provision of services for victims. This bill is a condensed version of a bill authored by Representative Mikulski to provide federal funding to shelters for battered women, which was unsuccessfully introduced into the House during each Congressional session since 1978 (Melling, 1984). At the time of this writing, the bill had been reduced in scope to $6 million in the first year, but was still alive and awaiting a joint vote in the House and Senate.

Fewer efforts need to be directed today, as compared to 10 years ago, toward convincing policymakers and service providers about the seriousness of wife battering as a problem. The data on the frequency and extent of this problem speak for themselves. Yet, despite our increasing awareness of wife battering, we are at an early stage in our understanding of how to intervene into this process. There must be continued efforts to discover how best to help batterers stop battering, help victims improve the quality of their lives and get beyond the battering, and to reduce the overall rates of this societywide problem.

The purpose of this chapter is to review what is known about the frequency of wife battering, to summarize theories on what causes wife battering, to describe current treatment modes, to identify some of the ethical and legal issues, and to highlight some promising future directions. We begin with a description and definition of wife battering.

GAYLA MARGOLIN, LINDA GORIN SIBNER, and LISA GLEBERMAN • Department of Psychology, University of Southern California, Los Angeles, CA 90089. Preparation of this chapter was supported by National Institute of Mental Health Grant IR01 36595.

GAYLA MARGOLIN
ET AL.

Wife battering, as a medical, legal, and societal problem, has a somewhat different description depending on the domain in which it is discussed. Wife battering comes to the attention of the medical profession when the injuries sustained by the woman require medical attention, or are severe enough to have caused death. From data on injuries and deaths, we can conclude that violence inflicted on a woman by her husband or boyfriend poses a serious health problem in the United States: 30% of female homicide victims are killed by their husbands or boyfriends (Federal Bureau of Investigation, 1982). More than one million abused women seek medical help for injuries caused by battering each year (Stark & Flitcraft, 1982). Further, in addition to the wounds inflicted on battered women, other disorders, some of which are self-inflicted, also tend to evolve during the course of an abusive relationship (Gayford, 1975). Battered women, compared to nonbattered women, are more likely to attempt suicide and to abuse drugs or alcohol (Stark, Flitcraft, & Frazier, 1983).

In the medical domain, the identification and appropriate treatment of battered women has been impeded by the reluctance of victims to admit the origin of the wounds and failure by physicians to recognize specific indicators of wife battering. According to Stark *et al.* (1983),

> where physicians saw 1 out of 35 of their patients as battered, a more accurate approximation is 1 in 4; where they acknowledged that 1 injury out of 20 resulted from domestic abuse, the actual figure approached 1 in 4. What they described as a rare occurrence was, in reality, an event of epidemic proportions. (p. 183)

Now, with the ninth revision of the *International Classification of Diseases: Clinical Modification* (ICD-9-CM), the syndrome finally has been given a label. "Battered spouse" and "battered woman" appear under heading 995.81, "Adult maltreatment syndrome." With this new label, emergency physicians can begin diagnosing the syndrome and using the term in their billing, and hospital records may begin to document systematically the existence of battered women ("Battered syndrome" now official, 1979).

Until 10 years ago, wife battering was given little recognition in the legal system, leaving battered women who sought legal protection from abuse with few options. One problem was that women did not report abuse. Dobash and Dobash (1979) found that of 109 women who reported a total of 32,000 assaults during their marriages, only 517, or less than 2%, were reported to the police. Another problem may have been that these women learned the futility of legal actions. Although assaults of a certain severity between strangers would automatically be classified as felonies, the same assaults between intimates might have been considered misdemeanors, if, indeed, an arrest were made at all. Rather than following traditional criminal procedures, officers had been trained to mediate the situations without making an arrest and may even have dissuaded the victim from pressing charges. Unfortunately, in some cases, this course of action contributed to the escalation rather than the containment of abuse. One study of domestic violence indicated that the police had been called at least once before in 85% of spouse assault and homicide cases. In 50% of these cases, the police had responded five times to family violence incidents prior to the homicide. (The Police Foundation, 1977, cited in the Attorney General's Task Force on Domestic Violence, 1984).

In the past few years, however, it has become increasingly common for states to enact specific legislation regarding wife battering and to treat wife battering as a crime.

For example, laws in 43 states now enable battered women to obtain civil protection orders without initiating divorce or other civil proceedings, as previously required. Thirty-three states have expanded police power to arrest in domestic abuse cases (Lerman & Livingston, 1983). The clearest and most comprehensive policy statement is found in the recent recommendations of the Attorney General's Task Force on Domestic Violence (1984). These recommendations state that (a) all complaints of family violence are to be reported as criminal offenses, (b) arrest is the appropriate response in situations involving serious injury or imminent danger to the victim, (c) the victim need not be required to sign a formal complaint before the prosecutor files charges unless mandated by state law, and (d) protection orders be readily issued and enforced. Thus, wife battering is beginning to be viewed, in the legal domain, as a serious criminal offense in which the victim's rights are to be protected and the perpetrator of the crime is to prosecuted.

Although medical and legal definitions and responses to this problem are important, many incidents of wife battering never reach either of these professions. It is, of course, very difficult to estimate exactly how frequent a problem wife battering is. Yet, from the data that are available, it appears that the majority of wife battering goes undetected, unreported, and untreated. The most widely cited data on the incidence of wife battering comes from the random nationwide survey of 2,143 husbands and wives conducted by Straus, Gelles, and Steinmetz (1980). Their data indicate that every year 3.8% or one out of 26 American wives get beaten by their husbands, for a total of almost 1.8 million annually. In terms of frequency, the Straus et al. (1980) data show that for one third of the wives, there was only one such severely violent attack within the year. Twenty percent of the husbands attacked their wives twice during the year and 47% of the husbands beat their wives three or more times during the year. The criteria for wife beating used by Straus et al. included kicking, biting, punching, hitting with an object, beating up, threatening with a knife or gun, and using a knife or gun. If the criteria are expanded to include any act of violence (e.g., throwing something at the spouse, pushing, grabbing, shoving, and slapping the spouse), then 12.1%, or about one in eight husbands, committed at least one such act within the year of the study. Similarly, a Louis Harris poll indicated that one in 10 female partners experienced some degree of spousal violence by their partners in the past 12 months (Schulman, 1979, cited in *Violence among Relatives and Friends: A National Crime Survey,* 1980). Hornung, McCullough, and Sugimoto (1981) found that 16% of women reported at least one incident of physical aggression in the previous year. Violence against women often predates marriage. O'Leary and Arias (1985) reported that at one month prior to marriage, 40% of their sample of 400 women were experiencing physical aggression.

A major question of interest has been whether the incidence of wife battering is related to specific demographic variables. However, conclusions are difficult to reach because of sampling problems and difficulties obtaining accurate data. There is clear evidence that wife battering knows no social or economic boundaries. Nonetheless, although it occurs in families across socioeconomic levels, it is somewhat more likely to occur in low-income, low-socioeconomic couples (Gelles & Cornell, 1985). A key factor appears to be the employment status of husbands, with wife battering more likely in unemployed, as compared to employed men, or in men with low job satisfaction (Gayford, 1975; Prescott & Letko, 1977). Another factor in interpreting results pertaining to social class is that by having more resources available, middle- and upper-class families may have ways of keeping their violence private.

A common theme running through the literature on wife battering is the difficulty of securing accurate estimates regarding incidence and frequency of this problem. As indicated previously, since most incidents of wife beating never come to public attention, any offical records of wife beating through the medical or criminal systems are gross underestimates. Even anonymous and/or confidential self-reports are subject to underreporting because of (a) sensitivity of the topic and embarrassment on the part of both the perpetrator and the victim to admit to wife battering; (b) acceptance of so-called normal violence and the failure to remember or label such events; and (c) reliance on married or cohabitating couples when many abusive couples have separated or divorced (Pagelow, 1979; Straus *et al.*, 1980). Further, several important definitional problems surrounding wife battering make it difficult to get accurate estimates of its frequency.

One definitional problem stems from the fact that wife battering often has been subsumed under the genderless category of spouse abuse or marital violence. One reason for this classification is the large number of couples in which both spouses engage in violent acts. Straus *et al.* (1980), for example, found that 16%, or approximately one out of six couples in the United States commits at least one violent act against his or her partner. Of these couples reporting violence, 49% of the cases reveal violence from both husband and wife. Overall, these investigators found approximately comparable rates of wife-to-husband and husband-to-wife violence. These data stand in contrast to the National Crime Survey data that indicated that between 1973 to 1977, men committed 95% of all assaults on spouses (U. S. Department of Justice, 1983, cited in "Wife Abuse: The Facts," 1984). Similarly, a survey of police cases of domestic violence for two cities in Scotland showed that, out of 1044 cases, 75.8% were directed against women whereas only 1.1% were directed against men (Dobash & Dobash, 1978).

As several investigators (Fleming, 1979; Straus *et al.*, 1980) have pointed out there are a number of problems in drawing parallels between wife battering and husband battering. Although sheer frequencies of violent acts may be approximately the same for husbands as for wives, the potential consequences of the violence by the wives is considerably less. Husbands tend to engage in more dangerous and injurious forms of violence. The greater size and strength of husbands make their behaviors more dangerous despite the fact that actions by both men and women may be described through the same labels (e.g., beating). Also, arguing that it is primarily women who are battered, Berk, Berk, Loseke, and Rauma (1983) concluded that "there is no inevitable correspondence between 'conflict tactics' (e.g., Straus, 1979) and the consequences of the 'conflict'" (p. 198). To obtain an accurate picture of the different roles of men and women in family violence, Fleming (1979) recommended assessing the intensity of the acts and the degree of damage inflicted on the victim, although she acknowledges that these are difficult constructs to operationalize.

Distinctions sometimes have been drawn between "one-way violence" and "mutual combat" (Gelles, 1974). In one-way violence, wives do not hit back because they are afraid that if they do, they will be hit even harder. In mutual combat, or what Gelles labels protective-reaction violence, the wife retaliates and hits back in self-defense or else stages a pre-emptive attack because she fears that her husband is about to hit her. Stark *et al.* (1983) also differentiate between battering and fighting. However, their definition leads us to be relatively unconcerned with the consequences of mutual combat. They maintain that

> whereas fighting may occur frequently without destroying the extended relations of family, community, or cultural life, "battering" appears only when persons have been forcibly isolated from potentially supportive kin and peer relations and virtually locked into family situations where their objectification and continued punishment are inevitable. (p. 195)

Definitional confusion regarding wife battering also stems from whether the label of wife battering is applied on the basis of specific violent behaviors or on a broader behavioral pattern. In some instances, wife battering has been operationally defined by the occurrence of violent acts, regardless of their context or intentionality (e.g., Straus *et al.*, 1980). Other investigators have attempted to describe a battering syndrome that takes into consideration a variety of emotional and relationship issues as well. According to Walker (1983), for example, battered women develop psychological sequelae that interfere with their ability to stop successfully the batterers' violence and that can be considered to constitute the battered women's syndrome. As she notes,

> Repeated batterings, like electrical shocks, diminish the woman's motivation to respond. She becomes passive. Secondly, her cognitive ability to perceive success is changed. She does not believe her response will result in a favorable outcome, whether or not it might. Next, having generalized her helplessness, the battered woman does not believe anything she does will alter any outcome, not just the specific situation that has occurred. (pp. 49–50)

Stark *et al.* (1983) elaborate this point when they describe "a paralyzing terror and overvaluation of male power" that trap the woman in an abusive relationship.

These definitional considerations illustrate the complex nature of wife battering. Violence may include verbal and psychological as well as physical acts of aggression. Even if violence is limited to physical acts, there still is the issue of whether or not milder forms of physical aggression should be differentiated from battering and whether or not mutual combat should be differentiated from the one-way attacks.

For the remainder of this chapter, the term *battered women* will be used to describe women who have experienced physically injurious behavior at the hands of men with whom they once had, or were continuing to have, an intimate relationship. No distinctions are made as to the exact nature of the relationship (i.e., married, cohabitating, separated, or divorced). Nor are distinctions made as to the severity of the physical assault; all forms of physical violence are included. Because mutual violence includes actions that are physically injurious to women, and because that often can be difficult to distinguish from one-way violence, mutual violence also will be considered below. This definition reflects our attitudes about the inappropriateness of any type of physical violence and the long-range significance of any such actions to both persons involved and to their overall relationship.

THEORIES REGARDING ETIOLOGY

There is a frustrating dilemma in attempting to summarize theories regarding the etiology of wife battering: although the list of theories is quite long, the empirical data in support of such theories is quite meager. Moreover, empirical investigations pitting one theory against another are almost nonexistent, thereby making it difficult to compare the relative utility of various theories. It also should be noted that wife battering is not necessarily a unitary phenomenon, although typically it is discussed as such. Snyder and Fruchtman (1981) recently identified five different types of abused wives, reflecting considerable variability in the women's individual histories, current relationships, and responses to abuse. Perhaps one reason why there are numerous theories and inconsistencies in the data is because we are trying to explain several different patterns of wife battering. Lacking a well-developed typology, we will present theories without tying them to specific types of wife battering. We will organize the theories, however, around three different levels of explanation: intrapersonal, interpersonal, and sociocultural.

In viewing wife battering from an intrapersonal level of analysis, it is assumed that one or both spouses possess certain characteristics that make them prone to wife battering. In the earlier literature, when investigators felt that they were dealing with an infrequent phenomenon, there was a tendency to look for pathological conditions either in the assaulter, the victim, or both. These studies also were very much affected by the populations sampled, for example, psychiatric case studies (Symonds, 1978), or prison populations (Faulk, 1974; Scott, 1974). Based on extreme samples, individual case studies, and in the absence of proper controls, the conclusions drawn reflected high levels of individual pathology. The wife beaters have been described as sadistic, passive-aggressive, addiction prone, pathologically jealous, pathologically passive and dependent (Faulk, 1974; Shainess, 1977; Snell, Rosenwald, & Robey, 1964), or suffering from neurological or biochemical disorders (Elliot, 1977; Schauss, 1982). Similarly, negative personality characteristics were assigned to battered women (e.g., masochistic, aggressive, immature) (Scott, 1974; Shainess, 1977; Snell *et al.*, 1964). This literature sparked considerable controversy for its underlying message about responsibility in wife battering. The conclusions drawn about pathological conditions in males tended to relieve them of responsibility for their actions whereas the conclusions drawn about females indicated that they were to blame for their own plight.

More recent studies have been more sensitive to issues of responsibility, particularly with respect to women. Although investigations still rely on pathological indexes, women's symptoms are viewed as sequelae of abuse, rather than comcomitants or precursors of abuse. These studies indicate, for example, that women who have been battered tend to suffer from depression, anxiety, alcohol abuse, and have elevated MMPI profiles (Douglas & Der Ovanesian, 1983; Hughes & Rau, 1984; Rosewater, 1984; Telch & Lindquist, 1984; Walker, 1984b).

There also has been a theoretical shift regarding men's responsibility for abuse. It was pointed out, for example, that many batterers are violent only toward their wives and only in the privacy of their own homes. Such findings undermine hypotheses regarding poor impulse control (e.g., Schechter, 1982). Although there is considerable evidence that batterers are prone to substance abuse (Fitch & Papantonio, 1983; Gayford, 1975; Peltoniemi, 1984; Rounsaville, 1978), that, too, has been brought into question as an explanation for the violence. There is little evidence that pharmacological properties of alcohol or drugs play a direct role in specific battery instances (Berk *et al.*, 1983; Taylor & Leonard, 1983).

Because wife battering increasingly has been viewed as a relatively common phenomenon, attention has focused on other, less pathologically oriented explanations. Several investigations have examined attitudinal factors. First, with respect to sex role attitudes, males have been described as conservative, rigid, and holding traditional and sex-stereotyped values (Davidson, 1978; Rosenbaum & O'Leary, 1981; Telch & Lindquist, 1984; Walker, 1979). Pairing traditional husbands with nontraditional wives may be a particularly violence-prone combination (Walker, 1984b; Whitehurst, 1974). Second, with respect to sex role identity, batterers, compared to nonbatterers, appear to be lower in masculinity, and are more likely to be categorized as undifferentiated (LaViolette, Barnett, & Miller, 1984; Rosenbaum, 1985). Third, attitudes regarding the acceptability of violence in intimate relationships also have proven quite enlightening. Data reported by Straus (1980c), for example, show that violent wives, as well as violent husbands, express more approval of violence than do nonviolent husbands and wives. Fourth, self-esteem has been implicated as being problematic for batterers (Gayford, 1975; Goldstein & Rosenbaum, 1985; Neidig, Friedman, & Collins, 1984; Walker, 1979) and, possibly, also for battered women (Carlson, 1977; Star, Clark, Goetz, & O'Malia, 1979; Walker, 1979). In considering these results, we should note, however, that there also are a number of insignificant findings, showing batterers and their victims to be no different from anyone else (e.g., Feldman, 1983; Neidig *et al.*, 1984).

On a behavioral level, research data portray the batterer as unassertive with his spouse (Rosenbaum & O'Leary, 1981). However, it is unclear whether this differentiates the violent partner from maritally discordant but nonviolent partners (Margolin, in press-b; O'Leary & Curley, 1986). Although not demonstrated empirically, it also has been suggested that these spouses have not learned how to acknowledge and express feelings other than anger (Ferraro, 1984; LaViolette *et al.*, 1984).

Integrating these findings, we can begin to formulate an overall picture of the batterer. Although the abuser tends to value traditional characteristics of masculinity (e.g., dominance, success), he actually feels quite inadequate in those respects. This leads to feelings of low self-esteem. His need to maintain an overadequate facade, coupled with the inability to express feelings of vulnerability, leaves the man susceptible to overreaction when he perceives a threat, particularly at home, the one domain where he believes he dominates and is in control.

The intrapersonal findings pertaining to battered women are even more varied than those regarding the batterers, making it difficult to formulate generalizations about their characteristics or functioning. In some descriptions, battered women appear anxious, low in ego strength and self-esteem, unable to cope, depressed, etc. In others, women appear no different than nonbattered women or, on occasion, have developed unusually high inner strength. Walker (1983), for example, reported that her sample of battered women perceived themselves as stronger, more independent, and more sensitive than other women. These data lead us to consider the warning by Wardell, Gillespie, & Leffler (1983), that perhaps the wrong question is being asked in the search for differences between battered and nonbattered women. These data exemplify "the tendency in the literature to isolate as deviant not only wife-beating but also beaten wives" (p. 71).

Interpersonal Levels

Interpersonal explanations focus on interactions of persons involved with each other, as well as with other persons with whom they have had contact. There are three main theories that fit this category: social learning, systems, and cycle. At this level of explanation, the theories are not specific to wife battering as distinct from other forms of family violence. The theories also draw on conflict literature more generally, viewing physical violence as one specific case of all forms of conflict between intimates.

Social Learning Theory. According to social learning theory, each individual's behavior is determined by his or her social environment, most notably his or her family members. Specific mechanisms whereby family members influence one another to perform violent behaviors are modeling, reinforcement, and coercion.

One of the most consistent findings regarding etiological characteristics of wife battering is the intergenerational transmission of violence. These findings indicate that one is more likely to be in a violent marital relationship if she or he had been exposed to violence as a child, either as a witness to interparental violence or as victim of parental abuse. A number of studies have shown a high frequency of violence in the families of origin of batterers (Gayford, 1975; Rosenbaum & O'Leary, 1981; Roy, 1977; Straus *et al.*, 1980). The most parsimonious explanation of the intergenerational transmission of violence, although not the only explanation, is modeling. Indeed, a large body of research has documented the role of modeling in the acquisition of aggressive behavior (Bandura, 1977; Parke & Slaby, 1983). According to this theory, witnessing aggressive models provides opportunities for acquiring and reproducing similar behaviors and, in some cases, producing nonimitative spontaneous forms of aggression. As suggested by Rosenberg (1984), the responses by battered women also may be a function of modeling, with women who choose avoidant, passive, and nonhelp-seeking responses having observed such responses in their families of origin.

In contrast to the modeling explanation, which revolves around interaction with one's family of origin, other social learning theory explanations involve interactions with the partner. Reinforcement describes the process whereby certain behaviors occur at a subsequently higher rate as a result of their producing a desired effect. In other words, a husband's battering would increase in frequency if it produces a desired outcome (e.g., compliance or submission on the part of the wife). As Pagelow (1981) described,

> There are usually no (or insufficient) punishments received and there may be (and from evidence gathered usually are) reinforcements. For example, some men may experience feelings of increased control and power, and the women may try harder to placate them or to remove all sources of irritation and stress, such as keeping the house cleaner, keeping the children quiet in their presence, and so forth—anything the men claimed led to the beating in the first place. (p. 45)

What might be operating for the wife is negative reinforcement, in which the termination of some stimulus leads to an increase in the frequency of the behavior that precedes this termination. The wife as victim may be negatively reinforced for making placating gestures or taking on the blame because that seems to make the physical attack cease.

Coercion refers to the overall process whereby intimates learn to control each other's behavior through the use of aversive or painful stimuli (Patterson & Reid, 1970). With the aggressor positively reinforced and the victim negatively reinforced, the overall interaction tends to escalate and intensify over time. In at least some couples in which bidirectional violence exists, the victimized person learns that coercion is effective in eliciting change and begins to aggress in return. Existent data are based on the general category of distressed, as opposed to abusive couples. These data do not directly test the coercive process but do demonstrate how aversive behaviors by one partner can alter the probability of the other person's behavior (Gottman, 1979; Margolin & Wampold, 1981; Revenstorf, Vogel, Wegener, Hahlweg, & Schindler, 1980).

Several cognitive features of the coercive process are elaborated upon when describing wife battering. Focusing on the abuser, Deschner (1984) describes the "last straw decision" in which the abuser makes a decision that the situation is so intolerable that violence is warranted. Focusing on the victim and borrowing from observations of Patterson (1982), Walker (1984b) discusses a "chaining" and "fogging" effect in battering. When battering is in its acute phase, aversive events occur so rapidly that control techniques usually available to the woman no longer are available or are not able to be used successfully.

Systems. A systems theory explanation of wife battering assumes that violence is a systemic product rather than a result of individual pathology (Straus, 1973). According to systems theories, all interdependent parts serve a role in maintaining the homeostatic balance of a system, as reflected in its current pattern of interaction. As Giles-Sims (1983) explains, "conceptualizing the battering relationship as a system means that we can look at the process of actions and reactions as a continuous causal chain, each reaction becoming in turn a precipitant" (p. 8). Integrating systems theory with a feminist perspective, Bograd (1982) cautions that

> the formulation that partners interact in specific patterned ways to maintain a violent marital system is *not* equivalent to the statement that each is equally responsible for the violence. Though one can caution that it is not pejorative to recognize that a woman (allegedly) plays a major role in her abuse (Lion, 1977), the fine line between supposedly neutral clinical recognition of systemic patterns and judgmental allocation of blame is often impossible to discern. (p. 74)

According to Gelles and Straus (1979), there are certain characteristics of families (e.g., the amount of time the family members spend together, the intensity of their involvement, the fact that they have impinging activities and needs, the right to influence inherent in families) that make them ripe for violence.

Other authors describe specific characteristics found in wife beating systems. Not surprisingly, it has been suggested that most battering relationships are characterized by poor communication, in which distortion and misinterpretation prevail (Walker, 1979) and in which feelings are expressed indirectly if at all. According to Traicoff (1982), violent couples (a) exist in closed systems, with tight boundaries between themselves and the outside world; (b) have inflexible family rules; (c) maintain a rule of secrecy, particularly with respect to the battering, and (d) have difficulty setting and maintaining limits. Hornung *et al.* (1981) report that status incompatibilities increase the risk of marital violence.

Systems theory also has provided explanations as to how battering becomes stabilized within a system or serves as the stimulus for disrupting a system. Giles-Sims (1983) reported that because most women are willing to forgive the first incident of violence, a positive feedback loop is set into motion, making it likely that the violence will reoccur. She further suggests that then a runaway process takes hold, in which each act of violence is cause for further revenge, which leads to further violence to the point where corrective action is of no avail. For some battered wives, at least the ones who eventually seek outside assistance, a critical incident occurs, resulting in a decision to accept new input and to make the family boundaries permeable to outside influence. The alternative sources of feedback outside the boundaries of the original system seem crucial in women's decision to leave the system.

Other Interpersonal Theories. Walker's (1979, 1984b) cycle theory of violence states that there are three distinct phases associated with wife battering. During the tension building phase, when there is a gradual escalation of tension through discrete action (e.g., name-calling, other intentionally hurtful actions, and/or physical abuse), the woman may maintain an unrealistic belief that she can control the man. During the acute battering incident, the batterer typically unleashes a barrage of verbal and physical aggression. Stage 3 seems to vary depending on whether the violence is new or well-established. In new relationships, the batterer may apologize profusely, and show kindness and remorse. Later in the relationship, Stage 3 may simply be characterized by the absence of tension or violence, which in itself may be reinforcing for the woman. Other interpersonal theories have examined threats to self with respect to loyalty and control (Ferraro, 1984), loyalty to one's family of origin (Cohen, 1984), and traumatic bonding, whereby battered women form strong emotional attachments under conditions of intermittent abuse (Dutton & Painter, 1981).

Sociocultural Explanations

GAYLA MARGOLIN
ET AL.

Sociocultural explanations examine historical, legal, cultural, and political factors that contribute to wife beating. Intrapersonal and interpersonal explanations alone do not explain why the family system, in particular, produces such high rates of violence and why women are the target of that aggression. Sociocultural explanations attempt to explain the legitimization of intrafamilial violence and the victimization of women (Straus & Hotaling, 1980).

Violence in the Family. Literature on the family generally emphasizes the extent of violence in our culture at large (e.g., governmental violence and media violence), but points to the family as the training ground for violence. Specifically, it is suggested that the family is the setting in which most people first experience physical violence. Although there are values and expectations promoting love, peace, and harmony within the family, there also exist norms permitting family members to hit or assault one another, particularly for purposes of childrearing (Straus, 1980a). As Straus (1977) pointed out, there are two lessons that are learned as a function of physical punishment.

> The first of these unintended consequences is the association of love with violence. The child learns that those who love him or her the most are also those who hit and have the right to hit. The second unintended consequence is the lesson that when something is really important, it justifies the use of physical force. (p. 202)

Straus proposes that these lessons are generalized beyond the parent–child relationship to the marital relationship.

Data suggest that these lessons are learned quite well. According to Stark and McEvoy (1970), approximately one quarter of the persons interviewed said they would approve of a husband or wife hitting each other under certain circumstances. Churchill and Straus (cited in Straus, 1980a) described an assault in which the female victim was knocked unconscious. Subjects reading the description were to indicate the severity of punishment that was warranted. Those who believed that the assailant was the husband meted out less severe punishments than subjects who believed that the assailant was a known male companion.

The analysis of the family as a particularly violent system often highlights the amount and types of stresses impinging upon that system. As noted earlier, Gelles and Straus (1979) examined various characteristics of the family that give rise to high levels of conflict. As Farrington (1980) stated it,

> In addition to those stresses that emanate from within the family are numerous events experienced by individual members in the ''external world,'' which are then brought back into the family setting. Although the family is commonly thought of as a place which family members can bring these external pressures and ''let off steam,'' this action may have overall negative consequences for the family as a whole.

Barling and Rosenbaum (1985) reported, for example, that the occurrence of stressful work events and their negative impact were associated significantly with wife abuse. Straus (1980b) suggested that stress does not directly cause violence; instead, this relationship between stress and violence is mediated by factors such as subscribing to male dominance norms and to the legitimacy of violence between intimates.

Violence against Wives. The analysis of violence in the family overall still does not explain why it is women who have been brutalized. For these answers, we turn to traditions that sanction violence against women and institutions that support male dominance. As many authors explain, patriarchial society fostered laws and practices that implicitedly and explicitedly approve of violence against women. Patriarchial society has taught men to dominate women and violence is one such way to maintain that dominance. As Dobash and Dobash (1979) state,

> men who assault their wives are actually living up to cultural prescriptions that are cherished in Western society—aggressiveness, male dominance, and female subordination—and they are using physical force as a means to enforce that dominance. (p. 24)

Patriarchial society also has promoted economic and legal conditions that maintain wife beating. Women have been kept economically dependent through an unequal division of labor and through lower earnings. Thus, they have had difficulty gathering the financial resources to leave their battering husbands or, if they have left, often they are driven back by their economic vulnerability. Further, with women being designated primary responsibility for childrearing and household responsibilities, they have been kept relatively isolated.

Policies in the legal system also have reflected male dominance. Earlier in history, laws actually granted husbands the right to chastise an errant wife. Although those laws have been changed, their message has lingered and the legal system still is reluctant to intervene in domestic disputes. As noted earlier, women have been discouraged at every step of the judicial process.

Based on this analysis, it would seem that the current move toward more egalitarian family structures should be an important solution to wife battering. In the long run, this may prove true. However, in the short run, during the transition, conflict may actually increase as men feel threatened by their loss of power (Brown, 1980). It is not enough that economic and resource structures become equalized. For violence to decrease, it appears that both husbands and wives have to accept and be comfortable with an egalitarian family structure.

Summary

In reviewing the three levels of explanation for wife battering, we find that the intrapersonal level has been the target of most of the empirical investigations, probably because those variables are easiest to operationalize and measure. But, as Straus (1977) concluded, "it is doubtful that more than 2 or 3% of all the wife-beating in the United States can be attributed to purely 'intra-individual' characteristics" (p. 195). The interpersonal level describes some of the relationship processes characteristic of battering couples but does not adequately explain why some spouses resort to violence whereas others are profoundly unhappy but still nonviolent. The same question can be raised in respect to sociocultural explanations: Why are some individuals and couple systems more prone to the negative influences of a patriarchal society? As we see in the following, most of the interventions for wife battering have been directed toward the intrapersonal and interpersonal levels although recently there has been increasing attention directed to societal actions as well.

INTERVENTION

As is obvious from the description of wife beating discussed thus far, interventions for the problem run the gamut from medical treatments, psychotherapy, criminal action, legal policy making, to public education. As with any problem, our ideas about etiology determine the interventions that are prescribed. In our presentation of interventions, we will address remedial treatments as well as some long-range preventive strategies.

Assessment

One of the major problems in treating wife battering is that it often goes undetected. Battered women frequently receive treatment for a variety of conditions associated with the abuse (e.g., depression, anxiety, marital problems) and yet the physical abuse goes undetected. The woman herself may not mention the battering, or may minimize, deny, or hide the fact that violence occurs in her relationship. It is not unlikely for the professional she encounters also to focus on other diagnosible conditions and to ignore the violence as a primary treatment issue (Bograd, 1982). Failure to recognize the violence is dangerous on two accounts: first, it maintains the violence-prone situation. Second, it may lead to an inappropriate treatment. Prescribing certain medications may be extremely dangerous, for example, given the risk of suicide in battered women and given the possibility of decreasing the woman's vigilance in a potentially lethal situation (Hilberman, 1980).

For women, the primary assessment concerns are to identify if abuse is occurring and then to determine what course of action is in order. Professionals who might encounter battered women must make specific inquiries into violence as part of routine intake procedures (King, 1981; Klingbeil & Boyd, 1984). Although it tends to be easier for the battered woman to discuss the abuse openly if professionals are straightforward and direct in their questioning, interviewers also need to be alert for subtle signs of wife battering (e.g., avoidance of discussing the marital relationship, the presence of fearfulness and terror, the description of the partner as jealous, possessive, or intrusive, and tremendous anxiety around the need to avoid upsetting the partner) (Walker, 1979).

To determine a course of action, the severity and potential fatality of the abusive situation must be assessed immediately. If the potential of suicide and homicide cannot be ruled out, then the focus must be directed to finding a safe place for the woman and her children. An assessment of concrete issues, such as where she will go later that day and that night are in order. In addition, her medical condition, emotional state, legal needs, and needs of her children must be addressed. This in itself may require professionals from several different disciplines. For a battered woman not in immediate danger, an evaluation still needs to be conducted to determine what type of assistance, if any, would suit her. Is she requesting some type of emotional support for herself or for her children? Does she want a referral for her husband, or for the two of them as a couple? Does she want financial and legal counseling to help her get out of the relationship? Anyone performing an assessment with a battered woman should make it clear that there are a variety of options to consider and not railroad the woman toward any one treatment choice.

Assessment with the batterer involves some of the same issues but from a different perspective. The way a batterer comes to the attention of professionals very often determines the course of his treatment but, even then, some distinctions are in order. An evaluation into the extent of his immediate dangerousness is necessary. If through interviewing the batterer it is clear that his wife or children are in immediate danger, then attempts should be made to try to convince the man of the negative consequences to him (e.g., arrest, fatal retaliation) and to his family if he does not control his violence. If it still appears that the woman is at risk, then actions are needed to block the batterer's violence (e.g., warning the spouse, counseling her to obtain a restraining order, involuntary hospitalization for the batterer).

When the batterer does not appear to be immediately dangerous to his wife, decisions still are necessary as to an appropriate course of action. Will contact with his wife exacerbate the probability of his violence? Is he voluntarily seeking assistance in controlling his violent behavior? Dutton and Browning (1984) distinguish between men who are violent in (a) many relationships, (b) only in relationships with women, and (c) only in one intimate relationship. Different treatments would follow from these different violence patterns.

Wife beating also should be evaluated with couples seeking therapy. Given the prevalence of the problem in couples at large, we can estimate that its prevalence is particularly high in couples who are distressed. Inquiries into what happens when the couple argues and specific questions regarding the occurrence of violence should be standard parts of the marital therapist's preliminary evaluation. As Margolin (in press-a) describes in detail, there are cognitive, affective, behavioral, and interpersonal dimensions to consider in understanding how anger escalates and turns into physical violence.

Victim Assistance Programs for Women

Medical Assistance. According to Klingbeil and Boyd (1984), the most significant contribution that the health care profession can provide to battered women "is the initial, accurate, and primary diagnosis that domestic violence has occurred" (p. 25). Hospital emergency personnel and office physicians also must be prepared to treat battered women for their physical injuries and for severe depression. Fleming (1979) recommended that women seek medical help whenever they are battered in case they have suffered internal damages of which they are unaware and also to establish a permanent medical record of the assault. She also suggests that the battered woman's chart be tagged to alert staff, that the woman be examined and interviewed alone, that she be asked directly if her injuries are the result of a beating, that she be given resource materials, and that she be admitted to the hospital as a safe refuge.

Legal Assistance. Legal counseling often is the next order of business. If the battered woman wants to file a criminal complaint against her husband, she most likely needs representation, either through a private attorney, community legal service, or a local legal-aid program. She may also need such assistance to extricate herself from the relationship, regardless of whether she presses charges.

Employment Assistance. Financial and employment assistance are very important for the battered woman. Melling (1983) reported on a survey conducted by the Employment Training and Small Business Project (funded by the National Coalition Against Domestic Violence; NCADV) that revealed that although many of the women in shelters were unemployed, 80% of the shelters did not provide any kind of employment training. Instead, women who needed employment training were referred to other agencies, such as CETA, the YWCA, Displaced Homemakers Centers, or Women's Resource Centers. The training that these women needed included GED, assertiveness training, vocational skills, job search and interviewing skills. Support services, such as child care and transportation, were identified as critical. Although the NCADV has provided money for a few model shelters to begin their own businesses and employment training programs, more generalized assistance of this type is essential.

Shelters. Although some of what shelters offer can be found outside of shelters, they offer several very important and unique functions: separation from the batterer, protection from outside influences, and security from the possibility that the batterer will force his way into the shelter and use violence to force a return home. In addition to the physical protection provided by shelters, they also provide battered women with the psychological safety necessary to regain a balanced perspective and to plan freely their futures (Bowker & Maurer, 1985). Shelters provide a whole milieu experience different from what the battered woman can receive anywhere else. She is surrounded by women who have suffered similar injustices, thereby allowing her to break free of her isolation. She also can benefit from role models in the staff, who, in many cases, also have been victims of abuse and have surmounted their victimizations.

According to Fleming (1979), the major philosophy of shelters is to provide a supportive, nonjudgmental atmosphere geared toward fostering independence and optimizing each woman's strength and abilities. Fleming lists the following range of services: childcare and children's services; aid in obtaining welfare; employment or financial assistance; accompaniment to the hospital, police, or courts; ongoing group counseling for residents, ex-residents, or nonresidents, and private therapy; stress reduction through meditation; transportation for outside appointments; legal aid; educational or vocational guidance; assistance and accompaniment to welfare offices and social security offices; assistance in getting housing; and survival-skill development, such as basic money management, parenting, nutrition, and driving. In some shelters, there are traditionally trained therapists, offering individual and group therapy. Others are run by peer counselors and paraprofessionals. Although some shelters limit their stay to 2 weeks, Bowker and Maurer (1985) recommend a stay of 2 to 3 months. In general, the need for shelters far exceeds their availability.

Mental Health Services. In the treatment of battered women, mental health services have received considerable criticism for reinforcing the family unit, looking for pathological explanations of the woman's behavior, blaming her, and focusing on intrapsychic factors rather than on survival skills. Although it can be argued, from a feminist perspective, that psychotherapy is an inappropriate intervention for battered women, battered women continue to turn to mental health professionals (Bograd, 1982). Further, many women suffer emotional sequelae to battering that demand attention and require psychological support to get beyond the victim role. Feminist, or at least nonsexist, approaches to therapy typically are recommended.

King (1981) suggested that to help women focus on their victimization,

> Practitioners should listen to their experiences and legitimize their feelings. Approaches that blame the woman for being assaulted, however subtlely, cause harm. Approaches that try to rescue the client reinforce her role as a victim. Expressions of anger should be encouraged and can be used constructively to initiate and implement change. (p. 8)

Although there is substantial agreement regarding the victim's need to feel and express anger, there also are recommendations that caution be exercised in the evocation of strong emotions too quickly and in the expression of such emotions toward the target (e.g., Walker, 1984b). Further, although assertion training has been recommended for battered women (e.g., Ball & Wyman, 1978), applying the training at home has been questioned because it may elicit further retaliatory and violent behavior (O'Leary, Curley, Rosenbaum, & Clarke, 1985).

Other goals include getting in touch with one's own strengths, increasing self-esteem, fostering self-reliance, regaining control of one's own life, and reducing isolation. The following specific procedures have been prescribed toward these goals: guided imagery, self-defense classes, anxiety control measures, systematic desensitization, and biofeedback to reestablish control over the body (King, 1981; Walker, 1984b). Cognitive restructuring also has been recommended to broaden choices, to correct faulty beliefs regarding the abusive relationship, to correct all-or-nothing expectations, and to reinforce that fact that no matter what, the beating was undeserved (Bedrosian, 1982; Walker, 1984b).

Because of battered women's isolation, group counseling often is the preferred therapeutic modality. Fleming (1979) recommended the following topics for group discussion: assertiveness, anger, self-esteem, self-image, automony and interdependence, self-definition, and problem solving. Specific techniques that she recommends include didactic methods, bibliotherapy, group discussion, role-playing, relaxation training, anger ventilation, and psychodrama. Lewis (1983) differentiated between groups for women who sever their relationships versus those who elect to stay. Women who sever the relationship first need a group that focuses on the immediate crisis and allow for mourning the loss of the marriage. The next stage, several weeks later, focuses on life-style changes as a result of the woman's independence. According to Lewis, in therapeutic interventions with battered women, it must be understood that the victim holds the decision to stay or leave the batterer and that problems confronting these women are unique to their current life situation.

Interventions with Batterers

Interventions with batterers occur either in the judicial realm (i.e., treating the assault strictly as criminal behavior), in psychotherapy or counseling (i.e., treating the battering as learned behavior), or as some combination of the two (i.e., court-mandated treatment is offered as one criminal justice response to wife battering).

Arrest. The most common recommendation for legal action is that batterers be prosecuted for their criminal actions. Sherman and Berk (1984) describe the first scientifically controlled test of the effects of arrest compared to attempts to counsel both parties or send assailants away from home for several hours. In the arrest condition, most suspects were kept in jail overnight although few actually received a formal sanction from a judge. Police records showed that the percentage of repeat violence over 6 months was 10%, 19%, and 24%, respectively, for arresting, advising, and sending the suspect away. Based on victims' reports, percentages of repeat violence over 6 months were 19%, 37%, and 33%, respectively, for the three conditions. This study demonstrates the importance of giving the police power to make an arrest in domestic violence cases without the signed complaint of a victim. Browne (1984) emphasized the importance of arresting first-time offenders, because they are the ones most deterred by the threat of prosecution, punishment, and potential damage to their reputation.

Psychoeducational Approaches. Although the primary goal for any psychotherapeutic and educational intervention is to stop the abuse, secondary goals include reducing anger and depression, changing attitudes about women's roles, and adopting new, nonsexist role behavior by the men (e.g., Saunders & Hanusa, 1984). Treatment programs that provide individual therapy, group therapy, and/or social support groups for violent men are of three general types: (a) programs developed specifically to help batterers, comprised soley of batterers; (b) programs that are part of a well-established community social service agency that serve batterers as well as other men; and, (c) battered women's programs that provide an adjunct treatment for the batterers.

Eddy and Myers (1984) summarized the services currently available to batterers in their survey of 54 treatments provided by agencies and organizations. Based on this survey, it appears that the majority of batterers enter programs through self-referral. Some come through referrals from agencies or professionals, and fewer, but still a substantial number, come through the judicial system. Batterers' groups and individual therapy were the therapy formats of choice for most programs. The three explanations of abuse found to be most closely linked with the goals and methods of these treatments were social learning of violent behavior, social skill deficits, and external factors, such as job stress, financial difficulties, and conflicts about children. The average number of actual intervention methods used by any one program was 12. Methods used by 75% or more of the sample included emotional awareness training, emotional expressiveness training, anger management, exploration of personal family histories, building social support systems, exploration of sex roles, problem-solving skills training, and communication skills training. Other methods used by 50% to 75% of the programs were client role-playing, stress management training, and separate support groups for the batterers' partners. Some programs evaluated the reoccurrence of violence during treatment, with self-report by the batterer as the primary monitoring procedure. Reports from the victim and from the police or probation officers also were used.

To meet the goal of helping batterers diffuse their anger, a variety of behavioral, cognitive, and affective strategies have been recommended. From a behavioral perspective, the objective is to impart skills, through assertiveness or relaxation training, that are incompatible with aggression (Saunders & Hanusa, 1984). From a cognitive perspective, the goal is to modify cognitions that accompany the beating. In other words, the batterer is trained to monitor, evaluate, and then challenge his interpretations and assumptions about his partner (e.g., Bedrosian, 1982). He is also taught to use self-talk to lessen rather than escalate his angry feelings (Saunders, 1982). The affective perspective helps the men focus on pain, hurt, sadness, fear, and loneliness that often precede anger and may be mistaken for anger (Adams & McCormick, 1982).

As Fleming (1979) pointed out, in working with batterers, it is essential to find a way to identify and empathize with them. The therapist must communicate acceptance of the person even though his violent behavior is unacceptable (Rosenbaum & O'Leary, 1986). In general, these men are likely to be quite apprehensive about seeking therapy and quite defensive about accepting responsibility for their violence. Thus, for individual therapy to proceed, it is first necessary to establish trust between the therapist and batterer. For group therapy, cohesion among the group members is critical.

Conjoint Therapy

Couples' therapy for wife battering is a very controversial topic. On the one hand, by virtue of seeing the couple together, there often is the implication that the couple is continuing as a unit and that the woman plays a role in maintaining her abuse. In addition, the woman may be reluctant to report the full extent of her abuse, of her terror, or of her desire to leave the relationship because of her fear of reprisal once the conjoint session is over. On the other hand, conjoint therapy is the treatment modality often sought and truly desired by some couples with a history of battering. Further, as previously indicated, battering frequently is associated with severely dysfunctional marital patterns. To reconcile these pros and cons of conjoint therapy for battering, Rosenbaum and O'Leary (1986) suggest an evaluation to determine whether the couple is an appropriate candidate for marital therapy. The first question to ask is whether the wife is safe. The second question is whether she is fully aware of alternative service delivery agencies for wife battering. The third question is whether the remediation of the marriage is a viable and realistic goal. In addition, to make it clear that the husband alone is responsible for his violent behavior, although the couple is mutually responsible for the marital discord, these investigators recommend an intervention specifically for the husband, either prior to or concurrent with conjoint marital therapy.

The first step in couples' therapy is to establish the ground rule that abusiveness is unacceptable under any circumstances. Further, to give this meaning, there must be consequences that, once established, will be carried through (Margolin, 1979). On the husband's part, this means accepting the notion that he is responsible for his behavior, regardless of any provocation he perceives, and that at any moment, he controls the choice not to be violent. On the wife's part, this means that she has made a commitment to herself no longer to tolerate violence and that she has worked out the details to know that, if need be, she can leave her husband and/or use legal channels. Other ground rules suggested by Rosenbaum and O'Leary (1986) are that spouses cannot come to a session in any state of intoxication or with any type of weapon, even a pocket knife.

As with the treatments for the batterer alone, the primary objective in conjoint therapy is to stop the abuse. Here, however, the goals might be stated somewhat more broadly to include all types of abuse and to improve conflict strategies in general.

Further, the unique factor that couples' therapy can contribute to these goals is the opportunity to identify and change repeating interactional cycles associated with abuse. Both partners can help to identify cues in themselves and one another that violence on the part of the husband may be forthcoming. That is, the husband can learn to monitor the emotions and anger-arousing cognitions that accompany his abuse. He can also learn to identify behaviors exhibited by the wife that trigger his anger, and experiment with alternative responses to those cues. Similarly, the wife can learn to monitor subtle nonverbal and cognitive cues in herself or in her partner that signal the escalation of conflict. If caught early enough, these cues can be used to trigger coping responses (e.g., rapid departure from the situation) rather than terrorized, self-blaming, or combative reactions. Once these patterns are identified, their disruption may require learning to take temporary time-outs from the relationship, self-talk to guide oneself through a coping response or to combat an irrational cognition, and using muscle relaxation or imagery techniques to reduce overall arousal (Bedrosian, 1982; Deschner, 1984).

Although disrupting anger and violence-producing interactions is the initial focus, conjoint therapists contend that by lessening the overall number of conflict areas and by improving the overall tone of the relationship, there will be less cause for conflict and violence. Strategies typically employed to accomplish these goals involve behavioral skills, such as training in problem-solving techniques, receptive listening, and assertion training to express relationship desires as well as to accept refusals from the partner (Deschner, 1984; Margolin, in press-b). These also involve strategies to enhance intimacy to bolster diffuse spouse subsystem boundaries (e.g., scheduling one-to-one enjoyable time, building a shared support system) (Bedrosian, 1982).

The therapist working with couples characterized by wife battering must be directive, helping the couple discuss the process of their conflict without repeatedly acting it out in therapy. Therapy that deteriorates into a blaming and ridiculing match may trigger violence outside of the session. The therapist must be particularly sensitive to what each spouse experiences. As in any marital therapy, the therapist must be aware of his or her alliances and attempt to balance them over time. As Bedrosian (1982) suggests, it might be best for the therapist to warn the couple early on that it will be necessary at times to antagonize one or the other through insistence on acceptance of personal responsibility. Geller (1982) warned against allowing spouses to become complacent about their situation. The therapist must mobilize the spouses' anxiety to help them overcome their natural resistance to change.

Legal Action

Widespread reforms for law enforcement, prosecutors, and judges recommended by the Attorney General's Task Force on Family Violence (1984) are likely to provide a major intervention into the problem of wife battering. Recommendations for law enforcement include establishing family violence as a priority response and requiring officers to file written reports on all incidents, establishing arrest as the preferred response, maintaining a current file of all protection orders valid in their jurisdiction, responding immediately to violations of protection orders, making protection orders available, and documenting violations of pretrial release conditions. Recommendations for prosecutors include organizing special units to process family violence cases, not requiring the victim to sign a formal complaint against the abuser, not requiring the victim to testify at the preliminary hearing, and restricting the defendant's access to the victim as a condition of setting bail or releasing the assailant on his own recognizance. For judges, the recommendations include considering a wide range of dispositional alternatives based on the consequences of the crime on the victim, making protection orders available on an emergency basis, establishing guidelines for expeditious handling of family violence cases, admitting hearsay evidence of family violence victims at the preliminary hearings, allowing expert witnesses on family violence to testify, and imposing conditions that restrict the defendant's access to the victim.

Public Education and Community Action

In the past 2 years, there have been a number of television broadcasts (both documentary and docu-drama) as well as newspaper and magazine articles that have addressed the problem of spouse abuse. Media attention that reaches several hundred thousand viewers serves several important functions. First, battered women in the audience learn that they are not alone and also learn where to turn for help in their own community. Second, battering men learn that their violent behavior is inappropriate and illegal, and has negative consequences. Third, others who are not directly affected by battering may become more sensitive to the problem and more attuned to friends and relatives who make vague references to battering. In general, increased public awareness and openness helps to dispel some of the secrecy which is a primary factor maintaining wife beating.

Efforts also are being directed toward reducing spouse battering in future generations by educating youngsters about the problem and by counseling children who have witnessed wife battering. Some high school classes in marriage and family living, for example, now address the problem of wife battering. Classes both emphasize the risks to young adults if they attempt to intervene on behalf of their mothers, and serve to make them more wary about their own dating relationships that may involve abuse.

The Attorney General's Task Force on Family Violence (1984) offers other suggestions for public awareness and community action. In addition to widespread public awareness campaigns, special efforts should be directed to all professionals who might counsel batterers or victims. These include medical personnel, mental health personnel, criminal justice personnel, attorneys, clergy, and teachers. Classes on wife battering and family violence more generally should be part of the core curriculum for relevant professionals; continuing education should be provided by professional organizations. Religious organizations and community service organizations also should address this problem with their members and staff. Recommended community actions that would directly benefit victims include 24-hour toll-free hotlines, drop-in crises centers, crisis nurseries, family educations centers, and additional shelters. It is recommended that battered women be put on priority lists for public housing. Finally, examples of how the private sector could provide low-cost resources and services to battered women include grocery stores donating food, taxi companies providing free emergency transportation, and businesses providing free mail listings of victim assistance programs.

Case Study

In this example, wife battering has been long-standing and severe, but over the past two years, has lessened in frequency and intensity. Sheila 41, and Mark 50, have been married for 17 volatile years. Physical violence has been part of their relationship since the second year of marriage, reoccurring approximately two to three times per year. Incidents generally consist of Mark throwing objects, pushing, slapping, hitting Sheila with a fist, and beating her up. Sheila usually does not defend herself although twice she retaliated, once by scratching Mark in the face and once by threatening him with a knife. In the past 2 years, physical aggression has been limited to threats and pushing.

This couple presented as part of a research project on marital conflict. Both spouses report low marital satisfaction but appear highly committed to having the marriage continue, particularly Mark. Both score in the average range on measures of self-concept and neither display psychopathology on the MMPI. Mark is college educated whereas Sheila has a 10th-grade education. Mark works as a self-employed salesman and Sheila works as a homemaker and mother. They have a middle-class income but describe themselves as barely able to pay their bills. Neither Sheila nor Mark were physically or verbally abused as children and there was no physical abuse or verbal abuse between their respective parents.

Mark and Sheila never have sought therapy, either individual or marital, nor are there any police or medical reports regarding the battering. Physical violence generally occurs in the context of an escalation of a verbal confrontation. Both Sheila and Mark are stubborn and opinionated; neither is willing to give in to the other in a conflict. Their interaction is riddled with harsh verbal abusiveness that, on occasion, leads to physical abuse. From the first violent incident to the most recent, the pattern of physical abuse has been consistent. Sheila and Mark both report that a physical confrontation is more likely when Mark is feeling more stress that usual (e.g., when he has had a difficult day at work). At these times, a nasty comment or a lack of consideration is more likely to send him into a rage. "A very touchy subject is family with Mark and when we first married and I gave my mother a present and I did not give his mother the identical thing, the identical color, the identical anything, he would go crazy."

The first incident of physical abuse occurred during their second year of marriage. According to Mark,

> Sheila had been snooping around somebody, I don't know who, and she said very bad things about my mother who was dying and she said to me something that hurt. "What are you worrying about? Your mother was always an imbecile." And this really hurt me. This is the only time I take 100% responsibility. I would have

done it to anybody. It's not the first time. I nearly killed someone for saying something bad about my father.

On a measurement of sex role attitudes, both Sheila and Mark score in the liberal, as opposed to traditional, range. This, however, does not coincide with Mark's verbalized attitude that, "If you don't act like a woman you don't expect to be treated like a woman." Basically, he subscribes to the notion that it is a wife's duty to respect her husband without question and, if she breaks this rule, then she is subject to her husband's wrath. Mark believes that Sheila controls whether or not she will be battered. "She is very smart in finding out what would make me lose my temper." Sheila concurs, "I can control things 100%. It is all in my attitude. I just ignore things that he says."

Sheila and Mark recently decided that it is important for them to control their physical confrontations for the sake of their two daughters. According to Sheila, "The children are very instrumental in stopping our fights. And when we have a fight now, they interfere, they tell us to stop." Mark adds, "I would hate for my children to grow up and when I'm gone to remember their father as somebody who was violent, someone who was a mean person." It appears, however, that without the calming influence of the children, Mark might resort to severe violence once again, particularly if he perceives a verbal attack. "I feel that I am always under control except when I can't find an answer. If you attack me and you are hitting below the belt, when I'm completely innocent, I'm going to retaliate. It would probably happen again, it most probably would."

The current lull in this couple's violence demonstrates that, indeed, they do have control. Nonetheless, by attributing his violence to Sheila's verbal attacks, Mark denies responsibility for, and control of, his actions. Sheila concurs with Mark's perspective. Although taking no responsibility for Mark's violence, she does report some sense of control. As such, she does not exhibit the fearfulness so often seen in battered women. Although it is likely that the pattern of wife beating described here is quite common, little is known about such couples because they rarely seek outside assistance. Sheils is not unhappy enough with the situation to change it nor does she seriously question the role of violence in a marriage.

LEGAL AND ETHICAL ISSUES

Legal Issues

The primary legal considerations are those already discussed regarding prosecution of the batterer and civil protection of the battered woman. Because there is a great deal of variability among the states, the reader is referred to Lerman and Livingston (1983), who have summarized what legislation currently exists or is pending for each state. Their summary considers provisions regarding protection orders, injunctions pending domestic relations proceedings, criminal laws, police interventions, and data collection and reporting.

There are, in addition, certain legal considerations for professionals working with batterers or their victims. There are no laws mandating the reporting of marital violence as there are for child abuse. However, if we generalize from the principle enunciated in the Tarasoff decision, it appears that a therapist is legally bound to take steps to protect a potential victim if the therapist has good reason to believe that a spouse is in imminent danger. Such steps could include warning the victim and helping her to seek protection, arranging an involuntary hospitalization of the batterer, or informing the police, although police cannot be counted on to act solely on the basis of a threat. These actions to ward off potential violence help to protect the victim but pose predicaments for the practitioner because it is very difficult to make accurate predictions regarding violence. False positives could disrupt the trust established in the therapeutic relationship and discourage the batterer from revealing his aggressive feelings. Yet, false negatives could result in bodily harm or even death.

Walker (1984a, b) has listed several other situations in which battered wives and involved professionals participate in litigation. If a battered woman decides to leave the relationship, she must contend with property settlements and custody decisions regarding her children. According to Walker (1984b), batterers tend to be particularly demanding and overpowering in the negotiations whereas battered women tend to be willing to settle for far less than their fair share, even at the expense of losing custody.

Walker (1984a) also described recent legal precedents surrounding cases in which a battered woman killed her abuser. Expert testimony, particularly from psychologists, has been used to help the judge and jury understand the battered wife syndrome, and to recognize the potential reprisals that these women face if they attempt to leave the situation or to reach out for help from family, friends, or police. Most courts that have been confronted with the question of admissibility of expert witnesses' testimony on the battered woman syndrome have accepted such testimony. The

> APA [American Psychological Association] concludes that the state of scientific knowledge is sufficient to permit qualified experts to form a reliable opinion whether a defendant was suffering from the syndrome and whether, as a result, she reasonably believed it was necessary to act in self defense. ("APA Issues Spouse Abuse Briefs," 1983, p. 3)

Although the actions committed by battered women do not always fit the exact definition of self-defense (e.g., using the least amount of force necessary to prevent imminent bodily harm), the battered wife syndrome, as a defense, incorporates the cumulative effects of repeated violence in self-defense as well as diminished-capacity considerations. Battered women who are on trial for killing their husbands are likely to elicit increasing attention and controversy over the next few years.

Ethical Issues

The primary ethical issue concerns how vigorously a therapist urges a battered woman to leave her marriage. In all individual and couple therapies, a therapist can exert tremendous control in encouraging a patient to remain in or leave an ongoing relationship (e.g., Margolin, 1982). When it is obvious that a woman is at risk for bodily harm, it is certainly the therapist's ethical responsibility to help that woman leave the relationship and find protection. Nonetheless, in some cases, the likelihood for repeated abuse is not self-evident, particularly if the batterer is willing to seek treatment. Further, the woman's desire to stay in the marriage is not always a product of fear. For many therapists working with battered women, it is a foregone conclusion that the most desirable outcome would be for the woman to terminate her marriage. This leads to a lot of disappointment due to the numbers of women who return to their battering relationships. Some therapists focus on other dynamics of the marriage, while not paying enough attention to violent aspects. These therapists may not encourage the woman to appraise fully whether or not she wants the relationship to continue. Aside from cases in which the dangerousness is obvious, the therapist must provide an atmosphere conducive to considering both alternatives of staying and of leaving and allow the client to come to this important decision at her own pace.

The second ethical issue concerns who is the therapist's client. When the batterer and the battered woman have conflicting goals, as is often the case, the therapist can find herself or himself in the awkward position of not being able to promote fully the welfare of both clients. The therapist may have to limit therapeutic contact to one of the spouses. Or, the therapist might have to expand therapeutic responsibility to include the children. As stated earlier, data indicate that children often experience emotional problems as a result of seeing their mother beaten and also have an increased likelihood of physical and emotional abuse themselves. Thus, unless the children have their own therapist, it is suggested that the mother's and/or father's therapist assume the responsibility of inquiring into the children's welfare and, if deemed necessary, helping to arrange for appropriate treatment for the children.

CURRENT RESEARCH STATUS

Incidence

Despite the difficulties conducting research into wife battering, three main types of research have evolved. First, there has been research on the incidence of wife battering. Straus *et al.* (1980), with a representative nationwide sample of 2,143 husbands and wives, and Hornung *et al.* (1981), with a random Harris polling of 1,793 Kentucky wives, present the most comprehensive and generalizable samples. Despite the strengths of these studies, they still are limited because the data are retrospective self-reports in which one partner reports on both spouses' actions.

Etiology

Second, there has been considerable research into factors associated with wife beating. The majority of this research has focused on intrapersonal, as opposed to interpersonal or sociocultural factors (e.g., batterers have witnessed abuse in their families of origin, have low self-esteem, tend to abuse alcohol, and suffer from low assertiveness). Unfortunate problems with much of this research are nonrandom samples and inadequate control groups. As such, although these factors characterize batterers, they may be equally likely to characterize other criminally deviant or psychologically deviant populations. Further, although this research suggests what factors may be important correlates of wife battering, it does not illuminate the necessary link between each variable and wife battering. Thus, we still need to determine the mediating factors between a history of abuse in one's family of origin and abuse in one's current marital relationship. As they now stand, these factors are not adequate explanations of what leads to wife battering.

In addition, Gelles (1980) identified three other shortcomings of this research. First, the literature suffers from the "woozle effect," in which research findings are repeatedly cited, without attention to the limitations of the research. Over time, the results of inadequate research studies eventually gain the status of truth, with no attention to the qualifications that the initial investigator noted. Second, data are reported regarding an association between a certain factor and wife beating, without any attention to the magnitude of that association. Third, the data samples for most studies on wife beating come from persons who have been publically identified as batterers or victims. Data on battered women come primarily from small, nonrepresentative samples of women who have sought refuge in shelters or who have volunteered to tell their personal stories. Batterers also tend to be persons publically identified as abusive, either through criminal charges or through their participation in treatment facilities. The public labeling of these subjects makes them quite different from the large number of batterers and battered women who, despite their experiences with violence, do not apply these labels to themselves let alone speak out on their experiences.

Treatment Outcome

There is a slowly growing body of research on treatment outcome for batterers (e.g., Gondolf, 1984; Grayson, Mathie, Wampler, Dennis, & Lynch, 1984; Purdy & Nickle, 1981; Rosenbaum & O'Leary, 1986; Saunders & Hanusa, 1984) and for abusive couples (e.g., Deschner, 1984; Geffner, Patrick, & Knowles, 1984; Margolin, 1979; Myers, 1984). What we know from this research is that individual or couple treatments for batterers appear to reduce or eliminate violent behavior in a substantial proportion of those treated. Because of the multiple interventions offered in any one treatment, we do not yet know the effective treatment variables.

Saunders (1984) discussed a number of dilemmas in conducting research with batterers. First, from a design perspective, (a) it is ethically unjustifiable to randomly assign batterers to a no-treatment control group; (b) random assignment to comparison groups often is impractical because of agency or justice system considerations; (c) long-term follow-up is made difficult by its intrusiveness, by the difficulty maintaining confidentiality, and by the practical problem of locating the men; and (d) base rates are difficult to obtain with low base rate behaviors such as battering. From a measurement perspective, there are questions about what to measure (e.g., frequency and severity of behavior) and who should be doing the reporting (e.g., male, female, or both partners). To improve research in this area, Saunders (1984) suggested studying the characteristics of those who drop out of treatment, examining what particular treatments are effective with what types of clients, and considering physiological recordings and behavioral role plays as two possible measurements.

Recommendations

With respect to subjects, it is suggested that emphasis be directed to nonclinical and noncriminal samples. In view of the documented high incidence of wife beating, we imagine that only the tip of the iceberg has been sampled thus far. It is suggested that, rather than try to make broad generalizations across all batterers and all women who are battered, we should focus, instead, on developing typologies. Certainly with a phenomenon as widespread as wife battering, there must be many different types of individuals affected by this problem. Further, such typologies should be developed with a view toward intervention. That is, we should begin to categorize people in a way that will influence decisions about their treatment. In addition to developing typologies, it is important to study examples of successful coping, such as persons who have witnessed violence in their families of origin but who have not exhibited violence themselves, or couples with a history of violence who stopped being violent. Even when there are general trends in the data (e.g., abuse tends to become more severe and more frequent over time), this does not characterize everyone. Also, we support Sherman's (1984) suggestion that future research relevant to wife beating be directed to modifiable, as opposed to static, variables. One of the most important goals should be to predict who is at risk for wife battering, and then to intervene in that process. Toward this end, longitudinal studies, such as the one currently underway by O'Leary and Arias (1985) are needed. Finally, it is suggested that research be developed to test theories and, by virtue of the complexity of the phenomenon of wife battering, these theories must be complex. Straus (1980b), for example, posited a variety of intervening variables that are likely to explain the relationship between stress and marital violence.

FUTURE DIRECTIONS

Wife beating takes an unfathomable toll on the lives of a multitude of individuals and also on society at large. Efforts to remedy this problem currently occur primarily through treatments designed to assist the battered woman or to help the batterer cease his battering. More information still is needed to know how well these treatments work and how to match specific treatments with specific individuals. In addition, efforts still need to be directed toward determining how to get batterers to acknowledge that they have a problem and seek treatment as well as how to help battered women actively eliminate battering from their lives. These directions, although crucial, are in themselves quite limited. Helping a battered woman leave her marriage, for example, may improve the quality of her life but may mean that another woman is soon to be battered by the same man. Even for the woman who leaves, there is no guarantee that she will escape further battering relationships. Furthermore, these efforts do nothing for the children who have witnessed violence between their parents.

The goal of reducing the overall incidence of wife battering can be achieved only through community-based prevention programs. Secondary prevention programs are needed to identify and give assistance to men at risk for battering and to couples at risk for bidirectional violence. Only through longitudinal research will we learn exactly what variables predict violence, that then would guide our efforts at secondary prevention. When available, such information would need to be brought to the public's attention so that at-risk individuals and couples could seek special assistance. The actual assistance probably would entail some of the components currently in treatment programs (e.g., training in anger management and conflict resolution).

Primary prevention interventions would be designed to aid the community at large, without singling out a special problem group. Primary prevention programs that focus on handling marital conflict, developing nonsexist roles and perspectives, and coping with anger could be offered through adult education programs. In addition, training of a similar sort can be made available to children and adolescents, which is the only way to affect the incidence of wife beating in the next generation. Once again, public awareness programs that increase everyone's consciousness about wife beating are the first step.

A key component of these communitywide prevention programs is adequate evaluation. Efforts must be made to obtain accurate data on the incidence of wife battering (through police and hospital records, and through random sampling) prior to initiating such programs, to introduce the programs in stages while monitoring the results, and to conduct long-term follow-ups. The results of instituting and evaluating model programs in a handful of communities could be used to direct the widespread implementation of such programs.

SUMMARY

In reviewing wife battering from a number of perspectives, it is evident that we still face many unanswered questions about this common, very serious problem. Although we have data suggesting the profile of a batterer, we still cannot predict who will become a batterer. Knowing what we do about the characteristics of women who are battered, we conclude that they are not a certain type of woman but potentially are every woman. The search into the etiology of wife battering must continue. However, given the immediate press for intervention, the best recommendations currently are for multidimensional treatments. In-depth assessments and attempting to tailor treatment to the individual are a luxury at this stage. The primary goal for everyone concerned with this problem is a reduction in the overall incidence of wife battering. Increasing attention on the part of professionals in many fields, coupled with more accurate diagnosis and more available referrals for treatment, is one important step. Increasing attention by the public at large, however, is at least as important. Heightened public awareness is likely to enable battered women to seek the support that they need to make decisions about their lives, and to convince batterers that wife beating is not sanctioned by society, is not a private matter, and is a crime.

REFERENCES

Adams, D. C., & McCormick, A. J. (1982). Men unlearning violence: A group approach based on the collective model. In M. Roy (Ed.), *The abusive partner: An analysis of domestic battering* (pp. 170–197). New York: Van Nostrand.

''APA issues spouse abuse briefs.'' (1983, Fall). *Division of child, youth, and family services newsletter, 6,* pp. 1, 3.

Attorney General's task force on family violence. (1984). Washington, DC: U.S. Government Printing Office.

Ball, P. G., & Wyman, E. (1978). Battered wives and powerlessness: What can counselors do? *Victimology: An International Journal, 2,* 545–552.

Bandura, A. (1977). *Social learning theory.* New York: General Learning Press.

Barling, J., & Rosenbaum, A. (1986). Work stressors and wife abuse. *Journal of Applied Psychology, 71,* 346–348.

''Battered syndrome'' now official. (1979, November). *Response to Violence in the Family,* p. 6.

Bedrosian, R. C. (1982). Using cognitive and systems intervention in the treatment of marital violence. In L. R. Barnhill (Ed.), *Clinical approaches to family violence* (pp. 117–138). Rockville, MD: Aspen.

Berk, R. A., Berk, S. F., Loseke, D. R., & Rauma, D. (1983). Mutual combat and other family violence myths. In D. Finkelhor, R. J. Gelles, G. T. Hotaling, & M. A. Straus (Eds.), *The dark side of families* (pp. 197–212). Beverly Hills, CA: Sage.

Bograd, M. (1982). Battered women, cultural myths and clinical interventions: A feminist analysis. *Women and Therapy, 1*(3), 69–77.

Bowker, L., & Maurer, L. (1985). The importance of sheltering in the lives of battered women. *Response to the Victimization of Women and Children, 8,* 2–8.

Brown, B. W. (1980). Wife-employment, marital equality, and husband-wife violence. In M. A. Straus & G. T. Hotaling (Eds.), *The social causes of husband-wife violence* (pp. 176–187). Minneapolis, MN: University of Minnesota Press.

Browne, A. (1984, August). *Making peace at home: Models for ending family violence.* Paper presented at the American Psychological Association, Toronto.

Carlson, B. E. (1977). Battered women and their assailants. *Social Work, 22,* 455–461.

Cohen, P. (1984). Violence in the family: An act of loyalty? *Psychotherapy, 21,* 249–253.

Commission on Professional and Hospital Activities. (1978). *The international classification of diseases, 9th revision, clinical modification.* Ann Arbor, Michigan.

Davidson, T. (1978). *Conjugal crime: Understanding and changing the wifebeating pattern.* New York: Hawthorn.

Deschner, J. P. (1984). *The hitting habit.* New York: Free Press.

Dobash, R. E., & Dobash, R. P. (1978). Wives: The appropriate victims of marital violence. *Victimology: An International Journal, 2,* 426–442.

Dobash, R. E., & Dobash, R. P. (1979). *Violence against wives: A case against patriarchy.* New York: The Free Press.

Douglas, M. A., & Der Ovanesian, M. (1983, December). *A comparative study of battered and nonbattered women in crisis.* Paper presented at the 17th Annual Convention of the Association for the Advancement of Behavior Therapy, Washington, DC.

Dutton, D. G., & Browning, J. J. (1984). Power struggles in intimate relationships. In G. Russell (Ed.), *Violence in intimate relationships.* New York: Spectrum.

Dutton, D., & Painter, S. L. (1981). Traumatic bonding: The development of emotional attachments in battered women and other relationships of intermittent abuse. *Victimology: An International Journal, 6,* 139–155.

Eddy, M. J., & Myers, T. (1984, August). *Helping men who batter: A profile of programs in the U.S.* Paper presented at the Second National Conference for Family Violence Researchers, Durham, NH.

Elliott, F. A. (1977). The neurology of explosive rage: The dyscontral syndrome. In M. Roy (Ed.), *Battered women: A psychosocial study of domestic violence* (pp. 98–109). New York: Van Nostrand.

Farrington, K. M. (1980). Stress and family violence. In M. A. Straus & G. T. Hotaling (Eds.), *The social causes of husband-wife violence* (pp. 94–114). Minneapolis, MN: University of Minnesota Press.

Faulk, M. (1974). Men who assault their wives. *Medicine, Science, & the Law, 14,* 180–183.

Federal Bureau of Investigation. (1982). *Uniform crime reports.* Washington, DC: U.S. Department of Justice.

Feldman, S. E. (1983). Battered women: Psychological correlates of the victimization process. *Dissertation Abstracts International, 44,* 1221–B.

Ferraro, K. J. (1984, August). *An existential approach to battering.* Paper presented at the Second National Conference for Family Violence Researchers, Durham, NH.

Fitch, F. J., & Papantonio, M. A. (1983). Men who batter: Some pertinent characteristics. *Journal of Nervous and Mental Diseases, 171,* 190–192.

Fleming, J. B. (1979). *Stopping wife abuse.* Garden City, NY: Anchor.

Gayford, J. (1975). Wife battering: A preliminary survey of 100 cases. *British Medical Journal, 1,* 195–197.

Geffner, R., Patrick, J., & Knowles, D. (1984, August). *Reducing marital violence: A new program that appears to work.* Paper presented at the American Psychological Association Convention, Toronto.

Geller, J. (1982). Conjoint therapy: Staff training and treatment of the abuser and the abused. In M. Roy (Ed.), *The abusive partner: An analysis of domestic battering* (pp. 198–215). New York: Van Nostrand.

Gelles, R. J. (1974). *The violent home: a study of physical aggression between husbands and wives.* Beverly Hills, CA: Sage.

Gelles, R. J. (1980). Violence in the family: A review of research in the seventies. *Journal of Marriage and the Family, 42,* 873–885.

Gelles, R. J., & Cornell, C. P. (1985). *Intimate violence in families.* Beverly Hills, CA: Sage.

Gelles, R. J., & Straus, M. A. (1979). Determinants of violence in the family: Toward a theoretical integration. In W. R. Burr, R. Hill, F. I. Nye, & I. L. Reiss (Eds.), *Contemporary theories about the family* (Vol. I, pp. 549–581). New York: The Free Press.

Giles-Sims, J. (1983). *Wife-battering: A systems theory approach.* New York: Guilford.

Goldstein, D., & Rosenbaum, A. (1985). An evaluation of the self-esteem of maritally violent men. *Family Relations, 34,* 425–428.

Gondolf, E. W. (1984, August). *Men who batter: How they stop their abuse.* Paper presented at the Second National Conference for Family Violence Researchers, Durham, NH.

Gottman, J. M. (1979). *Marital interaction: Experimental investigations.* New York: Academic Press.

Grayson, J., Mathie, V. A., Wampler, D., Dennis, M., Lynch, J. (1984, August). *In response to spouse abuse: A men's group.* Paper presented at the American Psychological Association Convention, Toronto.

Hilberman, E. (1980). Overview: The "wife-beater's wife" reconsidered. *American Journal of Psychiatry, 137,* 1336–1347.

Hornung, C. A., McCullough, B. C., & Sugimoto, T. (1981). Status relationships in marriage: Risk factors in spouse abuse. *Journal of Marriage and the Family, 42,* 675–692.

Hughes, H. M., & Rau, T. J. (1984, August). *Psychological adjustment of battered women in shelters.* Paper presented at the meeting of the American Psychological Association, Toronto.

King, L. S. (1981). Responding to spouse abuse: The mental health profession. *Response to violence in the family, 4*(5), 6–9.

Klingbeil, K. S., & Boyd, V. D. (1984). Emergency room intervention: Detection, assessment, and treatment. In A. R. Roberts (Ed.), *Battered women and the families* (pp. 7–32). New York: Springer.

LaViolette, A. D., Barnett, O. W., & Miller, C. L. (1984, August). *A classification of wife abusers on the Ben Sex-Role Inventory.* Paper presented at the Second Annual Conference on Research on Domestic Violence, Durham, NH.

Lerman, L., & Livingston, F. (1983). State legislation on domestic violence. *Response to Violence in the Family and Sexual Assault, 6*(5), 1–27.

Lewis, E. (1983). The group treatment of battered women. *Women and Therapy, 2*(1), 51–58.

Lion, J. R. (1977). Clinical aspects of wife battering. In M. Roy (Ed.), *Battered women: A psychosociological study of domestic violence* (pp. 126–136). New York: Van Nostrand.

Margolin, G. (1979). Conjoint marital therapy to enhance anger management and reduce spouse abuse. *American Journal of Family Therapy, 7*, 13–23.

Margolin, G. (1982). Ethical and legal considerations in marital and family therapy. *American Psychologist, 37*, 788–801.

Margolin, G. (in press-a). Conflict is not conflict is not conflict. *Proceedings of the 17th Banff International Conference of Behavior Sciences.* Beverly Hills, CA: Sage.

Margolin, G. (in press-b). Interpersonal and intrapersonal factors associated with marital violence. In G. T. Hotaling (Ed.), *Proceeding of the Second National Conference of Family Violence Researchers, Durham, NH.* Beverly Hills, CA: Sage.

Margolin, G., & Wampold, B. E. (1981). A sequential analysis of conflict and accord in distressed and nondistressed marital partners. *Journal of Consulting and Clinical Psychology, 49*, 554–567.

Melling, L. (1983). Employment training for battered women. *Response to Violence in the Family and Sexual Assault, 6*(6), 1–2.

Melling, L. (1984). Federal legislation for abuse victims. *Response to Violence in the Family and Sexual Assault, 7*(2), 5.

Myers, C. (1984, August). *The Family Violence Project: some preliminary data on a treatment program for spouse abuse.* Paper presented at the Second National Conference for Family Violence Researchers, Durham, NH.

Neidig, P. H., Friedman, D. H., & Collins, B. S. (1984, August). *Attitudinal characteristics of males who have engaged in spouse abuse.* Paper presented at the Second National Conference for Family Violence Researchers, Durham, NH.

O'Leary, K. D., & Arias, I. (1985, March). *Prevalence and development of physical aggression in marriage.* Paper presented at the 17th Banff International Conference on Behavior Sciences, Banff, Canada.

O'Leary, K. D., & Curley, A. (1986). Assertion and family violence: Correlates of spouse abuse. *Journal of Marital and Family Therapy 12*(3), 281–290.

O'Leary, K. D., Curley, A., Rosenbaum, A. S., & Clarke, C. (1985). Assertion training for abused wives: A potentially hazardous treatment. *Journal of Marital and Family Therapy, 11*, 319–322.

Pagelow, M. D. (1979). Research on woman battering. In J. B. Fleming (Ed.), *Stopping wife abuse* (pp. 334–349). Garden City, NY: Anchor.

Pagelow, M. D. (1981). *Woman-battering: Victims and their experiences.* Beverly Hills: Sage.

Parke, R. D.,& Slaby, R. G. (1983). The development of aggression. In E. M. Hetherington (Ed.), *Socialization, personality, and social development: Vol. 4, Handbook of child psychology* (pp. 547–641). New York: Wiley.

Patterson, G. R. (1982). *Coercive family processes.* Eugene, OR: Castalia.

Patterson, G. R., & Reid, J. B. (1970). Reciprocity and coercion: Two facets of social systems. In C. Neuringer & J. L. Michael (Eds.), *Behavior modification in clinical psychology* (pp. 133–177). New York: Appleton-Century-Crofts.

Peltoniemi, T. (1984, August). *Alcohol and family violence.* Paper presented at the Second National Conference for Family Violence Researchers, Durham, NH.

Prescott, S., & Letko, C. (1977). Battered women: A social psychological perspective. In M. Roy (Ed.), *Battered women: a psychosociological study of domestic violence* (pp. 72–96). London: Van Nostrand.

Purdy, R., & Nickle, N. (1981). Practice principles for working with groups of men who batter. *Social Work with Groups, 4*, 111–122.

Revenstorf, D., Vogel, B., Wegener, C., Hahlweg, K., & Schindler, L. (1980). Escalation phenomena in interaction sequences: An empirical comparison of distressed and nondistressed couples. *Behavioral Analysis and Modification, 4*, 97–115.

Rosenbaum, A. (1985). *Of men, macho, and marital violence.* Unpublished manuscript.

Rosenbaum, A., & O'Leary, K. D. (1981). Marital violence: Characteristics of abusive couples. *Journal of Consulting and Clinical Psychology, 49*, 63–71.

Rosenbaum, A., & O'Leary, K. D. (1986). Treatment of marital violence. In N. S. Jacobson & A. S. Gurman (Eds.), *Clinical handbook of marital therapy* (pp. 385–406). New York: Guilford.

Rosenberg, M. S. (1984, August). *Intergenerational family violence: A critique and implications for witnessing children.* Paper presented at the American Psychological Association Convention, Toronto.

Rosewater, L. B. (1984, August). *The MMPI and battered women.* Paper presented at the Second National Conference for Family Violence Researchers, Durham, NH.

Rounsaville, B. J. (1978). Battered wives: Barriers to identification and treatment. *American Journal of Orthopsychiatry, 48,* 487–494.

Roy, M. (1977). A current survey of 150 cases. In M. Roy (Ed.), *Battered women: A psychosociological study of domestic violence* (pp. 25–44). New York: Van Nostrand.

Saunders, D. G. (1982). Counseling the violent husband. In P. A. Keller & L. G. Ritt (Eds.), *Innovations in clinical practice: A sourcebook* (Vol. 1, pp. 16–29). Sarasota, FL: Professional Resources Exchange.

Saunders, D. G. (1984, August). *Issues in conducting treatment research with men who batter.* Paper presented at the Second National Conference for Family Violence Researchers, Durham, NH.

Saunders, D. G., & Hanusa, D. R. (1984, August). *Cognitive-behavioral treatment of abusive husbands: The short term effects of group therapy.* Paper presented at the Second National Conference for Family Violence Researchers, Durham, NH.

Schauss, A. G. (1982). Effects of environmental and nutritional factors on potential and actual batterers. In M. Roy (Ed.), *The abusive partner: An analysis of domestic battering* (pp. 76–90). New York: Van Nostrand.

Schechter, S. (1982). *Women and male violence: The visions and struggles of the battered women's movement.* Boston, MA: South End Press.

Scott, P. D. (1974). Battered wives. *British Journal of Psychiatry, 125,* 433–441.

Shainess, N. (1977). Psychological aspects of wife battering. In M. Roy (Ed.), *Battered women: A psycho-sociological study of domestic violence* (pp. 111–118). New York: Van Nostrand.

Sherman, L. (1984, August). *The Minneapolis police study.* Paper presented at the Second National Conference for Family Violence Researchers, Durham, NH.

Sherman, L. W., & Berk, R. A. (1984, April). The Minneapolis domestic violence experiment. *Police Foundation Reports,* pp. 1–8.

Snell, J. E., Rosenwald, J., & Robey, A. (1964). The wife-beater's wife. *Archives of General Psychiatry, 11,* 107–112.

Snyder, D. K., & Fruchtman, L. A. (1981). Differential patterns of wife abuse: A data-based typology. *Journal of Consulting and Clinical Psychology, 49,* 878–885.

Star, B., Clark, C. G., Goetz, K. M., & O'Malia, L. (1979). Psychosocial aspects of wife battering. *Social casework: The Journal of Contemporary Social Work, 6,* 479–487.

Stark, E., & Flitcraft, A. (1982). Medical therapy as repression: The case of the battered woman. *Health and Medicine, 1*(3), 29–32.

Stark, E., Flitcraft, A., & Frazier, W. (1983). Medicine and patriarchal violence: The social construction of a "private" event. In V. Navaro (Ed.), *Women and health: The politics of sex in medicine* (Vol. 4, pp. 177–209). New York: Baywood.

Stark, R., & McEvoy, J. (November, 1970). Middle class violence. *Psychology Today,* pp. 52–65.

Straus, M. A. (1973). A general systems theory approach to the development of a theory of violence between family members. *Social Science Information, 12,* 105–125.

Straus, M. A. (1977). A sociological perspective on the prevention and treatment of wifebeating. In M. Roy (Ed.), *Battered women: A psychosociological study of domestic violence* (pp. 194–238). New York: Van Nostrand.

Straus, M. A. (1979). Measuring intrafamily conflict and violence: The Conflict Tactics (CT) scales. *Journal of Marriage and the Family, 41,* 75–88.

Straus, M. A. (1980a). The marriage license as a hitting license: Evidence from popular culture, law, and social science. In M. A. Straus & G. T. Hotaling (Eds.), *The social causes of husband-wife violence* (pp. 39–50). Minneapolis, MN: University of Minnesota Press.

Straus, M. A. (1980b). Social stress and marital violence in a national sample of American families. *Annals of the New York Academy of Sciences, 347,* 229–250.

Straus, M. A. (1980c). Victims and aggressors in marital violence. *American Behavioral Scientist, 23,* 681–704.

Straus, M. A., Gelles, R. J., & Steinmetz, S. K. (1980). *Behind closed doors: Violence in the American family.* New York: Anchor Press.

Straus, M. A., & Hotaling, G. T. (1980). *The social causes of husband-wife violence.* Minneapolis, MN: University of Minnesota Press.

Symonds, M. (1978). The psychodynamics of violent-prone marriages. *American.Journal of Psychoanalysis, 38,* 213–222.

Taylor, S. P., & Leonard, K. E. (1983). Alcohol and human physical aggression. In R. G. Green & E. I. Donnerstein (Eds.), *Aggression: Theoretical and empirical reviews* (pp. 77–102). New York: Academic Press.

Telch, C. F., & Lindquist, C. V. (1984). Violent versus nonviolent couples: A comparison of patterns. *Psychotherapy, 21,* 242–248.

Traicoff, M. E. (1982). Family interventions from women's shelters. In J. C. Hansen & L. R. Barnhill (Eds.), *Clinical approaches to family violence* (pp. 105–116). Rockville, MD: Aspen.

Violence among relatives and friends. (1980, July). *Response to Violence in the Family.* p. 5.

Walker, L. E. (1979). *The battered woman.* New York: Harper & Row.

Walker, L. E. (1983). The battered woman syndrome study. In D. Finkelhor, R. J. Gelles, G. T. Hotaling, & M. A. Straus (Eds.), *The dark side of families* (pp. 31–48). Beverly Hills: Sage.

Walker, L. E. (1984a). Battered women, psychology, and public policy. *American Psychologist, 39,* 1178–1182.

Walker, L. E. (1984b). *The battered woman syndrome.* New York: Springer.

Wardell, L., Gillespie, D. L., & Leffler, A. (1983). Science and violence against wives. In D. Finkelhor, R. J. Gelles, G. T. Hotaling, & M. A. Straus (Eds.), *The dark side of families* (pp. 69–84). Beverly Hills, CA: Sage.

Whitehurst, R. N. (1974). Violence in husband-wife interaction. In S. K. Steinmetz & M. A. Straus (Eds.), *Violence in the family* (pp. 75–81). New York: Dodd, Mead.

Wife abuse: The facts (1984, January/February). *Response to Violence in the Family and Sexual Assault,* pp. 5–10.

6

Physical Abuse of Children

RAYMOND H. STARR, Jr.

INTRODUCTION

Cruelty toward and maltreatment of children has become a topic of much social concern during the past 20 years. The purpose of this chapter is to summarize the roots of this concern, analyze the magnitude of the problem, review current knowledge and, lastly, provide a framework for considering treatment, prediction, and prevention. Only physical abuse will be discussed; other forms of maltreatment such as sexual abuse, neglect, and institutional abuse are beyond the scope of this review. The terms *abuse* and *maltreatment* will be used synonymously and refer to inflicted trauma or injury by parents or other caregivers.

A research-based approach will be taken. Although we are far from understanding everything about physical abuse, research undertaken since 1970 provides a relatively clear picture. Information provided by such other approaches as clinical observation and philosophical analyses will be included where relevant.

HISTORY

Children have been maltreated since the dawn of creation. Numerous scholars have analyzed the history of child abuse in Western civilization (e.g., Bakan, 1971; deMause, 1974, 1980: Giovannoni & Becerra, 1979; Radbill, 1980; Williams, 1983) with a common conclusion that, the further back we trace the history of childhood, the less adequate child care was and the more likely children were to be abused, abandoned, traumatized, and murdered. Our concern about their well-being is relatively recent.

There are different theories as to the origins of our current, more compassionate view of children and their needs. DeMause (1980), for example, considered psychological factors to be of primary importance. Humane treatment of children is the outgrowth of the efforts of successive generations of parents to overcome abuse they received as children. The child maltreatment of earlier times was the product of the psychoanalytic mechanisms of projection and reversal that played key roles in abuse. DeMause sees a shift by many of

RAYMOND H. STARR, Jr. • Psychology Department, University of Maryland Baltimore County, Catonsville, MD 21228.

today's parents toward functioning in a different, empathic mode where parents can perceive and work to meet their children's needs. He reports finding no descriptions of parental empathy toward beaten children before the 18th century.

Bakan (1971) offered an explanation that is very different from that of deMause, one based on technological advancement. Child abuse is an evolution-based response to the need to balance population size with necessary resources. Three scientific advances are considered important precursors of our current concern about eliminating abuse: (a) the invention of the X-ray made professionals aware of the fact that parents could deliberately inflict injury on their children; (b) technology increased available resources; and (c) science has provided humane methods of birth control. Only with these modern advances is man free enough to work toward eliminating maltreatment.

MALTREATMENT IN EARLY TIMES

Infanticide was common from antiquity to 374 A.D. when it was outlawed in Rome in order to effect a population increase (deMause, 1974). It was socially acceptable, with children being tossed into rivers, placed in jars, and abandoned along roads. Girls were more likely to be abandoned than boys, illegitimate more than legitimate children, and later-born more than first-born offspring. Many of these practices continued into the 19th century. For example, living children were placed in the walls and foundations of new buildings to give them greater structural strength in Germany until 1843 (deMause, 1974).

The cessation of infanticide did not end inflicted infant death. Unwanted children were actively abandoned or left to die in the care of wet nurses or other surrogates. Prior to 1750 only 25% of children born in London lived to age 5 years (Kessen, 1965). Foundling homes were established in Britain by Thomas Coram, who tired of seeing dead and dying deserted infants on streets and dung heaps (deMause, 1974). But these homes did little to solve the problem of infant death. A total of 10,272 infants were admitted to a Dublin foundling home between 1775 and 1800. Only 45 survived (Kessen, 1965). Dead infants were still a common sight on streets in London in the 1890s (Rolph, cited in deMause, 1974). Many infants were placed in the care of wet nurses where they typically failed to thrive. An estimated 21,000 children were born in Paris in 1780. Only 700 of these were nursed by their mothers; 17,000 were sent out to wet nurses (deMause, 1974).

Children who survived were subjected to punishment, mutilation, and severe teasing. Adults frequently played catch with swaddled infants. A brother of Henry IV fell and died when being tossed between two windows (Graham, cited in deMause, 1974). Pemell (cited in de Mause, 1974) states that parents during the Renaissance would prevent illness in their newborn infants by burning them. Seneca saw nothing wrong with making children beggars through mutilation (deMause, 1974). Children in times past were routinely terrorized. They were exposed to corpses, witnessed hangings, and beaten so that they would remember what they had observed (deMause, 1980). Children in former times were often seen as innately evil (Kessen, 1965) and the terrorization of youth is seen by deMause (1980) as an effort to control this evil.

There were many, however, who worked to reform child care practices. As early as the fourth century, Christian theologians saw infanticide as a form of murder (Radbill, 1980). Overlaying (smothering children by lying upon them) was so common in medieval times that a 1224 British statute made it a crime for a woman to keep an infant in her bed (Radbill, 1980). In spite of all these efforts, child deaths were typically seen as accidents even where, today, we would suspect intentional abuse.

Our modern concern with child maltreatment is based on the English foundation of our legal and social system (Giovannoni & Becerra, 1979). From this we get the concepts of custody, parental obligation to protect children, and a societal obligation to protect poor people. Law related to poverty is particularly important, as it provided the basis for the removal of children from the homes of economically dependent parents. In such cases, maltreatment need not be present—mere poverty was sufficient to terminate parental rights. Regardless of whether a child was destitute, neglected, or delinquent, the remedy was the same: removal of the child. It is interesting to note that reformatories and orphanages were present before there were laws specifying the conditions for their use. In turn, challenges to the constitutionality of such laws came last (Schlossman, 1977).

The case of a Mary Ellen, a girl who was severely beaten by her stepmother, represents a major landmark in the development of our present system of protecting abused children. Although Mary Ellen was far from being the first abused child to be brought to the attention of authorities, her case was made famous by the intervention of Henry Bergh, the crusading founder of the Society for the Prevention of Cruelty to Animals, and his ability to generate press coverage. Mary Ellen's mother was convicted of assault and battery and was sent to prison (Williams, 1983). In the aftermath of this case, the Society for the Prevention of Cruelty to Children was founded and was given legal authority to intervene on behalf of children. Abuse cases of 100 years ago were similar to those reported today. The main difference is that action was faster. Child protection was the critical issue, not family privacy or parental rights (Williams, 1983).

Establishment of juvenile courts in the last part of the 19th century was the next major child protection change. Social workers, motivated by a desire to remove delinquents from the regular criminal justice system, were the major supporters of the new court system. The first law decriminalizing juvenile court proceedings and allowing judges to invoke the doctrine of *parens patriae* without considering due process issues was passed in Illinois in 1899 (Giovannoni & Becerra, 1979).

Efforts to protect children from maltreatment diminished by the early part of the 20th century; national attention was drawn to World War I and the Depression, funding for child protection agencies diminished, and competition and fighting between private agencies led to government intervention in child protection (Williams, 1983). Many services came to be provided by public agencies operating under the child welfare provisions of the Social Security Act (DeFrancis, 1973). The shift to public child welfare services emphasized the family as a unit rather than the child and, more importantly, meant a switch from primary prevention through improvement of rearing conditions for all children to an emphasis on the treatment of specific cases in need (tertiary prevention) (Williams, 1983).

The roots of our present concern with abuse go back to 1945, when an article suggesting that many of the injuries seen by pediatricians might be inflicted by their parents was published (Caffey & Silverman, 1945). Even when faced with what we would today state was undeniable evidence of parentally inflicted trauma, physicians 40 years ago sought to attribute injuries to strange, unknown diseases (Caffey, 1946). Although these and other publications clarified the role of parental actions in child injuries, public and professional attention were not drawn toward child abuse until 1962 when Henry Kempe coined the term *the battered child* to shock apathetic professionals (Kempe, Silverman, Steele, Droegemueller, & Silver, 1962).

Response was swift. A 1963 conference on battered children drafted model legislation. These and other efforts supported the role of publicly funded protective services agencies as the focal point for child abuse treatment (Kempe, 1978). Congressional response was equally swift with 11 of 18 child protection bills being passed the same year. All states enacted child protection laws by 1967. These efforts culminated in the 1974 passage of legislation establishing a central, federal agency: the National Center on Child Abuse and Neglect. Interestingly, the very need for such legislation is dramatic evidence of the resistance against guaranteeing humane care for children (Williams, 1983).

This section began with a brief discussion of theoretical views underlying our current concern. Regardless of which approach is more correct, we are at present in a time where child abuse is a topic of broad interest. However, developing a detailed understanding of the problem is a complex endeavor.

DEFINITION

The complexities of child abuse begin with the critical problem of definition. Definitions are determined by four factors: the intentionality of the act, the act's effect on a given child, the value judgment made about the act, and the standard on which the judgment is based (Garbarino & Gilliam, 1980). For example, practices seen as normal in one culture may be abusive in others (Korbin, 1980a). Thus, many African cultures practice scarification, (i.e., the cutting of the face or body to create scars, an act that would be considered abuse in Western societies). Alternatively, people in these cultures might view our use of orthodontia as barbaric. Child abuse must be examined in its cultural context. Most typically, acts that are seen as abusive represent idiosyncratic practices (Korbin, 1980a, 1981). Burning a child's hand in scalding water is abuse in the United States, but orthodontic treatment is not.

There have been many efforts at defining child maltreatment from early times. Early Christians, for example, defined infanticide as murder in the fourth century (Radbill, 1980). However, the difficulty in labeling maltreatment does not generally occur with such extreme events. Child care is provided along a continuum from optimal to devastatingly bad. Disagreement occurs in the gray area at the middle of this continuum (Besharov, 1978). The breadth of behaviors included in this area varies between cultures and within different groups in the same culture.

Definitions typically focus on physical abuse, which is usually seen as an act of commission where a parent or other caregiver does something injurious to a child. They vary as to the range of acts that are considered abusive, from a spanking to infanticide, and with regard to such other variables as intent to injure. Definitions have importance not only in a court or other legal settings, but as guides for detection, treatment, and prevention.

Legal definitions are typically vague. They do not specify the amount of injury considered as abusive and often use such terms as *mental suffering* and *unfit place* without specifically defining them (Giovannoni & Becerra, 1979). Some professionals believe that vague legislative wording is desirable, in that it allows flexibility in dealing with specific cases and for coping with different cultural norms. Others believe that vagueness can lead to due process violations and inconsistent handling of cases (Valentine, Acuff, Freeman, & Andreas, 1984).

The difficulties involved in developing a universal definition hinder our efforts to determine the incidence of maltreatment, study it, and develop effective prevention and treatment programs. It is ironic, however, that the very importance of maltreatment mitigates against the development of a universally agreed upon set of criteria for its definition (Giovannoni & Becerra, 1979).

Perhaps the most useful efforts at developing acceptable definitions are two surveys done by Gelles (1982) and Giovannoni and Becerra (1979). Both studies are sociological rather than diagnostic in focus and emphasize whether or not various caregiver acts are seen as normal or as child abuse. Gelles surveyed social service, educational, medical, and police personnel. Subjects were asked to indicate for each of 13 acts whether it was child abuse, was not abuse, or that they were undecided. Results indicated that reporting professionals do not use a single, universally accepted definition. The groups sampled used different operational definitions of abuse. There was greatest consensus when the act involved (a) direct harm (e.g., trauma, sexual abuse with injury, or willful malnutrition), (b) intent to injure (with an appreciation of the difficulty inherent in determining intent), or (c) intentionality without injury (e.g., locking in a dark closet). There was no agreement about those conditions that were not abusive. Thus, 38% of the sample believed injury due to inadequate parental precautions to be abuse, whereas 34% believed it nonabusive, and the remainder was undecided.

In their study, Giovannoni and Becerra (1979) argue that maltreatment is socially defined and must be considered in relation to the social contexts in which it occurs. They developed 78 pairs of vignettes about 13 categories of acts that might be considered physically or sexually abusive or neglectful. The incidents in each pair were differentiated as to whether or not a consequence was involved. For example, one pair in the physical abuse category involved a child being hit with a wooden stick by a parent. The two versions of the question varied in that the child suffered a concussion in one case and no consequence was specified in the other. Each respondent was given 60 randomly selected vignettes (but not both members of a given pair) to rate for seriousness on a 9-point arbitrary scale. The sample included lawyers, social workers, pediatricians, police officers, and 1,065 lay people.

The results for physical abuse support Gelles' (1982) finding of greater agreement for incidents involving more severe injury and disagreement for vignettes depicting less extreme punishments. Although ratings of professional and lay groups were similar for the most serious items (e.g., burning), they differed when injuries were less serious. In this latter case, professionals saw physical injuries and community members items related to drugs and delinquency as more serious. Within professions, Giovannoni and Becerra found that lawyers rated physical abuse and almost all other categories of mistreatment as less serious than the other three professions. This is most probably due to the fact that lawyers were reluctant to see maltreatment as present (''innocent until proven guilty'') and the relatively greater risks other professionals faced in not reporting a case.

Giovannoni and Becerra concluded that there is a need for greater specificity of the exact nature of the maltreatment on child abuse reporting forms. Their study shows that abuse and neglect are relatively meaningless terms and should be replaced in order to make informed policy and legal decisions affecting the lives of children. Such specificity is also important in studying the causes and correlates of maltreatment.

INCIDENCE AND REPORTING

We do not know the exact incidence of child abuse. This is only partly because of our inability to develop a definition that allows exact labeling of a given case as abuse or not abuse. The other critical factors are (a) abuse usually occurs in private, beyond public scrutiny, and (b) the failure of lay persons and professionals to report suspected maltreatment.

In 1983 approximately 1.5 million children from 1,007,658 families were reported to be abused and/or neglected in the United States (American Humane Association, 1985). Overall, 27.9% of reports dealt with physical abuse, 19.0% with abuse and neglect, and 45.7% with neglect only. Nonprofessionals reported 52% of cases. Most of these were friends, neighbors, or relatives. Professionals accounted for the remaining 48% of reports and are evenly divided among medical, school, law enforcement, and social services personnel. Most importantly for this chapter, 3.2% of reports were for major physical, 18.5% for minor physical, and 5.2% for unspecified injuries. For major and minor injuries, respectively, medical personnel reported 43% and 9% of cases, nonprofessionals 18% and 35%, school staff 12% and 23%, social services employees 10% and 10%, and law enforcement officers 7% and 10%.

The American Humane Association (1985) survey also examined case status. Overall, 52% of cases were closed after investigation. Less than half of reports (42%) resulted in the provision of protective services. Whereas nonprofessionals were the most likely to report cases, their reports were least likely to be confirmed upon investigation (36%). Approximately half of professionally reported cases were confirmed.

Reported cases of child abuse and/or neglect have increased 142% since the first systematic data were compiled in 1976 (American Humane Association, 1985). These figures are in spite of a decline in the child population of more than 5% during this period and a reluctance by professionals to report (Russell & Trainor, 1984). According to one study, approximately two out of three maltreatment cases known to professionals were not reported (Department of Health and Human Services, 1981). The type of maltreatment and source of reports have remained fairly constant from 1976 to present (Russell & Trainor, 1984).

The acknowledged underreporting of maltreatment means that we cannot rely solely on reported or adjudicated cases in order to estimate its full magnitude. Gelles (1978), in an improvement over earlier surveys and estimates (e.g., Gil, 1970; Nagi, 1977) of the incidence of child abuse, surveyed a random sample of households concerning violence between family members. Approximately 3.5% of the parents in his study admitted that they had acted in such a violent manner toward one of their children in the year prior to the survey that their actions could have caused injury. When these figures are extrapolated they indicate that, each year, between 1.4 and 1.9 million children are subjected to forms of violence that could potentially cause injury.

In addition to the efforts of the American Humane Association (1985) to understand reporting practices, a number of other studies have looked at reporting practices (e.g., Adams, Barone, & Tooman, 1982; Gelles, 1982; Hampton & Newberger, 1985; Morris, Johnson, & Clasen, 1985; Newberger, 1984). Gelles (1982), in the survey discussed in the definition section, asked the professionals surveyed about the factors that would lead them to report a case as child abuse. The most important was the physical condition of the child. Across professions, 55% said they would report on this factor alone. Physicians were least likely to report solely on physical condition (28%), even though it ranked first on their list of factors to consider. Between 50% and 67% of the other groups would report only on the basis of this variable. Across professions, the next most important factors leading to reporting were psychological state of suspected offender, psychological state of child, evaluation of caretaker's explanation for injury, and behavior of caretakers. Morris *et al.* (1985) examined physicians' reporting practices in more detail. They found that physicians' attitudes toward child discipline were related to reporting. Those favoring physical discipline were less likely to report maltreatment. Inappropriate discipline did not necessarily lead to reporting. Almost all (98%) of their subjects said that bruising a child with a belt was inappropriate, but only 48% said they would report a bruised child. Reasons for nonreporting were the low incidence of abuse in private practice patients, a fear of losing patients, a desire for absolute proof of inflicted injury prior to reporting, and a lack of confidence in community agencies.

There are additional problems with present reporting practices. Experience in Florida with a media public education campaign and a WATS reporting hot line suggests such programs may overload protective services staff (Carr, 1978). Nonprofessionals were the hot line's main users and, although the number of reports increased, the number of true abuse cases did not. Anonymous calls are the most problematic reports. They are typically for low risk situations (Adams *et al.,* 1982). For example, only 61 of more than 1,000 anonymous reports in the Bronx, New York represented new, substantiated cases. A few of these were serious, yet none was life threatening. Adams *et al.* (1982) conclude that anonymous reports are an undue burden on an overworked protective service system and should not be accepted. Alternatively, such reports could be screened using a triage model, with the more severe cases receiving attention first.

There are also problems with professional reporting sources. Hampton and Newberger (1985), using hospital reporting statistics, found dramatic underreporting of cases involving middle-class and white families. Low income and minority families are more likely to be reported by virtue of their personal characteristics, rather than their childrearing practices (O'Toole, Turbett, & Nalepka, 1983). Child abuse is less likely to be reported when the patient and hospital staff member have common personal characteristics (Pfohl, 1977). Indeed, Hampton and Newberger (1985) suggested that our system of reporting should be modified, and Newberger (1983) proposed deemphasizing reporting in favor of preventive strategies directed toward high-risk families and groups.

Difficulties in securing accurate reporting impede our efforts to find the true incidence of child maltreatment. At present we can only state that significant numbers of American children are injured by their parents or other caregivers each year, that many such incidents are not reported, and that biases exist as to which cases are reported and which are not.

CAUSAL THEORIES

Theoretical views of child abuse have become increasingly sophisticated over the past decade. Earlier views focused on unitary causal factors. For example, psychologically and medically oriented theorists examined parental psychological characteristics. Historically, we have tended to perceive most forms of deviance as the result of "sick" personalities (Garbarino & Gilliam, 1980). For example, Green (1978a) saw abuse as a consequence of unsatisfied parental dependency needs, a lack of impulse control, deficient self-concept combined with denial of underlying feelings, and a projection of this poor self-image onto the child. His approach is similar to deMause's (1974, 1980) explanation of abuse in prior eras. Other psychologically oriented theorists have focused on different sets of personality attributes with little consensus regarding the particular psychological characteristics that would lead to abuse (Gelles, 1973; Spinetta & Rigler, 1972).

Sociocultural theorists (e.g., Gelles, 1973; Newberger & Bourne, 1978), while stating that psychological factors cannot be omitted, emphasize such antecedents of abuse as isolation, stress, and unemployment. They argue that child abuse is the result of characteristics of our society and subgroups within it rather than specific personality patterns. Even when personality deviations are present, they are seen as the result of deviant social conditions (Bourne, 1979).

If abuse is the result of sociocultural factors, cross-cultural studies should clarify the variables of importance. Korbin (1981) stated that abuse must be considered in the context of the culture within which it occurs. Although culture affects the way abuse is defined, none of the cultures she surveyed sanctioned severe, inflicted, physical trauma. Korbin considered four factors important in determining whether a society maltreats children: (a) the value of children in the society, (b) whether some children are less valued than others (e.g., handicapped), (c) cultural expectations for child development and (d) the degree to which caregiving tasks are embedded in community and kinship structures. Korbin (1980a) concluded that the United States is at the extreme negative end of a cross-cultural continuum of caregiving practices.

Neither a psychological nor a sociocultural view fully explains the complexities of child abuse. Indeed, psychologically oriented professionals assign supporting roles to social factors with the reverse being true for those with sociocultural orientations. A full understanding of maltreatment can only be achieved through a more eclectic, ecological approach where the roles of different causal factors can be evaluated (Belsky, 1980; Garbarino, 1977a; Garbarino & Gilliam, 1980; Parke, 1982; Starr, 1978). Such an analysis has at its heart the developing child, placed in the context of interactions within a social environment that, in turn, is nested within the context of the overall culture within which the child lives. Furthermore, some theorists, supporting Bakan's (1971) views discussed earlier, have proposed combining ecological and evolutionary approaches (e.g., Burgess & Garbarino, 1983). The next section discusses research on all of these factors.

RESEARCH ON THE CAUSES AND CORRELATES OF ABUSE

This section will focus on research performed since 1973, the date when studies comparing abusive with matched, nonabusive samples became common. Earlier research has been discussed in detail elsewhere (see Starr, 1974). The retrospective nature of most of the modern studies limits our understanding of abuse. For example, they typically involve assessment of families currently under investigation for or known to be abusive. Thus, answers to questionnaires or even direct observation may be biased in order to create a more positive impression of a maltreating family. Other factors that further complicate our achieving a full understanding of physical abuse include the operational definition of child abuse used, control group selection procedures, and the reliability and validity of assessment instruments (Leventhal, 1981, 1982; Plotkin, Azar, Twentyman, & Perri, 1981). Ideally, our understanding of child maltreatment should be based on well-designed prospective studies. Unfortunately, there are few such studies, as they are expensive and difficult to conduct.

The two major prospective studies both recruited pregnant women and followed them for several years (Egeland, Deinard, Brunnquell, Phipps-Yonas, & Crichton, 1979; Vietze, Falsey, Sandler, O'Connor, & Altemeier, 1980; Vietze, O'Connor, Hopkins, Sandler, & Altemeier, 1982). Egeland *et al.* (1979) studied 267 high-risk mothers and infants divided into subsamples of 33 adequate care and 32 mistreating mothers. Most of their maltreated sample were neglected (25 cases) rather than abused (4 cases), with both present in 3 cases. Thus, their results have only suggestive implications for physical abuse. Vietze *et al.* (1982) interviewed 1,400 expectant mothers and followed up 273 predicted to be at high risk for maltreating and 225 women randomly selected from the entire sample. Overall, 70 children were maltreated, with 12 being physically abused (9 from the high risk group). Other aspects of these studies will be discussed in appropriate later sections.

This section summarizes our knowledge of parental, societal, child, and interactional factors as they contribute to physical abuse.

PSYCHOLOGICAL FACTORS

A number of psychological factors have been hypothesized to be correlated with abuse, including parental personality, intelligence, discipline history, and childrearing attitudes, knowledge, and expectations. However, to date, research has not indicated that there are any factors that are present in all abusing and absent in all nonabusing parents (Oates, 1979). Thus, the concept of role reversal in which parent and child switch roles (Helfer, 1980; Morris & Gould, 1963), although helping to understand and treat a given abusive parent, does not help us develop an overall understanding of maltreatment.

Personality

With regard to personality characteristics, it was initially thought child abusers were psychotic (Woolley & Evans, 1955). Spinetta and Rigler (1972), in the classic review of personality variables, concluded that the vast majority of abusive parents are not psychotic. The research surveyed reported 19 different personality traits as describing abusive parents. Only 4 of these were cited by more than one study (Gelles, 1973). Controlled research supports Spinetta and Rigler (1972). Spinetta (1978) found abusing parents were angrier, feared external threat and control, and attributed their feelings to their children. Wright (1976), using the MMPI, found significant differences between abuse and control groups for 2 of the 4 validity scales but none of the clinical scales. In a finding with implications for all retrospective studies, he reported his abuse sample appeared to be healthier on high face validity questions than on ones for which the socially desirable answers were less obvious. However, his suggestion that abusive parents respond in socially desirable ways has not been substantiated (Shorkey & Armendariz, 1985). Other studies have reported low self-esteem (Anderson & Lauderdale, 1982; Evans 1980) and depression (Evans, 1980; Kinard, 1982a; Lahey, Conger, Atkeson, & Treiber, 1984) among abusive parents. However, it is difficult to determine whether low self-esteem and depression are consequences of being reported and investigated for child maltreatment or are causal of the maltreatment. A larger study by Gaines, Sandgrund, Green, and Power (1978), comparing 80 abusive, 80 neglectful, and 80 control families, indicated that personality factors were not major correlates of maltreatment. Starr (1982), in a second large study (87 abuse and matched control families), although finding significant differences for two of five personality scales using the Psychological Screening Inventory (Lanyon, 1970), concluded that they probably do not represent true group differences. He examined a total of 249 variables of which only 16 (slightly more than would be expected by chance) were statistically significant. Indeed, it may be that significant differences are more likely to be found when a limited number of domains (e.g., personality only, stress only, physical health only) are investigated rather than in studies such as Starr's of a large number of variables across many domains. Thus, a particular variable that, examined in isolation from other variables, appears to differentiate maltreating from control groups, may become unimportant in the context of the complexities underlying human behavior as investigated in broader studies.

Egeland, in his prospective study, provides evidence that personality variables are correlated with maltreatment (Brunnquell, Crichton, & Egeland, 1981). Maltreating mothers were more suspicious, aggressive, and had lower self-esteem.

It is likely that the key factor in abuse is a relationship between emotional distress, rather than personality, and maltreatment. It has been hypothesized that people who are emotionally aroused are more likely to be aggressive toward others (Bandura, 1973; Baron, 1977; Berkowitz, 1974). This speculation has been supported in three laboratory studies of the psychophysiological responses of abusive and control parents to videotapes of aversive child behaviors (Disbrow, Doerr, & Caulfield, 1977; Frodi & Lamb, 1980; Wolfe, Fairbank, Kelly, & Bradlyn, 1983). Results suggest abusive parents are in a constant state of physiological arousal in response to child behaviors. Wolfe (1985) proposed that this responsivity may mediate aggression and explain the difficulty abusive parents have in controlling it.

Intelligence

In spite of the intuitive appeal of the hypothesis that abusive parents are less intelligent, there is little evidence supporting it. Starr (1982) found no IQ differences between his abuse and control groups. Although Brunnquell *et al.* (1981) found maltreating parents to be less intelligent, there were significant demographic differences between their good care and maltreating groups that could account for this difference. Although other studies also suggest that there is a relationship, the maltreatment studied is typically neglect rather than abuse; furthermore, these studies suffer from a variety of methodological flaws (Schilling, Schinke, Blythe, & Barth, 1982).

Intergenerational Transmission of Abuse

Probably the most common public conception of the cause of physical abuse is that parents who were abused as children grow up to be abusive adults. Surprisingly, few controlled studies have examined this hypothesis (see Jayaratne, 1977, for a review). Disbrow *et al.* (1977) found abusing parents were handled more negatively when they were children than were matched neglecting or control parents. Perry, Wells, and Doran (1983) reported more childhood maltreatment among abusive mothers, but not fathers. Almost half of the mothers interviewed in a third study reported being abused as children, compared to 6% of a contrast group of mothers of conduct-disordered children (Webster-Stratton, 1985). However, Starr (1982), in a detailed examination of parental punishment histories, found no differences between abuse and control samples. Two studies have examined the parenting practices of adults who were abused as children. In the first, Smith, Bohnstedt, and Grove (cited in Pagelow, 1984) found 3% of 313 abused children were suspected of abusing their own children. In a second study, Herrenkohl, Herrenkohl, and Toedter (1983) reported 56% of abusive parents were themselves maltreated as children compared to 38% of nonabusers. The presence of multiple rather than single abusive caregivers was positively correlated with growing up to be an abusing parent.

These findings may be due to differing methodologies or, as Straus (1980) suggested, to the age at which parents were physically punished and who punished the child. Parents who were physically punished most by their mothers when they were teens were less physically punitive toward their children. Parents whose fathers hit them when they were teens were more physically punitive toward their own offspring. In addition, parents who grew up in families characterized by high father-to-mother violence were 44% more likely to abuse their children (23% of high violence cases grew up to be abusive). Although exposure to violence as a child predisposes children to grow up to be abusers, the relationship is far from perfect. The majority of abused children do not grow up to be abusive parents (Hunter & Kilstrom, 1979; Miller & Challas, 1981; Straus, Gelles, & Steinmetz, 1980). Hunter and Kilstrom, in their prospective study, found more than 80% of families where a parent was abused as a child did *not* abuse their high-risk infants. These parents generally had a strong social network, good child care arrangements, were optimistic, and could cope with stress. Indeed, adults who are abused as children may grow up to eschew violence and work toward its elimination (McGuire, 1983).

Childrearing Skills, Attitudes, and Knowledge

The final, major, hypothesized psychological determinant of physical abuse is inadequate childrearing skills and attitudes. Child abuse is, by definition, the result of societally labeled deviant childrearing. Beyond this simple fact, the actual understanding of these inadequacies is complex. Investigators have focused on parental perceptions, expectations for the achievement of developmental milestones, childrearing attitudes, and choice of disciplinary techniques.

Retrospective studies of parental perceptions of their children generally show no difference between abuse and matched, control samples (e.g., Elmer, 1977; Milner & Wimberley, 1980; Rosenberg & Reppucci, 1983; Starr, 1982). An exception to this conclusion is the finding by Oates, Davis, Ryan, and Stewart (1979) that abusive parents, interviewed between one and three years after the abuse occurred, reported they did not enjoy caring for their child (34%) and perceived their children to have been below average or worse babies (45%). This retrospective report must be interpreted with caution due to distortion resulting from long-term recall of perceptions. Similarly, Rosenblatt (1980), comparing severely and mildly abused children, found that mothers of the more severely injured children saw their children more negatively. However, other differences between his two samples (e.g., child age), may account for these findings.

Temperament, although usually seen as a child characteristic, is typically measured by maternal interview rather than direct observation. Thus, temperament is also a measure of parental perceptions (Vaughn, Taraldson, Crichton, & Egeland, 1981). Mothers in the Egeland *et al.* (1979) excellent care group rated their infants as temperamentally easier than did inadequate care group mothers. Egeland *et al.* saw these differences as related to maternal personality rather than actual infant differences. Maltreated infants were also rated as temperamentally more difficult in a second prospective study (Vietze *et al.*, 1980). Retrospective studies report few significant temperament differences (Kotelchuck, 1982; Starr, 1982). This may be due to either the retrospective nature of these studies (prospective studies assessed temperament at 6 months of age or less), or to differences between the abused children who were the focus of the retrospective analyses and neglected children who constituted the majority of subjects in the prospective projects.

The most commonly examined area within this cluster is parental knowledge of developmental norms that are interpreted as expectations for the attainment of developmental milestones. Early, uncontrolled studies and clinical case reports suggested unrealistic expectations were a major cause of physical abuse (Spinetta & Rigler, 1972). Parents were thought to consider their children capable of age-inappropriate mature behavior (S. Feshbach, 1980). Results of prospective studies are contradictory. Egeland *et al.* (1979) found maltreating parents varied more from norms in their developmental expectations, whereas Altemeier *et al.* (1979) found a low correlation between developmental knowledge and maltreatment. Most retrospective studies find no differences in expectations when parents are asked to indicate the age they expect their child to perform various tasks (Gaines *et al.*, 1978; Kotelchuk, 1982; Kravitz & Driscoll, 1983; Rosenblatt, 1980; Smith & Hanson, 1975; Spinetta, 1978; Starr, 1982). Three studies report group differences (Disbrow *et al.*, 1977; Larrance & Twentyman, 1983; Perry *et al.*, 1983). The Perry *et al.* finding was the reverse of the hypothesized direction, with their abuse sample expecting developmental milestones to be reached at a later than normal age. The other two studies used methods other than the standard method discussed earlier. At present, we can state that abusive parents are not markedly deviant in their knowledge of normal developmental milestones. It may be, however, that this knowledge does not lead to the implementation of these expectations in everyday life.

Few studies have examined parental attitudes concerning childrearing. Evans (1980), in a limited investigation of punishment and reward oriented attitudes, found no abuse versus control-group differences. Rosenblatt (1980) found no differences in attitudes toward discipline and, using the Parental Attitude Research Instrument, found no group differences in overall factor scores. Starr (1982) found that one of the few differences between abuse and control samples in his study was for one of five childrearing attitude scales (Cohler, Weiss, & Grunebaum, 1970). The abuse sample saw childrearing as a simple, rather than a complex, task, thus providing partial support for the hypothesis that the unrealistic expectations present in abusive parents are for more complex variables rather than the age of achievement of developmental landmarks. Egeland, using the same measure, found major group differences (Egeland & Brunnquell, 1979) as did Disbrow *et al.* (1977) using another attitudinal measure.

Finally, a small number of studies have asked abusive parents about the disciplinary methods they actually use. Again, the conclusion is that retrospective reports of discipline used are similar in abuse and control families (Elmer, 1977; Starr, 1982; Susman, Trickett, Iannotti, Hollenbeck, & Zahn-Waxler, 1985; Webster-Stratton, 1985). Oates *et al.* (1979), in their limited study, reported more severe discipline practices in their abuse group, as did Disbrow *et al.* (1977). In the latter study, a more refined survey of discipline techniques was used in which parents were given a list of child behaviors and a list of handling options and were asked to indicate the option they would choose for each behavior. Thus, as was the situation for examining parental expectations, it may be that indirect measures need to be used to obtain valid responses.

SOCIAL FACTORS

The failure to find clear psychological causes of physical abuse has increasingly led researchers to examine the relation of social and demographic variables. Particular emphasis has been placed on stress, social isolation, and our societal acceptance of violence as a solution to interpersonal problems. Results of this research suggest that social factors play a critical, but not determining role in maltreatment. They still need to be considered in relation to personality, child variables, and the ways in which all three categories interact.

Stress

The effects of stress on human well-being have been a topic of increasing scientific study over the past 20 years. Stress has typically been measured in terms of the presence or absence of events deemed to be stressful using measures similar to Holmes and Rahe's Social Readjustment Rating Scale (Holmes & Rahe, 1967) rather than measures designed to examine individual differences in response to stress.

Results of most studies suggest that abusive families experience more of what Straus (1980) terms stressor stimuli. In the most convincing examination of the relation between stress and child abuse, participants in a national survey of family violence (Straus et al., 1980) were also surveyed about the presence or absence of stressful events (Straus, 1980). Reported stress within families was directly related to violence directed toward children. However, when this relationship was examined more thoroughly it was found to hold for fathers but not for mothers. Straus hypothesized that this result may be due to the relatively greater rate with which mothers use physical violence combined with their relatively lower rate of reporting of stressful events. He also examined the role of factors such as parental childhood punishment history, belief in the use of physical punishment, participation in an unrewarding marriage, and social isolation and found their presence or absence mediated the relationship between stress and maltreatment. Stress was found to differentiate good care from inadequate care families in one prospective study (Egeland, Breitenbucher, & Rosenberg, 1980). In particular, highly stressed mothers who were also anxious, aggressive, and low in succorance were more likely to neglect, and, in some cases, abuse their infants. Stress was significantly correlated with high maltreatment risk in a second prospective study (Altemeier et al., 1979).

Other studies, although they have examined stress, typically have failed to assess the roles of such mediating factors. Gaines et al. (1978), in their comparison of matched abusive, neglectful, and control families, found that stress was higher in the abuse than in the control group. However, significant variables in this study accounted for less than 12% of the discriminate space and stress was highest for the neglect sample, providing support to the conclusion that most parents who are under high levels of stress do not abuse children (Pagelow, 1984; Straus, 1980). Differences in stress levels were also reported by Conger, Burgess, and Barrett (1979), Elmer (1977), Oates et al. (1979), and Rosenberg and Reppucci (1983). One study reported no difference in the number of stressful events, but did find abusive parents reported the stressful events they experienced had a more negative impact on them (Perry, Wells, & Doran, 1983). This latter difference did not hold up when data for mothers and fathers were analyzed separately. Finally, two large retrospective studies (Kotelchuk, 1982; Starr, 1982) reported no differences in frequency of stressful events between abuse and control groups. In addition, Starr found no evidence of an increased frequency of stressful events close to the time of abuse. These data thus support the conclusion of Straus (1980) concerning the vagueness of the relation between stress and physical abuse and the need to assess mediating factors.

It is possible that the stress involved in physical abuse is situational and short-term rather than major and relatively long-lasting. In many cases, a glass of spilled milk can be a significant stressor and may precipitate abuse (Helfer, personal communication, 1978). An interesting laboratory study involving mothers and their children provides limited support for this contention (Passman & Mulhern, 1977). Mothers were subjected to one of two mild stressors: (a) an interruption by their child or (b) performing an ambiguous task. An examination of the relation of type of stress to child punishment indicated that both stressors were related to increased maternal punitiveness. Although the stress employed and the punishment used were mild, the results are supported by Herrenkohl and Herrenkohl (1981). The latter authors found a modest but significant correlation between early stress and maltreatment abusive parents experienced when they were children. The Herrenkohls also report that stressors experienced during childhood were also significantly related to the severity with which they disciplined their own children (E. C. Herrenkohl et al., 1983).

Poverty. Poverty is perhaps the single most studied stressor. Some authors suggest that child abuse is classless, occurring with equal incidence in all social classes, but underreported in the middle and upper echelons (see Pelton, 1978). What Pelton describes as the myth of classlessness is due to a number of factors, including a reluctance of physicians to report their private patients, increased scrutiny of poor families by social service professionals trained to suspect abuse, and a desire to see abuse as a psychiatric rather than a social problem, and so on.

Child abuse *is* class related. Almost half of all maltreating families receive public assistance, with no caretaker being employed in 40% of families (American Humane Association, 1985). Similarly, cases of infanticide, an act harder to conceal than nonfatal abuse, show a preponderance of children who were from poor families (Weston, 1980).

The most compelling evidence against the myth of classlessness comes from the Straus et al. (1980) national, stratified survey sample. They found an inverse relationship between income and parent-to-child violence. Families earning over $20,000/year were half as violent as those earning less than $5,999. It is important to note, however, that most families, even poor ones, do not abuse. Interestingly, a corollary examination of education and employment in relation to child abuse indicates some of the complexities involved in examining the role of social factors. For education, Straus et al. found that parents with a high school degree were most violent, those with either less than a 9th grade or who had some college were least violent. They hypothesize it may be more stressful to have a moderate amount of (as compared to little) education. Furthermore, male unemployment was related to high child abuse rates. However, the highest rate was for men who worked part time. It may be that the category of unemployed males includes those who have ceased looking for work and who find unemployment nonstressful, whereas part-time employees may be frustrated by an inability to find full-time jobs. This hypothesis is supported by the their finding that violence rates were the same for disabled fathers and those with full-time jobs. A disabled parent was likely to have adjusted to his inability to work competitively.

If recent unemployment and accompanying loss of income and stress are important factors in child abuse, then there should be a relation between employment data and child abuse (Steinberg, Catalano, & Dooley, 1981). Steinberg et al.'s cross-correlational analyses of changes in employment and child abuse over time in two metropolitan areas suggest that reported abuse increases when work force size declines, supporting the causal role of unemployment in maltreatment. This conclusion is supported by related analyses of census tract data for reported child abuse and economic conditions (Garbarino & Crouter, 1978).

Family Variables Inducing Stress. Finally, it has been proposed that such family variables as single parenthood or large numbers of children create stress and lead to subsequent maltreatment. Straus *et al.* (1980), although they studied only intact families in their national survey, suggested that stress would be higher in single-parent families because of the need for mothers to manage both income-generating and child-caregiving activities rather than sharing these tasks, and also to the stress induced during marital dissolution. Nationally, 40.3% of reported maltreatment cases (including neglect and sexual abuse) had single female headed households compared with 19% for all United States families with children under 18 (American Humane Association, 1985). Additional data suggestive of a relationship between abuse and single-parenthood comes from a retrospective study where a random sample of parents were interviewed about their punishment histories as children (Sack, Mason, & Higgins, 1985). They found frequencies were half as high among parents growing up in two-parent families. Abuse was more likely when the parental separation was due to divorce rather than death. Although these studies suggest a link between single parenthood and maltreatment, conclusive data are not available.

It has generally been thought that child abuse is highest in families with the largest numbers of children. Data for all forms of maltreatment indicate an average of 2.23 children per family compared with a national average of 1.89 (Russell & Trainor, 1984). More detailed evidence suggests that there is a complex relationship (Straus *et al.*, 1980). Straus *et al.* found that the rate of abuse was twice as high in families with two children than for those with only one. The rate peaked for five children families and then declined with the least violence in the largest families. They propose that this latter finding is due to the ability of older children in the largest families to help with child care and other household responsibilities. In addition, they report that economic stress caused by large numbers of children was related to abuse rates. The presence of each extra child increased the probability of abuse in the poorest but not the most economically advantaged homes.

Social Isolation

The importance of social networks has been studied for more than a century (Brownell & Shumaker, 1984). Most social scientists recognize that social support indirectly and directly influences physical and psychological well-being (Mitchell, Billings, & Moos, 1982). It is commonly concluded that such support serves to reduce the impact of stressful events (Brownell & Shumaker, 1984), and promotes a sense of identity, self-esteem, and physical well-being (Shumaker & Brownell, 1984). Social support provides help with child care, access to resources in times of stress or crisis, and allows interested outsiders to monitor what happens within the family (Garbarino, 1977b).

Similarly, some authors consider the presence of social isolation to be one of the key causal factors in child abuse (see Garbarino & Gilliam, 1980). The basic hypothesis is that a person with a strong, supportive social network has an increased ability to cope with stress. Social support can thus compensate for high levels of economic or other stressors. According to this view, poverty is both an economic and a social concept. The stress produced by social impoverishment may strengthen a family's predisposition to violence. This hypothesis was tested in a study comparing two neighborhoods matched for social class but differing markedly in reported abuse and neglect (Garbarino & Sherman, 1980).

Families in the low maltreatment neighborhoods had more extensive social networks, were more available to meet their children's needs, and were subjected to less stress. There was an attitude of competition rather than cooperation among the high-risk families.

Results of one prospective study also suggest abusive families are isolated (Altemeier *et al.*, 1979). High-risk status was significantly correlated with social isolation, which in turn was related to maltreatment. This finding is at best suggestive of a connection between isolation and abuse given the indirect nature of the relationship.

Numerous retrospective studies have examined the presence or absence of support networks in abusive and control or contrast families (e.g., Disbrow *et al.* 1977; Elmer 1977; Kotelchuck 1982; Oates *et al.* 1979; Starr, 1982). All provide varying degrees of confirmation for the hypothesis that abusive families lack social support networks. Kotelchuck (1982) described isolation as a major characteristic of his sample. Starr (1982), using many of the identical questions, provided partial confirmation of Kotelchuck's findings. In particular, in both studies, abusive mothers met less often with friends and relatives and *perceived* these meetings as not occurring often enough. Similarly, Milner and Wimberley (1980) found abuse group parents reported intense feelings of loneliness, and Disbrow *et al.* (1977) stated that abusive mothers felt trapped with their children, suggesting that there may be a psychological component to isolation.

Societal Acceptance of Violence

Violence toward children is normative in the United States. Most parents, regardless of social class, see slapping and spanking a 12-year-old as proper and appropriate (Straus *et al.*, 1980). Overall, 63% of parents surveyed were violent to their child on at least one occasion during the survey year. Although such corporal punishment is not presently considered to be child abuse in the United States, it is seen as part of a continuum of which abuse represents the extreme (N. Feshbach, 1980). Feshbach noted the paradox present in the legality of corporal punishment in schools combined with the requirement that teachers report the very maltreatment some feel that they commit. Educators in some states can punish children by means that would result in removal of children from the home if done by parents in other states (*Landeros v. Flood,* 1976, cited in Newberger & Bourne, 1978). Many authors consider the continued acceptance of corporal punishment in schools as key examples of the social acceptability of violence toward children in the U.S. (see Hyman & Wise, 1979).

Cross-cultural analyses support the proposition that childrearing practices in these countries lead to maltreatment (Korbin, 1980b). Thus, parents in Western countries are more likely to raise children in nuclear rather than extended households, and are lower in infant indulgence, starting child training at early ages. Korbin proposed that these caregiving practices, belonging as they do to the extreme end of the caregiving continuum, when combined with low levels of social support, lead to an increased risk of maltreatment. With the acceptance of violence in caregiving in the United States, it is relatively easier for a parent to overstep the bounds of acceptable care than it would be for a parent in a less violent society.

There are differences in violence rates among Western countries. A comparison of Sweden and the United States is a frequently cited example. In 1966 the right of Swedish parents to beat their children was rescinded (Swedish Information Service, undated). In 1979 this was extended to a ban on not only corporal punishment, but also other forms of humiliating treatment by a 259 to 9 vote in Parliament. The passage of the legislation was tied to surveys showing a drop in the belief that chastisement was needed for discipline from 53% in 1945 to 26% in 1978. The Swedish law was meant to establish a norm for parental conduct rather than to place all offending parents in prison (Solheim, 1982). The 1979 law was based on a belief in a caregiving continuum; if mild discipline is allowed, it opens the door for more severe punishment (Ekdahl, 1980). It was implemented with a massive, positive public education campaign designed to achieve voluntary compliance. The Swedish ban was not a sudden move; it was embedded in their culture, which places more emphasis on the role of government in family life and childrearing than has been the case in the United States (Carlsson, 1980).

CHILD FACTORS

Over the past 20 years there has been an increasing awareness of the effects that children have on their parents and on the caregiving they provide to them (Bell & Harper, 1977). Theories of child abuse have often considered child factors as important instigators of abuse (Burgess & Garbarino, 1983; Gelles, 1973; Parke, 1982; Parke & Collmer, 1975; Starr, 1978). As was the case with studies of parental characteristics, most studies of child variables are retrospective. Thus, it is difficult to state whether a given behavior exhibited by abused children is a cause or a consequence of maltreatment. Within this constraint, contributory child factors will be discussed first, followed by research on the sequence of maltreatment.

The Child's Role in Abuse

Variables believed to place children at increased risk of maltreatment include young age, prematurity, handicaps, difficult temperament, and behavioral or emotional difficulties. It is logical that children who differ from the norm should be at increased risk for maltreatment.

Child Age. Younger children appear to be at greater risk for physical abuse (Friedrich & Einbender, 1983). Such children spend more time with their caregivers and are more dependent on them, increasing the probability that their behavior might be frustrating. In addition, younger children are more likely to be injured by a blow of a given intensity and are less able to anticipate and avoid punishment. Nationally, 64% of abused children with major physical injuries and 37% of those with minor ones were less than 6 years old (American Humane Association, 1985). The corresponding figures for children over 11 years old are 16% and 30%, suggesting that young age is a risk factor for major but not minor injury. National survey data indicate that physical force is more often used against younger children (Straus *et al.*, 1980). Children less than 5 years old and 15- to 17-years-old were most likely to experience potentially injurious violence. Overall, 6.7% of 3- and 4-year-olds and 4.3% of older teens were subjected to such parental violence. No gender differences were found for younger children; boys and girls less than 9 years old were equally likely to experience violence. Older boys however, were more often subjected to violence than were older girls.

Perinatal Events and Birth Defects. Reviews of the literature suggest that prematurity and other handicapping conditions predispose children to maltreatment (Friedrich & Boriskin, 1976; Frodi, 1981; Nesbit & Karagianis, 1982). However, most of the relevant studies cited by these authors did not use matched control groups. With regard to prematurity, a comprehensive review of research found that the results of controlled studies were inconclusive (Starr, Dietrich, Fischhoff, Ceresnie, & Zweier, 1984). Results of one prospective study suggested that normal birth weight was the greater risk factor (P. Vietze, personal communication, June, 1983). Results of a second prospective study found a 6% prematurity rate in both a maltreated sample and a group of infants receiving high-quality care (Egeland & Vaughn, 1981). In a third prospective study, 3.9% of a sample of 255 premature infants were abused, a figure somewhat higher than would be expected, but not one suggesting premature infants are a major at-risk population (Hunter, Kilstrom, & Kraybill, 1978). Some retrospective studies and case-sibling comparisons find premature infants are overrepresented in abuse groups (Elmer, 1977; Herrenkohl & Herrenkohl, 1979; Lynch & Roberts, 1977, 1982; Starr *et al.*, 1982). Other such studies find no differences (Corey, Miller, & Widlack, 1975; Holman & Kanwar, 1975; Kotelchuck, 1982; Starr, 1982). The results of the previously cited studies are inconclusive. Case sibling assessments suggest that prematurity is a risk factor whereas prospective studies lead to a conclusion that it probably is not. As Egeland and Vaughn (1981) suggested, the vast majority of prematurely born infants are not later abused.

Results of studies examining the relation of perinatal problems to abuse are similarly inconclusive. Prospective studies suggest children who were later maltreated were at no greater perinatal risk (Egeland & Vaughn, 1981; Vietze, O'Connor, & Altemeier, 1983). This conclusion is supported by some retrospective studies (Benedict, White, & Cornerly, 1985; Gaines *et al.*, 1978; Kotelchuck, 1982; Starr, 1982; Starr *et al.*, 1982), but not by others (Elmer, 1977; Holman & Kanwar, 1975; Lynch, 1975; Lynch & Roberts, 1977, 1982; Nakou, Adam, Stathacopoulou, & Agathonos, 1982).

Studies of the relationship between congenital disorders and abuse lead to the conclusion that children with physical anomalies are not at increased risk. No relationship was found between handicaps and abuse in prospective studies (Egeland & Vaughn, 1981; Sherrod, O'Connor, Vietze, & Altemeier, 1984) and three retrospective evaluations (Herrenkohl & Herrenkohl, 1979; Starr, 1982; Starr *et al.*, 1982). An exception is a high incidence of handicaps reported by Lightcap, Kurland, and Burgess (1982).

Given the extensive literature concerning the major effects premature and handicapped children have on family functioning (see Murphy, 1982), it is surprising that such conditions are not clearly related to abuse. It may be that the diagnosis of a handicap leads to reduced parental expectations, increased tolerance of deviant behaviors, increased social support, and reduced likelihood of abuse (Martin, 1982; Martin & Beezley, 1974). The child with more subtle developmental abnormalities may be at greater risk for abuse (Martin, 1982; Martin & Beezley, 1974). This hypothesis is supported by results of prospective studies showing performance differences between high- and low-risk infants on the Brazelton Neonatal Behavioral Assessment Scale, which examines such subtle behavioral differences (Egeland *et al.*, 1979; Vietze *et al.*, 1983).

Child Health. Some investigators have reported unhealthy children are more likely to be abused, most likely because of added stress on parent–child relations. Lynch (1975), comparing abused children with siblings, found the abused group had significantly more major and minor health problems and illnesses in the first year of life. The siblings tended to be very healthy; only 3 of 35 siblings were in poorer health than the abused child from the same family. Lynch's findings are corroborated by Sherrod *et al*'s. (1984) prospective study. Infants who were later abused had more frequent infectious illness in the first 6 months of life. Other studies have failed to replicate these findings for either abused child versus sibling (Starr *et al.*, 1982) or abuse-control group comparisons (Kotelchuck,

1982). Thus, although poor child health may contribute to abuse, it is far from a determining factor.

137

PHYSICAL ABUSE OF
CHILDREN

Effects of Abuse on Children

Abused children have been described as having a number of cognitive, emotional, and social difficulties (see reviews by Aber & Cicchetti, 1982; Friedrich & Einbender, 1983; Frodi, 1981; Lamphear, 1985; Martin, 1976; National Center on Child Abuse and Neglect, 1979; Toro, 1982). Once again, because most of our knowledge is based on retrospective studies, we do not know whether these inadequacies were present prior to maltreatment and may have been causal, or are a consequence of maltreatment. However, this research does provide a guide for improving treatment for abused children.

Cognitive Deficits. A number of studies have found intellectual deficits in abused children (see Friedrich & Einbender, 1983; Hoffman-Plotkin & Twentyman, 1984). Studies typically report wide variance in the IQ of abused children. In one study the mean IQ for abused children was 92 with a standard deviation of almost 22 points (Martin, Beezley, Conway, & Kempe, 1974). However, the failure of some well-controlled retrospective studies (Starr, 1982; Starr *et al.*, 1982) and one prospective study (Egeland & Sroufe, 1981a) to find differences suggests that the negative relationship between IQ and abuse is far from universal. Results of one study suggest that intellectual deficits are greater with more severe maltreatment (Dietrich *et al.*, 1983).

The relationship of abuse to other cognitive areas has been less well studied. Morgan (1979) evaluated children in classes for emotionally disturbed children and found abuse-control differences on five ITPA subtests but not for the test profile. Communication deficits have also been reported by Perry, Doran, and Wells (1983). Abused children appear to do less well in school, but fare better than neglected peers (Kent, 1976). Neurological deficits and learning disabilities are frequently assumed to be overrepresented in abused samples (Martin, 1976). Limited controlled research suggests that this may be the case (Green, Sandgrund, Gaines, & Haberfeld, 1974).

Only through controlled, longitudinal research can we clearly determine the relationship between cognitive functioning and maltreatment. At present, data are suggestive of a relationship, but we do not know whether such findings indicate causes or consequences of abuse.

Social and Emotional Deficits. More attention has been directed toward the social and emotional behaviors of abused children from birth on. Some authors suggest that the deficits start with bonding failure related to early mother–infant separation (Lynch & Roberts, 1977). However the presence of such separations is not confirmed by Kotelchuck (1982) and Starr (1982). This latter finding is supported by the findings of one prospective study examining bonding failure (Egeland & Vaughn, 1981), but not by a second (O'Connor, Vietze, Sherrod, Sandler, & Altemeier, 1980). A prospective study of attachment formation in maltreated infants suggests bonding failure, although characteristic of neglect cases, is less likely to be found in abusive families (Egeland & Sroufe, 1981b).

It has been hypothesized that some infant attributes may predispose them to abuse (Frodi, 1981). Frodi suggested that infants who are seen as difficult based on their being different (e.g., premature) or having irritating cries create greater physiological arousal indicative of anger in their caregivers. This anger is likely to be expressed through abuse.

Thus, abusers exhibited greater physiological arousal to a crying baby than nonabusers (Frodi & Lamb, 1980). Given the lack of convincing evidence about a higher risk of abuse in handicapped infants discussed earlier, this hypothesis must be considered speculative.

A number of studies have performed global assessments of social and emotional status in abused and control children (see Aber & Cicchetti, 1982; Friedrich & Einbender, 1983). In general, they show that, although abused children typically have socioemotional deficiencies in a number of areas, there is no consistent behavior pattern that would allow labeling a child as abused. Indeed, when all of the various behavior problems used to describe abused children are considered, they constitute a listing of most of the children's entries in DSM-III. According to one report they also exhibit one behavior pattern not typically considered deviant: pseudo-mature behavior (Martin & Beezley, 1976). It is hypothesized that some children prematurely develop adult behavior in order to decrease their chance of being maltreated for more age-appropriate actions. Overall, it has been reported that abused children do not differ significantly from nonabused children from distressed families receiving treatment at a child welfare clinic (Wolfe & Mosk, 1983).

Many studies have focused on aggression in abused and nonabused children. They generally conclude that abused children are more aggressive in a variety of settings as assessed using a number of instruments and observational coding methods (George & Main, 1979, 1980; Green, 1978b, c; Herrenkohl & Herrenkohl, 1981; Hoffman-Plotkin & Twentyman, 1984; Kinard, 1980, 1982b; Main & George, 1985; Reidy, 1977; Wolfe & Mosk, 1983). More specifically, aggression during psychological testing may be related to severity of abuse (Kinard, 1982b), although Starr (1982) found no abuse-control group behavior differences during testing.

These differences in aggression have been found early in life. Abused toddlers reacted to distress in agemates with aggression, fear, and anger, whereas their nonabused peers exhibited concern (Main & George, 1985). Finally, abused children were the most threatening and aggressive family members in clinical settings (Reid, Taplin, & Lorber, 1981).

A variety of other social and emotional behaviors have been reported in abused compared to control children. These include external locus of control and decreased ability to comprehend social roles and label feelings (Barahal, Waterman, & Martin, 1981), more reality-based fear (Kinard, 1980), greater immaturity and decreased readiness to learn (Hoffman-Plotkin & Twentyman, 1984), depression (Green, 1978c; Wolfe & Mosk, 1983), and hyperactivity and anxiety (Wolfe & Mosk, 1983).

Thus, the picture that emerges is of verbal and physical aggression as a response to violent acts. Aside from this relatively specific reaction to abuse, there appears to be no typical maltreated child just as there is no typical abusive parent. There are, however, significant limitations to our knowledge concerning abused children. First, we are still uncertain about those child characteristics that might play a causal role in abuse and those that are a consequence of maltreatment. Second, most studies have significant methodological deficiencies, including inadequate control groups and investigator knowledge of group membership (Aber & Cicchetti, 1982).

Follow-up Studies

A number of studies have followed-up maltreated children in order to assess their long-term development (Elmer, 1977; Friedman & Morse, 1974; Kent, 1976; Morse, Sahler, & Friedman, 1970). Although these studies suffer from the limitations listed in the preceding paragraph, they have led to controversy. Kent (1976) compared abused, neglected, and nonmaltreated protective service (PS) cases at intake into the PS system and later, after at least 12 months of treatment. Approximately 80% of the maltreated children had been removed from their biological parents. Upon intake, the abused children had more problem behaviors, including aggressiveness. Follow-up results indicated that abuse sample aggression declined to the level of the neglect group but was still higher than that for the control group. Removal of the abused and neglected children from their homes also led to decreased withdrawal, improved peer relations, and general improvement in all problem behaviors. However, the foster homes were generally higher in social class than the biological homes, a factor that could account for some of Kent's findings.

The most controversial study is by Elmer (1977). She found few differences between abused, accidentally injured, and control children on follow-up. All three groups were not faring well. She concluded that the lower social class status of all the families in her study was a more important determinant of child development than abuse. These results are supported by Starr (1982), who found few differences between his abuse and control groups. Problems with Elmer's study include inadequate group assignment procedures and the possibility of abuse in the control and contrast groups (Aber & Cicchetti, 1982). However, Aber and Cicchetti are careful to note that Elmer's results should be considered tentative, not that they disagree with her conclusions. We can hope that better designed follow-up studies will clarify the sequelae of maltreatment.

PARENT–CHILD INTERACTION FACTORS

Many controlled studies have examined parent–child interaction patterns with a common conclusion that abusive parents differ from control ones, but abused children do not necessarily differ from control children. A recent review of 10 studies of parental behavior concluded that abusive parents show more aversive and fewer prosocial behaviors (Wolfe, 1985). Additional studies support this conclusion of parental interactional deficits (e.g., Dietrich et al., 1983; Herrenkohl, Herrenkohl, Toedter, & Yanushefski, 1984). Dietrich et al. found significant differences between families in which both abuse and neglect were present, those with only abuse or neglect, and a control group, on a factor labeled mutual engagement, which examined such variables as synchronization of feeding, maternal ease in caretaking, response to distress, sensitivity, and delight. Maternal variables were more important than infant ones. The authors concluded that relational variables are at the heart of the problem of infant maltreatment. Similarly, Herrenkohl et al. (1984) found that parents who were both neglecting and used harsh discipline practices (including abuse) used more negative and fewer positive behaviors and were rated as more hostile. Parents who used harsh discipline but were not neglectful had more negative global ratings. These findings thus support those of Burgess and Conger (1978), who reported more negative and less positive interaction in abusive families. In addition, the Herrenkohl et al. results support Elmer's (1977) conclusion of income-related risk. They found that parental interaction patterns were significantly related to income. Lower income parents were more parent-centered and rejecting of their children than upper income parents.

Not surprisingly, increased aggression is the most frequently observed behavior exhibited by abused children (Bousha & Twentyman, 1984; Burgess & Conger, 1977; George & Main, 1979, 1980; Herrenkohl et al., 1984; Reid et al., 1981). In particular, Reid et al. found that more aversive behaviors were directed toward mothers than fathers, and abused children were verbally and physically aggressive. They suggest that social learning plays a major role in the behavior of abused children. This is supported by Burgess and Conger, who reported similar interaction patterns in abused children and their parents. They touched each other less often than control family members, and the interactions among abused children were less reciprocal and more coercive.

George and Main (1979, 1980) found the interaction behaviors of abused children in a preschool setting were similar to those of rejected children from nonabusive families. Thus, there was avoidance of caregivers, a greater probability of aggression upon contact, and friendly approach was likely to be met with an indirect approach by the child. These findings suggest that parental rejection may be a critical factor in the behavioral patterns displayed by abused children. Another study comparing abused and nonabused children with a contrast group of behaviorally disturbed, hyperactive children found no differences between abuse and control groups, whereas the hyperactive children were more negative and noncompliant (Mash, Johnston, & Kovitz, 1983). The authors of a second study in which no child differences were found (Lahey et al., 1984) explain their findings by suggesting that the parental threshold for a punitive reaction to child misbehaviors is variable rather than fixed and is largely controlled by parental stress and emotional distress rather than child factors.

Additional dimensions on which abused children have been found to differ from control children include variables important in fostering mutuality in interactions (Dietrich et al., 1983), distortions in affective communication (Gaensbauer & Sands, 1979), and an overall higher level of negative behavior in harshly disciplined children (Herrenkohl et al., 1984). Results of two of these studies suggest there are more behavior problems in children who are both abused and neglected (Dietrich et al., 1983; Herrenkohl et al., 1984).

STUDIES OF IMMEDIATE PRECIPITATING FACTORS

Few studies have examined in detail the immediate precursors of abuse. One report found that child actions led to abuse in almost 57% of cases, drug or alcohol abuse in 13%, behavior generally considered socially inappropriate (e.g., stealing, running away) in 10%, with developmental problems accounting for the remainder of cases (Thomson, Paget, Bates, Mesch, & Putnam, cited in Herrenkohl, Herrenkohl, & Egolf, 1983). A second study also emphasizes negative child behaviors as immediate precursors of abuse (Kadushin & Martin, 1981). Behaviors included aggression (21%), stealing and lying (9%), and nine other less frequent child acts. The causal behavior was not specified in 16% of cases. Herrenkohl, Herrenkohl, and Egolf (1983), in the most detailed study to date found that, while events around mistreatment account for little of the total variance associated with abuse, child factors are contributors. Most of the child-related events associated with abuse are universal rather than unique or exceptional.

COMMENT

The preceding discussion of research on the causes and correlates of abuse supports the view that abuse is multiply determined with different variables being of importance in individual cases. However, the results of studies of parent-child interaction patterns discussed above and by Wolfe (1985), as well as the findings of studies of immediate precipitating factors, suggest that abuse represents a breakdown of the parent–child

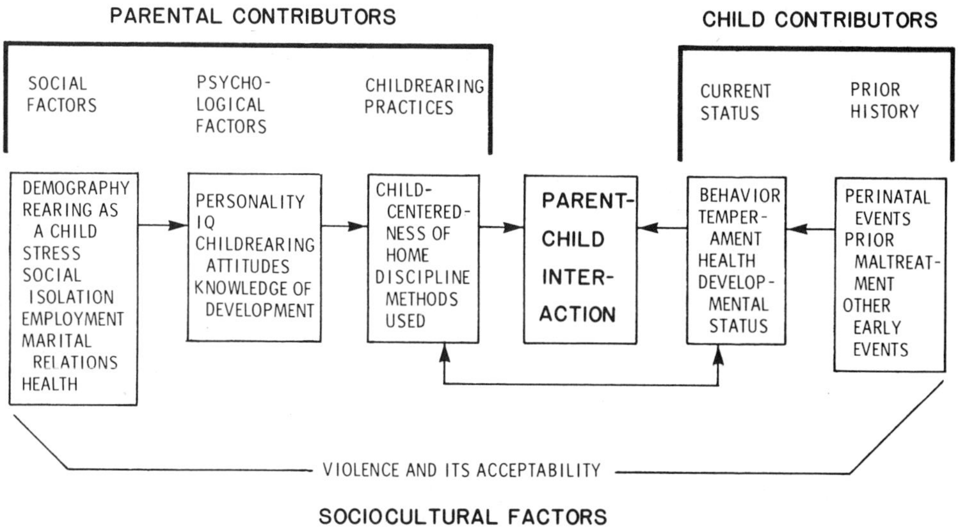

Figure 1. An ecological model of child abuse causation.

relationship. The role of parental psychological, social, child, and interactional variables is best interpreted using an ecological model (see Figure 1). This model emphasizes parent–child interaction patterns that are controlled by sociocultural, parental, and child contributors. The major sociocultural variable is the acceptability of violence in a society. There are three types of parental contributors: social factors, psychological factors, and childrearing practices. Social factors play a role in abuse only as they are filtered through parental psychological factors to determine childrearing practices. There are several specific aspects to each of the three parental contributors. These all influence each other (see Figure 2). Similarly, child contributors include the current status of the child and prior history variables that influence interactions through their effect on current status.

TREATMENT

Clinicians have focused their efforts on treating abusive parents and their children and have used a wide variety of methods. The most common therapeutic approach is social casework, which is frequently supplemented with parent-aides (lay persons who provide support and friendship and alleviate isolation), self-help or professionally led group therapy for parents, and crisis nurseries, child therapy, and foster care for children. Most families receive several different forms of treatment, with the average abusive family having three services (Shapiro, 1977).

A detailed discussion of treatment approaches is beyond the scope of this research-oriented chapter. A number of guides are available which detail commonly used therapeutic approaches with an emphasis on social casework (e.g., Ebeling & Hill, 1983; Faller, 1981; Helfer & Kempe, 1976; Kempe & Helfer, 1972; National Center on Child Abuse and Neglect, 1975; Pallone & Malkemes, 1984; Schmitt, 1978). In general, the goals of social services provided to families are strengthening the family to avoid a need for placement of the child outside the home (23% of cases), modifying personal functioning (22%), and modifying family relationships (20%) (Shyne & Schroeder, 1978).

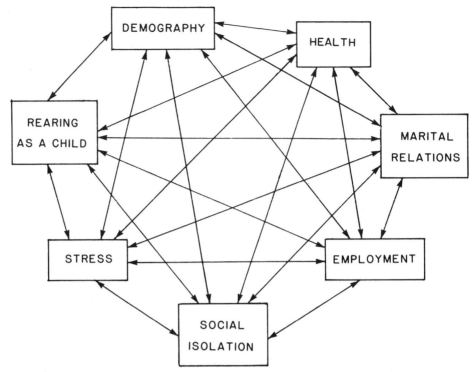

Figure 2. Sample interactions between variables within causal categories.

These conventional treatment approaches have been of only limited success. The best study of the effectiveness of various treatment approaches was an evaluation of 11 federally funded model demonstration treatment programs (Cohn, 1979a). Clinicians treating abuse and neglect cases were surveyed as to whether each of their cases had a reduced propensity for abuse or neglect. Approximately a third of the cases involved physical abuse. Positive results were found in only 42% of more than 1,700 cases. There was a severe recurrence of maltreatment in 30% of the cases during treatment with reabuse more common in serious cases (56% reincidence). The most effective treatment combination led to a 53% reduction in judged propensity for maltreatment. This was a program using conventional casework in conjunction with either a self-help group (Parents Anonymous) or a parent aide. Interestingly, these same cases were also the ones who were more likely to maltreat during the intervention period. Smaller case loads and longer treatment duration were also associated with greater improvement. The major conclusion is that it is unlikely that casework-based programs will be successful in more than half of treated cases. It remains to be demonstrated, however, what the baseline rate for improvement is in nontreated cases. If it is 5%, then the above results are quite good; if it is 35%, then they are far less impressive.

Three of the eleven treatment programs examined above also offered treatment to a total of 70 children (Cohn, 1979b). Cohn attributes the lack of child therapy to an emphasis on the role of the parent in abuse rather than on abuse as a result of deviant interactions, and the greater ease and lower cost of working with parents. As would be expected, the children had many problems. Over half of them were unable to give or receive attention, were unhappy, had deficits in attention span and self-concept, had inappropriate reactions to frustration, were deficient in interactions with adults and peers, and had parents who did not perceive or respond to their needs. Clinical staff judgments of improvement in these areas ranged from 41% for parental perception and response to needs, to from 59% to 79% for all but one of the child behavior problems. These results suggest that therapeutic efforts are more successful with children than with their parents. However, Cohn does not specify the duration of treatment or the time span between end of treatment and her follow-up evaluation. Similar improvements have been reported by Green (1978d). It should be remembered that the results of both of Cohn's reports are likely to be overestimates of treatment effectiveness because of possible positive biases resulting from clinical judgments of therapy effectiveness.

Success of treatment may also be related to parental satisfaction with services they receive. Pelton (1977) found social worker characteristics, particularly a willingness to go beyond the call of duty and an ability to be seen as friends rather than bureaucratic employees, were important in fostering parental satisfaction. Overall, 61% of the parents surveyed were satisfied and 30% had mixed opinions. However, the 45% of families who were unwilling to be interviewed may well have had more negative opinions and those who were interviewed may have cast their experiences in a more positive way to the male protective service system interviewer. Morse *et al.* (1970) found more negative parental feelings. None of their 13 parents felt the services were a success and 60% interviewed during a 3-year follow-up could not remember being helped. Given these findings, it is important that treatment programs develop ways of preventing high rates of worker turnover and burnout (Armstrong, cited in Sudia, 1981).

Findings of high rates of recurrence of abuse while in treatment and recidivism after treatment termination are additional indexes of the relative ineffectiveness of present agency-based treatment systems. Studies suggest that reabuse rates range from 20% (Johnson & Morse, 1968) to 60% (Skinner & Castle, 1969). The most comprehensive study of recurrence (indexed by repeated citations) found reabuse in 25% of families (Herenkohl, Herrenkohl, Egolf, & Seech, 1979). Because the families were in treatment, many incidents were not officially reported. Case record review found almost 70% of children had some reabuse during treatment. When closed cases were considered, 38% of these were reopened.

Sudia (1981) suggested that modifications in present treatment approaches would be beneficial. Some families should be considered not treatable (Wald, 1976). Agency priorities need to be shifted from a focus on meeting agency and staff needs toward meeting the needs of families. Giovannoni, Purvine, and Becerra (cited in Sudia, 1981) found caseworkers provided services that were most easily available, even though the families treated would benefit most from services they were unable to provide. There needs to be a better match between availability of and desire for specific services. Sudia suggested that effective treatment approaches will be those that provide a comprehensive approach to meeting the many needs of individual families.

Some investigators have designed such treatments using a behavioral perspective (e.g., Lutzker, 1984; Lutzker & Rice, 1984; Lutzker, Frame, & Rice, 1982; Lutzker, Wesch, & Rice, 1984; Wolfe, Kaufman, Aragona, & Sandler, 1981; Wolfe, Sandler, & Kaufman, 1981). Many other behaviorally oriented studies that are limited in scope have been undertaken (reviewed in Isaacs, 1982). For example, Reid *et al.* (1981) trained parents to reduce the total number of aversive child behaviors but did not attempt to modify other parental characteristics that might be associated with abuse. The approach taken by Wolfe and his associates is considerably broader. Wolfe, Kaufman, Aragona, and Sandler (1981) developed procedures designed to help parents better manage their children, resolve family conflicts and problems, control anger and aggression, and eliminate isolation through developing positive social contacts. In spite of limitations, their data suggest that the program was successful.

Lutzker's Project 12-Ways is the most comprehensive program. Based on an eco-behavioral approach (Lutzker, 1980), it provides training in 15 different areas that are matched to each family's needs. These are fostering the development of child skills; parent–child training, including compliance and other areas; stress reduction; assertiveness training; behavior management across settings; self-control; job finding; money management; leisure time activities; social support; alcoholism treatment or referral; home safety; health maintenance; intervention with unwed mothers; and marital counseling (Lutzker, 1984). The average number of treatment goals was three, with a range of from none (families terminating prior to the start of therapy) to 7. Over the first 4 years of the program, between 15% and 35% of cases were referred for physical abuse. The largest number (25% to 45%) were for child maltreatment prevention services. The major evaluation is a comparison of recidivism rates for families seen in 1980, 1981, and 1982. Project families were compared with matched samples of maltreating families who received only conventional protective services casework. Preliminary results suggest that Project 12-Ways was effective in lowering recidivism rates. Thus, an ecologically based treatment program focusing on improving parent–child relations shows promise as an alternative or supplement to conventional casework.

Treatment of abusive cases remains a problematic area. Present approaches are marked by high worker stress, inadequate funding, parental dissatisfaction, a lack of programming for children, and high recidivism. Current research suggests that programs designed to meet the needs of abusive families and to focus on parent–child relationships can be developed. However, it bears emphasizing that even the best treatment programs will not succeed with all families. These cases need to be identified and alternative means of protecting the children in them developed.

PREDICTION

Given the social importance of lessening the incidence and severity of child abuse, it is not surprising that a number of projects have evaluated the feasibility of primary and secondary prevention strategies. Secondary prevention strategies oriented toward detecting, and, to a lesser extent, working with families at risk for abuse will be discussed first followed by a review of primary prevention research.

Most work concerning secondary prevention has focused on the development of measures to detect families with a high probability of being abusive at a future time. A variety of strategies have been used in these studies, including retrospective analyses of research results comparing abusive and control families (Disbrow et al., 1977; Gaines et al., 1978; Kotelchuck, 1982; Starr, 1982), validation of predictive instruments using samples with known characteristics (Milner & Wimberley, 1979, 1980; Schneider, 1982), and prospective studies (Altemeier et al., 1979; Gray, Cutler, Dean, & Kempe, 1977, 1979; Murphy & Orkow, 1985).

Findings of retrospective studies using the results of controlled research to develop predictive equations that are validated by discriminant function analyses suggest measures with a sensitivity (% of abuse cases correctly classified) and specificity (% of control cases correctly classified) of approximately 75% can be developed. Thus, Starr (1982) found 73% of his abuse group could be correctly classified as abusive, and 67% of his control sample were classified as in the control group. He noted that although these are considered good results, between 24% and 33% of cases assessed using a questionnaire based on his results would be falsely labeled as potentially abusive and would need intervention services.

Studies of predictive questionnaires based on theoretical approaches to understanding abuse suggest this could be a fruitful way to detect high-risk families. Milner and Wimberley (1980) found that a psychologically oriented questionnaire had a sensitivity of 92% and a specificity of 100%. However, these are artificially high figures because their analyses involved assessing the predictive validity of their instrument against the sample used to collect their original data. Results validating questionnaires with independent samples are typically lower (Starr, 1982). Findings for the most widely used questionnaire, the Michigan Screening Profile for Parenting, are less positive. Schneider (1982) reports an average sensitivity of 80% and an average specificity of 70% across a variety of samples. However, this measure appears to be highly sensitive to social class differences with lower social class individuals being much more likely to be labeled as at risk. Such instruments need considerable improvement if they are to be of practical utility.

Results of three prospective studies demonstrate that abuse occurs much more frequently in high-risk families. Murphy and Orkow (1985) found 7% of 587 women interviewed during pregnancy were high risk based on responses to a 10-item checklist. Comparing these mothers with 100 low-risk mothers, their questionnaire had a sensitivity of 80% and a specificity of 89% for later abuse and neglect. The neglect or abuse rate was 10 times higher in the high-risk group. Although abuse was present in 10 children, they do not state how many of these cases were high and how many were low risk. In addition, comparisons of maltreating and nonmaltreating high-risk parents failed to indicate any factors that differentiated them from each other and might lead some to maltreat and others to provide more adequate care. Altemeier et al. (1979), in a study described earlier, found abuse was 11 times more frequent in their 273 high-risk families (4.4%) than in the remaining 1,127 families sampled (0.4%). In the third study, Gray et al. (1979) observed mothers during delivery of and interacting with their newborns. Based on these observations, their sample was divided into a low-risk and two high-risk groups. One at-risk group was provided with intervention including weekly public health nurse visits and the other with no additional services. Follow-up when children were between 17 and 35 months old showed 44% of high-risk and 8% of low-risk families had some indication of abnormal parenting. Overall, 8% of high- and no low-risk children had been reported to the central state child abuse registry. Quantitative analyses comparing the high risk intervention and nonintervention groups showed only one significant difference: a reduction in serious, inflicted injury. None of the children in the intervention group suffered injuries severe enough to result in hospitalization compared to 10% of the nonintervention sample. The services provided the intervention group appear to allow early detection and correction of abnormal parenting prior to the point of severe injury. Overall, the perinatal observations correctly predicted potential for abnormal parenting 76% of the time compared with 57% correct for a questionnaire that was also used. This approach had high sensitivity and low specificity.

Screening and prediction will be futile unless we have appropriate intervention methods (Altemeier et al., 1979), will provide the funds needed for their use, reduce the rate of false positives dramatically (Albee, 1980; Light, 1973; Starr, 1979), and can resolve ethical and legal problems including the rights of family privacy. Brody and Gaiss (1976), in an analysis of ethical issues in screening, discuss a number of these problems. Thus, programs would need to balance parental and child rights, individualize services, decide whether participation is mandatory or voluntary, provide full disclosure about the program if participation is voluntary, minimize coercion, and consider the negative effects of falsely labeling a parent as high risk (see Hobbs, 1975). In particular, we need to resolve due process and informed consent problems before predictive instruments can be widely used (Duquette, 1982). Specifically, the issue is whether parents should be told that the observations being made or the questions being answered may result in the provision of services, including being monitored for possible abusive behavior, even though they may not actually be abusive (Albee, 1980).

PRIMARY PREVENTION

Much of our current concern about child abuse focuses on primary prevention. In spite of this emphasis, there has been relatively little competent evaluation of prevention programs (Giovannoni, 1982; Helfer, 1982; Rosenberg & Reppucci, 1985) even though some emphasize the need for evaluation (e.g., Gray & DiLeonardi, 1982). Most prevention programs have not included an evaluation component and, because child abuse is a relatively low-base-rate behavior, such studies must be relatively large and are expensive to conduct (Cohen, Gray, & Wald, 1984). In spite of these difficulties, prevention is emphasized because of a humanitarian desire to eliminate abuse and our relative inability to develop effective treatment programs (Gabinet, 1983) and valid predictive instruments.

Preventive approaches have been proposed that are directed toward each of the parts of the ecological model presented in Fig. 1. Cohn (1983), drawing largely on the excellent work of Gray (1983a, b, c, d), sees a need for two types of community activity, community organization and public education, and eight types of prevention programs: support for new parents; parent education; screening and treatment; availability of appropriate child care; programs for victims of abuse to prevent its repetition; training in life skills for children and young adults; improved neighborhood supports and self-help groups; and services supporting families.

The current status of primary prevention has recently been reviewed by Rosenberg and Reppucci (1985), who concluded that health visitors, such as those used by Gray *et al.* (1979) in the study discussed in the preceding section, are probably an effective approach. The validity of other strategies has been neither demonstrated nor disproven. Rosenberg and Reppucci carefully analyze the research to date and suggest that there is a need to (a) require prevention programs to detail and measure objectively the relation between methods (stress reduction, for example) and goals (a reduction in abuse); (b) improve our knowledge of child abuse incidence and the use of service systems; (c) acquire more basic knowledge of the ecology of maltreatment so that prevention strategies could be directed toward those factors most closely related to abuse; (d) study the impact of child abuse prevention programs on the incidence of other deviant behaviors; (e) compare the effectiveness of different strategies; (f) include long-term follow-up; and (g) provide secure funding for programs and their evaluation.

SUMMARY

Eliminating child abuse will be difficult. First, we must continue to deal with reported cases. There are problems with our reporting system that were detailed earlier in this chapter. These lead to an overburdened system that is unable to investigate adequately reports and cannot provide appropriate treatment (Solnit, 1980). Some have even suggested that we need major reforms in child protection law (e.g., Stein, 1984). Second, we need to follow the recommendations of Rosenberg and Reppucci (1985) and develop effective prevention programs. Third, both of these measures must be integrated into a comprehensive child welfare policy rather than the present conglomeration of peacemeal programs (Kahn & Kamerman, 1980). This policy would have to resolve such difficult issues as the proportional allocation of funds between treatment and prevention programs (Giovannoni, 1982).

Child abuse came to be of national concern through a complex set of processes. In addition to events detailed in the history section of this chapter, abuse can be tied to the agenda setting process of Congress, the federal bureaucracy, state and local governments, and private social service and health agencies (Nelson, 1984). Nelson proposed that the present concern with abuse is the result of the availability of resources at the governmental level and labeling of child abuse as a social problem. Although abuse remains on the social service agenda at the present time, efforts need to be made to keep it from suffering the fate of many other major issues that have fallen from public interest: what Downs (1972) has called the issue attention cycle. The viability of child abuse as a social issue relies in part on our knowledge about it and about ways of treating and preventing it, and in part on continuing public and legislative concern about maltreatment. The purpose of this chapter has been to provide a summary of current knowledge to be used as a foundation for future research, prevention efforts, and social action.

ACKNOWLEDGMENT

The author thanks Professor Robert Deluty for his discerning review of a draft of this chapter.

REFERENCES

Aber, J. L., & Cicchetti, D. (1982). The socio-emotional development of maltreated children: An empirical and theoretical analysis. In H. Fitzgerald, B. Lester, & M. Yogman, (Eds.), *Theory and research in behavioral pediatrics* (Vol. 2, pp. 118–187). New York: Plenum Press.

Albee, G. W. (1980). Primary prevention and social problems. In G. Gerbner, C. J. Ross, & E. Zigler (Eds.), *Child abuse: An agenda for action* (pp. 106–117). New York: Oxford University Press.

Adams, W., Barone, N., & Tooman, P. (1982). The dilemma of anonymous reporting in child protective services. *Child Welfare, 61,* 3–14.

Altemeier, W. A., III, Vietze, P. M., Sherrod, K. B., Sandler, H. M., Falsey, S., & O'Connor, S. (1979). Prediction of child maltreatment during pregnancy. *Journal of the American Academy of Child Psychiatry, 18,* 205–218.

American Humane Association. (1985). *Highlights of official child neglect and abuse reporting 1983.* Denver CO: Author.

Anderson, S. C., & Lauderdale, M. L. (1982). Characteristics of abusive parents: A look at self-esteem. *Child Abuse and Neglect, 6,* 285–293.

Bakan, D. (1971). *Slaughter of the innocents: A study of the battered child phenomenon.* Boston, MA: Beacon Press.

Bandura, A. (1973). *Aggression: A social learning analysis.* Englewood Cliffs, NJ: Prentice-Hall.

Barahal, R. M., Waterman, J., & Martin, H. P. (1981). The social-cognitive development of abused children. *Journal of Consulting and Clinical Psychology, 49,* 508–516.

Baron, R. A. (1977). *Human aggression.* New York: Plenum Press.

Bell, R. Q., & Harper, L. V. (1977). *Child effects on parents.* Hillsdale, NJ: Erlbaum.

Belsky, J. (1980). Child maltreatment: An ecological integration. *American Psychologist, 35,* 320–335.

Benedict, M. I., White, R. B., & Cornely, D. A. (1985). Maternal perinatal risk factors and child abuse. *Child Abuse and Neglect, 9,* 217–224.

Berkowitz, L. (1974). Some determinants of impulsive aggression: Role of mediated associations with reinforcement for aggression. *Psychological Review, 81,* 165–176.

Besharov, D. (1978). *The abused and neglected child: Multidisciplinary court practice.* Philadelphia, PA: Practicing Law Institute.

Bousha, D. M., & Twentyman, C. T. (1984). Mother–child interactional style in abuse, neglect, and control groups: Naturalistic observations in the home. *Journal of Abnormal Psychology, 93,* 106–114.

Brody, H., & Gaiss, B. (1976, March). Ethical issues in screening for unusual childrearing practices. *Pediatric Annals,* pp. 106–112.

Brownell, A., & Shumaker, S. A. (1984). Social support: An introduction to a complex phenomenon. *Journal of Social Issues, 40*(4), 1–9.

Brunnquell, D., Crichton, L., & Egeland, B. (1981). Maternal personality and attitude in disturbances of childrearing. *American Journal of Orthopsychiatry, 51,* 680–691.

Burgess, R. L., & Conger, R. D. (1977). Family interaction patterns related to child abuse and neglect: Some preliminary findings. *Child Abuse and Neglect, 1,* 269–277.

Burgess, R. L., & Conger, R. D. (1978). Family interactions in abusive, neglectful, and normal families. *Child Development, 49,* 1163–1173.

Burgess, R. L., & Garbarino, J. (1983). Doing what comes naturally? An evolutionary perspective on child abuse. In D. Finkelhor, R. J. Gelles, G. T. Hotaling, & M. A. Straus (Eds.), *The dark side of families: Current family violence research* (pp. 88–101). Beverly Hills, CA: Sage.

Caffey, J. (1946). Multiple fractures in the long bones of infants suffering from Chronic Subdural Hematoma. *American Journal of Roentgenology, 56,* 163–173.

Caffey, J., & Silverman, W. A. (1945). Infantile cortical hyperostoses: Preliminary report on a new syndrome. *American Journal of Roentgenology, 54,* 1–16.

Carlsson, B. (1980). Violent childhood and the neglect of children's rights. In *The ombudsman and child maltreatment* (pp. 13–25). Stockholm, Sweden: Radda Barnen.

Carr, A. (1978). *Reported child maltreatment in Florida: The operation of public child protective service systems* (Report submitted to National Center on Child Abuse and Neglect, Department of Health, Education and Welfare, grant #90-C425). Unpublished manuscript, University of Rhode Island, Kingston.

Cohen, S., Gray, E., & Wald, M. (1984). Preventing a child maltreatment: A review of what we know. *Prevention focus* (Working paper No. 024). Chicago, IL: National Committee for Prevention of Child Abuse.

Cohler, B. J., Weiss, J. L., & Grunebaum, H. U. (1970). Child care attitudes and emotional disturbance among mothers of young children. *Genetic Psychology Monographs, 82,* 3–47.

Cohn, A. H. (1979a). Essential components of successful child abuse and neglect treatment. *Child Abuse and Neglect, 3,* 491–496.

Cohn, A. H. (1979b). An evaluation of three demonstration child abuse and neglect treatment programs. *Journal of the American Academy of Child Psychiatry, 18,* 283–291.

Cohn, A. H. (1983). *An approach to preventing child abuse.* Chicago, IL: National Committee for Prevention of Child Abuse.

Conger, R. D., Burgess, R., & Barrett, C. (1979). Child abuse related to life change and perceptions of illness: Some preliminary findings. *Family Coordinator, 28,* 73–78.

Corey, E. J. B., Miller, C. L., & Widlak, F. W. (1975). Factors contributing to child abuse. *Nursing Research, 24,* 293–295.

DeFrancis, V. (1973). Protecting the abused child. In *Child Abuse Prevention Act, 1973, Hearings before the Subcommittee on Children and Youth of the Committee on Labor and Public Welfare, United States Senate on S. 1191* (pp. 323–333). Washington, DC: U.S. Government Printing Office.

deMause, L. (1974). The evolution of childhood. In L. deMause (Ed.), *The history of childhood* (pp. 1–74). New York: Psychohistory Press.

deMause, L. (1980). Our forbears made childhood a nightmare. In G. J. Williams & J. Money (Eds.), *Traumatic abuse and neglect of children at home* (pp. 14–20). Baltimore, MD: Johns Hopkins University Press.

Department of Health and Human Services. (1981). *Study findings: National study of the incidence and severity of child abuse and neglect* (DHHS Publication No. OHDS 81-30325). Washington, DC: U.S. Government Printing Office.

Dietrich, K. N., Starr, R. H., Jr., & Weisfeld, G. E. (1983). Infant maltreatment: Caretaker-infant interaction and developmental consequences at different levels of parenting failure. *Pediatrics, 72,* 532–540.

Disbrow, M. A., Doerr, H., & Caulfield, C. (1977). Measuring the components of parents' potential for child abuse and neglect. *Child Abuse and Neglect, 1,* 279–296.

Downs, A. (1972). Up and down with ecology: "The issue attention cycle." *Public Interest, 32,* (Summer), 38–50.

Duquette, D. N. (1982). Protecting individual liberties in the context of screening for child abuse. In R. H. Starr, Jr. (Ed.), *Child abuse prediction: Policy implications* (pp. 191–204). Cambridge, MA: Ballinger.

Ebeling, N. B., & Hill, D. A. (Eds.). (1983). *Child abuse and neglect: A guide with case studies for treating the child and family.* Boston, MA: John Wright.

Egeland, B. & Brunnquell, D. (1979). An at-risk approach to the study of child abuse. *Journal of the American Academy of Child Psychiatry, 18,* 219–235.

Egeland, B., & Sroufe, A. (1981a). Developmental sequelae of maltreatment in infancy. *New Directions for Child Development, 11,* 77–92.

Egeland, B., & Sroufe, L. A. (1981b). Attachment and early maltreatment. *Child development, 52,* 44–52.

Egeland, B., & Vaughn, B. (1981). Failure of "bond formation" as a cause of abuse, neglect, and maltreatment. *American Journal of Orthopsychiatry, 51,* 78–84.

Egeland, B., Deinard, A., Brunnquell, D., Phipps-Yonas, S., & Crichton, L. (1979). *A prospective study of the antecedents of child abuse* (Final report, Grant No. 90-C-424, National Center on Child Abuse and Neglect). Minneapolis, MN: University of Minnesota.

Egeland, B., Breitenbucher, M., & Rosenberg, D. (1980). Prospective study of the significance of life stress in the etiology of child abuse. *Journal of Consulting and Clinical Psychology, 48,* 194–205.

Ekdahl, B. (1980). The Swedish law on physical punishment. In *The ombudsman and child maltreatment* (pp. 6–11). Stockholm, Sweden: Radda Barnen.

Elmer, E. (1977). *Fragile families, troubled children: The aftermath of infant trauma.* Pittsburgh, PA: University of Pittsburgh Press.

Evans, A. L. (1980). Personality characteristics and disciplinary attitudes of child-abusing mothers. *Child Abuse and Neglect, 4,* 179–187.

Faller, K. C. (Ed.). (1981). *Social work with abused and neglected children: A manual of interdisciplinary practice.* New York: Free Press.

Feshbach, N. (1980). Corporal punishment in the schools: Some paradoxes, some facts, some possible directions. In G. Gerbner, C. J. Ross, & E. Zigler (Eds.), *Child abuse: An agenda for action* (pp. 204–221). New York: Oxford University Press.

Feshbach, S. (1980). Child abuse and the dynamics of human aggression and violence. In G. Gerbner, C. J. Ross, & E. Zigler (Eds.), *Child abuse: An agenda for action* (pp. 48–60). New York: Oxford University Press.

Friedman, S., & Morse, C. (1974). Child abuse: A five-year follow up of case finding in the emergency department. *Pediatrics, 54,* 404–410.

Friedrich, W. N., & Boriskin, J. A. (1976). The role of the child in abuse: A review of the literature. *American Journal of Orthopsychiatry, 46,* 580–590.

Friedrich, W. N., & Einbender, A. J. (1983). The abused child: A psychological review. *Journal of Clinical Child Psychology, 12,* 244–256.

Frodi, A. M. (1981). Contribution of infant characteristics to child abuse. *American Journal of Mental Deficiency, 85,* 341–349.

Frodi, A. M., & Lamb, M. E. (1980). Child abusers' responses to infant smiles and cries. *Child Development, 51,* 238–241.

Gabinet, L. (1983). Child abuse treatment failures reveal need for redefinition of problem. *Child Abuse and Neglect, 7,* 395–402.

Gaensbauer, T. J., & Sands, S. K. (1979). Distorted affective communications in abused/neglected infants and their potential impact on caretakers. *Journal of the American Academy of Child Psychiatry, 18,* 236–250.

Gaines, R., Sandgrund, A., Green, A. H., & Power, E. (1978). Etiological factors in child maltreatment: A multivariate study of abusing, neglecting, and normal mothers. *Journal of Abnormal Psychology, 87,* 531–540.

Garbarino, J. (1977a). The human ecology of child maltreatment: A conceptual model for research. *Journal of Marriage and the Family, 39,* 721–735.

Garbarino, J. (1977b). The price of privacy: An analysis of the social dynamics of child abuse. *Child Welfare, 56,* 565–575.

Garbarino, J., & Crouter, A. (1978). A note on the problem of construct validity in assessing the usefulness of child maltreatment report data. *American Journal of Public Health, 68,* 598–600.

Garbarino, J., & Gilliam, G. (1980). *Understanding abusive families.* Lexington, MA: Lexington Books.

Garbarino, J., & Sherman, D. (1980). High-risk neighborhoods and high-risk families: The human ecology of child maltreatment. *Child Development, 51,* 188–198.

Gelles, R. J. (1973). Child abuse as psychopathology: A sociological critique and reformulation. *American Journal of Orthopsychiatry, 43,* 611–621.

Gelles, R. J. (1978). Violence toward children in the United States. *American Journal of Orthopsychiatry, 48,* 580–592.

Gelles, R. J. (1982). Problems in defining and labeling child abuse. In R. H. Starr, Jr. (Ed.), *Child abuse prediction: Policy implications* (pp. 1–30). Cambridge, MA: Ballinger.

George, C., & Main, M. (1979). Social interactions of young abused children: Approach, avoidance, and aggression. *Child Development, 50,* 306–318.

George, C., & Main, M. (1980). Abused children: Their rejection of peers and caregivers. In T. M. Field, S. Goldberg, D. Stern, & A. M. Sostek (Eds.), *High-risk infants and children: Adult and peer interactions* (pp. 293–312). New York: Academic Press.

Gil, D. G. (1970). *Violence against children.* Cambridge, MA: Harvard University Press.

Giovannoni, J. M. (1982). Prevention of child abuse and neglect: Research and policy issues. *Social Work Research and Abstracts, 18,* 23–31.

Giovannoni, J. M., & Becerra, R. M. (1979). *Defining child abuse.* New York: Free Press.

Gray, E. B. (1983a). Final report: *Collaborative research of community and minority group action to prevent child abuse and neglect: Vol. I. Perinatal interventions.* Chicago, IL: National Committee for Prevention of Child Abuse.

Gray, E. B. (1983b). *Final report: Collaborative research of community and minority group action to prevent child abuse and neglect: Vol. II. Culture-based parent education programs.* Chicago, IL: National Committee for Prevention of Child Abuse.

Gray, E. B. (1983c). *Final report: Collaborative research of community and minority group action to prevent child abuse and neglect: Vol. III. Public awareness and education using the creative arts.* Chicago, IL: National Committee for Prevention of Child Abuse.

Gray, E. B. (1983d). *Final report: Collaborative research of community and minority group action to prevent child abuse and neglect: Vol. IV. Community-wide education, information and referral programs.* Chicago, IL: National Committee for Prevention of Child Abuse.

Gray, E., & DiLeonardi, J. (1982). *Evaluating child abuse prevention programs.* Chicago, IL: National Committee for Prevention of Child Abuse.

Gray, J. D., Cutler, C. A., Dean, J., & Kempe, C. H. (1977). Prediction and prevention of child abuse. *Child Abuse and Neglect, 1,* 45–58.

Gray, J., Cutler, C., Dean, J. & Kempe, C. H. (1979). Prediction and prevention of child abuse and neglect. *Journal of Social Issues, 35,* 127–139.

Green, A. H. (1978a). Child abuse. In B. B. Wolman, J. Egan, & A. O. Ross (Eds.), *Handbook of treatment of mental disorders in childhood and adolescence* (pp. 430–455). Englewood Cliffs, NJ: Prentice Hall.

Green, A. H. (1978b). Psychopathology of abused children. *Journal of the American Academy of Child Psychiatry, 17,* 92–103.

Green, A. H. (1978c). Self-destructive behavior in battered children. *American Journal of Psychiatry, 135,* 579–583.

Green, A. H. (1978d). Psychiatric treatment of abused children. *Journal of the American Academy of Child Psychiatry, 17,* 356–371.

Green, A. H., Sandgrund, A., Gaines, R., & Haberfeld, H. (1974, May). *Psychological sequelae of child abuse and neglect.* Paper presented at the meeting of the American Psychiatric Association, Detroit, MI.

Hampton, R. L., & Newberger, E. H. (1985). Child abuse incidence and reporting by hospitals: Significance of severity, class, and race. *American Journal of Public Health, 75,* 56–60.

Helfer, R. E. (1980). Developmental deficits which limit interpersonal skills. In C. H. Kempe & R. E. Helfer (Eds.), *The battered child* (3rd ed., pp. 36–48). Chicago, IL: University of Chicago Press.

Helfer, R. E. (1982). A review of the literature on the prevention of child abuse and neglect. *Child Abuse and Neglect, 6,* 251–261.

Helfer, R. E., & Kempe, C. H. (Eds.). (1976). *Child abuse and neglect: The family and the community.* Cambridge, MA: Ballinger Publishing.

Herrenkohl, E. C., & Herrenkohl, R. C. (1979). A comparison of abused children and their nonabused siblings. *Journal of the American Academy of Child Psychiatry, 18,* 260–269.

Herrenkohl, E. C., Herrenkohl, R. C., & Toedter, L. J. (1983). Perspectives on the intergenerational transmission of abuse. In D. Finkelhor, R. J. Gelles, G. T. Hotaling, & M. A. Straus (Eds.), *The dark side of families: Current family violence research* (pp. 305–316). Beverly Hills, CA: Sage.

Herrenkohl, E. C., Herrenkohl, R. C., Toedter, L., & Yanushefski, A. M. (1984). Parent–child interactions in abusive and nonabusive families. *Journal of the American Academy of Child Psychiatry, 23,* 641–648.

Herrenkohl, R. C., & Herrenkohl, E. C. (1981). Some antecedents and developmental consequences of child maltreatment. *New Directions for Child Development, 11,* 57–76.

Herrenkohl, R. C., Herrenkohl, E. C., Egolf, B., & Seech, M. (1979). The repetition of child abuse: How frequently does it occur? *Child Abuse and Neglect, 3,* 67–72.

Herrenkohl, R. C., Herrenkohl, E. C., & Egolf, B. P. (1983). Circumstances surrounding the occurrence of child maltreatment. *Journal of Consulting and Clinical Psychology, 51,* 424–431.

Hobbs, N. (1975). *The futures of children.* San Francisco: Jossey-Bass.

Hoffman-Plotkin, D., & Twentyman, C. T. (1984). A multimodal assessment of behavioral and cognitive deficits in abused and neglected preschoolers. *Child Development, 55,* 794–802.

Holman, R. R., & Kanwar, S. (1975). Early life of the "battered child." *Archives of Diseases of Children, 50,* 78–80.

Holmes, T. H., & Rahe, R. H. (1967). The Social Readjustment Rating Scale. *Journal of Psychosomatic Research, 11,* 213–218.

Hunter, R. S., & Kilstrom, N. (1979). Breaking the cycle in abusive families. *American Journal of Psychiatry, 136,* 1320–1322.

Hunter, R. S., Kilstrom, N., & Kraybill, E. N. (1978). Antecedents of child abuse and neglect among premature infants: A prospective study in a newborn intensive care unit. *Pediatrics, 61,* 629–635.

Hyman, I. A., & Wise, J. H. (Eds.). (1979). *Corporal punishment in American education.* Philadelphia, PA: Temple University Press.

Isaacs, C. D. (1982). Treatment of child abuse: A review of the behavioral interventions. *Journal of Applied Behavior Analysis, 15,* 273–294.

Jayaratne, S. (1977, January). Child abusers as parents and children: A review. *Social Work,* pp. 5–9.

Johnson, B., & Morse, H. (1968). *The battered child: A study of children with inflicted injuries.* Denver, CO: Department of Welfare.

Kadushin, A., & Martin, J. (1981). *Child abuse: An interactional event.* New York: Columbia University Press.

Kahn, A. J., & Kamerman, S. B. (1980). Child abuse: A comparative perspective. In G. Gerbner, C. J. Ross, & E. Zigler (Eds.), *Child abuse: An agenda for action* (pp. 118–134). New York: Oxford University Press.

Kempe, C. H. (1978). Child abuse: The pediatrician's role in child advocacy and preventive pediatrics. *American Journal of Diseases of Children, 132,* 255–260.

Kempe, C. H., & Helfer, R. E. (Eds.). (1972). *Helping the battered child and his family.* Philadelphia, PA: J. B. Lippincott.

Kempe, C. H., Silverman, F. N., Steele, B. F., Droegemueller, W., & Silver, H. K. (1962). The battered child syndrome. *Journal of the American Medical Association, 181,* 17–24.

Kent, J. T. (1976). A follow-up study of abused children. *Journal of Pediatric Psychology, 1,* 25–31.

Kessen, W. (1965). *The child.* New York: Wiley.

Kinard, E. M. (1980). Emotional development in physically abused children. *American Journal of Orthopsychiatry, 50,* 686–696.

Kinard, E. M. (1982a). Child abuse and depression: Cause or consequence? *Child Welfare, 61,* 403–413.

Kinard, E. M. (1982b). Experiencing child abuse: Effects on emotional adjustment. *American Journal of Orthopsychiatry, 52,* 82–91.

Korbin, J. E. (1980a). The cross-cultural context of child abuse and neglect. In C. H. Kempe & R. E. Helfer (Eds.), *The battered child* (3rd. ed., pp. 21–35). Chicago, IL: University of Chicago.

Korbin, J. E. (1980b). The cultural context of child abuse and neglect. *Child Abuse and Neglect, 4,* 3–13.

Korbin, J. E. (1981). Conclusions. In J. E. Korbin (Ed.), *Child abuse and neglect: Cross cultural perspectives* (pp. 205–210). Berkeley, CA: University of California Press.

Kotelchuk, M. (1982). Child abuse and neglect: Prediction and misclassification. In R. H. Starr, Jr. (Ed.), *Child abuse prediction: Policy implications* (pp. 67–104). Cambridge, MA: Ballinger.

Kravitz, R. A., & Driscoll, J. M. (1983). Expectations for childhood development among child-abusing and nonabusing parents. *American Journal of Orthopsychiatry, 53,* 336–344.

Lahey, B. B., Conger, R. D., Atkeson, B. M., & Treiber, F. A. (1984). Parenting behavior and emotional status of physically abusive mothers. *Journal of Consulting and Clinical Psychology, 52,* 1062–1071.

Lamphear, V. S. (1985). The impact of maltreatment on children's psychosocial adjustment: A review of the research. *Child Abuse and Neglect, 9,* 251–263.

Lanyon, R. L. (1970). Development and validation of a psychological screening inventory. *Journal of Consulting and Clinical Psychology, 35,* 1–24.

Larrance, D. T., & Twentyman, C. T. (1983). Maternal attributions and child abuse. *Journal of Abnormal Psychology, 92,* 449–457.

Leventhal, J. M. (1981). Risk factors for child abuse: Methodologic standards in case-control studies. *Pediatrics, 68,* 684–690.

Leventhal, J. M. (1982). Research strategies and methodologic standards in studies of risk factors for child abuse. *Child Abuse and Neglect, 6,* 113–123.

Light, R. J. (1973). Abused and neglected children in America: A study of alternative policies. *Harvard Educational Review, 43,* 556–598.

Lightcap, J. L., Kurland, J. A., & Burgess, R. L. (1982). Child abuse: A test of some predictions from evolutionary theory. *Ethology and Sociobiology, 3,* 61–67.

Lutzker, J. R. (1980). Deviant family systems. In B. Lahey & A. Kazdin (Eds.), *Advances in clinical child psychology* (Vol. 3). New York: Plenum Press.

Lutzker, J. R. (1984). Project 12-Ways: Treating child abuse and neglect from an ecobehavioral perspective. In R. F. Dangel & R. A. Polster (Eds.), *Parent training: Foundations of research and practice* (pp. 260–297). New York: Guilford Press.

Lutzker, J. R., & Rice, J. M. (1984). Project 12-Ways: Measuring outcome of a large in-home service for treatment and prevention of child abuse and neglect. *Child Abuse and Neglect, 8,* 519–524.

Lutzker, J. R., Frame, R. E., & Rice, J. M. (1982). Project 12-Ways: An ecobehavioral approach to the treatment and prevention of child abuse and neglect. *Education and Treatment of Children, 5,* 141–155.

Lutzker, J. R., Wesch, D., & Rice, J. M. (1984). A review of Project 12-Ways: An ecobehavioral approach to the treatment and prevention of child abuse and neglect. *Advances in Behaviour Research and Therapy, 6,* 63–73.

Lynch, M. A. (1975). Ill-health and child abuse. *Lancet, 2,* 317–319.

Lynch, M. A., & Roberts, J. (1977). Predicting child abuse: Signs of bonding failure in the maternity hospital. *British Medical Journal, 1,* 624–626.

Lynch, M. A., & Roberts, J. (1982). *Consequences of child abuse.* New York: Academic Press.

Main, M., & George, C. (1985). Responses of abused and disadvantaged toddlers to distress in agemates: A study in the day care setting. *Developmental Psychology, 21,* 407–412.

Martin, H. P. (Ed.). (1976). *The abused child: A multidisciplinary approach to developmental issues and treatment.* Cambridge, MA: Ballinger.

Martin, H. P. (1982). The clinical relevance of prediction and prevention. In R. H. Starr, Jr. (Ed.), *Child abuse prediction: Policy implications* (pp. 175–190). Cambridge, MA: Ballinger.

Martin, H. P., & Beezley, P. (1974). Prevention and the consequences of child abuse. *Journal of Operational Psychology, 6,* 68–77.

Martin, H. P., & Beezley, P. (1976). Personality of abused children. In H. P. Martin (Ed.), *The abused child: A multidisciplinary approach to developmental issues and treatment* (pp. 105–111). Cambridge, MA: Ballinger.

Martin, H. P., Beezley, P., Conway, E. F., & Kempe, C. H. (1974). The development of abused children. *Advances in Pediatrics, 21,* 25–73.

Mash, E. J., Johnston, C., & Kovitz, K. (1983). A comparison of the mother-child interactions of physically abused and non-abused children during play and task situations. *Journal of Clinical Child Psychology, 12,* 337–346.

McGuire, R. (1983, March 28). Victim's vision. *US,* pp. 68–69.

Miller, D., & Challas, G. (1981, July). *Abused children as adult parents: A twenty-five year longitudinal study.* Paper presented at the National Conference for Family Violence Researchers, Durham, NH.

Milner, J. S., & Wimberley, R. C. (1979). An inventory for the identification of child abusers. *Journal of Clinical Psychology, 35,* 95–100.

Milner, J. S., & Wimberly, R. C. (1980). Prediction and explanation of child abuse. *Journal of Clinical Psychology, 36,* 875–884.

Mitchell, R. E., Billings, A. G., & Moos, R. H. (1982). Social support and well-being: Implications for prevention programs. *Journal of Primary Prevention, 3*(2), 77–98.

Morgan, S. R. (1979). Psychoeducational profile of emotionally disturbed abused children. *Journal of Clinical Psychology, 8,* 3–6.

Morris, J. L., Johnson, C. F., & Clasen, M. (1985). To report or not report: Physicians' attitudes toward discipline and child abuse. *American Journal of Diseases of Children, 139,* 194–197.

Morris, M. G., & Gould, R. W. (1963). Role reversal: A concept in dealing with the "battered child syndrome." *American Journal of Orthopsychiatry, 33,* 298–299.

Morse, C. W., Sahler, O., & Friedman, S. (1970). A three-year follow-up study of abused and neglected children. *American Journal of Diseases of Children, 120,* 439–446.

Murphy, M. A. (1982). The family with a handicapped child: A review of the literature. *Developmental and Behavioral Pediatrics, 3,* 73–82.

Murphy, S., & Orkow, B. (1985). Prenatal prediction of child abuse and neglect: A prospective study. *Child Abuse and Neglect, 9,* 225–235.

Nagi, S. Z. (1977). *Child maltreatment in the United States: A challenge to social institutions.* New York: Columbia University Press.

Nakou, S., Adam, H., Stathacopoulou, M. A., & Agathonos, H. (1982). Health status of abused and neglected children and their siblings. *Child Abuse and Neglect, 6,* 279–284.

National Center on Child Abuse and Neglect. (1975). *Child abuse and neglect: The problem and its management* (Vols. 1–3) (DHEW Publication No. (OHD) 75-30073, 75-30074, 75-30075). Washington, DC: U.S. Government Printing Office.

National Center on Child Abuse and Neglect. (1979). *Child abuse and developmental disabilities: Essays* (DHEW Publication No. OHDS 79-30226). Washington, DC: U.S. Government Printing Office.

Nelson, B. J. (1984). *Making an issue of child abuse: Political agenda setting for social problems.* Chicago, IL: University of Chicago Press.

Nesbit, W. C., & Karagianis, L. D. (1982). Child abuse: Exceptionality as a risk factor. *Alberta Journal of Educational Research, 28,* 69–76.

Newberger, E. H. (1984). The helping hand strikes again: Unintended consequences of child abuse reporting. *Journal of Clinical Child Psychology, 12,* 307–311.

Newberger, E. H., & Bourne, R. (1978). The medicalization and legalization of child abuse. *American Journal of Orthopsychiatry, 48,* 593–607.

Oates, M. R. (1979). A classification of child abuse and its relation to treatment and prognosis. *Child Abuse and Neglect, 3,* 907–915.

Oates, R. K., Davis, A. A., Ryan, M. G., & Stewart, L. F. (1979). Risk factors associated with child abuse. *Child Abuse and Neglect, 3,* 547–554.

O'Connor, S., Vietze, P. M., Sherrod, K. B., Sandler, H. M., & Altemeier, W. A., III. (1980). Reduced incidence of parenting inadequacy following rooming-in. *Pediatrics, 66,* 176–182.

O'Toole, R., Turbett, P., & Nalepka, C. (1983). Theories, professional knowledge, and diagnosis of child abuse. In D. Finkelhor, R. J. Gelles, G. T. Hotaling, & M. A. Straus (Eds.), *The dark side of families: Current family violence research* (pp. 349–362). Beverly Hills, CA: Sage.

Pagelow, M. D. (1984). *Family violence.* New York: Praeger.

Pallone, S. R., & Malkemes, L. C. (1984). *Helping parents who abuse their children: A comprehensive approach to intervention.* Springfield, IL: Charles C. Thomas.

Parke, R. D. (1982). Theoretical models of child abuse: Their implications for prediction, prevention, and modification. In R. H. Starr, Jr. (Ed.), *Child abuse prediction: Policy implications* (pp. 31–66). Cambridge, MA: Ballinger.

Parke, R. D., & Collmer, C. W. (1975). Child abuse: An interdisciplinary analysis. In E. M. Hetherington (Ed.), *Review of child development research* (Vol. 5, pp. 509–590). Chicago, IL: University of Chicago Press.

Passman, R. H., & Mulhern, R. K. (1977). Maternal punitiveness as affected by situational stress: An experimental analogue of child abuse. *Journal of Abnormal Psychology, 86,* 565–569.

Pelton, L. H. (1977). *Child abuse and neglect and protective intervention in Mercer County, New Jersey: A parent interview and case record study.* Unpublished manuscript, Bureau of Research, New Jersey Division of Youth and Family Services, Trenton, NJ.

Pelton, L. H. (1978). Child abuse and neglect: The myth of classlessness. *American Journal of Orthopsychiatry, 48,* 608–617.

Perry, M. A., Doran, L. D., & Wells, E. A. (1983). Developmental and behavioral characteristics of the physically abused child. *Journal of Clinical Child Psychology, 12,* 320–324.

Perry, M. A., Wells, E. A., & Doran, L. D. (1983). Parent characteristics in abusing and non-abusing families. *Journal of Clinical Child Psychology, 12,* 329–336.

Pfohl, S. (1977). The discovery of child abuse. *Social Problems, 24,* 310–323.

Plotkin, R. C., Azar, S., Twentyman, C. T., & Perri, M. G. (1981). A critical evaluation of the research methodology employed in the investigation of causative factors of child abuse and neglect. *Child Abuse and Neglect, 5,* 449–455.

Radbill, S. X. (1980). Children in a world of violence: A history of child abuse. In C. H. Kempe & R. E. Helfer (Eds.), *The battered child* (3rd ed., pp. 3–20). Chicago, IL: University of Chicago Press.

Reid, J. B., Taplin, P. S., & Lorber, R. (1981). A social interactional approach to the treatment of abusive families. In R. B. Stuart (Ed.), *Violent behavior: Social learning approaches to prediction, management, and treatment* (pp. 83–101). New York: Brunner/Mazel.

Reidy, T. J. (1977). The aggressive characteristics of abused and neglected children. *Journal of Clinical Psychology, 33,* 1140–1145.

Rosenberg, M. S., & Reppucci, N. D. (1983). Abusive mothers: Perception of their own and their children's behavior. *Journal of Consulting and Clinical Psychology, 51,* 674–682.

Rosenberg, M. S., & Reppucci, N. D. (1985). Primary prevention of child abuse. *Journal of Consulting and Clinical Psychology, 53,* 576–585.

Rosenblatt, G. C. (1980). *Parental expectations and attitudes about childrearing in high risk vs. low risk child abusing families.* Saratoga, CA: Century Twenty One.

Russell, A. B., & Trainor, C. M. (1984). *Trends in child abuse and neglect: A national perspective.* Denver, CO: American Humane Association.

Sack, W. H., Mason, R., & Higgins, J. E. (1985). The single-parent family and abusive child punishment. *American Journal of Orthopsychiatry, 55,* 252–259.

Schilling, R. F., Schinke, S. P., Blythe, B. J., & Barth, R. P. (1982). Child maltreatment and mentally retarded parents: Is there a relationship? *Mental Retardation, 20,* 201–209.

Schlossman, S. L. (1977). *Love and the American delinquent: The theory and practice of "progressive" juvenile justice.* Chicago, IL: University of Chicago Press.

Schmitt, B. D. (Ed.). (1978). *The child protection team handbook: A multidisciplinary approach to managing child abuse and neglect.* New York: Garland STPM Press.

Schneider, C. J. (1982). The Michigan Screening Profile of Parenting. In R. H. Starr, Jr. (Ed.), *Child abuse prediction: Policy implications* (pp. 157–174). Cambridge, MA: Ballinger.

Shapiro, D. (1977). *Identification of factors associated with the discontinuation of parental abuse and neglect.* Unpublished manuscript, Child Welfare League of America, New York.

Sherrod, K. B., O'Connor, S., Vietze, P., & Altemeier, W. (1984). Child health and maltreatment. *Child Development, 55,* 1174–1183.

Shorkey, C. T., & Armendariz, J. (1985). Personal worth, self-esteem, anomia, hostility and irrational thinking of abusing mothers: A multivariate approach. *Journal of Clinical Psychology, 41,* 414–421.

Shumaker, S. A., & Brownell, A. (1984). Toward a theory of social support: Closing conceptual gaps. *Journal of Social Issues, 40*(4), 11–36.

Shyne, A. W., & Schroeder, A. G. (1978). *National study of social services to children and their families: Overview.* Unpublished manuscript, Westat, Inc., Rockville, MD.

Skinner, A. E., & Castle, R. L. (1969). *78 battered children: A retrospective study.* London: National Society for the Prevention of Cruelty to Children.

Smith, S. M., & Hanson, R. (1975). Interpersonal relationships and child-rearing practices in 214 parents of battered children. *British Journal of Psychiatry, 127,* 513–525.

Solheim, J. S. (1982). A cross-cultural examination of use of corporal punishment on children: A focus on Sweden and the United States. *Child Abuse and Neglect, 6,* 147–154.

Solnit, A. J. Too much reporting, too little service: Roots and prevention of child abuse. In G. Gerbner, C. J. Ross, & E. Zigler (Eds.), *Child abuse: An agenda for action* (pp. 135–146). New York: Oxford University Press.

Spinetta, J. J. (1978). Parental personality factors in child abuse. *Journal of Consulting and Clinical Psychology, 46,* 1409–1414.

Spinetta, J., & Rigler, D. (1972). The child abusing parent: A psychological review. *Psychological Bulletin, 77,* 296–304.

Starr, R. H., Jr. (1974). *Child abuse: A controlled study of social, familial, individual, and interactional factors* (Grant no. 90-C-426). Washington, DC: National Center for Child Abuse and Neglect, DHHS.

Starr, R. H., Jr. (1978). The controlled study of the ecology of child abuse and drug abuse. *Child Abuse and Neglect, 2,* 19–28.

Starr, R. H., Jr. (1982). A research-based approach to the prediction of child abuse. In R. H. Starr, Jr. (Ed.), *Child abuse prediction: Policy implications* (pp. 105–134). Cambridge, MA: Ballinger.

Starr, R. H., Jr., Ceresnie, S. J., Dietrich, K. N., Fischhoff, J., Schumann, B., & Demorest, M. (1982, August). *Child abuse: A case-sibling assessment of child factors.* Paper presented at the meeting of the American Psychological Association, Washington, DC.

Starr, R. H., Jr., Dietrich, K. N., Fischhoff, J., Ceresnie, S., & Zweier, D. (1984). The contribution of handicapping conditions to child abuse. *Topics in Early Childhood Special Education, 4,* 55–69.

Stein, T. J. (1984). The Child Abuse Prevention and Treatment Act. *Social Services Review, 58,* 302–314.

Steinberg, L. B., Catalano, R., & Dooley, D. (1981). Economic antecedents of child abuse and neglect. *Child Development, 52,* 975–985.

Straus, M. A. (1980). Stress and child abuse. In C. H. Kempe & R. E. Helfer (Eds.), *The battered child* (3rd ed., pp. 86–103). Chicago, IL: University of Chicago Press.

Straus, M. A., Gelles, R. J., & Steinmetz, S. K. (1980). *Behind closed doors: Violence in the American family.* Garden City, NY: Anchor Books.

Sudia, C. E. (1981). What services do abusive and neglecting families need? In L. H. Pelton (Ed.), *The social context of child abuse and neglect* (pp. 268–290). New York: Human Sciences Press.

Susman, E. J., Trickett, P. K., Iannotti, R. J., Hollenbeck, B. E., & Zahn-Waxler, C. (1985). Child-rearing patterns in depressed, abusive, and normal mothers. *American Journal of Orthopsychiatry, 55,* 237–251.

Swedish Information Service. (undated). *The "anti-spanking" law: Text of the law and background.* New York: Swedish Consulate General.

Toro, P. A. (1982). Developmental effects of child abuse: A review. *Child Abuse and Neglect, 6,* 423–431.

Valentine, D. P., Acuff, D. S., Freeman, M. L., & Andreas, T. (1984). Defining child maltreatment: A multidisciplinary overview. *Child Welfare, 63,* 497–509.

Vaughn, B., Taraldson, B., Crichton, L., & Egeland, B. (1981). The assessment of infant temperament: A critique of the Carey Infant Temperament Questionnaire. *Infant Behavior and Development, 4,* 1–17.

Vietze, P., Falsey, S., Sandler, H., O'Connor, S., & Altemeier, W. A. (1980). Transactional approach to prediction of child maltreatment. *Infant Mental Health Journal, 1,* 248–261.

Vietze, P., O'Connor, S., & Altemeier, W. (1983, April). *Continuity in mother-infant interaction in families with maltreated infants.* Paper presented at the meeting of the Society for Research in Child Development, Detroit, MI.

Vietze, P. M., O'Connor, S., Hopkins, J. B., Sandler, H. M., & Altemeier, W. A. (1982). Prospective study of child maltreatment from a transactional perspective. In R. H. Starr, Jr. (Ed.), *Child abuse prediction: Policy implications* (pp. 135–156). Cambridge, MA: Ballinger.

Wald, M. S. (1976). State intervention on behalf of "neglected" children: Standards for removal of children from their homes, monitoring the status of children in foster care, and termination of parental rights. *Stanford Law Review, 28,* 623–706.

Webster-Stratton, C. (1985). Comparison of abusive and nonabusive families with conduct-disordered children. *American Journal of Orthopsychiatry, 55,* 59–69.

Weston, J. T. (1980). The pathology of child abuse and neglect. In C. H. Kempe & R. E. Helfer (Eds.), *The battered child* (3rd ed., pp. 241–271). Chicago, IL: University of Chicago Press.

Williams, G. R. (1983). Child protection: A journey into history. *Journal of Child Clinical Psychology, 12,* 236–243.

Wolfe, D. A. (1985). Child-abusive parents: An empirical review and analysis. *Psychological Bulletin, 97,* 462–482.

Wolfe, D. A., & Mosk, M. D. (1983). Behavioral comparisons of children from abused and distressed families. *Journal of Consulting and Clinical Psychology, 51,* 702–708.

Wolfe, D. A., Kaufman, K., Aragona, J., & Sandler, J. (1981). *The child management program for abusive parents: Procedures for developing a child abuse intervention program.* Winter Park, FL: Anna Publishing.

Wolfe, D. A., Sandler, J., & Kaufman, K. (1981). A competency-based parent training program for child abusers. *Journal of Consulting and Clinical Psychology, 49,* 633–640.

Wolfe, D. A., Fairbank, J., Kelly, J. A., & Bradlyn, A. S. (1983). Child abusive parents' physiological responses to stressful and non-stressful behavior in children. *Behavioral assessment, 5,* 363–371.

Woolley, P. V., & Evans, W. A. (1955). Significance of skeletal lesions in infants resembling those of traumatic origin. *Journal of the American Medical Association, 158,* 539–543.

Wright, L. (1976). The "Sick but Slick" syndrome as a personality component of parents of battered children. *Journal of Clinical Psychology, 32,* 41–45.

7

Child Victims of Sexual Abuse

DAVID A. WOLFE, VICKY V. WOLFE, and CONNIE L. BEST

INTRODUCTION

Attitudes about the occurrence of sexual behavior between adults and children have shown considerable changes throughout history. Whether such behavior was considered abuse has been dependent on societal values of the particular period, with different cultures considering adult–child sexual relations to be normal, immoral, criminal, or psychopathological (P. B. Mrazek, 1981a). Over the last several generations, North American culture has viewed adult–child sexual relations primarily from the perspective of the adult's social deviance, which has prompted legal and psychiatric definitions and interventions for such behavior. However, only within the past 25 years has the concern about sexual child abuse focused on the needs of the child victims, leading to a significant shift from adult psychopathology to more of a child protection orientation.

By the late 1960s all states and provinces in North America had at least two statutes that dealt with sexual abuse (Fraser, 1981): a *criminal statute* (i.e., classification of certain acts as being crimes against the state, punishable by a fine and/or jail term), and a *child protection statute* (i.e., sexual acts between children and caretakers that are potentially injurious to the child's health, safety, and welfare). The latter statute (which is the more common route followed in most sexual abuse investigations) carries no criminal penalties and instead allows for placement of children in foster care and/or termination of parental rights. Unfortunately, enforcement of such statutes often is restricted by problems in defining the specific sexual activity that is to be prohibited, and by procedural problems related to the victim's ability to testify and the community's lack of support for the prosecution of offenders who are family members (Fraser, 1981).

As a partial function of the shift in policy and attention, the topic of sexual abuse has reemerged with prominence in national magazines (e.g., Magnuson, 1983) and newspapers (e.g., Timnick, 1985) that highlight the extent and type of sexual victimization of children being discovered among different agents of child socialization. This attention has been accompanied by a surge of sexual abuse reports throughout North America: a 500%

DAVID A. WOLFE and VICKY V. WOLFE • Department of Psychology, University of Western Ontario, London, Ontario, Canada N6A 5C2. CONNIE L. BEST • Department of Psychiatry and Behavioral Sciences, Medical University of South Carolina, Charleston, SC 29471.

increase (from 319 to 1,593) in identified cases between 1977 and 1980 in Canada (Committee on Sexual Offenses Against Children and Youth, 1984), and a 566% increase (from 1,362 to 7,705) in the United States (Russell & Trainor, 1984). It would be premature to attribute these rapid increases in sexual abuse reports to any particular cause(s), and researchers are uncertain as to whether or not such figures are indicative of an increase in actual abusive incidents, an increase in public awareness and reporting, or inconsistency in defining childhood sexual abuse (see NCCAN, 1981).

In this chapter we will review the characteristics associated with sexual abuse and explore the possible reasons for increased reporting and societal concern for the problem. The latter part of the chapter offers a conceptual model for understanding the emergence of psychological problems among child victims, followed by procedural suggestions for assessment and treatment.

DESCRIPTION OF THE PROBLEM

Defining Sexual Abuse

Although there is a strong consensus favoring the development of a broad-scope definition of child sexual abuse, no criteria or guidelines have been widely accepted (P. B. Mrazek, 1981a). The definition of child sexual abuse has been primarily approached from the standpoint of two overlapping considerations, reflecting the inappropriateness of sexual behavior between adults and children, as well as the type of relationship between the victim and the perpetrator (i.e., extrafamilial or intrafamilial abuse).

Regarding the inappropriateness of adult–child sexual contact, a definition that is commonly applied in legal and social interventions with children emphasizes sexual experiences that occur between children or youth (usually considered to be under age 16) and older persons (often defined as more than 5 years older: Finkelhor, 1979a). The type of act is usually not a critical factor in defining abuse, in that most definitions agree that any form of sexual contact between an adult and child is inappropriate. This judgment is based on the premise that a dependent, developmentally immature child should not be involved in sexual activities that they do not fully comprehend or to which they are unable to give consent (P. B. Mrazek, 1981a). Finkelhor (1979b) adds to this position by emphasizing that prohibition of adult–child sexual experiences should be grounded on the ethical position that because children are incapable of full and informed consent, such behavior cannot be sanctioned by our moral standards. A distinct advantage of this ethical position is that it absolves the victim (and concerned adults) of the need to prove that harm resulted from the abuse, and it further clarifies that sexual freedom does not apply to individuals who are incapable of giving consent (due to their developmental immaturity).

The relationship between the victim and the offender has also been used to distinguish between different types of sexual abuse. *Intrafamilial* abuse, or incest, refers to any type of exploitative sexual contact occurring between relatives (no matter how distant). Although a genetic relationship is implied by this definition, incest often is considered to include any individual who assumes a parental or familial role in the child's life, such as a stepparent, foster parent, or adoptive parent (Russell, 1983). *Extrafamilial* child sexual abuse, on the other hand, refers to all other perpetrators, who may be either a familiar (e.g., babysitter, neighbor, childcare worker) or unfamiliar person to the child.

The Child Abuse Prevention and Treatment Act of 1974 is the most widely adopted statute definition of child sexual abuse. The Act operationally defines the problem as

The obscene or pornographic photographing, filming, or depiction of children for commercial purposes, or the rape, molestation, incest, prostitution, or other such forms of sexual exploitation of children under circumstances which indicate that the child's health or welfare is harmed or threatened thereby. (NCCAN, 1979)

One of the main problems with such a definition, however, is that it can be open to debate or conflict during an adversarial procedure (i.e., criminal action against the alleged offender), because the definition implies that the child must, in some way, be harmed or threatened. An additional concern voiced by some parents is that normal physical contact with their child (e.g., bathing, dressing) could be misinterpreted as exploitative or abusive, and protection against false accusations (e.g., by ex-spouses) could be troublesome (P. B. Mrazek, 1981a). These issues currently remain unresolved by the legal and social working definitions of sexual abuse, and further clarification will undoubtedly become necessary as this topic becomes the subject of greater scrutiny.

Incidence and Prevalence

Estimates of the incidence (i.e., new cases reported each year) and prevalence (i.e., total cases existing in the population at a given time) of childhood sexual abuse vary considerably, based on differences in reports received from studies of adult populations (such as therapy clients) or current cases reported to child protective services. Estimates of incidence and prevalence derived from both informational sources will be presented, followed by a discussion of their discrepancies.

The National Center on Child Abuse and Neglect has been systematically compiling records of child abuse cases reported to state departments of social services across the United States for over a decade. These data represent a conservative estimate of sexual abuse because they are based on actual cases that have been investigated and confirmed, thereby missing an unknown portion of undetected abuse. Nevertheless, they reflect the most complete and thorough compendium of data available, and provide a foundation by which to examine other sources of information regarding abuse. Extrapolating from these data, estimates of the national incidence rate of reported child sexual abuse in the United States range from 0.7 (NCCAN, 1981) to 1.4 (American Humane Association, 1984) victims per 1,000 children in the population.

In contrast, epidemiological and retrospective studies of nonclinical populations provide estimates of incidence rates from a broader sample of the population, generally contacted through anonymous surveys and interviewing techniques. This approach is particularly appropriate with sexual child abuse because epidemiological studies reveal that only 2% to 6% of child victims ever report the abuse to a responsible adult (see Finkelhor, 1979a; Russell, 1984), and even fewer are reported to government agencies. Typically, epidemiological researchers interested in understanding the incidence or prevalence of childhood sexual abuse have framed their inquiry within a more broad or general definition of sexual misconduct than is commonly employed by child welfare departments (e.g., unwanted sexual contact, in the former, in comparison to physical evidence or corroborating reports, in the latter). One of the most widely recognized studies was conducted by Finkelhor (1979a), who surveyed 795 students from several colleges to ask about the occurrence of unwanted sexual experiences during childhood (ranging from exposure and fondling to forcible rape). He found that 19.2% of the women and 8.6% of the men in his college sample reported being sexually victimized by someone within or outside of the family before the age of 17 years. A similar study conducted by Russell

(1983), based on a random survey of 930 adult women in the general population, indicated that 16% of the women reported at least one experience of intrafamilial abuse before the age of 18 (12% before the age of 14). In addition, 31% of her sample reported at least one incident of abuse by someone other than a family member before the age of 18 (20% before age 14).

These prevalence data based on random surveys of college students and the general population are buttressed by findings from the Los Angeles *Times* telephone survey of 2,627 adults chosen randomly from across the United States in July, 1985 (Timnick, 1985). Participants were told that their confidential views of the problem of sexual abuse and their own childhood experiences were of interest to the researchers in understanding the prevalence and impact of sexual abuse. The findings revealed that 27% of the women who participated in the survey and 16% of the men said they had been molested as children (which corresponds to an estimate of 22% of the combined male and female child population). Although the majority of these molestations were isolated incidents, 39% of the victims of sexual intercourse during childhood reported recurrences of the abuse. A similar finding was reported in Canada based on an analysis of research literature, interviews with victims and professionals, and statistics from reported abuse cases (Committee on Sexual Offenses Against Children and Youth, 1984). The committee concluded that at some point in their lives about one in two females and one in three males have been victims of one or more unwanted sexual experiences, and that 80% of these unwanted acts had been first committed when the person was a child or youth.

Epidemiological Characteristics of Child Sexual Abuse

Critical Features of Sexual Abuse

Child's Age and Sex. Based on findings reported from ongoing clinical investigation and treatment services, Courtois (1980) estimated that sexual abuse typically begins when the child is between 4 and 12 years of age. It is noteworthy, as well, that the ages of 4 and 9 are described as particularly high-risk years (Gelinas, 1983; Timnick, 1985). The child's naiveté and sexual curiousity at a younger age, and the exploitation of the older child's loyalty, desire to please, and trust of the adult are suspected reasons linking the child's age to the onset of victimization. Sexual abuse is usually terminated by ages 14 or 15 because of the child's disclosure, threats of disclosure, or behavioral symptomatology (such as running away from home) that leads to the discovery of abuse (Courtois, 1980; Finkelhor, 1984).

Findings from national incidence reports (Russell & Trainor, 1984) and large-scale epidemiological studies (e.g., Conte & Berlinger, 1981) support the conviction that these children are a distinct subgroup relative to other forms of child maltreatment. For example, sexually abused children average 10.5 years of age at the time of discovery, which is significantly older than abused or neglected children (who tend to be preschool-aged or younger, on average). There is also a more proportionate racial distribution among sexual abuse victims (75% white, 15% black, 10% other), and the families of the victims are less likely to be receiving public assistance and to be single-headed households than families of other child victims (Russell & Trainor, 1984). Most notably, a disproportionate sex ratio of approximately 85% female victims exists among sexual abuse reports. Despite the present consensus that girls are more likely to be abused than boys, however, a discrepancy may exist between officially reported male and female victimization, in part because of cultural stereotypes that influence reporting decisions (i.e., boys should not seek help for their problems; fear that others may associate the abuse with homosexuality; Finkelhor, 1981).

Relationship to the Perpetrator. Studies of adult perpetrators of sexual abuse reveal a preponderance of male offenders (92%, Farber, Showers, Johnson, Joseph, & Oshins, 1984; 97%–98%, NCCAN, 1979; 93%, Timnick, 1985). These findings hold true for male as well as female victims, whereas reports of mother–child incest are believed to be extremely rare (Finkelhor, 1981; Russell, 1983). Furthermore, a well-established consensus favors the conclusion that the offender, whether a family or non-family member, is often a familiar person to the child. For example, Conte and Berlinger (1981) found that the offender was a family member among 47% of their 583 children seen for evaluation and treatment, and in another 42% of the cases the offender was not related but was known to the child. Russell's (1983) prevalence study of adults indicated that 77% of the perpetrators of intrafamilial abuse were uncles, brothers, or grandfathers, and 23% were natural fathers or stepfathers. Moreover, the respondents in this study indicated that only 15% of the extrafamilial sexual abuse experiences were committed by strangers. These figures reveal quite dramatically that a child is in greater jeopardy of sexual abuse by familiar adults than by strangers in the community at large (see Becker, this volume, for greater detail concerning adult perpetrators of sexual abuse).

Type and Severity of Abuse. Several studies provide percentage estimates reflecting the proportion of lesser to more severe forms of abuse. It should be noted that these estimates vary, however, in accordance with the research methodology (i.e., college samples, hospital samples, telephone surveys). Finkelhor (1980), for example, found that the most frequently reported experience (mentioned by 40% of his college-based sample) involved fondling of the child's or adult's genital area. In contrast, Farber *et al.* (1984) found that 54% of the females ($n = 81$) and 47% of the males ($n = 81$) in their hospital sample had been subjected to anal or vaginal intercourse, and approximately one third of the females and one quarter of the males had experienced fondling (based on medical records of abused children). Findings similar to the latter study regarding type and severity of abuse were revealed by the recent L.A. *Times* random survey of adults, where sexual intercourse was reported to be involved in 55% of the experiences and 36% of the victims reported fondling.

To further an understanding of the types and seriousness of abusive acts, Russell (1983) categorized her sample of adult female victims of child sexual abuse into three types: very serious (e.g., forced or unforced vaginal penetration, cunnilingus, anal intercourse), serious (e.g., digital vaginal penetration, touching of unclothed breasts), and least serious sexual contact (e.g., forced kissing, intentional touching of clothed areas of body). Based on these categorical definitions, 23% of her incest cases were classified as very serious, 41% serious, and 36% least serious. Russell (1983) also noted that in incest cases stepfathers tend to commit the most serious forms of abuse, and younger relatives (e.g., brothers, cousins) commit the least serious. This categorical system assists in understanding the difference in severity of abusive experiences, which has implications for predicting the victim's recovery and long-term adjustment (e.g., Friedrich, Urquiza, & Beilke, 1986; Steele & Alexander, 1981).

Use of Bribery and Intimidation. Although the most extreme forms of coercion involving physical violence or imminent danger are considered to be rare (Finkelhor, 1982; P. B. Mrazek, 1983), in most cases of sexual abuse some method for procuring compliance and secrecy is involved. Bribery methods such as money, food, beer, or cigarettes are occasionally used. However, the most frequently reported tactics involve intimidation (e.g., threats or implied threats), particularly to insure secrecy (e.g., 44%, Farber *et al.*, 1984; 55%, Finkelhor, 1980; 41%, Russell, 1983). Physical violence has been estimated to accompany approximately 20% of the incidents (e.g., 22%, Farber *et al.*, 1984; 18%, Timnick, 1985), and is believed to increase with the age of the child (see Gelinas, 1983). However, because the majority of abusive acts involve a person who is known to the child, less overt and more deceptive methods of procurement (e.g., bribes, threats, use of authority status, reassurance) seem to predominate.

Vulnerability Factors

Several factors have been identified through retrospective studies of adults and current studies of child victims that assist in understanding the factors that increase a child's vulnerability to sexual abuse. From Finkelhor's (1979a) survey of 795 college students, eight vulnerability factors were identified that reflect the features most significantly associated with sexual abuse. These included the presence of a stepfather, the separation of the child from his or her natural mother, the mother's failure to complete high school, the mother's punishment of the child's sexual curiosity, the father's lack of physical affection toward the child, a family income under $10,000/year, and the child's limited friendships. For respondents who reported none of these factors, a history of childhood sexual abuse was virtually absent. Among those with 5 or more factors, however, two-thirds had been sexually victimized. Gruber and Jones (1983) conducted a similar study of vulnerability factors with 41 delinquent youths, 20 of whom had a known history of sexual abuse. Controlling for delinquent behavior and associated family patterns, these investigators found that poor parental marital relations, a child living with a step or foster father, and a poor relationship with mother were strong discriminators of abused and nonabused delinquents.

Researchers have also found that sexual abuse of one child is often associated with incestuous relations among other family members. For example, Meiselman (1978) and Russell (1983) have reported that over 30% of their incest cases reported that the offender had also abused one or more other relatives. Commenting on this issue, P. B. Mrazek (1983) observed that previous incestuous experience or knowledge of its occurrence within the family of origin may be the most important factor in the perpetuation of incest across generations. Overall, the previously cited studies suggest that children are at greater risk of sexual abuse in accordance with the degree to which they are supervised by sexually opportunistic men, have mothers who are relatively unpowerful in their relationships and thus fail to protect their child, or have mothers who have difficulty fostering a healthy mother–daughter relationship, thus decreasing the likelihood of early disclosure and prevention of abuse.

Behavioral and Emotional Symptoms Associated with Child Sexual Abuse

At present, little research in the area of sexual abuse is available to document the mechanisms or processes that interfere with the abused child's development, although it is evident that such interference does occur in some cases (Browne & Finkelhor, 1986). Research investigations of the impact of sexual abuse on the child's emotional and behavioral adjustment have generally been conducted with either small groups of agency-referred abused children or samples of a broad spectrum of adults who provide retrospective reports of their experiences. Unfortunately, limitations to both of these methods of inquiry prevent the drawing of firm conclusions, because known cases of abused children may not be representative of the majority of incidents, and reports from adults may be biased due to selection criteria and subsequent events. In addition, with these samples it is often difficult to determine the impact of abuse on children because of the numerous intervening variables that may accentuate or attenuate the symptomatology. The harmful effects of sexual abuse may stem not only from the abusive actions, but could result as well from the traumatic interruptions and confusion that emanate from the disclosure of abuse and its aftermath. That is, concurrent or subsequent to the discovery of sexual abuse the child may experience disruption in his or her family situation, stressful legal procedures, and criticism or blame from family members (Gomes-Schwartz & Horowitz, 1981; see later section). As well, the child's family environment may have been quite unstable or chaotic prior to the discovery of sexual abuse, and the impact of chronic, disruptive family conditions on the child's development cannot readily be separated from the impact of abuse or trauma *per se* (Fromuth, 1986; Steele & Alexander, 1981; D. A. Wolfe, 1987).

A dispute over the severity and nature of sexual abuse has existed for many years in the absence of empirical enquiry, leading to widely discrepant viewpoints that attempt to explain the associations between childhood sexual abuse and subsequent adjustment. One viewpoint argues that a sexual experience with an adult during childhood may be unpleasant or traumatic at the time, but that most children recover unscathed (e.g., Bender & Grugett, 1951; Gagnon, 1965). On the other hand, a strong position in favor of viewing child sexual abuse as similar to adult rape (in terms of its impact on the victim) has received support in the theoretical and clinical literature (Burgess & Holmstrom, 1974). Finkelhor's (1979a) interpretation of this theoretical and moral controversy, in the acknowledged absence of empirical data, highlights the fact that child sexual abuse is obviously harmful to some people, although the exact traumagenic factors are not clear.

Initial Effects. Clinical reports of the initial effects of sexual abuse on the child's behavior have highlighted a number of concerns related to anxiety and fears, guilt and depression, problems in sexual and interpersonal adjustment, and learning and behavior problems at school (see reviews by Browne & Finkelhor, 1986; P. B. Mrazek & D. A. Mrazek, 1981). Anxiety and fear are perhaps the most commonly reported problems in clinically based studies of child victims. Such children have shown problems related to sleeping alone and nightmares (Peters, 1976), fear of contacts with adults (James & Nasjleti, 1983; Kinsey, Pomeroy, Martin, & Gebhard, 1953), compulsive bathing (Burgess & Holmstrom, 1974), and nonspecific symptoms of anxiety, such as increased agitation and nervous behavior (Meiselman, 1978). Closely related to these anxious symptoms are reports that the child may display signs of guilt and shame, feelings of grief and loss, and a sense of stigma based on his or her experience (Adams-Tucker, 1982; Browning & Boatman, 1977; Justice & Justice, 1979). The presence of somatic complaints, such as fatigue, loss of appetite, aches and pains, and the sudden onset of bedwetting, headaches, and changes in sleeping and eating patterns may also accompany these related internalizing problems (Browne & Finkelhor, 1986; Lewis & Sarrell, 1969).

Burgess, Hartman, McCausland, and Powers (1984), in discussing the reactions of children involved in sex rings and pornography, related the children's behavior following exposure of the exploitation as being similar to patterns found with adult victims of posttraumatic stress disorder. That is, some of the children exhibited intrusive thoughts, flashbacks, vivid memories and dreams of retaliation, diminished responsiveness to others, hyperalertness, moodiness and crying spells, reduced trust of others, withdrawal from peers, and school refusal. Interestingly, when parents of these children were asked (after the fact) to report on symptoms observed in their children prior to exposure of the abuse, the symptoms were more vague and ill-defined (e.g., somatic complaints, genital concerns, acting out, and abrupt changes in their behavior), suggesting that the exposure of the abuse may, in itself, be a very traumatic event for the child.

Recent efforts to quantify the extent of these internalizing-type symptoms with sexually abused children support the clinical reports noted earlier, based on objective measures and ratings by clinicians. Similar to clinically based studies, a significant proportion of these internalizing problems consisted of fears and fear-related avoidance behavior. For example, Anderson, Bach, and Griffith (1981) found that 40% of their crisis center sample suffered from extreme fears, and DeFrancis (1969) also found a high rate of fear symptoms among 83% of victims referred for assessment prior to court. Focusing on age and developmental differences, the Tuft's New England Medical Center (1984) found major fears or anxiety to be present in 20% of preschool-aged children, 45% of school-aged children, and 36% of the adolescents who had been sexually abused. In a large-scale investigation using a standardized parent-report questionnaire of child behavior problems (the Child Behavior Profile: Achenbach & Edelbrock, 1983), Friedrich *et al.* (1986) found that 46% of the female victims ($n = 61$) and 35% of the males ($n = 24$) were significantly above the norm (T-score ≥ 70) on internalizing problems. Moreover, regression analyses predicting child internalizing symptoms revealed that female children who were abused frequently and severely by a perpetrator who was emotionally close to them exhibited the greatest elevations in internalizing behavior. In the aggregate, these recent empirical studies support the contention that sexual abuse negatively affects the child's level of anxiety, distress, and emotional well-being, and that these effects vary partially as a function of the context and severity of victimization.

In addition to internalizing symptomatology, a number of reports have also noted the presence of externalizing behavior problems, such as aggression and delinquency (Browne & Finkelhor, 1986; P. B. Mrazek & D. A. Mrazek, 1981). Friedrich *et al.* (1986) found that 36% of the males and 39% of the females in their study displayed significant externalizing problems. A longer duration of abuse, a close relationship between the child and the perpetrator, more time elapsed since onset and reporting, and the sex of the child (males more than females) were significant predictors of increased externalizing symptoms in this study. Elevated symptoms of anger and hostility were also reported by the Tuft's (1984) investigation, in which 45% to 50% of the 7- to 13-year-olds showed significant problems in these areas.

The tendency to find coexistence of child sexual abuse and delinquency has led a number of authors to infer that sexual assault may lead to, or cause, subsequent delinquent activity (Browning & Boatman, 1977; DeFrancis, 1979). Gruber and Jones (1981) argued, however, that alternative explanations to that relationship need to be considered: (a) youths involved in delinquent activity (by their own actions) may be more prone to sexual assault than other groups of youths, and (b) the same environments that tend to be associated with a higher likelihood of delinquency may also produce a greater than typical risk of sexual assault against youths who were raised in such environments. That is, involvement in delinquent behavior could be relatively common among these youths even if they were not sexual assault victims. Further empirical confirmation of this hypothesized relationship between family functioning and child symptomatology must be obtained before conclusions that rule out other explanations (e.g., peer influences, predisposition for delinquent behavior, school failure, etc.) can be more firmly established.

Another developmental problem that has been associated with sexual abuse concerns the child's sexual adjustment. Heightened sexual activity, such as compulsive masturbation, precocious sexual play, knowledge of sexual matters inappropriate to age and developmental level, and overt sexual acting-out toward adults had been associated with abuse, and may be detected even in very young children (Adams-Tucker, 1982; James & Nasjleti, 1983; Justice & Justice, 1979; Meiselman, 1978). James and Nasjleti (1983) found that sexually abused children not only expressed more overt sexuality, but also tended to express coexisting themes of sexuality and violence in their artwork, written schoolwork, language, and play. Yates (1982) suggested that sexually abused children become eroticized as a result of their sexual victimization, and described from case examples how young sexually abused children were easily aroused by a variety of circumstances (e.g., sitting on an adult's lap, playground activities). Yates (1982) argued that sexually abused children may have difficulty distinguishing sexual arousal from physical or psychological closeness, which may lead to the inappropriate expression of sexuality and associated adjustment problems (e.g., rejection, peer problems). Although empirical studies of sexualized behavior are rare with this population, at least one study found that the more frequent the abuse by a greater number of perpetrators, the more likely the child was to demonstrate sexualized behavior (Friedrich *et al.*, 1986).

Long-Term Effects. The clinical and empirical literature is generally supportive of the proposition that childhood sexual abuse is detrimental to the psychological development of the person over time. Moreover, these long-term effects are similar in nature to those discovered in the short term (P. B. Mrazek, 1983). The majority of reports indicate that long-term effects are manifested in problems related primarily to negative self-esteem, interpersonal problems, and marital and sexual satisfaction (Browne & Finkelhor, 1986).

Interpersonal and emotional problems, including marital conflict, social isolation, parenting difficulties, anxiety attacks, nightmares, sleeping difficulties, and suicidal ideation appear most commonly in studies of adults who were childhood victims of sexual abuse (Browne & Finkelhor, 1984, 1986; Goodwin, McCarthy, & Divasto, 1981; Herman, 1981; Justice & Justice, 1979). Sexual adjustment problems in adulthood have also been noted, such as nonorgasmia, sexual disinterest, or sexual discomfort (Becker, Skinner, Abel, & Cichon, 1986; McQuire & Wagner, 1978). There is also evidence obtained from retrospective studies of adult prostitutes that sexual child abuse is related to juvenile and adult prostitution (e.g., 55% of a sample of 136 prostitutes had been child victims of sexual abuse, James & Meyerding, 1977; 60% of a sample of 200 prostitutes, Silbert & Pines, 1981). Similar findings of sexually abusive childhood experiences have been reported as well for adult male sex offenders (e.g., Groth, 1979).

These preliminary studies must be accompanied by the caveat that child sexual abuse does not inevitably lead to later disturbances in development and interpersonal relationships. Differences in later adjustment, for example, have been accounted for by variables related to the emotional responses evoked at the time of the abuse (i.e., feelings of fear, panic, and apprehension at the time of abuse were associated with greater maladjustment on standard measures of adult personality; Tsai, Feldman-Summers, & Edgar, 1979). Such emotional responses, in turn, have been theoretically and empirically linked to three main factors that appear to mediate the victim's long-term adjustment: the severity of the abuse, available emotional and social support, and the victim's attributional style regarding unpleasant event(s) (Janoff-Bulman & Frieze, 1983). For example, adults who were less plagued by repetitive, intrusive thoughts and continued negative emotions stemming from childhood sexual abuse have been differentiated from those who were in greater distress on the basis of their supportive marital relationship, a positive relationship with their mother during childhood, and academic and/or career success (see Gold, 1986; Seidner & Calhoun, 1984; Silver, Boon, & Stones, 1983; Tsai *et al.,* 1979, for research studies with adults; see Peterson & Seligman, 1983, for a discussion of attributional styles following victimization experiences).

In sum, preliminary evidence seems to support the position that the resources of the victim (in terms of his or her support network and attributional style for coping with stressful events) may account for a significant proportion of variance in determining the long-range outcome of childhood sexual abuse. It should also be acknowledged, however, that biases undoubtedly exist in these research samples because of their retrospective nature, the fact that the subjects (in many cases) had sought treatment, and the over-reliance on clinical impressions and case reports because of the small research base that has been developed to date. Until longitudinal, comparative data are available, conclusions regarding the more subtle or pervasive aftereffects of these experiences must be cautiously drawn.

A CONCEPTUALIZATION OF SEXUAL ABUSE TRAUMA AND RECOVERY

The development of assessment and therapeutic strategies for the sexually abused child is a complex task that requires knowledge of the symptoms a child may exhibit, as well as knowledge of the diversity of treatment approaches available to meet the needs of the child and family. This section will present a conceptual model of the traumatic impact of sexual abuse in order to guide efforts aimed at formulating assessment and intervention goals. Issues regarding the importance of coordinating professional services in working with sexually abused children will also be addressed. This information will be followed by suggestions for assessing and treating the child's symptomatology arising from the traumatic impact of sexual abuse and its aftermath.

The processes by which a child may be harmed by sexual abuse are not well understood and presently must be conceptualized along hypothetical dimensions. The traumagenic impact of sexual abuse likely is not limited to the abusive incident(s) alone, but rather appears to be linked to sequential events coexisting with different stages of the child's traumatization. With this sequential and interdependent nature of sexual abuse in mind, a conceptual model of sxual abuse traumatization and recovery was developed by Wolfe and Wolfe (1987). Three phases of involvement that the sexually abused child typically experiences are delineated by this model: (a) Sexual victimization and pre-disclosure phase, (b) disclosure crisis phase, and (c) recovery and adjustment phase. Each phase may be accompanied by factors related to the nature of the abuse (e.g., the seriousness and frequency of abuse, the child's relationship with the offender), characteristics of the child and family (e.g., child's age and developmental stage, child's vulnerability to bribery or threats, family isolation from the community, poor marital relationship) and community attitudes and resources (e.g., cultural tolerance of sexual exploitation of children, efforts toward teaching children about victimization and avenues for disclosure, reactions to protect the child at the point of disclosure, adaptability of the criminal justice system for managing cases with child witnesses).

This conceptual model posits that the child's development of either adaptive or maladaptive behavior patterns will, to a certain extent, reflect the interplay of stress and support factors that have occurred in the past and/or are currently exerting a crucial influence on the child. For example, a school-aged girl who has been forced by her step-father to submit to fondling and who perceives that her mother will not act to stop the abuse (because of poor communication, previous attempts on the child's part to discuss the behavior with her mother, etc.), often has no source of information or support by which to disclose her concerns and receive help. Such a child is highly vulnerable to continued and escalated victimization and is more susceptible, according to this model, to negative psychological sequelae, such as symptoms of fear, anxiety, depression, and peer relationship problems. A contrasting sequence of events highlights an alternative scenario: a child who has been forced to engage in sexual acts with a relative or person known to the family, who has a good channel of communication with his or her parents, and who has been informed of the inappropriateness of such behavior and how to report it is viewed as being less vulnerable to continued sexual abuse and less susceptible to psychological trauma and symptomatology. In the latter example, the child is surrounded by protective factors that serve to counteract or diminish the traumagenic impact of sexual victimization.

A similar interplay of stress and support factors that may affect the child's short- and long-term adjustment continues during the remaining two phases of involvement, in which family reactions to the disclosure (e.g., belief and acceptance of the child's report) and community actions taken to protect the child (e.g., removal of the offender from the home, court testimony) become potent factors influencing the child's recovery.

Psychological Processes Underlying Child Maladjustment

Whereas the previous conceptualization of sequential events affecting the child's adjustment helps to establish the temporal dimension and interaction of persons and events, functional relationships are needed to explain the connection between the circumstances of sexual abuse and the major adjustment problems noted among the child victims. The psychological processes that are suspected to underlie the abused child's development of fears and anxieties, inappropriate sexual conduct with peers, negative self-concept, and so on, may be somewhat different than those associated with other clinical-child populations where victimization was not involved.

In reference to a child's psychosexual development (i.e., sex roles, sexual behavior, and sexual identity), this critical interpersonal dimension may be interrupted or impaired by sexual abuse through the psychological processes of social learning. The sexually abused child may learn, for example, that sexual behavior can be used as a tool for manipulating others, particularly if he or she has received rewards or special privileges for sexual behaviors (Finkelhor & Browne, 1985). Similarly, the psychological processes of modeling may be operative, in which the child is taught, through repeated exposure to sexual demands, that the use of authority, promises of rewards, or threats of punishment are often successful in gaining sexual compliance and achieving control in relationships. As a consequence of such learning experiences, the child who is sexually exploited by an adult may justify such actions against others in the future, leading to sexually inappropriate behavior with his or her peers or with other adults. This line of reasoning is linked to the emerging reports that a relatively high percentage of adult sex offenders have histories of sexual victimization (e.g., Groth, 1979) and that abused children are overrepresented among juvenile and adult prostitutes.

The emergence of specific or pervasive fears and anxieties among sexually abused children (e.g., fear of the perpetrator, worry about the discovery by others, fear that they have committed an unpardonable sin), and the development of a negative self-concept has implicated the importance of psychological processes associated with conditioned fear responses and cognitive appraisals of the abuse. Although abusive episodes may vary considerably with regard to the degree of fear evoked in the child, pronounced fear responses appear to be commonly associated with abusive experiences and the aftermath of discovery (Browne & Finkelhor, 1986; P. B. Mrazek, 1983; Steele & Alexander, 1981). In the presence of elevated symptoms of fear and anxiety (e.g., increased cardiovascular activity, feelings of apprehension or punishment, etc.), the child's response may readily generalize to other stimuli, including some that are only remotely associated with the original fearful situation (e.g., fear of babysitters, walking to school, older males, etc.).

Sexual abuse may also create a passive response style in some children, similar to that described in the revised learned helplessness model. This model states that persons who have a tendency to make internal, global, and stable attributions about negative life events will develop a more passive and self-defeating response style when confronted with new situations (Abramson, Seligman, & Teasdale, 1978; Peterson & Seligman, 1983). For example, a child who is offered a reward for participation in sexual acts, or one who offers little resistance, may develop internal attributions about the event (e.g., "I'm to blame for what happened"). Such attributions have been linked in clinical-adult victimized populations (e.g., rape victims; Baker & Peterson, 1977) to the development of a negative self-concept, guilt, and self-blame. In a similar fashion, a child who was threatened or coerced by the perpetrator may come to believe that he or she will remain vulnerable to future maltreatment (e.g., "the world is a dangerous place," "bad things always happen to me," "adults can't be trusted"). According to such theoretical reasoning, therefore, sexual abuse may impair a child's development of psychosexual, emotional, and interpersonal behavior through psychological processes that are known to be potent influences in other circumstances (e.g., the etiology of anxiety, depression, and/or sexual dysfunction).

The Coordination of Professional Services

Children may be referred for psychological assessment and treatment by a range of childcare professionals, including child protective service workers, medical and mental health practitioners, educators, or criminal justice officials. The degree of involvement of each profession will vary according to the specific aspects of each case, and it becomes important to coordinate the roles of the different service providers available to the child to ensure that the services are not duplicated or overlooked. Each of these referring sources may have unique assessment concerns, such as the child's credibility as a witness, the type of protective services needed, or the symptomatic patterns of behavior shown by the child.

Whereas the overall goal of each profession is to be an advocate for the child, their specific roles may differ significantly and may, at times, be antagonistic. For example, Bander, Fein, and Bishop (1982) pointed to the contrast between the necessary actions of police and protective service workers, whose primary responsibilities are required during the initial discovery of the abuse, with the role of subsequent mental health professionals who become involved with the child and his or her family following the initial crisis period. Whereas the former agents must focus their action on the protection of the child and the prosecution of the perpetrator (a very intrusive and stressful function), the latter agents may advocate for the reunion of the family in order to deal therapeutically with the family issues. Potential role conflict can occur when the plan of the child protection advocates contradicts the therapist's desire to work with the entire family system and to remove or reduce pressures from the criminal justice and/or social service systems. In contrast, coordinated efforts can yield fruitful results that are otherwise less likely to occur. For example, coordination of mental health and criminal justice professionals can change the potentially traumatic event of providing court testimony into an experience in which the child gains a sense of mastery and control over the events in his or her life.

Because the involvement of multiple systems and agencies is typically the rule rather than the exception, effective treatment of the sexually abused child must be approached from a multidisciplined, multisystem orientation to minimize resistance and interference. Therefore, the development of a treatment plan that advocates the contributions of each professional representative should be (a) cognizant of all systems involved, (b) aware of potential sources of resistance between the systems that may arise and be prepared to work toward the resolution of the resistance, and (c) be able to appreciate the unique contributions each system has to offer.

ASSESSMENT AND TREATMENT OF SEXUAL CHILD ABUSE VICTIMS

The task of assessment varies according to the sequence of events to which the sexually abused child typically is subjected (i.e., events associated with separate phases of involvement). For example, during the predisclosure phase the child may be referred for assessment because of unusual or atypical behaviors of unknown origin (e.g., fears or phobias, anxiety, concern about personal harm or sexual matters). The examiner must be sensitive to the possibility of undisclosed sexual abuse in such circumstances, and act accordingly to assist the child in revealing the nature of his or her distress. Once abuse has been disclosed by the child or discovered by an adult, reasons for referral often focus on the child's adjustment, his or her credibility as a witness, circumstances of the abuse, and treatment recommendations. During the recovery phase of involvement, the assessment purpose becomes more focused on the child's overall adjustment in relation to school, peers, family, and self, in addition to the determination of therapeutic efforts. Assessment objectives and procedures pertinent to each of these three phases of involvement will be presented, accompanied by an overview of treatment recommendations that may be initiated to assist in the child's recovery.

Predisclosure: Professional Awareness of Sexual Abuse Signs

Detecting cases of sexual abuse that have not been discovered requires a broad understanding of social background factors that increase a child's vulnerability (e.g., social isolation and disadvantage; family relationship problems), in addition to child response patterns that may be indicative of sexual abuse. Brenner (1984) summarized the clinical literature regarding behaviors that occur most frequently among children who have been sexually abused, which aids in organizing an assessment strategy to verify the occurrence of abuse. These behaviors are organized into five categories to assist in identification of patterns: (a) development of new fears, such as fears of sleeping alone, dark places, strangers, or particular adults; (b) changes in usual behavior patterns, such as loss of appetite, bedwetting, increased irritability, sleep disturbances, or sudden worry about keeping clean; (c) overt expressions of sexuality, such as precocious sexual activity, compulsive masturbation, excessive interest in sex, or seductive behavior with peers and adults; (d) changes in school performance, such as not being able to concentrate, sudden decline in performance, hints to teachers about sexual activity or fears, or refusal to participate in previously enjoyed activities; and (e) strained relationship with parents, in which the child talks of running away from home, is overprotected, or is not allowed to bring friends into the home. Although these behaviors may be indicative of sexual abuse, no pattern of behavior is necessary or sufficient evidence of abuse *per se* without additional verification from the child or other evidential sources.

Interviewing a preschool-aged or older child about possible sexual victimization is a procedure that has not been standardized or widely discussed in the literature. Sgroi (1982) emphasized the importance of establishing the child's familiarity with the examiner and the setting prior to broaching the topic, through activities such as play, drawing, and discussions of favorite topics. For children older than 5 or 6 years, a recommended procedure is to allow the child an opportunity to raise the topic of sexual abuse spontaneously, by discussing fears, worries, and positive and negative events that have recently occurred (e.g., D. A. Mrazek, 1981; Sgroi, 1982). The examiner should also follow-up these general probes with more specific inquiry regarding particular experiences or events that may have made the child feel uncomfortable, afraid, or "bad." The interviewer may, for example, ask "Has any adult touched you in places that made you feel uncomfortable?" "Has anyone ever threatened to hurt you if you didn't do what you were told?" Such inquiry should be guided by the child's level of anxiety, and he or she should be reassured of their innocence and safety. The examiner may also wish to conduct this interview in the accompaniment of a familiar person who can serve as comfort and support for the child, such as a social worker, parent, or older sibling.

Disclosure and Crisis Intervention

The period surrounding the disclosure or discovery of sexual abuse clearly represents a crisis situation for the child or adolescent and other family members. Commonly, the child has been misled by the offender to trust or accept his or her behavior as being acceptable or desirable (although the child may have ambivalent or negative emotions about this rationale), and therefore the sudden discovery and termination of the abuse itself can be confusing, upsetting, and traumatic to the child. Demands are then immediately placed on the child and his or her family, such as the separation of the child from family members, arrest of the alleged perpetrator, medical examinations, repeated interviews by different individuals who require the recall of unpleasant events, and involvement in court processes. Emerging findings from studies of children who have recently disclosed such traumatic events offer support for the position that their symptomatology increases dramatically once the crisis of disclosure has begun (e.g., Burgess *et al.*, 1984).

Once a child discloses an episode of sexual abuse to a professional, that individual is legally required to report the abuse to the local child protective services agency. As part of the process of reporting the abuse, the child's reasons and motives for disclosure should be explored, along with his or her expectations for what will follow. The child should be informed of the professional's responsibility and intention to report the abuse, as well as the sequence of events that might result from the disclosure. Children sometimes have false expectations about what will occur, at times expecting terrible consequences from the family and offender, at other times having unrealistic fantasies that disclosure of the abuse will correct a multitude of problems within his or her family. These unrealistic expectations and fears should be clarified with the child and assurances made that the ensuing sequence of events will have the goal of protecting the child and serving his or her best interests.

It is important to recognize that children's reactions to the disclosure of sexual abuse vary considerably. Some children who do not display or report any problems following disclosure may develop problems at a later point in time. Conversely, some children who show significant adjustment problems early on may begin to improve rapidly once the disclosure has been made. The process of disclosure itself may lead to stress-related symptoms (e.g., sleep problems, school decline, enuresis, peer problems) that may decrease rapidly once the child's situation has been stabilized. Therefore, the assessment of the child's adjustment is an ongoing concern that involves the monitoring of clinical symptomatology, as well as an assessment of the child's strengths and coping resources vis-à-vis immediate and long-term changes in his or her family situation.

An adult's belief of the child's allegations is often one of the first issues facing the child, and the manner in which this is handled can significantly affect his or her degree of traumatization and fear (James & Nasjleti, 1983; Sgroi, 1982). A strong consensus, derived from clinical case studies and arguments based on norms of sexual development, maintains that children very rarely make up stories about being sexually abused (Faller, 1984; Kerns, 1981; Melton, 1985; D. A. Mrazek, 1981; Sgroi, 1982). Nevertheless, the child's story may not be supported by a credible adult, and often is vehemently denied by the offender (and his or her spouse), which adds to the stress on the child. Therefore, it has become recommended practice for professionals to accept the child's allegations at face value for the purpose of mounting an investigation (Kempe & Kempe, 1984).

Assessment of Crisis Adjustment. Unfortunately, the lack of assessment technology that has been designed and validated especially for this population currently limits the specificity of information available to the researcher/clinician. Readily available standardized instruments for assessing childhood problems are suitable for obtaining a general understanding of the extent of problems expressed by the child and his or her caregivers, yet there is a pressing need for further adaptation and refinement of assessment tools for sexually abused children (Wolfe & Wolfe, 1987).

The following overview of assessment procedures highlights some of the available approaches to assessing the child's crisis adjustment, with an emphasis on emotional and behavioral symptomatology that may impede the child's recovery from the trauma. These assessment procedures are most applicable to children aged six or older; younger children should be approached with considerably less structure and with greater reliance on adult informants and clinical observation during age-appropriate activity (e.g., see Broder & Hood, 1983, for suggestions regarding pediatric assessment techniques). This approach is outlined in conjunction with the previous conceptual model that emphasizes the child's attributions for the event(s) and his or her conditioned fear reactions and heightened anxiety preceding or following disclosure. Readers interested in further information for assessing the details of alleged sexual abuse, such as the use of anatomically correct dolls, videorecorded testimony, and interview procedures are referred to Sgroi (1982) and Wolfe and Wolfe (1987).

An assessment of the child's self-perceived fear, anxiety, and affective functioning is a necessary concern for understanding his or her level of discomfort and distress during the crisis and recovery periods of involvement. For school-aged children, fear and anxiety can be referenced through self-report methods that provide a comprehensive sampling of fear-evoking stimuli (both tangible and intangible) and self-perceptions of distress. The use of norm-referenced instruments is especially beneficial for two reasons: the child is given a private opportunity to respond to a wide range of potentially troublesome symptoms in a format that is usually less stressful than a clinical interview, and the results can provide a broad-scale comparison of the child's overall crisis adjustment in reference to age- and sex-based normative data. Subsequently, the clinical interviewer can probe further with the child to determine the functional components of his or her reported distress.

The *Fear Survey Schedule for Children—Revised* (FSSC-R: Ollendick, 1978; Scherer & Nakamura, 1968), for example, is an 80-item questionnaire to assist in rating the child's fear in relation to a number of common and uncommon stimuli or events (e.g., fear of small animals, medical procedures, injury, failure, death, and the unknown). Other available instruments that provide information about the child's level of distress and anxiety may also be considered, such as the *State–Trait Anxiety Inventory for Children* (Spielberger, 1973), the *Children's Depression Inventory* (Kovacs, 1983), and the *Children's Manifest Anxiety Scale—Revised* (Reynolds & Richmond, 1978). It is necessary to follow-up these self-rated fears and worries with specific inquiry regarding their origin, intensity, and the child's typical response, in order to determine their debilitating nature. Furthermore, even though the child's score on one of these measures may not fall into the clinical range, these instruments allow for a survey of the child's individual distress that may lead to the discovery of singly important fears (e.g., pregnancy, homosexuality, parental rejection) that warrant attention.

In addition, children and adolescents who have been abused may have developed specific fears associated with abuse-related stimuli that are not included on a fear survey. To detect these patterns, the child should be asked about common, everyday activities that they engage in (e.g., dressing, bathing, walking to school, playgrounds, babysitters, going to bed, etc.) that might provoke anxiety or fear. Because the child may recognize the irrationality of certain atypical fears (such as fear of undressing or bathing) the examiner must probe in a very cautious and sensitive manner to avoid unintentionally conveying to the child the inappropriateness or unimportance of their distress. The examiner may facilitate this assessment by reassuring the child that he or she has spoken to many other children about similar problems and discovered that others have fears and worries that are difficult to express initially, and that the child will be allowed ample opportunity to express his or her thoughts and feelings without pressure or blame.

Beyond the assessment of specific internalizing or externalizing symptoms displayed by sexually abused children, an understanding of the child's attributions for the traumatic event(s) may provide information pertinent to the planning for treatment and recovery. Drawing from the literature on rape victims and child sexual abuse victims (who were assessed during adulthood), it has been found that persons who believe that they were responsible in some way for their own victimization and who feel that they have little control in preventing similar exploitation in the future are considered to be at higher risk for maladjustment and continued distress. In contrast, those who attribute the event to factors unrelated to their own ability or characteristics (e.g., parental drinking, marital problems, a ''crazy'' person) often show more rapid recovery and elimination of symptoms, and are assumed to have resolved the crisis dilemma (Janoff-Bulman & Frieze, 1983; Seidner & Calhoun, 1984; Silver *et al.*, 1983). These attributional styles can be assessed in children through open-ended discussion of their beliefs and attitudes about the experience, once the crisis period of adjustment has begun to subside. The child should be encouraged to express his or her thoughts about what happened, and attempt to resolve the ambiguity that may still remain concerning why an adult exploited and abused him or her. V. V. Wolfe, D. A. Wolfe, and LaRose (1986) developed the *Children's Impact of Traumatic Events Scale* for the purpose of assessing a child's beliefs and reactions to victimization experiences in a structured and comprehensive manner. In addition to determining a child's attributions about the abuse, feelings of helplessness, stigmatization, and betrayal are assessed, as well as the presence of intrusive thoughts related to the abusive circumstances.

Intervention Goals and Modalities. Stabilization of the child's routine activities (such as living arrangements, school, contact with familiar persons and possessions) and the reduction of stress-inducing events is a major goal to be achieved during the aftermath of disclosure. This goal may be approached through efforts designed to help the child cope with current events (e.g., assistance with court proceedings, medical and psychological assessments, involvement of supportive adults), as opposed to attempts at modifying long-standing problems in his or her family or social relationships. Crisis intervention efforts aimed at helping the child to accept rapid changes in his or her living situation, to overcome excessive feelings of guilt and blame, and to understand the intrusive events that are occurring are appropriate short-term goals to aid the child's recovery. In accordance with the child's developmental level and his or her progress in readjusting to the changes following disclosure, specific skills training may be introduced gradually to assist the child in coping with these stressors, such as relaxation training, the use of positive coping statements, and the use of imagery and positive practice (see Karoly, 1981; Meichenbaum, 1977). In essence, the goal during the crisis phase of involvement is to provide the child with successful coping experiences that serve to counteract previous experiences of helplessness by reframing the difficult changes the child faces into challenges that may result in self-mastery and improved self-confidence.

Individual therapy with the child can be initiated during the crisis period following disclosure of sexual abuse. Under these circumstances, therapy would concentrate on providing immediate emotional support to the child and protection of the child's welfare. Referred to as total life support therapy (Porter, Blick, & Sgroi, 1982), the therapist must be prepared to provide emotional support and to assist victims with interviews by police, medical personnel, child protective services, and agents of the legal system. If the child remains in the home the provision of emotional support is an essential concern, especially if the child's parent(s) does not accept the allegations. Establishment of a therapeutic relationship, therefore, is often based on the therapist's ability to assist the child in obtaining resources during the days following disclosure. Individual therapy with the child may continue throughout the short- and long-term phases of treatment. The "damaged goods syndrome" (i.e., the child feels that he or she is "broken" or permanently damaged by the abuse), and feelings of betrayal, fear, depression, and low self-esteem can be addressed during individual sessions with the child, depending on the circumstances and psychological status of the child (further discussion of therapeutic procedures during the recovery phase of involvement is presented later in this chapter).

Assisting the Child with Court Procedures. During the immediate aftermath of sexual abuse disclosure, a number of potentially critical issues may arise concerning the child's testimony in the courtroom. The child may be expected to relate his or her experiences to several different agencies, and the complexity of the court system is likely to be confusing (e.g., plea bargaining, grand juries, possible acquittal of perpetrator).

Accordingly, the mental health professional may provide any or all of the following roles in the courtroom (Berliner & Barbieri, 1984): (a) provide input regarding the child's credibility, (b) prepare the child emotionally and psychologically for the stress of court testimony, (c) serve as an expert witness about child sexual abuse and children's testimony, and (d) educate the court (i.e., judges, prosecutors) about psychological issues concerning children's testimony (e.g., developmental limits to answering questions, concrete vs. abstract reasoning abilities, the effects of court procedures on children's emotional well-being). Therefore, an overview of these issues and procedures regarding the professional's role in the courtroom will precede the remaining discussion of assessment and therapeutic objectives during the recovery phase.

Credibility and emotional stability/strength are two assessment issues that dominate judicial concerns with the sexually abused child. Major credibility questions that are likely to surface in the courtroom include the child's accuracy of memory, ability to discern fantasy from reality, and his or her record of honesty, as well as normative concepts of children's morality, suggestability, ability to make eyewitness identification, and ability to relate the sequence of events/dates of molestations. In contrast to credibility issues, an assessment of the child's emotional response in relation to criminal justice system involvement is often required in order to determine the reliability and validity of the testimony and the possible harm or strain to the child in providing firsthand information. The child's fear of causing harm to the family, guilt for the perpetrator's punishment, feelings of futility, unpreparedness, and worry about being believed often dominate the child's ability to withstand the stress of courtroom testimony.

Recent interventions for helping the child victim deal with court procedures have been reported that merit the attention of researchers, clinicians, and members of the legal profession. For example, courtroom procedures may be modified by limiting press coverage and by using a one-way mirror to hide the child's view of the perpetrator while relaying testimony (this procedure will maintain, as well, the defendent's right to a face-to-face confrontation). The use of videotaped testimony and the assignment of special proscecutors who are familiar with sexual abuse may also reduce the stress on the child.

Whereas the previously mentioned changes may require considerable legal changes, preparing the child for court is a form of intervention that can be initiated with minimal delay or intrusion. This involves a discussion with the child of the specifics of the trial, the meaning of the charges, the probability and procedures of plea bargaining, the number of times the child might appear in court, and particular problems involved in the case (i.e., lack of evidence, expected postponements, etc.). School-aged children may also be taught about court procedures by acquainting the child with the courtroom and players through the use of drawings, dolls in a dollsize courthouse, visits to a courtroom, the use of mock trials, and role playing. Although it is not appropriate to advise the child witness as to what to say, it is appropriate to help him or her think through answers to probable direct- and cross-examination questions (this should be done in conjunction with the prosecutor). Courtroom etiquette may also be rehearsed, such as the importance of telling the truth, speaking clearly and loudly, being courteous and properly dressed, and only answering the question that has been asked. Interested readers are advised to review procedures of cognitive-behavioral intervention developed with other clinical-child populations (e.g., Kendall & Braswell, 1985; Meichenbaum, 1977), which may also help the child to prepare for stressful encounters, to confront one issue at a time, to cope with feelings of being overwhelmed, and to use self-statements that reinforce his or her attempts at coping. It is particularly important to approach the child's participation in court as a mastery experience for the child and to focus on the child's performance of civic duties (i.e., to tell the truth, to help society control crime, etc.), rather than focusing on the outcome of the trial.

Recovery and Adjustment Phase

The assessment and modification of family relationships is a critical step toward promoting the child's recovery following the disclosure of sexual abuse (Alexander, 1985; P. B. Mrazek & Bentovim, 1981; Sgroi, 1982; Wolfe & Wolfe, 1987). This is a potentially overwhelming task that implicates both dyadic and systemic relationships that may be directly or indirectly involved in the perpetuation of abuse within the family. Such a task requires careful planning and the gradual understanding of the temporal and functional relation between negative family processes (e.g., inappropriate forms of child punishment, poor communication, marital discord) and sexual abuse.

The task of family assessment may be approached initially by obtaining a thorough family history relevant to (a) family disorganization prior to the abuse, (b) family violence or criminal activity, (c) previous marital discord or family relationship problems, (d) previous mother–child relationship difficulties, and (e) previous stressful events faced by the family and how these events were managed. In addition to reports from family members, the social worker's information and perspective concerning previous assessments, home-based observations, and changes within the family system provide crucial direction throughout this phase of the assessment process.

Family Assessment Issues. To provide structure and direction to the task of assessing families where incest has occurred, we have developed an assessment strategy that focuses on two primary areas: dyadic relationships (e.g., marital and parent–child relations) and general family relationship patterns (Wolfe & Wolfe, 1987). Each of these areas will be discussed from an assessment viewpoint, with the objective in mind of identifying areas of change that may facilitate the child's recovery and readjustment following abuse.

The extent to which marital conflict is overt and commonplace has important implications for the child's adjustment. Results of studies involving children of divorce (e.g., Emery, 1982; Hetherington, Cox, & Cox, 1976; Rutter, 1983) and children of battered women (e.g., Jaffe, Wolfe, Wilson, & Zak, 1986; D. A. Wolfe, Jaffe, Wilson, & Zak, 1985) indicate that externalizing problems (e.g., aggression, delinquency, noncompliance) often surface during the course of marital conflict and often persist well beyond the point of family separation, especially among boys. Thus, self-report instruments for assessing marital relationship problems, such as the *Marital Adjustment Test* (Locke & Wallace, 1959) or the *Dyadic Adjustment Scale* (Spanier, 1976) can be useful for assessing a couple's overall satisfaction and specific problem areas within the marriage. Detailed assessment of the couple's satisfaction with their sexual relationship may also be warranted, particularly with couples who decide to continue their relationship and who wish to have custody of the abused child. The *Sexual Interaction Inventory* (LoPiccolo & Steger, 1974) is well suited for this purpose, for it is a multidimensional inventory reflecting sexual functioning as well as sexual satisfaction. Whereas all of the previously mentioned instruments have repeatedly been shown to possess adequate reliability and validity with clinical populations, it must be noted that their value in identifying problem areas within incestuous families has not as yet been empirically established.

Direct observation methodology also has not been used to date with sexually abusive families, although such procedures offer promising insights regarding the dynamics of family processes underlying major problem areas. Several important issues may be addressed through formal and informal observational procedures, such as the extent of positive and negative exchange within the family (which may relate to the development of child behavior problems: Patterson, 1982; Prinz, Foster, Kent, & O'Leary, 1979), individual responses of family members to the child's expression of negative affect or emotion (which may relate to the development of internalizing, overcontrolled behavior patterns; Arthur, Hops, & Biglan, 1982), and the extent to which family members acknowledge the child's assertions (which may relate to the passive response style of learned helplessness: Peterson & Seligman, 1983; Wolfe & Wolfe, 1987). Unfortunately, direct observational systems for assessing interaction patterns of children who exhibit internalizing problems (the most common symptomatology related to sexual abuse) have not kept pace with the expansion of methods designed to assess conduct problem children and their families (cf. Karoly, 1981). For this reason, researchers interested in family interactional data must adapt existing systems or develop new coding procedures that include definitions of affective responding, such as happy, warm/caring, irritated, depressed, sarcastic, etc. (see Arthur *et al.*, 1982, for an exemplary system used with depressed adults).

In addition to assessing interactions during everyday activities, the investigator may find it useful to observe parent–child interactions during conflict resolution and problem-solving tasks (Prinz *et al.*, 1979; Robin & Weiss, 1980). The parent and child (or entire family) are presented with a challenging problem to discuss (e.g., planning a weekend together, deciding chores and household responsibilities, etc.), and observations of cooperation, defensive behavior, humor, disruption, and problem solving may be conducted in the context of such realistically structured family communication.

Intervention Goals and Modalities. The primary therapeutic goal addressed during the recovery period involves the resolution of problems that resulted from the abuse itself, or any traumatization that occurred as a result of the disclosure of the abuse. Reestablishment of the family unit or the redefinition of the child's family situation (e.g., supervised visits with the offender) is often a concurrent goal during this phase (Giarretto, 1982). Several specific psychological treatment needs of the sexually abused child have been identified by Porter *et al.* (1982), which generally involve more long-standing problems within the family system that require different therapeutic approaches than those initiated during the crisis phase. These treatment needs have been referred to previously (see Behavioral and Emotional Symptoms Associated With Sexual Child Abuse) and therefore will be mentioned here only briefly. They include the child's feelings of guilt and responsibility for the sexual activity that took place, as well as feelings of betrayal for disclosing the abuse or upsetting family members; fears associated with the episodes, culminating in sleep disturbances, school disruption, avoidance of particular persons or places, etc.; symptoms of depression, associated with self-harm, lack of initiative, lowered self-esteem, and/or poor social skills with peers; anger toward the abuser or other family members who failed to protect or intervene, coupled with an inability to trust others or to express his or her feelings in a direct manner; and the child's failure to complete normal developmental tasks, especially those involving the development of healthy peer relationships and sexual identity and expression.

Individual psychotherapy or counseling with sexual child abuse victims represents a strategy that is particularly useful for establishing a supportive relationship with a positive adult role model. The objectives in undertaking a one-to-one therapeutic approach are to improve the child's ability to relate to adults in a trusting manner, to encourage the development of positive self-esteem, and to establish the child's sense of control over events in his or her life. These objectives may be accomplished, for example, through the therapeutic channels of modeling (i.e., providing the child with examples of problem-solving and interpersonal expression via adult and peer models), rehearsal (i.e., establishing weekly objectives that assist in strengthening self-confidence, social skills, etc.), and cognitive restructuring (i.e., challenging the child's beliefs about the causes and blame for actions that were beyond his or her control). Individual therapy also provides opportunities to investigate the child's attributions regarding the abuse and the child's perceptions of control regarding future events (e.g., self-awareness and protection; self-efficacy). The child's social skills with peers, feelings about sexuality, relationships with family members, and similar areas of developmental progress may be monitored over several months in order to assist the child in recovering from the far-reaching consequences associated with sexual abuse.

Dyadic counseling involving other family members is another common modality of therapy with abuse victims (Deaton & Sandlin, 1980; Giarretto, 1982; Porter *et al.*, 1982). Typically, the sexually abused child and his or her mother are seen together in order to reestablish or initiate a sound mother–child relationship. This focus is derived from several presumptions concerning the child's perception of mother's role in the abuse (which are, at this time, tenable yet untested therapeutic foundations). The child may feel that mother knew about or condoned the abuse and did not act to stop it. This feeling may be accompanied by fear and worry that mother did not believe his or her story, or may be expressed as anger for failure to respond in a helpful manner. Associated with these concerns surrounding the discovery of the abuse may be a history of related fears and mother–child relationship problems, such as the child's view of the mother as ineffectual or noncaring, and real or self-perceived blame of the child for the major disruptions that have occurred in the family. On the other hand, a mother may not understand the behavioral and emotional problems that the child may be experiencing and how these problems relate to the mother–child relationship. For example, the mother may perceive the child's increased difficulties in school to be a function of the child's inherent laziness or carelessness, and fail to consider the impact of events on the child that may lead to an inability to concentrate or to derive satisfaction from schoolwork. The first direction for mother–child dyadic therapy, therefore, is to educate the mother about the effects of abuse on children and about possible concerns the child may have. Mothers should be encouraged to discuss their responsibility for the abuse with the child, and to express their concern for ensuring that further abuse does not happen. Concurrently, the therapist may clarify for the child his or her mother's source of heightened anxiety, irritability, worry, etc., in that she also has been a victim of the abuse.

When fathers or father-figures are the perpetrators, dyadic therapy may be of benefit to assist in mending the father–child relationship which is considered to be a critical therapeutic goal for the child (P. B. Mrazek & Bentovim, 1981; Sgroi, 1982). This approach to attaining the goal of recovery, however, is appropriate only when the father admits his responsibility. In cases where the father is unwilling to accept full responsibility, or has been legally advised not to participate in therapy (because this may be construed as an admission of guilt), dyadic therapy is necessarily omitted. Many role boundaries are obviously broken when an adult initiates sexual contact with a child, and the result is confusion and turmoil on the part of the child and other family members. The use of a clarification conference, whereby the roles and responsibilities of each family member are clarified for the benefit of the child's recovery, is a particularly valuable intervention strategy for most incest victims (Ralston, 1984). Porter *et al.* (1982) also recommend that the perpetrator should explain to the child that the perpetrator is responsible for the abuse and accepts all blame for the misconduct and any subsequent disruptions and difficulties (such as family separation).

Separately or in conjunction with individual and dyadic therapy, family therapy may be a useful treatment modality where many of the psychological needs of the sexually abused child can be addressed. However, this therapeutic approach also relies on the acceptance by both parents of their responsibility for the abuse. Feelings of guilt and depression resulting from the abuse and its aftermath, anger toward the parents, confusion over blurred role boundaries, and issues of the child developing a sense of self-mastery and self-control can be approached within the context of family therapy. The family unit may also be strengthened by emphasizing the expression of feelings that may be common to all members, such as anger at the system, feelings that their private lives have become public (stigmatization), feelings of concern and care toward one another, and the development of greater trust. Family therapy may also be advantageous in treating the covictims of sexual abuse within the family, such as siblings and parents who were physically and emotionally disrupted by the disclosure of the abuse. For example, incarceration, financial hardship, parental separation, and out-of-home living arrangments may follow from the aftermath of sexual abuse, and siblings of the victimized child often need an avenue through which to discuss their concerns about events and challenges facing all family members.

Peer group counseling represents a preferred mode of treatment for older children and adolescents (Porter *et al.*, 1982), especially once the immediate crisis situation and turmoil (e.g., court hearings, family disruption) have subsided. Because abused children often experience guilt and lowered self-esteem, support from others who have had similar experiences tends to lessen the impairment and confusion (Adams-Tucker & Adams, 1984; P. B. Mrazek, 1981b). Peers may serve to validate the victim's self-worth and provide insights into family process and readjustment. The group may also facilitate the acquisition of social skills and the accomplishment of developmental tasks (e.g., grooming, dress, relating to peers of the same or opposite sex) that were delayed or altered by the victimization. Group members who have progressed beyond the initial phases of involvement serve as positive role models for other members, providing motivation and important guidance to the child or adolescent seeking to recovery from the aftermath of sexual abuse disclosure and trauma.

FUTURE DIRECTIONS IN RESEARCH AND PREVENTION

Child sexual abuse has been the focus of concerted research effort only recently, and progress in this area lags behind the investigation of physical abuse by perhaps as much as 15 to 20 years (P. B. Mrazek, 1981a; D. A. Wolfe, 1987). At this point researchers are primarily interested in establishing the extent and nature of the problem that sexual abuse poses for its child victims, which requires time-consuming studies of incidence data reflecting demographic and descriptive information about these children and their families. However, now that an understanding of the severity and impact of sexual abuse is beginning to emerge into a field of empirical enquiry (e.g., Browne & Finkelhor, 1986; Finkelhor, 1984), researchers interested in the more specific psychological phenomena associated with this problem must surmount the methodological concerns that have existed in studies to date. These concerns include (a) the definition of child sexual abuse and the samples used, (b) reliance on case reports, (c) the choice of outcome measures and criteria for adjustment, and (d) drawing causal inferences without controlling for other pathological influences (P. B. Mrazek & D. A. Mrazek, 1981).

Regarding definitional concerns, studies have seldom differentiated between the widely disparate types of sexual abuse, which requires clarification in terms of the extent of sexual contact, age and developmental maturity of the child, degree of relatedness between victim and perpetrator, affective nature of the relationship, age difference between the victim and perpetrator, and the length of the abuse (P. B. Mrazek & D. A. Mrazek, 1981). Perhaps even more than in the case of physical abuse, the clarification of the extent and nature of the victim's experiences is essential because the impact on the child appears to covary with factors associated with the abusive episodes (e.g., threats, bribery, relationship to the offender). Similarly, the samples employed in the research have been comprised of very different subgroups (i.e., victims whose abuse has recently been discovered, "deviant" populations of adults, and college students). Retrospective data from adults, in particular, have often been used for judging psychological trauma stemming from childhood, although this approach is fraught with difficulties (e.g., selective memory bias, distortion of events, current interest in abuse victims).

Moreover, much of the information available on the effects of sexual abuse is based on clinical case material, and thus general findings cannot be established. Although these case reports assisted in establishing the importance of this new area of research, few studies have gone beyond this approach to control for the vast number of interfering factors that are contained in such reports. This state of affairs is reminiscent of physical abuse in the 1960s and early 1970s, when the emphasis in research and public opinion was on the dire consequences and deviancy of this form of behavior in the family, and the research was based on incidence data and case reports (e.g., Spinetta & Rigler, 1972). In terms of measurement and outcome criteria, few studies have used any standardized outcome measures of cognitive or psychological functioning, and have instead relied on the psychiatric interview, case histories, medical records, etc. Criteria for adjustment, accordingly, have lacked specificity and accuracy, and often conclusions are worded in general terms (e.g., the individual exhibits a "major disturbance of interpersonal relationships"). Finally, cause and effect relationships cannot be established on the basis of the methodological approaches considered to date. This impairs our ability to distinguish the effects of the abuse itself from the associated circumstances, such as a difficult home life, disruption in family cohesiveness following the exposure of abuse, criminal justice involvement, etc. A variety of possibilities exists for explaining the associations between childhood sexual abuse and later adult adjustment, and controlled, longitudinal studies are necessary before more firm conclusions can be reached.

In addition to studies on the impact of abuse, investigations related to successful treatment and prevention approaches with this population seem warranted. One promising direction for future research efforts that emerges from the available findings is the potential importance of early preventative activities for children and their families. The majority of sexual abuse incidents appear to result from the exploitation of the child's naiveté and innocence surrounding privacy and appropriate sexual conduct. Coupled with the assumption that many children initially enjoy the attention of adults whom they already know (in the absence of coercion or threats), it is evident that one direction for prevention involves the education of children in awareness of their right to privacy and self-discretion. This issue is not as straightforward as it may seem at first, however, because teaching children to discriminate between appropriate and inappropriate touching is a sensitive topic to many parents and school officials.

Programs designed to prevent physical and sexual child abuse have begun to emerge recently in community and educational settings. Child abuse prevention activities have ranged from nationwide public awareness campaigns to locally sponsored educational programs for adults and children. Programs aimed specifically at the prevention of childhood sexual abuse, however, must deal with sensitive issues that have traditionally been avoided by community and educational institutions (because of the disguised and intrafamilial nature of most sexual abuse). The task of informing young children of potential misdeeds by adults whom they trust and depend on, without frightening or alarming the child unnecessarily, is very difficult. Prevention objectives must be formulated on the basis of the child's current developmental level, community and educational resources and support available, and realistic assumptions regarding family privacy and the child's ability to modify inappropriate family patterns (Wolfe, MacPherson, Blount, & Wolfe, 1986).

Several evaluative studies have recently demonstrated improvements in children's knowledge and awareness of possible actions to take in the event of potential or actual abuse following exposure to educational programs. In one study, preschool- and school-aged children were exposed to a 3-hour program teaching common sexual abuse prevention concepts (e.g., the difference between OK and not-OK touches; Conte, Rosen, Saperstein, & Shermack, 1985). Relative to the control group, children who received the prevention training significantly increased their knowledge of prevention concepts. Similar findings were reported by D. A. Wolfe *et al.* (1986), in which brief skits and focal discussion in the classroom were used to teach sexual abuse prevention concepts. Both groups of researchers caution, however, that some of the children had difficulty learning prevention concepts of an abstract nature. Additionally, the issue of whether or not a child would actually benefit from the information taught in these programs if faced with a potentially abusive situation has not as yet been determined, because the outcome criteria are knowledge based. Programmatic revisions based on these early findings may lead to critical improvements for broadening the scope and impact of educationally based child abuse prevention in future studies, such as the provision of developmentally appropriate information, extended training/educational sessions, and rehearsal of appropriate responses to threatening situations. Readers interested in materials for sexual abuse prevention are advised to consult the review of books for parents and children by Schroeder, Gordon, and McConnell (1986).

SUMMARY

In this chapter we have explored many of the characteristics of sexually abused children and their families, with an emphasis on the child's psychological recovery from abuse by persons with whom the child is familiar. Although sexual abuse has been in existence for centuries, society's definition and condemnation of the harm of adult–child sexual relations continues to evolve among lawmakers and mental health professionals. Delays in documenting the significant impact of sexual abuse on its victims are believed to have existed, in part, because of the lack of physical injuries or evidence of physical assault, and the difficulty of specifying the relative importance of factors that are either directly or indirectly associated with the abuse (such as the child's relationship with the offender, the type and severity of the abuse, the use of bribery and intimidation, family reaction to disclosure, etc.).

The available literature on sexual child abuse is currently dependent to a large extent on case reports of children seen by clinicians and studies of adult incest "survivors."

Despite the methodological limitations, the problems shown among a significant proportion of these children and adults have been found repeatedly across a number of studies. Such a confluence of findings regarding the child's fears and anxieties, impaired self-esteem, guilt, depression, and peer relationships supports the conclusion that sexual abuse and its aftermath represent traumatic events that can have a long-ranging impact on the child's subsequent development. A major influence of the literature, however, is that the negative impact of sexual abuse is not universal. Rather, the impact varies across individuals and relates to the degree of associated stressful life events and available supports for assisting the child's recovery.

A conceptual model was presented herein that highlights the major events occurring at different phases of the child's involvement (i.e., predisclosure, disclosure crisis, and recovery). Accordingly, it was argued that the sexually abused child may undergo major life crises or trauma during the time preceding and following the disclosure of the abuse, which may permeate the child's view of him or herself and others for a significant period of time. Psychological processes of social learning, such as the modeling of inappropriate sexual conduct or the development of conditioned fears and anxieties associated with the abuse, were used to explain the development of symptomatology among sexually abused children.

Assessment and therapeutic strategies for assisting the child and his or her family also appear to vary in accordance with the sequence of events to which the child is subjected. This chapter presented an assessment strategy that involves the child's overt behavioral and emotional problems and self-reported attributions for the event(s), in addition to assessment of family patterns and reactions. The most commonly employed therapeutic approaches involving individual, dyadic, family, and peer-group counseling were discussed, and it was concluded that these services may provide critical support and clarification that fosters the child's recovery from abuse. Moreover, innovative approaches for helping the child deal with the stress of courtroom procedures, as well as school- and community-based programs aimed at making children more aware of their safety and privacy, were presented as promising directions for research and prevention.

REFERENCES

Abramson, L. Y., Seligman, M. E. P., & Teasdale, J. D. (1978). Learned helplessness in humans: Critique and reformulation. *Journal of Abnormal Psychology, 87,* 49–74.

Achenbach, T., & Edelbrock, C. S. (1983). *Manual for the Child Behavior Checklist and Child Behavior Profile.* Burlington, VT: University of Vermont.

Adams-Tucker, C. (1982). Proximate effects of sexual abuse in childhood: A report on 28 children. *American Journal of Psychiatry, 139,* 1252–1256.

Adams-Tucker, C., & Adams, P. (1984). Treatment of sexually abused children. In I. R. Stuart & J. G. Greer (Eds.), *Victims of sexual aggression: Treatment of children, women, and men* (pp. 57–74). New York: Van Nostrand Reinhold.

Alexander, P. C. (1985). A systems theory conceptualization of incest. *Family Process, 24,* 79–88.

American Humane Association. (1984). *Highlights of official child neglect and abuse reporting—1982.* Denver, CO: Author.

Anderson, S. C., Bach, C. M., & Griffith, S. (Sept., 1981). *Psychosocial sequelae in intrafamilial victims of sexual assault and abuse.* Paper presented at the Third International Conference on Child Abuse and Neglect, Amsterdam.

Arthur, J. A., Hops, H., & Biglan, A. (1982). *LIFE (Living in Familial Environments) coding system.* Unpublished manuscript, Oregon Research Institute, Eugene, OR.

Baker, A. L., & Peterson, C. (1977). Self-blame by rape victims as a function of the rape's consequences: An attributional analysis. *Crisis Intervention, 8,* 92–104.

Bander, K., Fein, E., & Bishop, G. (1982). Child sex abuse treatment: Some barriers to program operation. *Child Abuse & Neglect, 6,* 185–191.

Becker, J. V., Skinner, L. J., Abel, G. G., & Cichon, J. (1986). Level of post-assault sexual functioning in rape and incest victims. *Archives of Sexual Behavior, 15,* 37–49.

Bender, L., & Grugett, A. (1951). A follow-up report on children who had atypical sexual experiences. *American Journal of Orthopsychiatry, 22,* 825–837.

Berliner, L., & Barbieri, M. K. (1984). The testimony of the child victim of sexual assault. *Journal of Social Issues, 40,* 125–137.

Brenner, A. (1984). *Helping children cope with stress.* Lexington, MA: D. C. Heath.

Broder, E. A., & Hood, E. (1983). A guide to the assessment of child and family. In P. D. Steinhauer & Q. Rae-Grant (Eds.), *Psychological problems of the child in the family* (pp. 130–149). New York: Basic Books.

Browne, A., & Finkelhor, D. (1984, August). *The impact of child sexual abuse: A review of the literature.* Paper presented at the 2nd National Conference for Family Violence Researchers, Durham, NH.

Browne, A., & Finkelhor, D. (1986). Impact of child sexual abuse: A review of the literature. *Psychological Bulletin, 99,* 66–77.

Browning, D., & Boatman, B. (1977). Incest: Children at risk. *American Journal of Psychiatry, 134,* 69–72.

Burgess, A. W., Hartman, C. R., McCausland, M. P., & Powers, P. (1984). Response patterns in children and adolescents exploited through sex rings and pornography. *American Journal of Psychiatry, 141,* 656–662.

Burgess, A. W., & Holmstrom, L. L. (1974). *Rape: Victims of crisis.* Bowie, MD: Robert Brady.

Committee on Sexual Offenses Against Children and Youth. (1984). *Sexual offenses against children in Canada: Summary.* Ottawa: Supply and Services Canada.

Conte, J. R., & Berlinger, L. (1981). Sexual abuse of children: Implications for practice. *Social Casework, 62,* 601–606.

Conte, J. R., Rosen, C., Saperstein, L., & Shermack, R. (1985). An evaluation of a program to prevent the sexual victimization of young children. *Child Abuse & Neglect, 9,* 319–328.

Courtois, C. A. (1980). Studying and counseling women with past incest experience. *Victimology: An International Journal, 5,* 322–334.

Deaton, F. A., & Sandlin, D. L. (1980). Sexual victimology within the home: A treatment approach. *Victimology: An International Journal, 5,* 311–321.

DeFrancis, V. (1969). *Protecting the child victim of sex crimes committed by adults.* Denver, CO: American Humane.

Department of Health & Human Services (1981). *National Study of the incidence and severity of child abuse and neglect.* Washington, DC: U.S. Government Printing Office.

Emery, R. E. (1982). Interparental conflict and the children of divorce. *Psychological Bulletin, 92,* 310–330.

Faller, K. C. (1984). Is the child victim of sexual abuse telling the truth? *Child Abuse & Neglect, 8,* 473–481.

Farber, E. D., Showers, J., Johnson, C. F., Joseph, J. A., & Oshins, L. (1984). The sexual abuse of children: A comparison of male and female victims. *Journal of Clinical Child Psychology, 13,* 294–297.

Finkelhor, D. (1979a). *Sexually victimized children.* New York: Free Press.

Finkelhor, D. (1979b). What's wrong with sex between adults and children? Ethics and the problem of sexual abuse. *American Journal of Orthopsychiatry, 49,* 692–697.

Finkelhor, D. (1980). Risk factors in the sexual victimization of children. *Child Abuse & Neglect, 4,* 265–273.

Finkelhor, D. (1981). The sexual abuse of boys. *Victimology: An International Journal, 6,* 76–84.

Finkelhor, D. (1982). Sexual abuse: A sociological perspective. *Child Abuse & Neglect, 6,* 95–102.

Finkelhor, D. (1984). *Child sexual abuse: New theory and research.* New York: The Free Press.

Finkelhor, D., & Browne, A. (1985). The traumatic impact of child sexual abuse: A conceptualization. *American Journal of Orthopsychiatry, 55,* 530–541.

Fraser, B. G. (1981). Sexual child abuse: The legislation and the law in the United States. In P. B. Mrazek & C. H. Kempe (Eds.), *Sexually abused children and their families* (pp. 55–73). New York: Pergamon Press.

Friedrich, W. N., Urquiza, A. J., & Beilke, R. (1986). Behavioral problems in sexually abused young children. *Journal of Pediatric Psychology, 11,* 47–57.

Fromuth, M. E. (1986). The relationship of childhood sexual abuse with later psychological and sexual adjustment in a sample of college women. *Child Abuse & Neglect, 10,* 5–15.

Gagnon, J. (1965). Female child victims of sex offenses. *Social Problems, 13,* 176–192.

Gelinas, D. J. (1983). The persisting negative effects of incest. *Psychiatry, 46,* 312–332.

Giarretto, H. (1982). A comprehensive child sexual abuse treatment program. *Child Abuse & Neglect, 6,* 263–278.

Gold, E. R. (1986). Long-term effects of sexual victimization in childhood: An attributional approach. *Journal of Consulting and Clinical Psychology, 54,* 471–475.

Gomes-Schwartz, B., & Horowitz, J. (1981, July). *A model for assessing factors contributing to trauma in child sexual abuse*. Paper presented at the National Conference for Family Violence Researchers, Durham, NH.

Goodwin, J., McCarthy, T., & Divasto, P. (1981). Prior incest in mothers of abused children. *Child Abuse & Neglect, 5*, 87–96.

Groth, N. A. (1979). *Men who rape*. New York: Plenum Press.

Gruber, K. J., & Jones, R. J. (1981). Does sexual abuse lead to delinquent behavior? A critical look at the evidence. *Victimology: An International Journal, 6*, 85–91.

Gruber, K. J., & Jones, R. J. (1983). Identifying determinants of risk of sexual victimization of youth: A multivariate approach. *Child Abuse & Neglect, 7*, 17–24.

Herman, J. L. (1981). *Father–daughter incest*. Cambridge, MA.: Harvard University Press.

Hetherington, E. M., Cox, M., & Cox, R. (1976), Divorced fathers. *The Family Coordinator, 25*, 417–428.

Jaffe, P., Wolfe, D. A., Wilson, S., & Zak, L. (1986). Similarities in behavioral and social maladjustment among child victims and witnesses to family violence. *American Journal of Orthopsychiatry, 56*, 142–146.

James, B., & Nasjleti, M. (1983). *Treating sexually abused children and their families*. Palo Alto, CA: Consulting Psychologists Press.

James, J., & Meyerding, J. (1977). Early sexual experiences and prostitution. *American Journal of Psychiatry, 134*, 1381–1385.

Janoff-Bulman, R., & Frieze, I. H. (1983). A theoretical perspective for understanding reactions to victimization. *Journal of Social Issues, 39*, 1–17.

Justice, B., & Justice, R. (1979). *The broken taboo*. New York: Human Sciences Press.

Karoly, P. (1981). Self-management problems in children. In E. J. Mash & L. G. Terdal (Eds.), *Behavioral assessment of childhood disorders* (pp. 79–126). New York: Guilford Press.

Kempe, R. S., & Kempe, C. H. (1984). *The common secret: Sexual abuse of children and adolescents*. New York: W. H. Freeman.

Kendall, P. C., & Braswell, L. (1985). *Cognitive-behavioral therapy for impulsive children*. New York: Guilford Press.

Kerns, D. L. (1981). Medical assessment of child sexual abuse. In P. B. Mzarek & C. H. Kempe (Eds.), *Sexually abused children and their families* (pp. 129–141). New York: Pergamon Press.

Kinsey, A. C., Pomeroy, W. B., Martin, C. E., & Gebhard, P. H. (1953). *Sexual behavior in the human female*. Philadelphia, PA: Saunders.

Kovacs, M. (1983, April). *The Children's Depression Inventory: A self-rated depression scale for school-aged youngsters*. Unpublished manuscript, University of Pittsburgh.

Lewis, M., & Sarrell, P. M. (1969). Some psychological aspects of seduction, incest, and rape in childhood. *Journal of the American Academy of Child Psychiatry, 8*, 606–610.

Locke, H. J., & Wallace, K. M. (1959). Short-term martial adjustment and prediction tests: Their reliability and validity. *Journal of Marriage and Family Living, 21*, 251–255.

LoPiccolo, J., & Steger, J. (1974). The Sexual Interaction Inventory: A new instrument for assessing sexual dysfunction. *Archives of Sexual Research, 3*, 585–595.

Magnuson, E. (1983, Sept. 5). Child abuse: The ultimate betrayal. *Time*, pp. 16–18.

McQuire, I. S., & Wagner, N. N. (1978). Sexual dysfunction in women who were molested as children: On response patterns and suggestions for treatment. *Journal of Sex and Marital Therapy, 4*, 11–15.

Meichenbaum, D. (1977). *Cognitive-behavior modification: An integrative approach*. New York: Plenum Press.

Meiselman, K. C. (1978). *Incest: A psychological study of causes and effects with treatment recommendations*. San Francisco: Jossey-Bass.

Melton, G. B. (1985). Sexually abused children and the legal system: Some policy recommendations. *The American Journal of Family Therapy, 13*, 61–67.

Mrazek, D. A. (1981). The child psychiatric examination of the sexually abused child. In P. B. Mrazek & C. H. Kempe (Eds.), *Sexually abused children and their families* (pp. 143–154). New York: Pergamon Press.

Mrazek, P. B. (1981a). Definition and recognition of sexual child abuse: Historical and cultural perspectives. In P. B. Mrazek & C. H. Kempe (Eds.), *Sexually abused children and their families* (pp. 5–16). New York: Pergamon Press.

Mrazek, P. B. (1981b). Group psychotherapy with sexually abused children. In P. B. Mrazek & C. H. Kempe (Eds.), *Sexually abused children and their families* (pp. 199–208). New York: Pergamon Press.

Mrazek, P. B. (1983). Sexual abuse of children. In B. B. Lahey & A. E. Kazdin (Eds.), *Advances in clinical child psychology* (Vol. 6, pp. 199–215). New York: Plenum Press.

Mrazek, P. B., & Bentovim, A. (1981). Incest and the dysfunctional family system. In P. B. Mrazek & C. H. Kempe (Eds.), *Sexually abused children and their families* (pp. 167–178). New York: Pergamon Press.

Mrazek, P. B., & Mrazek, D. A. (1981). The effects of child sexual abuse: Methodological considerations. In P. B. Mrazek & C. H. Kempe (Eds.), *Sexually abused children and their families* (pp. 235–245). New York: Pergamon Press.

National Center on Child Abuse and Neglect (1979). *Child sexual abuse: Incest, assault, and sexual exploitation* (DHEW Publication No. OHDS 79-30166). Washington, DC: U.S. Government Printing Office.

National Center on Child Abuse and Neglect. (1981). *Study findings: National study of the incidence and severity of child abuse and neglect* (DHHS publication No. OHDS 81-30325). Washington, DC: U.S. Government Printing Office.

Ollendick, T. H. (1978). Reliability and validity of the Revised Fear Survey Schedule for Children (FSSC-R). *Behaviour Research and Therapy, 21,* 685–692.

Patterson, G. R. (1982). *Coercive family process.* Eugene, OR: Castalia.

Peters, J. (1976). Children who are victims of sexual assault and the psychology of offenders. *American Journal of Psychotherapy, 30,* 398–412.

Peterson, C., & Seligman, M. E. P. (1983). Learned helplessness and victimization. *Journal of Social Issues, 39,* 103–116.

Porter, F. S., Blick, L. C., & Sgroi, S. M. (1982). Treatment of the sexually abused child. In S. Sgroi (Ed.), *Handbook of clinical intervention in child sexual abuse* (pp. 109–145). Lexington, MA: Lexington Books.

Prinz, R. J., Foster, S. L., Kent, R. N., & O'Leary, K. D. (1979). Multivariate assessment of conflict in distressed and non-distressed mother-adolescent dyads. *Journal of Applied Behavior Analysis, 12,* 691–700.

Ralston, L. (1984). *Intra-family sexual abuse: A community system approach to a family system problem.* Unpublished manuscript (available from the Sexual Abuse Treatment Project, Department of Psychiatry, Medical University of South Carolina, Charleston, SC, 29425).

Reynolds, C. R., & Richmond, B. O. (1978). What I think and feel: A revised measure of children's anxiety. *Journal of Abnormal Child Psychology, 6,* 271–280.

Robin, A. L., & Weiss, J. G. (1980). Criterion-related validity of behavioral and self-report measures of problem-solving communication skills in distressed and non-distressed parent-adolescent dyads. *Behavioral Assessment, 2,* 339–352.

Russell, A. B., & Trainor, C. M. (1984). *Trends in child abuse and neglect: A national perspective.* Denver, CO: American Humane.

Russell, D. E. H. (1983). The incidence and prevalence of intrafamilial and extrafamilial sexual abuse of female children. *Child Abuse & Neglect, 7,* 133–146.

Russell, D. E. H. (1984). The prevalence and seriousness of incestuous abuse: Stepfathers vs. biological fathers. *Child Abuse & Neglect, 8,* 15–22.

Rutter, M. (1983). Stress, coping, and development: Some issues and some questions. In N. Garmezy & M. Rutter (Eds.), *Stress, coping, and development in children* (pp. 1–41). New York: McGraw-Hill.

Scherer, M. W., & Nakamura, C. Y. (1968). A fear survey schedule for children (FSS-FC): A factor-analytic comparison with manifest anxiety. *Behavior Research and Therapy, 6,* 173–182.

Schroeder, C. S., Gordon, B. N., & McConnell, P. (1986). Books for parents and children on sexual abuse prevention. *Journal of Clinical Child Psychology, 15,* 178–185.

Seidner, A. L., & Calhoun, K. S. (1984, July). *Childhood sexual abuse: Factors related to differential adult adjustment.* Paper presented at the Second Annual National Family Violence Research Conference, Durham, NH.

Sgroi, S. (1982). *Handbook of clinical intervention in child sexual abuse.* Lexington, MA: Lexington Books.

Silbert, M. H., & Pines, A. M. (1981). Sexual child abuse as an antecedent to prostitution. *Child Abuse & Neglect, 5,* 407–411.

Silver, R. L., Boon, C., & Stones, M. H. (1983). Searching for meaning in misfortune: Making sense of incest. *Journal of Social Issues, 39,* 81–102.

Spanier, G. B. (1976). Measuring dyadic adjustment: New scales for assessing the quality of marriage and similar dyads. *Journal of Marriage and the Family, 38,* 15–28.

Spielberger, C. D. (1973). *State-Trait Anxiety Inventory for Children.* Palo Alto, CA: Consulting Psychologists Press.

Spinetta, J. J., & Rigler, D. (1972). The child-abusing parent: A psychological review. *Psychological Bulletin, 77,* 296–304.

Steele, B. F., & Alexander, H. (1981). Long-term effects of sexual abuse in childhood. In P. B. Mzarek & C. H. Kempe (Eds.), *Sexually abused children and their families* (pp. 223–234). New York: Pergamon Press.

Timnick, L. (1985, August 25). 22% in survey were child abuse victims. *Los Angeles Times,* p. 1.

Tsai, M., Feldman-Summers, S., & Edgar, M. (1979). Childhood molestation: Variables related to differential impacts on psychological functioning in adult women. *Journal of Abnormal Psychology, 88,* 407–417.

Tuft's New England Medical Center, Division of Child Psychiatry. (1984). *Sexually exploited children: Service and research project.* Final report for the Office of Juvenile Justice and Delinquency Prevention. Washington, DC: U.S. Department of Justice.

Wolfe, D. A. (1987). Child abuse and neglect. In E. J. Mash & L. G. Terdal (Eds.), *Behavioral assessment of childhood disorders* (2nd ed.). New York: Guilford.

Wolfe, D. A., Jaffe, P., Wilson, S., & Zak, L. (1985). Children of battered women: The relation of child behavior to family violence and maternal stress. *Journal of Consulting and Clinical Psychology, 53,* 657–665.

Wolfe, D. A., MacPherson, T., Blount, R., & Wolfe, V. V. (1986). Evaluation of a brief intervention for educating school children in awareness of physical and sexual abuse. *Child Abuse & Neglect, 10,* 85–92.

Wolfe, V. V., & Wolfe, D. A. (1987). The sexually abused child. In E. J. Mash & L. G. Terdal (Eds.), *Behavioral assessment of childhood disorders* (2nd. ed.). New York: Guilford.

Wolfe, V. V., Wolfe, D. A., & LaRose, L. (1986). *The Children's Impact of Traumatic Events Scale* (CITES). Unpublished manuscript available from the authors at the Department of Psychology, The University of Western Ontario, London, Ontario, Canada, N6A 5C2.

Yates, A. (1982). Children eroticized by incest. *American Journal of Psychiatry, 139,* 482–485.

8

Incest

JUDITH V. BECKER and EMILY M. COLEMAN

DESCRIPTION OF THE PROBLEM

The definition and societal perspective of incest varies from culture to culture. Most cultures, however, do prohibit sexual relations and marriage between nuclear family members, such as between fathers and daughters, mothers and sons, or brothers and sisters. Some cultures encourage sexual intimacy between family members and do not consider it incest. For those readers interested in further information about cultural attitudes toward incest, Robin Fox's *The Red Lamp of Incest* (1980) offers an excellent discussion of the topic.

Although American society has strong taboos against incest, legal definitions of the problem vary across states. The major relevant laws regulating sexual activity between individuals can be found in the criminal or penal codes. Clinicians are advised to be aware of the statutes and laws in their individual states regarding sexual activity. All 50 states now have laws forbidding sexual activity between adults and children. The American Bar Association's National Legal Resource Center for Child Advocacy and Protection has published a monograph (1980) related to criminal statutes involving sexual offenses against children. It is a useful source of information for the clinician.

In the New York State Penal Code, sexual offenses involving children may be considered misdemeanors or felonies, depending on the ages of the victim and the offender, the degree of force, and the degree of physical injury sustained (New York Criminal Procedure Law, *Graybook,* 1982). State laws vary considerably and may or may not include genital fondling, oral sex, and other sexual behaviors as criminal offenses. In determining incest, many states consider the age of the victim and the nature of the relationship between the victim and the perpetrator. However, the psychiatric definition for some cases of incest as prescribed by the *Diagnostic and Statistical Manual of Mental Disorders—Third Edition* (DSM-III, American Psychiatric Association, 1980) under the psychosexual disorders, specifically, under pedophilia, focuses on another factor: "The essential feature is the act or fantasy of engaging in sexual activity with pre-pubertal

JUDITH V. BECKER • Sexual Behavior Clinic of the New York State Psychiatric Institute, New York, NY 10032, and Department of Clinical Psychology in Psychiatry of the College of Physicians and Surgeons, Columbia University, New York, NY 10032. **EMILY M. COLEMAN** • Sex Offender Program, The Franklin County Mental Health Center, Franklin County, MA.

children as a repeatedly preferred or exclusive method of achieving sexual excitement''
(p. 271). This definition is rather limited in that it would exclude those perpetrators who
may prefer and have sex with adults, but also involve themselves sexually with children.
A considerable number of adult sexual incest perpetrators engage in sexual activities with
their wives and also relate sexually with their children. Thus, although the behavior may
meet the legal criteria for incest within a state, it might not be criteria for a psychiatric
diagnosis.

EPIDEMIOLOGICAL FINDINGS

The social problem of incest has been clouded by many myths. Initially, it was
believed that incest was limited to certain geographical areas (e.g., Appalachia) and to
only lower socioeconomic families. Incest was thought to occur only once or twice and
not to be an ongoing pattern. The belief that dysfunctional family dynamics cause incest
has been a prevailing theory for many years. Often, the mother is blamed for the occurrence of incest because she was ''cold'' or depressed or not available sexually to her
husband. An alternative formulation has been that a sexually provocative child may entice
the parent into being sexual with her or him. In reviewing early writings in the area, it is
intriguing to note how people other than the perpetrator are seen as causal and responsible
for incest.

The exact incidence of incest is unknown because of inadequate reporting and the
lack of reliable statistics. Prevalence figures on child sexual abuse are available from a
variety of sources. The National Center on Child Abuse and Neglect (U. S. Department of
Health and Human Services, 1981) notes that child sexual abuse is not limited by racial,
ethnic, or socioeconomic boundaries, but is to be found in all strata of society. In its
report, the Center lists varying figures for the incidence of child sexual abuse, ranging
from 800 to 1000 per million; there are an average of 500,000 cases per year for girls
under 14 years of age alone. In the largest survey conducted to date, Kinsey, Pomeroy,
Martin, and Gebhard (1953) questioned 5,940 adult females about their sexual experiences. Twenty-four percent of the adult females reported that they had been childhood
victims of various types of sexual contact with adult males. These experiences ranged
from ''hands off'' sexual experiences, such as exhibitionism, to forced sexual intercourse.

Finkelhor (1979) surveyed 530 female and 266 male students at six New England
colleges and universities. The sample came largely from intact, middle-class family
backgrounds. Twenty-eight percent of the women and 23% of the men admitted to a
sexual experience with a relative. The highest incidence of incest occurred between
brothers and sisters.

Recently, Russell (1983) surveyed a probability sample of 930 women residents of
San Francisco who were 18 years of age and older. The definition of sexual abuse used
was, ''any kind of exploitive sexual contact that occurred between relatives, no matter
how distant the relationship, before the victim turned 18 years old'' (p. 136). Sixteen
percent of the sample reported at least one experience of intrafamilial sexual contact
before the age of 18, and 12% had been sexually abused by a relative prior to age 14.
Thirty-one percent of the women reported that they had been victims of extrafamilial
sexual abuse.

Russell (1984) assessed the percentage of victims who were victimized by biological versus stepfathers. Fathers who were biological or adoptive parents represented 2.3% of the perpetrators. Seventeen percent of the perpetrators were stepfathers. Mothers, both biological and adoptive, accounted for .1% of the abusers.

In summary, although the actual incidence is unknown, recent data indicate that incest is not a rare phenomenon, and that the majority of perpetrators are male. Unfortunately, investigations are hampered by ambiguous categories of perpetrators; distinctions are not made between fathers and stepfathers. This chapter will focus primarily on father or stepfather and daughter incest, because this category appears most often in legal reports and clinical studies.

ORIGIN OF THE INCEST TABOO

Various theories have arisen to explain the origins of the incest taboo. The major theories can be categorized into biological, psychological, familial, and feminist. The biological theory stresses the harmful effects of inbreeding. Specifically, the incest taboo insured the survival of the species by prohibiting relatives from engaging in sexual relations. Therefore, it was hypothesized that deformed or recessive genes would not proliferate (Lindsey, 1967).

Offering a psychological explanation, Freud (1913/1950) noted that the taboo prohibits family members from engaging in unconscious sexual desires. Freud believed that sons wanted to be sexual with their mothers and daughters with their fathers.

It is of clinical interest that Freud (1896/1962) wrote a paper which at the time was considered controversial. The article, "The Etiology of Hysteria," is based on 18 clinical cases in which his patients reported being victims of sexual molestations and violence, the majority of which occurred within their families. Freud postulated that the trauma caused by the abuse was the basis of hysteria. Subsequently, Freud repudiated his theory and concluded that the memories that his patients recalled were fantasies and not real-life events. Perhaps because of Freud's repudiation of his seduction theory, clinicians have been unwilling until recently to take seriously the reports of sex abuse presented by their clients. (The interested reader is directed to J. Masson's book, *The Assault on Truth: Freud's Suppression of the Seduction Theory,* for further reading on the subject.)

The familial view of the incest taboo rests in the belief that the taboo distinguishes roles within the family. Without it, there would be role confusion and family disruption. The taboo creates order, unity, and cooperation among family members (Murdock, 1949).

Herman (1981a) proposed a feminist analysis of incest. According to this perspective, the incest taboo establishes the father as the ultimate and absolute authority figure in the family and promotes a patriarchal social structure that oppresses women. Males in society restrict access to certain women, thereby asserting their authority and domain. Herman (1981b) pointed out that father–daughter incest is a paradigm of female sexual victimization in which the female is powerless. It is this vulnerability (made possible by such unequal relationships) that sets the stage for incest victimization. "The father, in effect, forces the daughter to pay with her body for affection and care which should be freely given" (p. 4).

These theories are helpful in attempting to understand the nature and existence of the incest taboo. However, evidence to support these theories is lacking or equivocal.

JUDITH V. BECKER
and EMILY M.
COLEMAN

Social scientists and clinicians investigating incest have examined a number of variables, including socioeconomic factors, family and marital dysfunctions, and characteristics of the father, mother, and children.

Weinberg (1955), reporting on 203 cases of father–daughter incest, found that 55% of the families came from the lower socioeconomic class, 19.2% were middle-class, and 5.9% were from the "comfortable" socioeconomic level. In a study of 26 cases of paternal incest in Northern Ireland, Lukianowicz (1972) found that it primarily occurred among working-class families living in cramped quarters in industrial towns.

Contrary to such findings, Herman (1981) reported that half of the 40 Caucasion women they assessed were working class, and the other half were from middle-class families. Fifty-seven percent were between the ages of 18 to 25, and their religious backgrounds were representative of their geographic areas. These incest victims were described as being "to all appearances an ordinary group of women" (p. 67).

In a study of 400 families referred to the Santa Clara California Treatment Center for Incest, Giarretto (1978) noted that a broad spectrum of occupations were represented, including blue-collar, semiprofessional, and professional positions. The average income was similar to other nonincest families residing in the community. Westernmeyer (1978), reporting on 32 patients with histories of incest, found that educational level and social class were not skewed toward either end of the socioeconomic spectrum.

The dysfunctional family system has been stressed by many researchers as causal in the occurrence of incestuous behavior. Thorman (1983) contended that although no single correlational factor is present in every incestuous family system, there are deficiencies in specific areas: (a) lack of strong correlation between the parents, (b) mothers who are physically or psychologically absent, (c) reversed mother–daughter roles, (d) unequally distributed power between husband and wife, (e) conflict resolved through scapegoating, (f) family effect not supportive of family members, (g) lack of autonomy among family members, (h) confused communication, and (i) socially isolated family members who are unable to cope with stress.

Justice and Justice (1979) acknowledged that incest has the potential to occur in any family. However, whether incest occurs depends on a number of factors, including the personalities of the individuals involved, their situations, setting, and circumstances, and the changes or crises that recently have occurred in their lives.

A major confounding factor in viewing family dysfunction as the cause of incest is that the families are evaluated after incest occurs. Family dysfunction may be a result of incest rather than its cause. Incest may occur because the husband or stepfather is a pedophile who attempts to isolate the family, places the daughter in the role of an adult, and ignores the wife (who is consequently physically or psychologically absent). It is noteworthy that the family, and not the perpetrator, generally has been the target of intervention in cases of incest.

CHARACTERISTICS OF THE PERPETRATOR

Weinberg (1955) stated that incest culminates a long sequence of personal experiences and attitudes. These are used as criteria for classifying male incest offenders into personality types: (a) the endogamic orientation, a type who confines his sexual objects to family members because he does not have social or sexual contacts with women outside the family; (b) the pedophilic perpetrator who is psychosexually retarded and socially immature; and (c) the perpetrator who engages in indiscriminate promiscuity and tends to be pyschopathic.

Gebhard, Gagnon, Pomeroy, and Christenson (1965), using a prison sample, compared the incest offender with a non-sex-offender prison group. The offender group was subdivided by age of victim: victims younger than 12 years of age and victims older than 12 years of age. Differences were found in those offenders whose victims were older than 12; these men were shy, introverted, and dependent. Eight men (12%) were described as alcoholic, and 20% to 30% were frequent drinkers.

Incestuous fathers have been described as individuals suffering from personality disorders by Anderson and Shafer (1979) and Kirkland and Bauer (1982). The latter researchers compared MMPI scores of 10 incestuous fathers and stepfathers with those of a control group of nonincestuous fathers. Incestuous cases were drawn from the adult diversion program of the El Paso County, California, Department of Social Services. Control subjects were fathers from the same county, who were matched for age, race, education, age of daughter, and relationship to child (stepparent vs. biological parent). More pathological scores for incestuous fathers were observed on the psychopathic deviate, psychasthenia, and schizophrenia scales. These scales reflect chronic insecurity, social aberration, and acting-out behavior. The findings are limited, however, by the small sample size, nonrandom sampling, and lack of a deviant nonsexual offender comparison group.

Few studies conducted to date have employed large samples, control groups, and instruments with known psychometric properties to examine possible differences between incest offenders and nonincest offenders. Furthermore, data may be unreliable or invalid because patients may often be reluctant to reveal information. They may fear incarceration and/or be concerned that their sentences or therapy might be lengthened if they were honest in their disclosures.

Recently, investigators have attempted to classify child molesters on the basis of their erotic preference pattern. Abel, Mittleman, Becker, and Cunningham-Rathner (1983) questioned child molesters who volunteered for either assessment or treatment. In an attempt to secure reliable information from the sexual perpetrators, an elaborate system of confidentiality was developed that included coding all files. In addition, a Federal Certificate of Confidentiality was obtained that prohibited any city, county, state, or federal agency from accessing these records. Of those offenders whose victims were younger than 14 years of age, the mean number of molestations was 166.9, and the mean number of victims was 75.8. The mean number of pedophilic acts committed was 51.3 and 83.4 on related male and female children, respectively. These data suggest that the frequency of child molestation is much higher than previously suggested in the literature.

Also, of the incest perpetrators who involved themselves sexually with female children related to them, 44% molested female children not related to them, 11% molested male children not related to them, 18% raped, 18% committed exhibitionism, 9% engaged in voyeurism, 5% in frottage, 4% in sadism, and 21% had other paraphilias. The majority (59%) of the child molesters had the onset of this deviant sexual interest pattern during adolescence.

This early onset tends to refute the theory that family disruption causes men to relate sexually to children. A more plausible explanation may be related to the presence of a child who resides in the house of the age and sex to which the perpetrator is attracted.

JUDITH V. BECKER
and EMILY M.
COLEMAN

Empirical support for the presence of deviant sexual interest patterns in incest offenders is found in psychophysiologic evaluation data. Abel, Becker, Murphy, and Flanagen (1981) attempted to determine whether pedophiles are etiologically different from incest offenders. Using psychophysiologic assessment, 27 sexual deviates were assessed. This group included six cases of heterosexual incest, 10 heterosexual pedophiles, and 11 subjects with other sexual deviations. The incest offenders showed a significant amount of arousal to 2-minute audiotapes describing sex acts with female children other than their own. This pattern is consistent with responses of the majority of incest offenders seen in the authors' clinical work. These data support the hypothesis that the choice of victim relates to the availability of the child within the home.

Information concerning personality characteristics of incest offenders is sparse. However, a burgeoning research literature indicates that a substantial number of incest perpetrators evidence a deviant sexual arousal pattern. Readers interested in a comprehensive review of the area of pedophilia are referred to Quinsey (1977, in press).

CHARACTERISTICS OF THE MOTHER

Several authors have discussed characteristics of mothers of incest victims. In an evaluation of 26 families where incest occurred, Lukianowitz (1972) found that none of the mothers were psychotic. Rather, they were described as normal, hard-working, and suffering women. Further, there was evidence that 10 of the mothers were fully aware of the incest, but elected to remain silent. These women were extremely dependent and desperate to maintain their marriages. Herman and Hirschman (1981) compared 40 women who had incestuous relationships with their fathers to 20 women whose fathers had been seductive but not overtly incestuous. Mothers of the incest victims were described as chronically ill, disabled, and more often absent for some period of time. Also, mothers in the incestuous families had more pregnancies and children. In their survey of 112 families in which incest occurred, Justice and Justice (1977) found that mothers (a) sought role reversal with their daughters, (b) were sexually frigid, (c) tended to be weak and submissive, (d) took a mothering role with their husbands, (e) were tired and worn out, and (f) were indifferent.

Unfortunately, research on characteristics of mothers of incest victims has included small sample sizes, lacked comparison groups, or has relied on retrospective data or clinical impressions. In addition, findings are confounded by the fact that these characteristics may be a result rather than a cause of living with an incest perpetrator.

CHARACTERISTICS OF THE VICTIM

Female victims of incest have been reported from prepubescent children (Lukianowitz, 1972) to pubertal (Maisch, 1972) and midadolescent (Weinberg, 1955). The majority of investigations conducted on victims show that they are not extraordinary.

A number of researchers have examined the victim's role in incest. A classic study is an effort by Bender and Blau (1937), which describes victims as seductive and charming. More recently, however, de Young (1982) delineated the importance of other variables, such as the child's ability to say "no," and need for affection. Because the child is not in a position to give consent to incest, she can never be considered responsible for the act.

The literature dealing with incest can be divided into treatment of the perpetrator, victim, and family. A limited number of treatment-outcome studies have been carried out to date. Those that are available fall into the following categories: (a) family therapy or martial therapy, (b) individual and group insight-oriented therapy, and (c) behavior therapy (Dixon & Jenkins, 1981).

Family Therapy

The assumption underlying the use of family therapy in cases of incest is that poor communication, or a breakdown of roles are etiological factors in the disorder (Eist & Mandel, 1968; Gutheil & Avery, 1977).

Therapists disagree about the most efficacious form of family therapy. Molnar and Cameron (1975) reported that incestuous behavior was not eliminated through family therapy and recommend that intervention include removal of the child from the home, and individual therapy for family members.

Other clinicians contend that it is disadvantageous to separate family members (Machotka, Pittman, & Flomenhaft, 1967). If a family member (i.e., perpetrator) is removed, the victim may feel guilty for having disclosed the sexual abuse. Further, the victim may be held responsible by other family members for having "driven" the father out of the home.

In cases where the child is removed, the experience may serve to further victimize the child. She may feel that she is being punished for having disclosed the abuse. On occasion, victims have been placed in detention centers or other facilities until appropriate foster care placements can be found. Placement in such settings may heighten the trauma experience by the victim.

Giaretto, Giaretto, and Sgroi (1978) described a community-based treatment program for families in which incest has occurred. Based on his experience with more than 600 of these families, Giarretto (1978) stated that the primary emphasis of the program should be to maintain family integrity. In addition, he feels that the authority of the criminal justice system is essential in treating incest cases. Program dropouts largely have been those men who were not under criminal justice system supervision. The treatment program combines individual therapy with group therapy and self-help groups. The victimized child frequently is permitted to select whether she wishes to remain with her family or be placed in a foster care setting. Therapy begins with counseling of the daughter, then individual counseling of the mother, and joint mother–daughter counseling. If there are other siblings, they join in counseling with the mother and victim. The perpetrator receives individual counseling, and the couple receives marital therapy. The father is finally placed in family counseling. This is supplemented with participation in self-help groups known as Daughters United and Parents United. Giaretto (1978) reported that no recidivism has been reported in the more than 600 families treated and finally terminated. Unfortunately, data regarding length of follow-up or recidivism rates are not provided.

Individual and Group Therapy

Sgroi (1982) indentified 10 major problem areas and symptoms in working with sexually abused children. The traditional model of treating sexual assault victims with insight-oriented counseling is not very helpful in working with very young children who have been incest victims because of their limited communication skills. Stember (1980) recommended the use of art therapy as a medium that enables child victims to express emotions they are unable or unwilling to verbalize. Naitove (1982) suggested that in addition to art therapy, children can express their feelings through dance, drama, and poetry.

Peters (1976) discussed the implementation of psychoanalysis and hypnosis in the treatment of incest victims. For further reading on nontraditional treatment approaches, *Sexually Abused Children and their Families* (Mrazek & Kemp, 1981) and *Handbook of Clinical Intervention in Child Sexual Abuse* (Sgroi, 1982) are highly recommended.

Peters and Rothke (1972) utilized group psychotherapy in treating probationed sex offenders at Philadelphia General Hospital. Offenders were required to attend at least 16 therapy sessions. The mean number of weeks of therapy received was 26.2. The investigators report a 2-year follow-up comparing arrest rates and change in attitude in 92 treated offenders with 75 retrospectively matched subjects who received probation supervision. Re-arrests for sex crimes in the treated groups was 1% and 8% for the comparison group.

Salzman's (1972) psychodynamic approach to sex deviations involves understanding the underlying personality distortions that have produced the deviant behavior. Therapy focuses on a detailed presentation of the offender's current functioning to identify areas of anxiety and ways that these anxieties are handled.

Costell and Yalom (1972) described a group therapy strategy based on the curative factors of the group process and strategies to facilitate impulse modification and control. Unfortunately, all of these reports have either relied on self-reported recidivism rates, or have lacked experimental control.

Behavior Therapy

Abel, Blanchard, and Becker (1977) have identified the common elements of behavioral treatment for sexual perpetrators. This form of intervention has consisted of (a) reducing deviant sexual arousal patterns, (b) developing an age-appropriate consensual arousal pattern, (c) social and assertiveness skills training, (d) eliminating cognitive distortions, and (e) remediating deficits in sexual knowledge.

A considerable body of data are being accrued on the use of behavioral treatment in sexual deviations. However, due to space limitations, only those studies involving incest offenders will be discussed. In one of these, Harbert, Barlow, Hersen, & Austen (1974) employed covert sensitization in the treatment of a 52-year-old incestuous male. Follow-up assessments were conducted at 2 weeks, 3 months, and 6 months. Assessment included use of a penile plethysmograph and Sex Interest Card Sort. Although there was some increase in deviant sex arousal at 2 weeks and 3 months, no deviant arousal was evident at a 6-month follow-up.

Brownell and Barlow (1976) utilized covert sensitization in the treatment of a 34-year-old incestuous pedophile. At an 11-week follow-up, the patient indicated no deviant sexual interest. Using variations of covert sensitization, Levin, Barry, Ganiaro, Wolfinsohn, and Smith (1977) treated a 39-year-old male who had engaged in incest. A 10-month follow-up demonstrated that control over the deviant sexual interest pattern had been achieved.

Recently, Abel, Mittelman, Becker, Cummingham-Rathner, and Rovleau (in press) carried out a multicomponent behavioral intervention for 192 child molesters, a percentage of whom were incest offenders. All patients were treated on an outpatient basis. They participated in 30 therapy sessions of 1½ hours each and were evaluated after therapy, and at 6- and 12-month follow-ups. Results indicate that incest offenders had extremely low rates of recidivism.

Behavioral techniques for victims include cognitive therapy, systematic desensitization, and stress management techniques. These strategies have the potential for alleviating some of the sequelae (e.g., fears, self-destructive behavior, sleeping and eating problems) that develop secondary to an incestuous relationship. The authors, however, have found only one article in the literature concerning behavioral intervention with an incest victim. In this effort, Becker, Skinner, and Abel (1982) applied contingency management in the treatment of a 4-year-old victim of sexual assault.

CASE MANAGEMENT

The clinician should be aware of the laws in her or his state regarding the reporting of cases of intrafamilial child abuse. Knowledge of what families can expect once a case has been reported also is crucial. If the clinician is requested to assess the family and make recommendations for intervention, adherence to the following procedures is recommended.

The Disclosure

In the initial interview, one or both parents may deny that child sexual abuse actually occurred, or the parent(s) may blame the child. The perpetrator will be extremely concerned about possible action by the criminal justice system, particularly incarceration. Consequently, he may minimize or deny involvement out of fear of arrest. The mother may be concerned about the father's being removed from the home and imprisoned. She also may be concerned about the emotional and financial impact this may have on the family. As a result, the mother may report that she believes the father's account of the situation.

From a clinical standpoint, it is important to keep in mind that a psychological profile of an incest offender has yet to be developed. Thus, assessment is somewhat difficult. The authors have evaluated incest offenders from all races, professions, and socioeconomic classes. They do not fit into any single category on the basis of demographic or personality characteristics.

If parents blame the child, they need to be educated about the fact that children cannot consent to sexual relations with adults. Children do not understand the nature and consequences of sexual activity with an adult. When both parents blame the child, consider separation of the child from the family (because of the danger of further emotional, physical, or sexual abuse) must be considered.

In some cases, the nonoffending parent believes the child, and is aligned with the child, but the perpetrator denies or minimizes the abuse. The clinician might then recommend that the perpetrator be removed from the home until he receives appropriate treatment.

In other cases, the perpetrator accepts responsibility for the sexual abuse and there is within the family a nonabusing adult relative or other adult who can protect the child. The clinician may then recommend that the family stay intact. However, a contract would be arranged indicating that for the course of therapy, the perpetrator would never be left alone with the child.

The child should be involved as much as possible in decision making regarding return to the home or placement with relatives, friends, or a foster care facility.

The Issue of False Accusations

Recently, there has been considerable concern about false accusations of child sexual abuse. Yet, Giaretto (1978) reported that in 600 families seen for incest, fewer than 1% of the cases were found to be based on false accusation. These data indicate that children very rarely falsely accuse parents of sexual abuse. However, because false accusations have occurred, the clinician should be aware of the symptoms of sexual abuse that children experience.

Interviewing the Child

Sgroi (1982) lists 20 behavioral indicators of possible sexual abuse. Those include:

> Overly compliant behavior; acting out aggressive behavior; pseudomature behavior; hints about sex activity persistent and inappropriate sex play with peers or toys or with themselves, or sexually aggressive behavior with others; detailed and age-inappropriate understanding of sexual behavior; arriving at school early and leaving late with few, if any, absences; poor peer relationships or inability to make friends; lack of trust, particularly with significant others; non-participant in school and social activities; inability to concentrate in school, sudden drop in school performance; extraordinary fears of males; seductive behavior with males; running away from home; sleep disturbances; regressive behavior; withdrawal; clinical depression; suicidal feelings. (pp. 40–41)

Sgroi (1982) emphasized that the child should receive a complete physical examination to assess any trauma to the genitals or rectal area. Although the previously listed signs or symptoms are not exhaustive, they may serve as markers for the clinician in conducting an evaluation.

Sgroi (1982) also made a number of recommendations for interviewing a sexually abused child. First, it should not be assumed that the particular report of abuse was the initial episode. Children often use a different vocabulary to describe their genitalia and sexual behaviors that occurred. Anatomically correct dolls or drawings are useful to help children communicate what occurred.

Second, children may have been threatened with further harm if they disclosed all or certain portions of the abuse. Consequently, the clinician should interview the child on several occasions under conditions where the child feels safe. When it is clear that no more harm is coming to her or him, the child may more fully disclose the extent of the abuse.

Third, it should not be assumed that all children will be impacted to the same degree or show the same symptomatology. Children vary in response to incest. Their age, the length of time the abuse occurred, and extent of force and pain inflicted must all be taken into account. Separation from the family may serve as a further stressor for the child. If peers have learned of the abuse and do not respond in a supportive manner, further trauma may result.

Finally, the ciminal justice and court procedures may serve as a stressor. Although many states are revising their laws and practices regarding child witnesses, many children have been and continue to be further victimized by an insensitive criminal justice system.

In evaluating the child victim, the clinician should proceed with sensitivity and employ psychological assessment instruments that are appropriate for the child's developmental level. The child should be interviewed over many sessions and evaluated using several behavioral rating scales to assess changes in behavior before and after the incest occurred. To the authors' knowledge, an assessment package specific to incest victims, and with demonstrated psychometric properties, has yet to be developed.

Evaluating the Offender

The authors utilize a number of assessment procedures with incest offenders. First, a history of the deviant sexual interest pattern is taken in a structured clinical interview. The perpetrator is asked about the first time he had fantasies about being sexual with his child, when he first was sexual with her, what the behavior involved, and whether verbal or physical coercion was used. It is important to question the perpetrator about all possible sexual deviations, because most have been involved in other deviant sexual behaviors.

In addition to the sexual history, a standard psychiatric interview, including mental status exam, is needed to screen out psychotic perpetrators or those at low levels of cognitive functioning. A cognitive-behavioral treatment program would not be appropriate for these individuals. A battery of psychometric questionnaires is recommended:

1. The Sexual Interest Card Sort (Abel & Becker, 1986a) is a self-report scale of arousal to all paraphilias.
2. The Cognition Scale (Abel & Becker, 1986b) measures the perpetrator's cognitive distortions justifying the incest.
3. The Beck Depression Scale (Beck, 1978) is a self-report of depression. Many perpetrators are anxious and depressed as a result of the disclosure of incest.
4. The Derogatis Sexual Functioning Inventory (Derogatis, 1980) provides information on 10 areas of sexual functioning, including knowledge of sexuality, body image, sex drive, and gender role.
5. The Adult Self-Expression Scale (Gay, Hollandsworth, & Galassi, 1975) is a measure of assertiveness.

A comprehensive assessment also should include psychophysiological evaluation of sexual arousal patterns. A mercury strain gauge (Laws & Osborn, 1983) measures the perpetrator's erection response while he sees or listens to a variety of stimuli (audio, video, slides) in a private laboratory setting. Stimuli should cover the gamut of paraphilias, and also include adult consenting cues. It is helpful to give instructions to suppress arousal to some cues in order to evaluate the perpetrator's degree of control. Instructions not to suppress, or to react normally, also are given to other cues. (The clinician interested in establishing a laboratory is referred to Laws & Osborn, 1983.)

Because of the frequent denial of perpetrators, use of psychophysiological assessment is crucial. There is evidence that small changes in erection response (less than 10%) may still be valuable in determining arousal patterns (Earls & Marshall, 1983). However, it is not conclusive in all cases; the possibility of false negatives still exists. Pedophiles have been known to fake their sexual responses in the laboratory (Laws & Holman, 1978). It also is important to assess any organic problems or medication effects that may interfere with the individual's erection response.

At the conclusion of the evaluation, a feedback or debriefing session is conducted with the perpetrator. At this time, the results, (including psychophysiological measures) are discussed with the patient. Any discrepancies between his self-report and the laboratory measures are examined. Treatment recommendations are based on these evaluation results.

A Cognitive-Behavioral Treatment Model for the Incest Perpetrator

A treatment strategy that has proven successful with incest offenders is the cognitive-behavioral model based on social learning theory. According to this approach, incest offenders involve themselves sexually with their children because they have a sexual interest in the child. Consequently, treatment strategies are used that will decrease or eliminate that sexual interest. Although a variety of behavioral techniques have been demonstrated to be effective in single case studies, two cognitive-behavioral techniques are particularly useful: covert sensitization (Barlow, Leitenberg, & Agras, 1969; Cautela, 1966) and satiation (Marshall, 1979; Marshall & Barbaree, 1978; Marshall & Lippens, 1977).

Covert sensitization directly attacks deviant sexual urges by associating those urges with aversive social consequences. The majority of incest offenders do not consider the consequences of their behavior at the time that they have a deviant sexual urge, because these thoughts might deter them from commiting the offense. Therapy involves teaching the incest offender to associate the consequences of his behavior with the precursors of engaging in sexual contact with a child. By the frequent pairing of aversive consequences with sexually deviant fantasies, the deviant fantasy acquires negative characteristics and consequently becomes less pleasurable and erotic to the offender.

During treatment sessions, the therapist assists the patient in building a covert chain. Specifically, the offender learns that his sexual behavior with a child is the final link in a long chain of events. It is critical that the patient be able to identify all the links in his chain that lead up to his engaging in sexual behavior with a child. A typical chain might include the following events: (a) a wife leaving the house to go grocery shopping, leaving the offender alone with a child; (b) drinking or engaging in other behavior that lessens his control; (c) having fantasies about engaging in sexual behavior with a child; (d) masturbating or somehow stimulating himself to those fantasies; (e) approaching the child and actually engaging in sexual contact with the child. It is important for the offender to realize that the sexual behavior does not just occur ''out of the blue'' as is frequently heard from offenders. Understanding the precursors of incest facilitates the individual's development of control at various points along the chain.

Once the precursors have been identified, the patient is taught how to develop fantasies and images that are aversive to him. Aversive scenes may include imprisonment, loss of one's job or professional license, severing of family ties, and trauma to the victim and her family. Each patient is instructed to make a 15-minute covert sensitization tape during which he associates the consequences with the precursors to engaging in sexual behavior with a child. Offenders are requested to make a minimum of ten 15-minute tapes. The therapist then listens to the tape to insure that the session has been conducted and to determine whether the covert exercise is being carried out correctly.

The goal of satiation is to reduce and ultimately eliminate the offender's deviant sexual fantasies. Satiation involves the pairing of deviant sexual fantasies with masturbation for 55 minutes after orgasm. Therapy consists of having the offender masturbate in private to nondeviant adult fantasies until ejaculation occurs or for a maximum of 5 minutes. At the point of either ejaculation or at ''the switch point,'' the individual switches and for the remainder of the session masturbates to deviant sexual material (i.e., sex with children). This technique reinforces the nondeviant fantasies by associating a pleasurable activity, orgasm and ejaculation, with consensual sexual fantasies about adults. It also makes the deviant fantasies extremely boring and aversive by requiring that the patient repeat the fantasies over and over again for at least 55 minutes while he continues to masturbate after ejaculation.

For those patients who decline to masturbate for physical, religious, or ethical reasons, the procedure can be followed without masturbation. Each patient is required to engage in 20 hours of satiation exercises. Therapists listen to the tapes to insure that the offender is complying with the therapy.

A third treatment utilized to decrease deviant sexual interest is cognitive restructuring. In assessing over 500 adult sexual offenders, a significant proportion of whom were incest offenders, it became clear that they have inappropriate thoughts about the acceptability of engaging in sexual behavior with children. For example, many sexual offenders stated that they engaged in sex with their children because they wanted to show them how much they loved them, or that they were concerned that their children would learn about sex from other children and that it would be inaccurate information. These cognitive distortions give the offender permission to engage in a deviant sexual activity. It is important that the therapist confront these cognitive distortions. This goal is accomplished by having the therapist role play the part of a child molester who uses the various cognitive distortions. The patient is then asked to assume the role of a probation officer, family member, or policeman in an attempt to confront his own cognitive distortions. Research indicates that a number of sexual perpetrators themselves have been molested as children. Having the offender recount his own molestation and its impact on him helps him develop empathy, and thereby confronts his cognitive distortions.

Another cognitive-behavioral treatment strategy for incest perpetrators is communication skills training. Inability to express feelings, make requests, and resolve conflicts is common among incest families. However, it is unclear whether this communication difficulty is a cause, effect, or merely correlational with incest. The term *dysfunctional family,* so often applied to the incest family, is primarily defined by the inability to communicate among family members.

Family therapy that includes supporting and teaching all family members to express their feelings, particularly concerning the incest, is crucial if the family is to be reunited and/or maintained. Before family therapy occurs, however, communication skills training can be offered to the offender independent of his family. He is thus provided with a less emotionally charged opportunity to learn these skills. Communication skills include social skills (initiating, maintaining, and ending conversations), assertion (expressing intimate feelings and making requests), and conflict resolution skills. Essentially, the client acquires these skills through role-playing in which learning techniques, such as shaping and positive reinforcement of appropriate behavior, are utilized. Communication skills training is particularly effective in a group therapy format. As with all therapeutic interventions, the need to practice and apply skills outside of the treatment session is emphasized.

Sex Education

Sexual misconceptions can contribute to insecurity regarding one's own sexuality. Concern about adequate penis size is ubiquitous among sex offenders, as is a corollary sexual myth that an erect penis is necessary to satisfy a sexual partner. The unfortunate equating of sex with penile-vaginal intercourse can result in considerable performance anxiety, a major cause of sexual dysfunction. It is important that offenders have accurate information regarding male and female anatomy, sexual response cycles, and sexual behavior and attitudes. This knowledge can reduce the offender's feelings of sexual inadequacy and result in a more satisfying sexual relationship with his partner.

Communication of sexual desires also is emphasized in sex education. The skills previously learned in social and assertion training are transferred to expression in the sexual arena. Embarrassment regarding sexual words and needs must be overcome because without assertive expression of sexual likes and dislikes, a satisfying sexual relationship is unlikely.

Case Illustration

Mr. B. is a 40-year-old Caucasion male who sexually molested both his natural son and daughter. He was referred by a child protective agency after the incest was disclosed by his children. Mr. B. admitted incest and was very motivated to become involved in treatment in order to be reunited with his family. The psychiatric interview revealed no other psychopathology and no evidence of drug addiction, psychosis, or sociopathy. Mr. B. was of above average intelligence and articulate, although he lacked insight into his sexual deviance. He had a stable and successful business for the past 10 years.

Mr. B. reported that his first pedophilic act occurred at age 21 when he fondled the breasts of the 10-year-old daughter of a friend. The molestation did not occur again and was not disclosed to anyone. Mr. B., however, continued to use this occurrence as a primary masturbatory fantasy. At age 23, he married and denies any other sexual contact with children until he fondled his 9-year-old son's penis. The deviant sexual behavior quickly escalated to include mutual masturbation approximately once a month over the next 2 years. When his younger daughter was 9 years old, he began fondling her breats and genitals. This followed the same pattern as with his son, and soon progressed to mutual masturbation at a frequency of twice a mongth for the next 4 years. During the last 2 years, he was involved with his son and daughter together. No physical force was used, but affection, toys, and trips were contingent upon their sexual involvement with him. His sexual relationship with his wife, originally very satisfying to both, gradually diminished in frequency, although he did not evidence any sexual dysfunction. Mr. B. also had been sexually involved with adult men intermittently since adolescence.

Assessment results indicated Mr. B. to be depressed and anxious because of the disclosure of the incest, separation from his family, and the possibility of criminal charges. The Derogatis Sexual Functioning Inventory showed below average knowledge of sexuality and a rigid gender role, as is frequently found among sex offenders. Laboratory assessment using the penile plethyomograph indicated low overall arousal.

Table 1. Percent Erection Response—Case B

Stimulus cues	Pretreatment	Post—10	Post—20
Young female incest	21%	4%	4%
Adult female	7%	4%	7%
Young female-initiated sex	14%	4%	0%

However, Mr. B.'s highest arousal was to adult males and to mutually consenting sex with young girls.

Mr. B. entered group therapy and proved to be a motivated and diligent client who followed through with the treatment regimen. Following five sessions of covert sensitization and five sessions of masturbatory satiation, laboratory evaluation revealed decreased arousal to young girls and maintained arousal to adults (see Table 1). This more appropriate arousal pattern was maintained at the conclusion of social and assertion skills training. At this writing, Mr. B. has completed sex education and is involved in cognitive restructuring therapy. Upon completion of that treatment component, the entire evaluation will be conducted again to determine therapeutic progress and further treatment needs. Family therapy is of course required if the family is to be reunited. At a minimum, continued follow-up care will be required.

FAMILY ISSUES

A detailed description of treatment of incest victims will not be reviewed here. The reader is referred to Chapter 7 for a discussion of the management of victims.

If the family in which incest has occurred elects to remain together as a unit, the clinician is advised to assess what, if any, stressors within the family may have affected the father's ability to control his deviant sexual interest pattern. Specifically, were there any mental or sexual problems? Was there difficulty with role boundaries? Was the daughter placed in a position by both parents in which she was asked to assume the role of an adult?

Family members should be apprised of behaviors in the past that served as precursors for the father engaging in sexual contact with a child. A case example involves a family in which the father worked days and the mother worked an evening shift. The father would have a beer or two after the mother left for work. He would then watch TV while reclining on the sofa. He then would ask his daughter to sit next to him and begin to fondle her. Recommendations given to this family involved (a) therapy for the perpetrator to help him control his interest in pubescent children; (b) altering of parents' work hours so that the father is not left alone with the child; (c) not allowing the father to consume alcohol when in the presence of a child because this serves to weaken his control; and (d) not permitting father to be alone in a room in close physical proximity to the child.

Each family situation will vary, as will the precursors to the behavior. It is imperative that the clinician identify the precursors and stressors so that the family members are informed and can target those behaviors.

Those families that elect to separate should also receive counseling. Issues to be addressed include (a) a clear understanding that the child was not responsible for the incest; (b) supervision of the perpetrator if he is to have visitation, until such time as the treating clinician determines it is unlikely that such visits will be harmful to the child.

All family members are affected in one way or another by the occurrence and/or disclosure of incest. The clinician must assess the impact on all family members.

LEGAL AND ETHICAL ISSUES

Clinicians in their training are taught to honor confidentiality. In cases of incest clients, however, the law dictates that for the protection of the child, a disclosure of incest cannot be kept confidential. To do so would constitute a violation of the law by the clinician.

This situation, however, can present a catch 22 to incest perpetrators who want to seek therapy to help them gain control of their deviant sexual interest pattern. By disclosing the behavior they are at risk for arrest and incarceration. There is no simple solution to this dilemma. Of primary importance, however, is that regardless of whether our society decides to incarcerate a perpetrator or allow him to receive probation, therapy should be made available to him.

Frequently, the criminal justice system will request an opinion from a clinician regarding sentencing options for an incest offender. Clinicians will differ on their degree of comfort in making such recommendations. One option is to specify treatment needs without rendering an opinion concerning sentencing options. Other clinicians may choose to consider the following issues in making a recommendation for outpatient versus institutional placement: (a) the degree of force or coercion used by the offender; (b) recognition of the presence of a psychosexual disorder; (c) willingness to participate in therapy; (d) degree of control over the problem—specifically, can the patient be allowed to remain in society while undergoing treatment or is his control so tenuous that he is likely to reoffend; (e) family members' feelings as to what would be a just resolution.

FUTURE DIRECTIONS

As is clear from the previous writing, considerable research remains to be conducted to understand, treat, and prevent incest. Studies carried out to date have only begun to provide such crucial information. This preliminary research has been hampered by small sample sizes with little or no follow-up. Yet, incest occurs with such alarming regularity and is so widespread in our society that there clearly are a sufficient number of cases to study. Invaluable data would be provided by simply following incest perpetrators, victims, and families over time. Recidivism rates for incest perpetrators appear to be lower than for other sex offenders. Is it possible that disclosure without specific treatment is devastating enough that the perpetrator does not reoffend? Other basic research questions concern the differences and similarities among incest offenders, nonsexual offenders, and nonoffenders. Such information can only be provided by dependent measures that are reliable, valid, and uniform. Often research results are difficult to interpret because of the variability in dependent measures. Coordination of research by, for example, utilization of the same instruments and pooling of data, although difficult to engineer, would be a potentially heuristic approach.

Once basic knowledge is obtained regarding incest, more sophisticated research designs evaluating the contributions of specific treatment components can be implemented. This includes the evaluation of behavioral treatment strategies, psychodynamic interventions, and family therapy. It is important to consider treatment attrition rates in considering possible therapeutic approaches. Follow-up assessment over 5- to 10-year periods of those clients completing and dropping out of therapy is essential.

Finally, research pertaining to prevention of incest is needed. The various theories regarding the etiology of this disorder suggest directions that future investigation might take, for example, can incest be prevented by teaching families better communication and conflict negotiation skills? How important is confrontation of sexist attitudes and unequal relationships in preventing incest? Although incest has been a problem since the beginning of human history, comparatively little methodologically adequate research has been conducted. Answering such questions requires empirically sound investigative effort and is a measure of our commitment as a society to reducing and ultimately eliminating incest.

Abel, G., & Becker, J. V. (1986a). *Sexual Interest Card Sort*. Unpublished assessment instrument.

Abel, G., & Becker, J. V. (1986b). *Cognition Scale*. Unpublished assessment instrument.

Abel, G., Blanchard, E. B., & Becker, J. V. (1976). Psychological treatment of rapists. In M. J. Walker & S. L. Brodsky (Eds.), *Sexual assault: The victim and the rapist* (pp. 99–115). Toronto: Lexington Books.

Abel, G., Becker, J. V., Murphy, W. & Flanagan, B. (1981). Identifying dangerous child molesters. In R. B. Stuart (Ed.), *Violent behavior: Social learning approaches to prediction, management and treatment* (pp. 116–137). New York: Brunner/Mazel.

Abel, G., Mittleman, M., Becker, J. V., & Cunningham-Rathner, J. (December, 1983). *The characteristics of men who molest young children*. Presented at the World Congress of Behavior Therapy, Washington, D. C., 1983.

Abel, G., Mittleman, M., & Becker, J. V., Cunningham-Rathner, J., & Rouleau, J. (In press). *Sex offenders: Results of assessment and recommendations for treatment*.

American Bar Association (1982). *Child sexual abuse and the law*. National Legal Resource Center for Child Advocacy and Protection. Washington, D. C.

American Psychiatric Association (1980). *Diagnostic and statistical manual of mental disorders* (3rd ed.). (DSM-III). Washington, DC: Author.

Anderson, L., & Shafer, G. (1979). The character disordered family: A community treatment model for family sexual abuse. *American Journal of Orthopsychiatry, 49*, 436–445.

Barlow, D. H., Leitenberg, H., & Agras, W. S. (1969). The experimental control of sexual deviation through manipulation of the noxious scene in covert sensitization. *Journal of Abnormal Psychology, 24*, 596–601.

Beck, A. T. (1978). *Depression inventory*. Philadelphia, PA: Center for Cognitive Therapy.

Becker, J. V., Skinner, L. J., & Abel, G. (1982). Treatment of a four year old victim of sexual assault. *The American Journal of Family Therapy, 10*, 41–46.

Bender, G., & Blau, A. (1937). The reactions of children to sexual relations with adults. *Journal of Orthopsychiatry, 7*, 500–518.

Brownell, K. O., & Barlow, D. H. (1976). Measurement and treatment of two sexual deviations in one person. *Journal of Behavior Therapy and Experimental Psychiatry, 7*, 349–354.

Cautela, J. R. (1967). Covert sensitization. *Psychological Record, 20*, 459–468.

Costell, R., & Yalom, I. (1972). Institutional group therapy. In H. L. P. Resnick & M. E. Wolfgand (Eds.), *Sexual behaviors: Social, clinical and legal aspects* (pp. 305–330). Boston, MA: Little, Brown.

De Young, M. (1982). *The sexual victimization of children*. Jefferson, NC: McFarland.

Derogatis, R. L. (1980). Psychological assessment of psychosexual functioning. In J. K. Meyer (Ed.), *Psychiatric clinics of North America* (Vol. 3, No. 1, pp. 113–131). New York: W. B. Saunders.

Dixen, J., & Jenkins, O. (1981). Incestuous child sexual abuse: A review of treatment strategies. *Clinical Psychology Review, 1*, 211–222.

Earls, C., & Marshall, W. (1983). The current state of technology in the laboratory assessment of sexual arousal patterns. In J. Greer & I. Stuart (Eds.), *The sexual aggressor: Current perspectives on treatment* (pp. 336–362). New York: Van Nostrand Reinhold.

Eist, H., & Mandell, A. (1968). Family treatment of ongoing incest behavior. *Family Process, 7*, 216–232.

Finkelhor, D. (1979). *Sexually victimized children*. New York: The Free Press.

Fox, R. (1980). *The red lamp of incest*. New York: E. P. Dutton.

Fradkin, L. (1974). Incest in middle class differs from that processed by police. *Psychiatry News, 2*, 3–10.

Freud, S. (1962). The etiology of hysteria. In *The complete psychological works of Sigmund Freud*. Translated by James Strachy, Standard edition. London: Hogarth Press. (Originally published 1896).

Freud, S. (1913/1950). *Totem and taboo* (James Strachy, Trans.). New York: W. W. Norton & Co., Inc. (Originally published 1913).

Gay, M. L., Hollandsworth, J. G., & Galassi, J. P. (1975). An assertiveness inventory for adults. *Journal of Counseling Psychology, 22*, 340–344.

Gebhard, P. H., Gagnon, J. H., Pomeroy, W. B., & Christenson, C. V. (1965). *Sex offenders: An analysis of types*. New York: Harper & Row.

Giarretto, H. (1978). Humanistic treatment of father–daughter incest. *Journal of Humanistic Psychology, 32*, 20–25.

Giarretto, H., Giarretto, A., & Sgroi, S. (1978). Coordinated community treatment of incest. In A. Burgess, A. N. Groth, L. L. Holmstrom, & S. M. Sgroi (Eds.), *Sexual assault of children and adolescents* (pp. 231–240). Boston, MA: Lexington Books.

Gutheil, T. G., & Avery, N. C. (1977). Multiple overt incest as family defense against loss. *Family Process, 16*, 105–116.

Harbert, T. L., Barlow, D. H., Hersen, M., & Austen, J. B. (1974). Measurement and modification of incestuous behavior: A case study. *Psychological Reports, 34,* 79–86.

Herman, J. (1981a). Father–daughter incest. Cambridge, MA: Harvard University Press.

Herman, J. and Hirschman, L. (1981b) Families at risk of father–daughter incest. *American Journal of Psychiatry 138,* 967–970.

Justice, B., & Justice, R. (1979). *The broken taboo: Sex in the family.* New York: Human Sciences Press.

Kinsey, A. C., Pomeroy, W. B., Martin, C., & Gebhard, P. H. (1953). *Sexual behavior in the human female.* Philadelphia, PA: W. B. Saunders.

Kirkland, K. D., & Bauer, C. A. (1982). MMPI traits of incestuous fathers. *Journal of Clinical Psychology, 38,* 645–649.

Laws, D. R., & Holman, M. L. (1978). Sexual response faking by pedophiles. *Criminal Justice and Behavior, 5,* 343–356.

Laws, D. R., & Osborn, C. (1983). How to build and operate a behavioral laboratory to evaluate and treat sexual deviants. In J. Greer & I. Stuart (Eds.), *The sexual aggressor: Current perspectives on treatment* (pp. 293–335). New York: Van Nostrand Reinhold.

Levin, S. M., Barry, S., Gambaro, S., Wolfensohn, L., & Smith, A. (1977). Variations of covert sensitization in the treatment of pedophilic behavior: A case study. *Journal of Consulting and Clinical Psychology, 45,* 896–907.

Lindsey, G. (1967). Some remarks concerning incest, the incest taboo, and psychoanalytic theory. *American Psychologist, 22,* 1051–1059.

Lukianowitz, N. (1972). Incest: Paternal incest. *British Journal of Psychiatry, 120,* 301–313.

Machotka, P., Pittman, F., & Flomenhaft, K. (1967). Incest as a family affair. *Family Process, 6,* 98–116.

Maisch, H. (1972). *Incest.* New York: Stein & Day.

Marshall, W. L. (1979). Satiation therapy: A procedure for reducing deviant sexual arousal. *Journal of Applied Behavior Analysis, 12,* 10–22.

Marshall, W. L., & Barbaree, H. E. (1978). The reduction of deviant arousal. *Criminal Justice and Behavior, 5,* 294–303.

Marshall, W. L., & Lippens, K. (1977). The clinical value of boredom: A procedure for reducing inappropriate sexual interests. *Journal of Nervous and Mental Disease, 165,* 283–287.

Masson, J. (1984). *The assault on truth: Freud's suppression of the seduction theory.* New York: Farrar, Straus & Giroux.

Molnar, G., & Cameron, P. (1975). Incest syndromes: Observations in a general hospital psychiatric unit. *Canadian Psychiatric Association Journal, 20,* 373–377.

Mrazek, P. B., & Kempe, C. H. (1981). *Sexually abused children and their families.* New York: Pergamon Press.

Murdock, G. P. (1949). *Social structure.* New York: Macmillan.

Naitove, C. (1982). Arts therapy with sexually abused children. In S. Sgroi (Ed.), *Handbook of clinical intervention in child sexual abuse.* Lexington, MA: Lexington Books.

New York Criminal Procedure Law, 1982–1983 Graybook. (1983; Bender Pamphlet Edition). New York: Matthew Bender.

Peters, J. J. (1976). Children who are victims of sexual assault and the psychology of offenders. *American Journal of Psychotherapy, 30,* 398–421.

Peters, J. J., & Roether, H. (1972). Group psychotherapy for probationed sex offenders. In H. L. P. Resnik & M. E. Wofgand (Eds.), *Sexual behaviors: Social, clinical and legal aspects* (pp. 255–266). Boston, MA: Little, Brown.

Quinsey, V. L. (1977). The assessment and treatment of child molesters. *Canadian Psychological Review, 18,* 204–220.

Quinsey, V. L. (in press). Men who have sex with children. In D. Weisstub (Ed.), *Law and mental health: International perspectives.* New York: Pergamon Press.

Russell, D. (1983). The incidence and prevalence of intrafamilial and extrafamilial sexual abuse of female children. *Child Abuse and Neglect, 7,* 133–146.

Russell, D. (1984). The prevalence and seriousness of incestuous abuse: Stepfathers vs. biological fathers. *Child Abuse and Neglect, 8,* 15–22.

Salzman, L. (1972). The psychodynamic approach to sex deviations. In H. Resnik & M. Wolfgang (Eds.), *Sexual behaviors: Social, clinical and legal aspects* (pp. 207–226). Boston, MA: Little, Brown.

Sgroi, S. (1982). *Handbook of clinical intervention in child sexual abuse.* Lexington, MA: Lexington Books.

Stember, C. J. (1980). Art therapy: A new use in the diagnosis and treatment of sexually abused children. K. McFarlane (Ed.), *Sexual abuse of children and adolescents: Selected readings.* National Center on Child Abuse and Neglect, Washington, D. C.

Thorman, G. (1983). *Incestuous families*. Springfield, IL: Charles C Thomas.

U. S. Department of Health and Human Services, National Center on child Abuse and Neglect. (1981). *Child sexual abuse*. Washington DC: Author.

Weinberg, S. K. (1955). *Incest behavior*. New York: Citadel Press.

Westermeyer, J. (1978). Incest in psychiatric practice: A description of patients and incestuous relationships. *Journal of Clinical Psychiatry, 39,* 643–648.

9

Marital Rape

MILDRED DALEY PAGELOW

INTRODUCTION

"Rape is rape no matter who is the perpetrator of the crime."

Del Martin, testifying in support of California's spousal rape law, 1979.

"[A] female slave has (in Christian countries) an admitted right, and is considered under a moral obligation to refuse to her master the last familiarity. Not so the wife: however brutal a tyrant she may unfortunately be chained to—though she may know that he hates her, though it may be his daily pleasure to torture her, and though she may feel it impossible not to loath him—he can claim from her and enforce the lowest degradation of a human being, that of being made the instrument of an animal function contrary to her inclinations."

John Stuart Mill, *The Subjection of Women*, 1869.

DESCRIPTION OF THE PROBLEM

The terms *marital rape* and *spousal rape* are most often used in reference to acts that are in reality *wife rape*. Is this because there is a presumption that the spouse who perpetrates rape is as likely to be a wife as a husband? It appears there is an assumed mutuality of sexual "ownership" and sexual aggression, considering the gender-neutral wording of California's rape statutes. For example, Penal Code 261 and Penal Code 262 refer only to a "person" or a "spouse" as victim or perpetrator of rape. Theoretically, it may be possible, but highly unlikely, for a wife to rape her husband. It is more likely that the gender-neutral language was used for political purposes (cf. Russell, 1982, p. 9), considering the difficulty of garnering support for legislation identified as women's issues.

Despite attempts to be nondiscriminatory in our language, when we write about or research marital or spousal rape, in reality we are addressing the problem of *wives raped by husbands*. And the issue is not that of bedroom quarrels over sex or what Finkelhor and Yllo (1985) term the "sanitary stereotype" of romantic lovers' quarrels. The recently acquired knowledge we have gained about rape between nonmarried persons is equally

---

MILDRED DALEY PAGELOW • Department of Sociology, California State University, Fullerton, CA 92634.

applicable in the case of marital rape: rape is a violent act, in which the weapon used is sex, intended to humiliate, degrade, and control the victims. The rape trauma syndrome is now a generally accepted phenomenon, but for wives the trauma may be even more severe. As Finkelhor (1984) said, "Rape is traumatic not because it is with someone you don't know, but because it is with someone you don't want—whether stranger, friend or husband." Finkelhor insists that marital rape victims suffer greater and longer term trauma than other rape victims. Raped wives suffer a profound sense of betrayal and entrapment. The betrayal results in a lost ability to trust others, and the feeling of entrapment, arising from repeated rapes, causes long-term anxiety and fear.

Marital rape is one of the least discussed and researched problems in the family violence field, probably in large part because of the extreme sensitivity most people feel about it. Victims of marital rape are more reluctant to discuss it with researchers than other violent acts they suffered, such as battering by husbands or rapes by strangers (Russell, 1982). There is the sense of shame and self-blame that persists, even years afterward, not only because society has placed the burden of making marriages successful on wives, but also because psychological abuse precedes and accompanies physical abuse. Social isolation is a common denominator in all types of family violence (Pagelow, 1984), and particularly in marital rape, which is a noncrime in almost half the states in the union. Raped wives have no outraged kin or social system to validate their victim status, thus they tend to blame themselves (Finkelhor, 1984).

Beyond the reluctance of victims to reveal their intensely personal violation, there is also the unwillingness of the public to consider wife rape a problem other than within a sexual context. As one Catholic prelate began his newspaper column:

> Rape in marriage! When I first heard the phrase some years ago I laughed—not because it was funny, but because it struck me as being goofy. How could a husband rape his own wife? Did he not have a right to sexual intercourse with her as a result of the marriage bond? . . . Wasn't he merely helping her to perform her wifely duties? I remember being taught . . . that when two people got married they surrendered themselves to each other. It was a mutual giving and taking so that a wife's body (sexually speaking) was no longer her own to do with as she pleased, nor was the husband's body his own. Because it was mutual it always struck me as fair. (Adamo, 1984)

Father Adamo had high ideals of marriage, but he has since come to the realization that in some cases, sex is not an act of love but an act of violence deserving the name of rape. On the other hand, some people prefer to think of marital rape as merely another bothersome feminist issue and prefer to brush it aside as a nonproblem (Finkelhor, 1984). For example, the President of the New York Criminal and Civil Courts Bar Association, Sidney Siller, had this to say in his *Penthouse* article, "'Wife Rape'—Who Really Gets Screwed" (1982, p. 104):

> Angry and apparently desperate for new issues following the crushing defeat of the Equal Rights Amendment, women's libbers, in their search for power under the guise of equality, are now focusing their attention on what they term "wife rape." . . . this means that your wife can accuse you of rape at any time during your marriage . . . [and] that charge can lead to your arrest, prosecution, and incarceration. Your protection against this conjugal lie is absolutely nil. It's her word against yours.

Siller (1982) also quoted some legislators who objected to proposals to strike the marital exemption clause (a subject that is discussed later) from Florida's rape laws, calling the issue a "bedroom crusade." One representative complained that the Bible did not give the state permission to "meddle" in bedrooms, "deciding what you can do and what you can't do.'' Because the state has always had great interest in what couples do or do not do in bedrooms (O'Donnell, 1980), these men obviously felt threatened by the notion of wives gaining the legal right to charge their husbands with rape.

Marital rape is far more than what Siller (1982) referred to as ''sheer nonsense''; it has more to do with anger, power, pain, and suffering than sex. Research shows that the closer the prior association of rapist and victim, the more violent the assault tends to be (Black, 1979; Landau, 1976; Queen's Bench Foundation, 1976; Russell, 1975). Marital rape is often accompanied by extreme violence involving bondage, torture, and mutilation, and it sometimes culminates in murder (Calkins, 1981; Donovan, 1985; Egner, 1980).

Researchers have carefully designed their studies to eliminate any cases that might be construed as misunderstandings or frivolous quarrels about sex. To fit researchers' definitions of rape, it had to be clear that the sexual contacts were unwanted by the victims. Yet because they were sensitive to women's reluctance to describe aggressive sex with spouses as rape, they phrased their questions in less threatening terms. Russell (1982) asked respondents if they had any ''unwanted sexual experiences'' with husbands or former husbands; Finkelhor and Yllo (1985) asked if a spouse had ever used physical force or threat to try to have sex; and the questionnaire used by Hanneke, Shields, and McCall (1985) asked if the wives had experienced sexual violence. Some researchers were more direct: one asked if husbands had ever pressured them to have sexual relations and if their husbands had ever raped them (Frieze, 1980); another asked: ''Were you ever sexually assaulted by him? (Forcible rape *is* an assault)'' (Pagelow, 1980, 1981, 1984).

In the largest study of rape to date using a probability sample of 930 adult women, Russell (1982) defined rape by the reported presence of physical coercion or fear of physical coercion. Another study, concentrating on marital rape (Finkelhor & Yllo, 1985), adopted the same definition. Sexual assaults accomplished by other types of coercion were categorized as experiences of unwanted sex. Researchers must decide whether or not the actions being described fit their definitions of rape, and their decisions tend to be conservative. For example, when one of Russell's (1982) respondents stated that she had been raped by her husband but probing revealed that no actual force or fear of force had occurred, that case was not counted as rape. However, wives were more likely to minimize the assaults by saying they were only ''like rape'' or that the kicking and pushing did not ''really hurt.'' One woman said: ''He started pushing me around, threw me on the bed and slapped me. He broke my beads and ripped my shirt. I don't think it was really violence'' (Russell, 1982, p. 48).

Interviews with victims revealed many cases of extreme violence, sometimes in the presence of their children or even involving children in the rapes. Other rapist-husbands tried to muffle their victims' screams by shoving their faces into pillows (Finkelhor & Yllo, 1985; Russell, 1982). Russell's (1982) sample admitted they had been subjected to many types of abuses, ranging from forced vaginal intercourse to beating, bondage, group sex, inserting objects in their vaginas, urolagnia, bestiality, and oral and anal rape. Similarly, Finkelhor and Yllo's (1985) interviews revealed rapes ranging from ''force only'' to extreme cases of brutality, including a gang rape arranged by a husband, and a child-hostage situation. The most common type of sexual abuse, besides penile-vaginal intercourse, was forced anal intercourse (one third of the women they interviewed mentioned their husbands had either assaulted or attempted to assault them in the anus). One wife had a six centimeter gash ripped in her vagina by her husband trying to '''pull her vagina out.' '' Obviously, these are not mere ''lovers' quarrels.''

MILDRED DALEY
PAGELOW

Many people believe that wife rape occurs infrequently, and then only among the lower classes by drunken, perverted husbands. Russell's (1982) rigorously designed study obtained a representative sample of women who were personally interviewed in depth to determine how many had been sexually abused by strangers, family members, and husbands. Russell noted:

> The study . . . is the only study of wife rape in the United States to be based on interviews with a random sample of women. *Fourteen percent (14%) of the 930 women interviewed who had ever been married had been raped by a husband or ex-husband*. . . . it suggests that at least one woman out of every seven who has ever been married has been raped by a husband at least once, and sometimes many times over many years. (1982, pp. 1–2)

In addition, the number of incidents of rape and attempted rape of all types of assailants is by far the highest for husbands and former husbands: 979 total number of incidents, compared to 237 incidents by acquaintances and 344 by lovers or former lovers (Russell, 1982, p. 67). Leaving out attempted rapes and narrowing analysis to completed rapes only, Russell found that women reported more rapes by husbands and former husbands (almost twice as many as rapes by acquaintances), the highest number of incidents of rape, and the highest percentage of all categories (Russell, 1982, p. 65).

Despite optimal interview conditions and rigorously trained interviewers, the 14% of ever-married women reporting rape by husbands or former husbands very likely provided an underestimate of marital rape in this country. Many women found it extremely difficult to discuss forced sex by spouses, even when the abuse had occurred many years earlier. Some said enough to indicate they had been raped by their husbands, but refused to answer any more questions. Russell (1982) commented, ''it seems that honest disclosure of unwanted sexual experiences in marriage was more difficult for many women than disclosure of sexual abuse by all other categories of people, including victims of incestuous abuse'' (p. 39).

Studies of woman battering most frequently are the sources of empirical evidence of wife rape, with the exception of Russell's and a few others (Doron, 1980; Hanneke *et al.*, 1985). Based on her research experience on rape, Russell (1980a) very early challenged the notion that marital rape is just another form of abuse suffered by battered wives:

> Although ongoing intimate heterosexual relationships that are violent often involve both rape and beating, it is also important to recognize that the issues of wife rape and wife beating can be quite separate in many marriages, and that wife rape is not merely one more abuse suffered by the already battered woman. (1982, p. 21)

Russell's own study showed that, out of the 644 ever-married women, there were 75 husbands (12%) who battered their wives but did not rape them; 24 husbands (4%) who raped their wives but did not batter them; and 63 other husbands (10%) who did both. By comparison, the Hanneke *et al.* (1985) study, using a variety of techniques to obtain a sample of 439 ever-married or cohabiting women, found that 117 (62%) were ''battered only,'' eight (4%) were ''raped only,'' and 64 (34%) were ''raped and battered.'' Combining the last two categories in both studies, it shows that Russell found 14% of the wives had been raped by their husbands, whereas Hanneke *et al.* found 38% wife victims of rape. The much higher rates of violence in the Hanneke *et al.* study may be due to several factors, one of which was their sampling techniques and another was their data collecting instrument, which provided ''very detailed lists of individual sexual and non-sexual behaviors'' from which respondents were asked to select the behaviors they had ever experienced (Hanneke *et al.,* 1985).

The study by Finkelhor and Yllo (1983, 1985) cannot provide a direct comparison, because it was designed to investigate marital rape, not other forms of marital violence. Their sample was not a victim population and there was no attempt to obtain a ''battered only'' category. They obtained their sample through a variety of methods, but the majority of respondents were clients at a family planning clinic in New England. Fifty women consented to in-depth interviews and 10% of a larger sample of 326 women answered yes to a questionnaire item about sex by force or threat of force.

These researchers categorized their interview responses as ''force-only rapes,'' ''battering-rapes,'' and ''obsessive rapes'' (Finkelhor & Yllo, 1985). They found that the battering type is most common, in which the husband uses sex to humiliate and degrade his wife and to dominate her in a generally abusive relationship, which they compare to Groth and Birnbaum's (1979) anger rapes. About 40% of their interviewed wives described what they called ''force-only rapes,'' or rape in an otherwise nonviolent context, which generally occurs when husbands are attempting to gain a sense of control over the type and frequency of their sexual intercourse. They compare this type to Groth and Birnbaum's power rapes. Least common are obsessive rapes (compared to what Groth described as sadistic rapes). These not only include sexual sadism but fetishism, and frequently involve anal intercourse. As one writer put it, ''many men apparently consider anal sex 'the quintessential sexual act' by which to humiliate a woman'' (Mettger, 1982).

Most other discussions of marital rape come from studies of woman battering (Bowker, 1983a; Dobash & Dobash, 1979; Frieze, 1980; Pagelow, 1980, 1981, 1984; Shields & Hanneke, 1983; Walker, 1979). Bowker (1983a) attempted to answer the question raised by Russell: Are rape and battering distinct phenomena, or is marital rape the extreme end of a continuum of violence against wives? In-depth interviews with 146 victims of marital violence revealed that 23% had experienced marital rape, whereas the others did not. Differences found between the sexually violent and the nonsexually violent couples were the wives' higher marital dissatisfaction and the couples' value dissimilarities, but it was not possible to specify the direction of the causal influence (Bowker, 1983a). Raped wives were also more likely to divorce their husbands. On the basis of his data, Bowker (1983a) concluded the following: ''there is no distinct syndrome that differentiates raping marriages from nonsexual battering marriages''; helping professionals might anticipate that marital rape is a factor in the lives of some couples; ''raped wives may need even more extensive support services than other battered wives''; and marital rape may damage marriages so extensively that its occurrence signifies the termination of the relationships (pp. 351–352).

Shields and Hanneke (1983) also investigated to see if marital rape is a distinct phenomenon or not. Do victims perceive the act of rape as different from nonsexual acts of violence? If they perceive the violence as rape, could that be viewed as the ''ultimate attack''? These researchers postulated that marital rape may be more stressful than nonsexual battering because of victims' contradictory ideas about their sexual rights and obligations in marriage. On the other hand, the idea of living with a rapist may be too painful, so victims may redefine sexual aggression in nonsexual terms, as being part of the overall violence. Shields and Hanneke's sample of 92 wives of violent men, obtained through a variety of sources, reported that: ''*46 percent of the women had experienced marital rape*'' (1983, p. 136).

MILDRED DALEY
PAGELOW

When marital rape occurs in violent marriages, it seems to have a more profound negative effect on the victim's self-esteem, their attitudes toward men, and sex with their husbands (Finkelhor & Yllo, 1985; Shields & Hanneke, 1983). A combination of sexual and nonsexual violence seems to be at the highest level on a continuum of wife abuse, because these victims have experienced more severe forms of nonsexual violence and stronger reactions (Bowker, 1983a; Russell, 1982; Shields & Hanneke, 1983). Wife rape, like nonmarital rape, appears to be mainly an act of violence and aggression in which sex is a method used to humiliate and hurt.

Thirty-four percent of a self-selected sample of 137 battered women admitted they had been raped (Frieze, 1980). After completing interviews to obtain a matched control group of 137 women for comparison purposes, Frieze found that 35% ($n = 48$) of the controls had also been physically assaulted by their husbands. These were designated as the battered-control group, and the balance were nonbattered controls (Frieze, 1980). To the rape question, in addition to the 34% of battered wives, 6% of the battered controls and 1% of the nonbattered controls said yes. In response to a less threatening item, "Sex is unpleasant because he forces you to have sex," 43% of the battered women, 13% of the battered controls, and 2% of the nonbattered controls agreed (Frieze, 1980). Despite the fact that forced sex is legally defined as rape, some women were obviously unwilling to admit they had been raped by their husbands but did admit to the less threatening term "force."

A great many wives are subjected to unwanted sexual contact through force or coercion, in addition to other types of physical battering; Finkelhor and Yllo (1985) noted that battered women report marital rape rates clustering between 33% and 50%, in studies done in different places, at different times, and using different questions. Pagelow's (1981) investigation of woman battering was not designed to see if rape in marriage is a distinct phenomenon; marital rape was assumed to be one of many forms of violent attacks on wives. There was no attempt made to discover whether or not any of the surveyed women went to shelters to escape marital rape alone. But the topic of rape was raised by many wives during interviews, and the survey instrument yielded data in response to an item that asked, "Were you ever sexually assaulted by him? (Forcible rape *is* an assault)" (Pagelow, 1981, p. 257). The purpose of the wording was to first introduce the less threatening term "sexual assault," but the word "rape" was included to make clear the point of the question for the women who responded to the self-administered questionnaires.

Although 25 women did not answer the rape question, over one third (37%) replied yes. The next item asked "about how often?" Out of the 119 women who said they had been sexually assaulted by their batterers, 110 told how many times it had occurred. Almost three out of four (74%) said they had been raped more than once; and 10% indicated that sex was always on demand and they felt they had no choice but to submit. Findings that rape usually occurs on a repetitive basis is consistent with other research. Of the researchers who note frequency rates of sexual assault for their samples, the following mentioned that rape occurred more than once: Frieze (1980), 59%; Shields and Hanneke (1983), 83%; and Russell (1982) 71%. Finkelhor and Yllo (1985) said only that for the majority of the women they interviewed, rape was a repeated occurrence.

It is somewhat surprising that so many women admitted they had been raped, because at the time they and the women in the Pagelow (1980) sample gave their responses, the law in most states did not acknowledge marital rape. On the other hand, many other wives did not identify sexual assault with rape, regardless of whether it was done by force, threat of force, or their own fears. It is clear that the 37% rate for marital rape in the Pagelow sample is an underreport of its occurrence. During interviews and discussion, many of the women who said they had not been raped explained that they submitted to sexual demands in order to prevent beatings, not because they wanted sex. Anal sex was mentioned several times, always in the context of repulsion and disgust and amid speculation on why men would find this ''unnatural'' and ''horrible'' sexual activity to be so desirable. Some women mentioned fighting back, but they did not connect this with rape or attempted rape. Most submitted to sex due to threats or their own fears. Wives who *denied* they had been raped wrote statements like the following:

> ''No, not exactly—it wasn't part of the assault. This was our general sex life.''
> ''On a few occasions I felt afraid of a beating if I refused him.''
> ''I gave in before it reached the rape stage.''
> ''If he beat me at other times when I was trying to please him, I knew better than to refuse sex.''
> (Pagelow, 1984, p. 430)

Fear and coercion are obvious in many cases, such as one wife who said to Dobash and Dobash, ''I didn't refuse him—I was too scared to refuse him.'' (1979, p. 14). The question of consent simply does not occur to many wives. One woman who said she had never been raped always submitted to sex against her will. She was terrified of having sex with her husband because:

> ''he beat me only during intercourse. He would start choking me once he mounted me; sometimes he choked me so long I passed out. When I'd come to, he was finished. One time I know he almost killed me because my neck was terribly bruised afterward.'' (Pagelow, 1984, p. 431)

As Russell (1982) noted, many women who were not included in her marital rape category ''saw it as their 'duty' to submit to sexual intercourse with their husbands, even when they had no desire for sex or were repulsed by the idea'' (p. 58). During an interview, one older woman revealed her acceptance of a ''wife's duty'' to take care of her husband's needs, sexual or otherwise. She seemed to assume the blame for her unhappy marriage because of her inability to respond sexually to her husband, saying:

> ''I guess some of our problems came from the fact that I never knew much about sex, and I never enjoyed having him touch me that way. Maybe some of it came from the fact that the first time I ever had sex was when he raped me—I was so ignorant! It hurt and I hated him, and then when I got pregnant and had to be his 'wife,' I never could learn to feel good when he touched me.'' (Pagelow, 1984, p. 431)

Some survey items asked about the frequency and quality of sexual intercourse between the wives and their spouses (Pagelow, 1981). Of the women responding to the frequency question, 59% indicated that sexual relations occurred either often or very, very often, and to the question on quality, 77% said their sex life was either about average or extremely unsatisfying. An open-ended question asked why they were unsatisfied, and 50 women said they did not want sex because it was forced, or their husbands were rough and/or brutal. These data support Walker's (1979) conclusions when she says:

> The violence and brutality in the sexual relationship between assaultive couples seem to escalate with time. As marital rape becomes more frequent, loving, tender sex becomes more rare. When brutality is at its height in other areas of the marriage, it seems as if more coercive techniques need to be used in order for sex to happen at all. Almost all of the women in this sample report being sexually abused by their men. The concept of marital rape is not acceptable under the law in most states, although most married women could describe instances where it occurred. Most men feel that their wives' sexual availability is guaranteed by the marriage license. (p. 126)

Walker notes that this progression of violence occurs also among unmarried co-habitees, a feature also found in the Pagelow study, in which 20% of the survey consisted of women not married to the men who battered and/or raped them. For some women, sexual encounters with their spouses had always had at least an element of force and violence, but for most, their sexual intimacy had begun almost ideally, characterized by gentleness and loving playfulness. Women whose husbands' violence remained nonsexual had the most difficulty in severing their relationships because their satisfying sexual relationships served as a positive reinforcement. Even though they had sought safety from violence in a shelter, 23% recalled their sexual relations as extremely satisfying. But for the many whose sex lives had deteriorated as the violence increased, or for those whose husbands used both sexual and nonsexual violence, they could only agree with Walker when she says, "Good sex often turns into assaultive behavior after awhile." (1979, p. 112). But why? What could cause so many men to batter sexually and rape their wives—women who are frequently also the mothers of their children?

FACTORS THAT PROMOTE MARITAL RAPE

There are some social and economic factors transferred from antiquity through to the present that promote marital rape, and there are other, more individual factors, that are firmly grounded in contemporary life in the United States. In this section, causes of male sexual aggression against wives are explored. First, it is necessary to look at the history of marriage, its foundations in the patriarchy, and the ideology according to which a wife's body belongs to her husband. As a consequence, this background leads to the second factor, the establishment of the marital exemption clause into rape laws. The third is the social and economic disadvantaged position of women, which operates to keep them tied to men regardless of the quality of their lives. The fourth factor is the violence of American society and its rape culture, which provided the spawning ground for pornography to fuse violence and sex into a mutation of aggressive masculine sexuality.

Historical Foundations

One reason it has taken so long for scientists to address the various types of family violence and to bring to public scrutiny the pain and suffering some family members bring upon others is the demand for family privacy. Some of the insistence for maintaining family privacy is based on the historical establishment of patriarchal marriage and common law rights and privileges. Under the patriarchy, men are undisputed heads of their households and other family members are subordinate to them and must obey their wishes and commands without question. The patriarch has absolute rights and power over wife and children. The autocratic patriarchal family structure under British law is described in this way: "The child's duty was that of 'unquestioning obedience,' the wife's to 'submit' and 'defer' to her husband's rule" (May, 1978, p. 138). The patriarchal family structure and common law are part of the English heritage adopted in the United States (Davidson, 1977; Dobash & Dobash, 1979). Common law refers to decisions based on customs of the people or what judges believe their communities feel is correct (Davidson, 1977). Once decisions are reached in courts of law, they become part of the legal fabric of society and influence other decisions often for many years before they are successfully usurped.

One British judge reached a decision that affected many thousands of lives and took centuries even to be challenged. Weitzman (1981) began her book on marriage contracts by stating that, "Blackstone, the renowned English legal scholar, described marriage under the common law of England as the merger of husband and wife into a single identity." Clearly, the one who remained was the husband. The woman's identity as an individual citizen ceased at the moment she became a wife, and was submerged into her husband's until the very moment she became a widow (Stannard, 1977). British and American law refused even to acknowledge that women were persons (Sachs & Wilson, 1978; Schulder, 1970). Blackstone had decreed that the "very being" of a woman was suspended during marriage, with the result that only the husband remained thereafter (Kanowitz, 1969). Under common law, wives had no right to sell, sue, or contract without their husbands' approval. As recently as 1966, there was a case of a Texas wife who defaulted on a loan taken out in her name only; the bank had granted the loan without obtaining her husband's signature. The Supreme Court upheld the common law of coventure, and the bank lost its suit to collect. Dissenting Justice Black stated:

> This rule has worked out in reality to mean that though the husband and wife are one, the one is the husband. This fiction rested on [the] . . . notion that a married woman, being a female, is without capacity to make her own contracts and do her own business. (Black, cited in Schulder, 1970, p. 165)

This merger of two persons into one has been defended for centuries as the rationale for immunity from testifying against a spouse in court, suing a spouse, or why there was no legal recognition of the concept of marital rape. How, the reasoning went, if two persons are one, could a person be forced to testify against him or herself? How could one sue one's own self? Or rape one's own body? "The reasoning followed that since the husband and wife were legally one, the law would not allow one person to sue himself. This view of the merging of the spouses was primarily a political move to settle property claims." (Calvert, 1974, p. 90).

The concept of spousal immunity may have been motivated by economic factors favoring husbands, but it also protected husbands from suits for battery and rape. Women were still excluded from suing husbands for abuse even whey then began to gain some rights with the passage of the *Married Women's Property Acts* during the American Civil War period. Spouses could not sue each other for personal injuries supposedly to protect "domestic tranquility." Kanowitz (1969) noted: "A husband could beat his wife mercilessly . . . but the law in its rectitude denied her the right to sue her husband because such a suit, it claimed, could destroy the peace of the home" (p. 78). As many scholars have noted since, when a husband is beating or raping a wife, how much "peace" is in that home, anyway?

The Marital Exemption in Rape Laws

Legal policies based on common law and the patriarchy have served to give husbands support for the notion that their wives—and their bodies—belong to them. Spousal exemption clauses, which protect husbands from prosecution for wife rape, were inserted in the rape laws of most states, and remained unchallenged until very recently. Marital immunity stems from the clause that defines rape as nonconsensual sexual intercourse by a man with a female not his wife. The result is that as long as husbands can rape wives with impunity from the law, women do not own their own bodies (Pagelow, 1977).

In most countries of the world and almost half the states in the United States, women still cannot refuse their husbands sexual access to their bodies. Traditional marriage vows call for a wife's promise to "love, honor, and obey," and the legal contract insures the husband's rights to sexual intimacy so that if a husband desires sex with his wife, she has an obligation to cooperate. Outside of marriage, however, a man who forces sexual intimacy on a nonconsenting woman can be charged with rape. One writer noted:

> Rape is an act of violence which subjects the victim to physical and emotional humiliation besides pain, fear, and not infrequently serious injury. It is recognized by the law as a crime, one of the most serious known. This same act however, if perpetrated within the marriage, is no offense and carries no sanctions; it is merely the exercise of the husband's right in pursuance of the marriage contract. (Mitra, 1979, p. 558)

Rape is considered a serious violent crime, and penalties have ranged all the way to execution. But a number of feminist scholars insist that rape laws were instituted to protect male privilege (Brownmiller, 1976; Freeman, 1981; Kurman, 1980). They insist that the severe penalties for rape serve as "punishment for the defilement of another man's property rather than a form of protection for women or a recognition of women's rights over their own bodies" (Smart, 1977). If rape laws were for the protection of women, it would make no sense to make an exception for a man who rapes his wife (LeGrand, 1973). Conversely, if rape laws are to protect men's property from other men, then they would exclude property owners with a clause defining rape as "forced sexual intercourse with a female *not the wife* of the perpetrator." They do contain such a clause. "The law in most states protects a man from prosecution for the rape of his wife. The marital 'right' to rape one's wife is expressed in state criminal statutes." (Mettger, 1982, p. 1). What is the legal basis for this marital exemption?

The British common law precedent is traced to the 17th century Chief Justice Sir Matthew Hale. Geis (1980, pp. 1–2) explained:

> The major figure in shaping this law was Sir Matthew Hale, whose dictum on the subject occupies but four lines in his encyclopedic *Historia Placitorum Coronae,* published posthumously in 1736. They read: "But the husband cannot be guilty of a rape committed by himself upon his lawful wife, for by their mutual matrimonial consent and contract the wife hath given up herself in this kind unto the husband which she cannot retract."

Hale's brief statement and the doctrine it established, *irrevocable consent,* have no legal basis, according to legal scholars (Mettger, 1982). Although Hale offered no citations to support the rule, it was accepted because it "was congruent also with views prevailing in the social system of the time about women, about sexual assault, and about marriage" (Geis, 1980, p. 3). Despite its flaws, it became part of American common law, and "eventually was incorporated, either implicitly or explicitly, into state and federal criminal law as a 'marital exemption' which grants a husband immunity from prosecution for raping his wife" (Mettger, 1982, p. 2). Geis says there was "an unquestioning acceptance of the Hale dictum" in American case law (1978).

History shows that Hale was viciously misogynistic, but his attitudes were supported by the more general views about women's place in marriage. Blackstone had already set forth the principle of matrimonial unity: in marriage, the man and woman become one. In addition, patriarchal marriage decreed that wives are the property of their husbands.

Under common law, a wife could not refuse to have sex with her husband, but Hale's dictum was not introduced into court until 1888 in the Clarence case (Geis, 1978; Kurman, 1980). In this case, the issue was not wife rape but whether or not Clarence had committed fraud by concealing the fact that he had gonorrhea when he had intercourse with his wife. In finding Clarence guilty of inflicting harm and assault causing harm, "the trial court reasoned that Clarence's 'fraud' in concealing his medical condition from his wife had vitiated her consent to intercourse, and that the infection that she subsequently contracted represented bodily harm'' (Geis, 1978, p. 287).

Although wife rape did not occur in this case, the prosecution raised this irrelevant issue by claiming that Clarence would have been guilty of raping his wife if she had known about the gonorrhea, had refused consent, and he had persisted with force. This claim aroused comments from several judges that according to Geis (1978, p. 288)

> amounted to little more than stray, unfocused observations. But later, these inconclusive musings would come to serve as a major basis for more fixed judicial views upholding Lord Hale's statement on the inviolability of the husband's right of sexual access to his spouse.

The Hale dictum of irrevocable consent still influences many lives today. Yet non-violent people have difficulty understanding how some men could force unwanted sexual activity on their wives:

> It is mind-boggling for a woman to be raped by the man she expected to show true love for her. Such dread deeds are almost blasphemous—the act that God designed to enable man and wife to manifest their love is twisted into an act of hatred. Rape in marriage may be the ultimate sex sin. It's time it was dragged out of the closet. (Adamo, 1984)

We now know that rape in marriage is a common occurrence that has just recently been ''dragged out of the closet,'' and there are many people who would like to shove it back. The marital exemption in rape laws has been under attack since the 1970s, and slowly, state by state, it has been eliminated or modified by about half of them. But for many years, and for countless wives who were and are victims of rape, there was no recourse for legal sanction, based on the dictum uttered by the same judge who produced the now infamous ''cautionary instructions'' for rape juries: '''it must be remembered . . . that it [rape] is an accusation easily to be made and hard to be proved, and harder to be defended by the party accused, tho never so innocent' '' (Hale, cited in Geis, 1978, p. 286).

Rape laws have great symbolic importance for husbands and wives, but for many repeatedly raped wives, a more important question is, How can they stop the violence? Bowker's (1983b) research shows that raped wives were more likely to obtain divorces than nonsexually abused wives. In the Finkelhor and Yllo (1985) study, 76% of the interviewed women were divorced or separated, in fact, only 6% were still living with the men who had raped them. Permanent dissolution of their marriages appears to be the method of choice for raped wives to stop the abuse. But because all the studies show that the vast majority of raped wives suffered multiple sexual assaults, obviously they did not take those drastic steps immediately. The next section explains not only why many raped wives delay breaking up their families, but also why their rapist husbands know this will be the case.

Economic Disadvantages of Formerly Married Women

When a man rapes his wife, he has to have some inner confidence that his victim will neither report the rape to police nor leave him. Wives' economic dependence on their husbands contributes to marital rape, and both spouses are aware of this fact. Even if a wife threatens that she will leave if he ever is sexually aggressive again, this is unlikely to prevent future attacks because he knows that her limited economic prospects will keep her tied to him. In her latest book, Weitzman (1985) reported a 73% drop in divorced women's and their children's standard of living at the same time that there is a 42% increase for their divorced husbands.

Women who are victims of marital rape are most often also victims of nonsexual battering, as research previously cited shows (Hanneke *et al.*, 1985; Finkelhor & Yllo, 1985; Russell, 1982). As such, they share in common the problems faced by all battered women trying to establish an independent lifestyle. Abused wives are most often socially isolated, denied freedom of movement, and jealously watched by their abusers whenever they are outside the home—the last thing the husbands want is for their wives to leave them. The resource the women lack the most is economic independence. One way to ensure that is to control tightly the family finances. Wives of abusive men, even wealthy women, frequently have no cash or credit cards, or credit in their own names (Martin, 1976), they are often ignorant of money management, and may have no or limited marketable job skills. Their economic dependence on the men who abuse them puts them (and their children) in a vulnerable position. Even when a wife is gainfully employed, she may have no decision-making power on how her own earnings are spent; in some cases, wives are accompanied by their abusive husbands on payday so the checks are turned over to them immediately (Dobash & Dobash, 1979; Martin, 1976).

Fleming describes the economic control in these terms: "In violent marriages, the husband invariably controls the family finances—usually with an iron hand. It is the rare victim who has more than a few dollars she can call her own" (1979, p. 83). Cases abound in which abused wives were forced by their circumstances to hide coins over a period of years until they could accumulate enough to pay bus fares to escape out of town with their children (Eisenberg & Micklow, 1977; Fleming, 1979; Pagelow, 1981).

Leaving a husband, despite his abuse, may be a difficult choice for any woman. Intact couple families enjoy a higher standard of living than single parent families, but when the single parent is a woman, their income is likely to be half or less what it is expected to be when both husband and wife are present. In rounded figures, it costs a woman (depending on her skin color) between about $11,000 and $13,000 to live in a household without a husband present, and the income lost is more than she can expect to receive at paid employment. Conversely, a male householder loses approximately 23% of the family income, or it costs about $5,000 per year to live without a wife present (U.S. Bureau of the Census, 1983a).

Employment leading to economic independence for women is not always a possibility, because regardless of education and job skills, women consistently have higher unemployment and underemployment rates than men. When employed, women tend to cluster in lower paid job categories, their opportunities for advancement are more restricted, and they suffer higher layoff rates. Wives with less than 12 years of education can expect to earn only 56% of what husbands with the same education can earn. Even when women have earned college degrees or had postgraduate education, they can expect to earn almost $2,000 *less* than men who are high school dropouts. The median income for women with 4 or more years of college is $8,360 less per year than men with the same level of education (U.S. Bureau of the Census, 1980).

Even if they are well educated, wives may have been out of the employment market for so long that their skills are outdated, or they may have no marketable skills. On the other hand, employed wives often have to terminate their jobs to prevent their husbands from finding them to punish them or force them to return home. Women in career positions can suffer serious damages to their future earning potential when outraged husbands stalk them at their places of employment. Finding new jobs can be difficult, especially when the women are older, not particularly attractive, minority group members, or burdened with preschool youngsters, because of the lack of adequate and inexpensive child care facilities in this country.

Despite some gains of the women's movement, in the 26-year period from 1955 to 1981, white women employed full time, year round in 1981 received proportionately less compared to white men than they received in 1955. And although black women received more in 1981 relative to black men, they still only receive about 55% the median income of white male workers (U.S. Bureau of the Census, 1983a). A black woman may have less economic dependency on a black man, but she is even more disadvantaged in the job market than a white woman. Income rates are higher for individuals and lower for family members. In 1978 the overall poverty rate for families in the United States was ten percent, but among families headed by women, the rate was much higher: 24 percent of white, 51 percent of black, and 53 percent of Spanish origin female householders lived below the official poverty level (Rawlings, 1980). By 1980, the family poverty rate was still ten percent, but for female-headed families the rate was 50 percent, and for black female-headed families the rate was 70 percent (U.S. Bureau of the Census, 1983b).

Not all raped and battered wives have children, but mothers of dependent children have compelling reasons for staying tied to abusive men. The men often are loving fathers or if not, at least they provide for the children financially. The women have been socialized to believe that an intact home is better for their children than having no father, and to sacrifice their own self-interest for their children. The mothers feel compelled to endure their fear and pain ''for the sake of the children.'' They often do not recognize the harm being done and do not decide to leave until they realize that their children are also victims of violence, directly or indirectly (Pagelow, 1982).

If they are lucky, their children are in good health and old enough to attend school, but many children in abusive homes suffer from chronic illnesses or various handicaps (Pagelow, 1981). But if they leave, where will they go and how will they provide for themselves and their children? They may fear retaliation and hesitate to go to court to attempt to get child and spousal support, but when they do, awards are often less than adequate.

There were approximately 15 million mothers and children under the age of 18 living in families with no husband/father present in 1979 (U.S. Bureau of the Census, 1981). Some fathers contribute to family support after separation or divorce to help maintain their families above the poverty level. However, of the 7.1 million women with one or more children under 21 in 1979, 41% of these mothers were never awarded child support payments and had to depend on other sources. Of those who were awarded child support, the majority received less than the full amount or nothing. Fewer than one out of four mothers can depend on receiving court-awarded child support payments on a regular basis. The overall average payment in 1978 was $1,800, about 20% of their mean total money income (U.S. Bureau of the Census, 1981).

Whether or not a mother is awarded and receives child support payments, as well as the amount of such payments, is strongly correlated with socioeconomic characteristics. In other words, an educated white woman from an affluent background with employment skills is in the best position to receive support. A woman who occupies the opposite end of the spectrum is in the least favorable position and the more children there are, the less likely the mother will receive child support payments. Children under 18 living in their mother's households are extremely likely to be poor:

> The poverty rate among children living in families maintained by women was much higher than for children in families overall (51 percent versus 16 percent). Among children in Spanish-origin

and Black families maintained by women, the rates were 69 and 66 percent, respectively, compared with 40 percent for their White counterparts. (Rawlings, 1980, p. 34)

When a woman leaves her abuser, her economic standard of living very likely takes a drastic drop. If she has dependent children, she must take into consideration the lives and welfare of her children, who have roughly one chance out of two of dropping below the poverty level (two out of three for minority children). Is it any wonder that many women remain with their rapist husbands for many years, sometimes until the children are grown and have left home? Repeatedly, raped wives say that they stayed for many years because they doubted they could support themselves and their children without their abusive husbands' financial support. Is there any question that those husbands were aware of this fact and took full advantage of it?

Economic dependence helps explain why so many wives find themselves unable to take the one step that will terminate marital rape—leaving. But because rape is a violent act that not all men can or will commit—even some husbands who batter and otherwise physically abuse their wives—what could cause a man to rape his wife? Factors outside the marital union encourage or enable men to rape women. It is generally understood that the United States has a higher violent crime rate than other industrialized nations, but is there something in our society that encourages a rape mentality among men?

American Violence and Its Rape Culture

What would cause a man to rape a woman who is his wife and frequently the mother of his children? Going one step farther, we might ask what would cause a man to rape any woman? "Marital rape, like stranger rape, is not an act of sexual desire but an expression of power and hostility" (Mettger, 1982, p. 13). Russell (1982) saw male sexual aggression inside and outside marriage as an issue that stems from two serious and predominantly male problems: male violence and predatory male sexuality. Males constitute 90% of the perpetrators of violent crimes, and according to Russell (1982):

> Wife rape is equally a manifestation of a male sexuality which is oriented to conquest and domination, and to providing masculinity; masculinity unfortunately is defined in terms of power, superiority, competitiveness, control, and aggression. A "real man" is supposed to get what he wants, when he wants, particularly with his wife, and even more particularly, in his sexual relations with her. (p. 357).

Men rape their wives for a number of reasons: in retaliation for perceived wrongs or for punishment—to frighten, humiliate, punish, and degrade (Finkelhor & Yllo, 1985). They also rape to assert power and strength, prove their virility, and overcome their feelings of being unloved (Groth & Birnbaum, 1979). Another reason is entitlement (Bart, 1981; Finkelhor & Yllo, 1985). Husbands often view their wives as their property, thus they feel entitled to do whatever they wish with their wives' bodies, with or without their consent. The marital exemption in rape laws gives tacit approval to the entitlement notion. These laws infer that what goes on in private between husbands and wives is none of the state's business.

Entitlement ideas also stem from the fact that some religions have emphasized that wives should obey and submit to their husbands (Finkelhor & Yllo, 1985). The justification for a chain of command has recently been challenged as a distortion of scripture to support domestic violence:

> Wives are told to continually submit to terrible situations because they belong to their husbands. . . . One case involved marital rape. The wife was told by the pastoral counselor that her

body belonged to her husband and therefore he had a right and she should just submit. (Scanzoni, cited in Carter, 1982, p. 35)

221

MARITAL RAPE

Wives clearly lack freedom of choice when refusal to engage in sexual intimacy is considered to be a sin against God. Although he now rejects "the archaic attitude of absolute ownership," one Catholic prelate writes: "I was taught to instruct wives in particular that it was sinful to deny the husband sex except for serious reasons, and that an unloving wife could drive her husband to drink or masturbation or adultery—and those sins would be on her soul" (Adamo, 1984).

An important feature of marital rape is that it is safe for a man to rape his wife. Malamuth (1981) has conducted many studies on men's "proclivity to rape," which he defines as "according to the *relative* likelihood for men to rape under various conditions" (p. 139). His studies found that *not being caught* increased college male's willingness to rape, which again increased (to 51%) if they were assured of *no punishment*. The significance of these findings relative to wife rape cannot be overlooked. About a third to half of all males tested indicate some interest in committing rape if they can get away with it, and there could be no safer targets than their wives.

Malamuth (1981) believes "average men" have a proclivity to rape under certain circumstances. In his laboratory experiments, Malamuth has used written scenarios of rape scenes, or shown R-rated films that imply that women welcome violence and that rape is justified. The scenarios depict rape after rejection by a casual date, and 51% of male college students indicate they might be willing to rape under those circumstances. What about men who believe their wives have rejected them? Russell (1984), suggested: "one wonders how much the percentage might increase if the story were about a man who forced intercourse on his wife after she had declined his sexual advances for over a week" (p. 224).

Malamuth used R-rated movies in his studies, not "hard-core porn," yet they feature the rape myths (victims deserve, invite, desire, and/or enjoy rape) that are prevalent in pornography. In recent years, images of violent sex have flourished in movies, advertisements, popular music, and television so that they are available to all, not limited to pornography users. But at the same time, pornography has become increasingly explicit and violent. As the availability of pornographic materials has increased, so have violent crimes, including rape and femicide. Of the many publications available, the three leading magazines sell in the millions. According to Russell (1982), *Playboy, Penthouse,* and *Hustler* have "circulations of 5.7 million, 4.7 million, and 1.6 million, respectively," but circulation rates are tripled to determine total readership.

All pornography is not blatantly violent, but as Stoller noted, "An essential dynamic in pornography is hostility" (1975, p. 88). Feshbach and Malamuth (1978) stated; "one exposure to violence in pornography can significantly influence erotic reactions to the portrayal of rape" (p. 116). Russell (1980b) agreed with Malamuth that many men possess a proclivity to rape, but she noted that inhibitors to rape are first, the possibility of being caught (social control); second, that it is socially unacceptable behavior (social norms); and third, the view that it is immoral and brutal (conscience).

Analysis of the contents of 428 adults-only paperbacks published between 1968 and 1974 showed there were 4,588 sex episodes, 20% involving completed rape (Bart & Jozsa, 1980). It was also found that the number of rapes increased in each year's publications; 6% involved incest; the victims' fear and terror transformed into orgasmic passion; and less than 3% had negative consequences whereas some were rewarded. These portrayals serve to reduce inhibitions: rapists do not get caught (social control); normal men rape, thus it is socially acceptable (social norms); and women really enjoy being raped (conscience).

Finding an association between marital rape and pornography does not justify a conclusion that rape is *caused* by a husband's exposure to pornography, but Russell (1982) believes that "at minimum, it *does* have some effect." Undoubtedly, some men would rape their wives with or without the encouragement of pornography, and many other men are consumers of pornography without raping. The question is, How many men—who might not otherwise be inclined to rape—accept messages from pornographic material indicating that women like to be dominated and raped? What effect does it have on men who feel that their old methods have not worked in the past, therefore why not try something new? For example, reports of the rape trial of an Orange County, California man state that after months of marriage counseling, the wife made an appointment with a divorce attorney and began looking for an apartment.

> On the day of the alleged attack, she . . . told [her husband] she was moving out, the prosecutor said. That night . . . [the wife] was watching the Miss American beauty pageant on a television in a bedroom while [her husband] was watching an X-rated movie in the family room. [Her husband] allegedly entered the bedroom, threw her on the bed and bound her. [He] also ripped off her clothing and began taking nude photos of her. . . . He then sexually assaulted her. (Brown, 1981, p. 6)

The time period of greatest danger for an abused woman is when she leaves or threatens to leave her husband (Pagelow, 1984). This is a crisis point for domineering husbands who fear losing control of their women, and they are more likely to increase their violence by extreme battering and/or raping, or even killing their wives. Battered women in Frieze's (1980) study were more likely to be sexually assaulted, and over two thirds of the Finkelhor and Yllo (1985) sample "were raped in the waning days of a relationship." A combination of the two factors—a wife about to leave him and the X-rated movie—may have stimulated the husband into the bondage, rape, and photographing of his wife.

One of the cases presented by Finkelhor and Yllo (1985) of an "obsessive rapist" included pornography, bondage, rape, and photographs taken of the victim. Although numerically few were found in their study, the behavior of obsessive rapists was bizarre and possibly life threatening. Not only were they involved in pornography, but they also "tried to get their wives to participate in making or imitating it." Sexual sadism and many cases of anal rape also occurred in this category. One man not only collected all types of pornography, but he wrote pornographic short stories, and kept index cards grading each wife rape of the previous few months (Finkelhor & Yllo, 1985).

Many women in the Pagelow (1984) study mentioned that their husbands tried to get them to perform sexual acts they found objectionable, particularly anal sex, which is abundantly featured in pornography. Some associated these requests with pornography; others did not. In-depth interviews with women who spoke of marital rape or sexual abuse of their children revealed that many had husbands who seemed obsessed with pornography. The following case appears to have a direct connection between sexual assault and pornography: a battered farm wife found a closed room in the barn while she was looking for her husband. She described her discovery this way:

> "I was so shocked, I didn't know what to make of it. It was a room with all kinds of big pictures on the walls, and crazy pieces of equipment, like whips and such. It wasn't like the rest of the barn—this was kind of like a shrine, or a temple, or something, you know? I don't remember if there were candles or not, but it had that feeling. I stood there stupefied, and when the shock got less, I started looking at those pictures. They were all—like women being bound up, whipped—

with metal and chains and things, and some had men doing things to them. All of a sudden, I remembered that *he* [her husband] had tried to do some of those things to me, or tried to get me to do! There was a big dog in one, too! He must of been coming to this place to get psyched up before raping me. Then I *knew* I had to get away from him!'' (Pagelow, 1984, p. 435)

One woman staying at a shelter asked for a personal interview. She began by saying that she had lived with her husband, a man who had studied for the priesthood, for 3 years before they married. Their sex life at first, she said, ''was great!'' But when they impulsively got married in Las Vegas:

''That night we attended a show where they had a contest, inviting the women in the audience to get up on the stage and do a strip act. My husband wanted *me* to get up there but I refused. We went back to our hotel but he was sulking; he left me on our wedding night and stayed out all night. After that, our sex life was awful: he either beat me first and then raped me or he would make me dress up in those terrible clothes like garter-belts and trashy things so he could make himself believe I was a whore so he could fuck me. He had to pretend I was a whore so he could hate me before he could have sex! I think I began hating him from our wedding night on.'' (Pagelow, 1984, p. 431)

This woman made no direct reference to pornography, but the materials her husband brought home for his sexual fantasies are usually found in ''sex shops.'' Many wives are totally unaware of their husbands' consumption of pornography. Millions of dollars are spent each year in sex shops that pander directly to consumers, and there is a growing mail-order business that sends materials to offices or post office boxes. Many rapists are discovered by police to have pornographic materials in their possession. Commander James Bannon of the Detroit Police Department is cited by Diamond (1980, p. 201) as saying: ''often we find that the man is trying to enact a scene in some pornographic pictures.''

Russell asked the women in her sample the question, ''Have you ever been upset by anyone trying to get you to do what they'd seen in pornographic pictures, movies or books?'' (1982, p. 84). Out of the total sample of 930, 10% answered yes, but of the victims of wife rape, 24% said yes. Activities that the wives directly connected to their husbands' interest in pornography included sadomasochism, group sex, inserting objects in their vaginas, oral intercourse, anal intercourse, urolagnia, and bestiality (1982). One woman is quoted as saying:

''My old man and I went to a show that had lots of tying up and anal intercourse. We came home and proceeded to make love. He went out and got two belts. He tied my feet together with one, and with the other he kinda beat me. . . . But when he tried to penetrate me anally, I couldn't take it, it was too painful. . . . He did stop, but not soon enough to suit me.'' (Russell, 1980b, pp. 226–227)

Clearly, there is an association between pornography and sexual abuse of women, including wife rape, but there is no way to determine if it is a causal connection. Exposure to violent sex scenes increases men's proclivity to rape, and it increases even more when they believe they will not be caught or punished (Malamuth, 1981). Rape and incest can be committed with an almost guaranteed probability of not being caught or punished in a man's own home.

ASSESSMENT AND TREATMENT

Although there are relatively few studies of marital rape, effects on victims found in various reports are remarkably consistent: trauma is severe and long lasting (Finkelhor & Yllo, 1985). Shields and Hanneke (1983) compared reactions of victims who were nonsexually assaulted to victims who suffered sexual and nonsexual abuse, and found significant differences. One test found that "the more often the women had been raped, the lower was her self-esteem, the more negative were her attitudes toward her own marriage, the more psychosomatic reactions she experienced, and the more likely she was to have attempted suicide" (Shields & Hanneke, 1983, pp. 140–141). Moreover, they found that the incidence of reactions "increase significantly during victimization and *continues to increase even after the relationship has ended*" (1983, p. 144, emphasis added). Bowker (1983a,b) found more negative attitudes toward their own marriages, and a greater likelihood for divorce among wives who suffered both types of assaults. Russell (1982) found that two raped wives had been so upset at the abuse that they had attempted suicide, and several other women were afraid of being killed by their husbands, indicating long-term fears. There is abundant evidence showing:

> The consequences of wife rape are often very severe, and that wife rape is not infrequently accompanied by life-threatening violence. In fact, wife rape appears to be the most traumatic form of rape by intimates, and many factors cause wife rape often to be more traumatic than rape by strangers and other non-intimates; for example, the sense of betrayal, the disillusionment, the fact that it frequently contaminates the entire marriage, and the additional fact that wife rape is often repeated, sometimes for years on end. (Russell, 1982, p. 359)

Only a small minority of raped wives had been raped only once (Finkelhor and Yllo, 1983, 1985; Frieze, 1980; Pagelow, 1980; Shields & Hanneke, 1983). Most people believe that rape by a stranger is far more traumatic than marital rape because they focus on sexual aspects of rape but:

> It touches a woman's basic confidence in forming relationships and trusting intimates. It can leave a woman feeling much more powerless and isolated than if she were raped by a stranger. Moreover, a woman raped by her husband has to live with her rapist, not just a frightening memory of a stranger's attack. . . . Most of the women we interviewed were raped on multiple occasions. (Finkelhor & Yllo, 1983, pp. 126–127)

Sexually abused children and wives share some commonalities, one of which is helplessness of the victims and their inability to prevent, avoid, or escape sexual exploitation by more powerful persons. Another similarity is that the sexual assaults are committed by close family members, people they have loved and trusted. A child victim of sexual assault by a stranger is more likely to receive love, concern, and family support than when she accuses an adult in her own family (MacFarlane, Jenstrom, & Jones, 1980). Reactions to complaints of rape by a wife are likely to follow the same pattern. A woman raped by an acquaintance or stranger is much more likely to receive sympathy, concern, and assistance from her family and the community.

Violence accompanying rape tends to increase with the degree of intimacy of the prior association of rapist and victim (Bart, 1981; Black, 1979; Queen's Bench Foundation, 1976; Russell, 1975). When Bart (1981) studied the difference between rapes and attempted rapes, she found that women were more likely to be raped when (a) they were attacked by men they knew, particularly if they had a prior sexual relationship with them, (b) the only strategy they used was talking or pleading, (c) the assault took place in their homes, (d) their primary concern was not being killed or mutilated, and (e) there was a threat of force. Husband rapists are more likely to succeed in their rape attempts than stranger rapists (Russell, 1982). One woman had successfully fought off two rapists but was raped later by her own husband (Bart, 1981). Two women in the Pagelow study had been raped by strangers and afterward raped by their husbands as punishment for succumbing to strangers (or supposedly wanting them); both wives were hospitalized after the rapes by their husbands.

Raped wives suffer from the rape crisis syndrome that now is familiar to most professionals who come in contact with rape victims. The symptoms include humiliation, shame, disjointedness, anger, inability to concentrate or express themselves, or withdrawal (Bard & Ellison, 1974). The trauma suffered by marital rape victims are at least as severe as those suffered by women raped by strangers. The husband who violates his wife's body against her will is also her socially designated protector, with whom she shares intimate sexual relations. He took an oath before witnesses to "love, honor, and cherish" her, and frequently, he is the father of her children.

Implications for treatment from research findings are that caregivers in the medical, psychological, and social services and others must become sensitized to the special problems of raped wives. Therapists, physicians, nurses, and social workers need to develop awareness that clients who present certain symptoms may not be totally honest, and may be hiding the true cause of their distress (Weingourt, 1985). Battered women hesitate to reveal their victimization (Hilberman & Munson, 1978), and raped wives are even more hesitant, but do so when questioned by empathetic, nonjudgmental professionals. Helping professionals first must become aware that wife rape occurs with great frequency, and secondly, be sensitive to the symptoms. Next, they need to ask about it, couching their questions in gentle, nonthreatening terms. Finally, when it has been determined that marital rape has occurred at least once, they can then use their professional skills to assist victims, plus advising them about community resources to help them and protect them from further abuse.

Bowker (1983a) also advises professionals working with battered wives not to overlook the possibility that their clients might have suffered marital rape; these women may need even more extensive support services than other abused wives. Helping professionals should anticipate rape when there is extensive marital conflict, furthermore: "marital rape may damage many marriages so extensively that helping professionals may prefer to help the couple plan lives apart rather than to help them stay together" (Bowker, 1983a, p. 352). There is a "negative prognosis for the continuation of the marriage even if the violence ceases, and a similarly negative prognosis for the quality of those marriages that hold together" (Bowker, 1983a, p. 351).

ETHICAL AND LEGAL ISSUES

Most researchers believe that rape laws exempting husbands from prosecution promote marital rape because through them: "men are taught that they can rape their wives, and women are taught that they have no right to say 'no' " (Russell, 1982). Changes have occurred in rape laws since the 1970s, spearheaded by feminists who were joined by law and order groups (Russell, 1982). "Conservatives support changes in evidentiary requirements for rape because they desire to see more criminals more readily convicted" (Geis, 1978, p. 293).

But conservative legislators balk at any attempt to eliminate the marital exemption clause, even citing the Bible for support (Schulman, 1980). The District of Columbia City Council passed a sexual-assault bill that removed the husband's exemption from rape charges, but the Moral Majority, led by Senator Denton, succeeded in overturning the new law (*Ms.*, 1982). Federal law was modernized to allow rape charges by a wife if there was a "violent" component (Geis, 1980), but there was intense opposition:

The Senate Judiciary Committee placed the provision in the bill over the strong objections of Committee member Jeremiah Denton (R-AL) and the Moral Majority, which feels it is ''too hard on husbands accused of raping their wives,'' according to a *New York Times* article last November. Denton . . . told his fellow committee members that while he considers sexual abuse in marriage a ''hideous crime,'' he does not believe a husband guilty of ''a little coercion'' should be placed in the same category as a criminal rapist. ''Dammit,'' he declared, ''when you get married you kind of expect to get a little sex'' (Mettger, 1982, pp, 2, 13).

Objections from some politicians make it appear that they have a personal interest in maintaining a husband's ''license to rape.'' For example: ''But if you can't rape your wife, who can you rape?'' (California State Senator Bob Wilson, cited in Schulman, 1980).

Despite some fierce opposition, one after another, states are changing their laws so that husbands can be prosecuted for rape. By 1980, only three states, New Jersey, Oregon, and Nebraska, had completely abolished the marital rape exemption, and it was partially striken by five other states (Russell, 1982). And by 1982, two more states had followed suit and two others joined the partial exemption states. In the meantime, 13 other states expanded the marital privilege to include cohabiting men (Mettger, 1982), and five states granted partial immunity to men who had previously had consensual sex with a woman. This was called the ''voluntary-social-companion'' exemption: ''This in effect sanctions 'date rape' '' (Finkelhor & Yllo, 1985, p. 149).

It would be futile to attempt to present here the current status of state marital rape laws, because as Finkelhor and Yllo note, ''some laws are in transition, some are vague and have not been subjected to judicial interpretation, and in some states contradictory implications can be drawn from different statutes'' (1985, p. 140). In addition, by the time this reaches publication, the data undoubtedly will be outdated. Recent sources for information on marital rape exemption laws are Finkelhor and Yllo (1985), and Russell's book (1982), which contains a state-by-state summary. The authors of these two books note the contributions in marital rape law data gathering and analysis by Joanne Schulman, staff attorney at the National Center on Women and Family Law in New York, and Laura X, director and founder of the National Clearinghouse on Marital Rape in Berkeley, California. Changes in rape laws will continue to occur, but as of this time, only a little over half the states allow the prosecution of a husband for rape while they are still living together. Others contain partial exemptions (prosecution only if court papers were filed to end the marriage or the couple do not cohabit). Only one or two states still have an absolute marital exemption that protects the husband from prosecution until the very day a divorce decree becomes final.

Arguments against striking the exemption included claims that it would be difficult to enforce; it would undermine the family; victims are sufficiently provided redress under current laws; and it would lead to a virtual flood of complaints by vindictive wives. This has not happened in the states that have changed their laws. Oregon dropped the exemption in 1977 without such a deluge (there were only four cases up to 1982), although one, the Rideout case in Salem, did generate extensive publicity. This was the first trial in American history in which a man had been charged, indicted, and tried for raping his nonestranged wife, and the husband was acquitted (Footlick, 1979; Fox, 1979). The first spousal rape conviction took place in Salem, Massachussets, on September 21, 1979. In the Chretien case, the wife had filed for divorce in 1978 although the divorce was not yet final, and the couple had been living apart when the husband broke into his wife's home (*Response,* 1979; *Time,* 1979).

As for the claim that marital rape laws would be difficult to enforce, there were 42 cases of rapes by husbands in California from 1980–1981, and out of the 30 cases that were prosecuted, 89% resulted in convictions. This is much higher than nonmarital rape cases, but the ones that went to trial were made up almost entirely of well-documented and brutal crimes. The National Clearinghouse on Marital Rape carefully collected and summarized these cases (see Appendix B, Finkelhor & Yllo, 1985, for their analysis).

Despite opponents' claims that striking the marital exemption would destroy the family, that has not happened in other countries where there has been no exemption for years. Some countries do not follow the Anglo-Saxon common law tradition. Poland has allowed husbands to be prosecuted for rape since 1932 (before the Communist take-over), and other communist block countries such as the USSR and Czechoslovakia, all allow such prosecution (Geis, 1980). Israel, Sweden, Norway, and Denmark also have no marital exemption. Sweden's law has stood since 1965 without doing any of the mischief opponents claim such laws will generate (Geis, 1980).

It is important to many people that the marital exemption be stricken from rape laws because, "As long as husbands can rape wives with impunity from the law—women do not own their own bodies" (Pagelow, 1977). Striking the marital *privilege to rape* will be a signal to some possessive and violent men that their wives are *not* their property; that their wives are full citizens under the law; and that men are responsible before the law for their private actions. Del Martin (1979), in her testimony before lawmakers considering a spousal rape bill said, "In effect existing law legalizes and condones rape in marriage." Society's values are expressed in its laws: "It is no small oversight that four-fifths of this country's states have sexual assault laws which fail to criminalize rape when the man's victim is his wife. A state that fails to act in this regard gives its consent" (Chase, 1982, p. 22). Still, the nationwide organizing and lobbying to get the marital exemption eliminated from rape laws has helped educate and inform the public that "rape is not a husband's marital right; . . . women *are* raped by their husbands; that rape is a violent rather than sexual act; that it is an abhorrent act for which the state will take severe punitive measures" (Chase, 1982, p. 21).

FUTURE DIRECTIONS

The research on marital rape cited here is largely responsible for bringing the issue out of the closet, and forcing an unwilling public to face a form of violence many people would prefer remained hidden. But the American media, always interested in the subjects of sex and violence, brought marital rape out of research labs and academia, and featured it on television, radio, magazines, and newspapers. Few people now can call the idea "goofy."

There are limitations in the current research, conducted when most states did not recognize marital rape as a crime. Other limitations are largely due to the sensitivity of the subject matter: no matter how carefully designed, researchers will encounter high refusal rates; another possible bias could result from the tendency of respondents to answer in socially desirable ways. More and larger studies are needed, not only on victims but also on perpetrators. It will be even more difficult to get wife rapists to talk to researchers than wife beaters, but the difficulty of drawing samples is not an insurmountable problem for dedicated researchers. As battering men interviewed by researchers can be considered the "cream of the crop" of wife beaters (Pagelow, 1984), so too will rapists who seek therapy and consent to interviews. But we can learn much from them that will enable helping educators and other professionals design effective programs.

MILDRED DALEY
PAGELOW

Legislation

Legal changes have come slowly over the past 20 years or so, and they will continue to occur as informed people lobby their legislators. This route has perhaps been the most successful method to date for combatting the problem of wife battering and rape. But as the marital exemption clause has been eliminated from many states' rape laws, some states have extended protection to unmarried men who cohabit with their victims or even some boyfriends under the name of a voluntary-social-companion exemption. Concerned advocates for human and civil rights will strengthen their efforts to organize and change laws that discriminate against victims.

Education

Changes have occurred and will continue as people learn about the problems faced by raped wives. Attorneys will begin to alert divorcing women to the particular danger of marital rape they face at this crisis point in their lives. Therapists and other mental health professionals will learn that "the unspoken and unacknowledged grievance plaguing many wives is that their husband sexually assaults them" (Finkelhor, 1984). Religious counselors will begin to stress the mutuality of marital responsibilities, and speak of a compassionate diety who knows that sex without love and tenderness "kills romance and undermines the marriage" (Adamo, 1984). Physicians will become aware that "it is not a simple matter for some women to avoid sex postoperatively, even though their recovery urgently requires it" (Finkelhor, 1984). Emergency room personnel will become aware that battered wives should receive a sensitive yet thorough physical examination to determine the extent of their injuries, and carefully document the medical evidence. Law enforcement and the courts will begin to take seriously the complaints of abused wives who show signs of the rape trauma syndrome, and act accordingly.

Socialization Changes and Redefinition of Masculinity and Feminity

As employment fields open up and opportunities for advancement increase for females as mandated by law, young women increasingly will begin early to prepare themselves for gainful employment so they will have the protection of economic independence. As the pressure builds for comparable worth, some time in the future men's and women's wages may begin to reach parity, and women will marry and remain with their husbands out of choice, not of necessity.

A new and nonviolent image of masculinity can be promoted by Americans who become sensitized to the prevalence of merging sex and violence in the media and other features of our culture. They will demand a reduction of these distorted images of sexuality by consumer activism, organizing, and boycotting. The debate rages on about whether or not to initiate legislation to control (censor) pornography and both sides raise strong arguments. With research showing an association between violent sexual images and proclivity to rape, and with pornography's prevalence and easy availability, it would be easy to argue for some types of control. But a more critical issue is why it enjoys such popularity in the first place. Because a society's repressive sexual attitudes and pornography are positively correlated, it seems that rather than trying to limit the supply of what many people obviously want, it might be wiser to begin a reeducational program to promote different sexual attitudes.

This could begin by massive educational efforts both for children and adults to take sex out of the closet. If young boys, in particular, were taught that tender, loving sex with willing partners is more masculine than violent, degrading practices of domination and control associated with *machismo,* there might be far fewer men inclined to rape to assert masculinity.

All these measures could help reduce the incidence of marital rape. For those who truly care about the future of the family, one of their first tasks should be to begin reducing marital rape—the great destroyer of family life. And for those who still believe that stranger rape is more serious and traumatic than husband rape, Finkelhor (1984) summed it up this way: ''when you are raped by a stranger you have to live with a frightening memory. When you are raped by your husband you have to live with your rapist'' (p. 4).

SUMMARY

This chapter first attempted to establish the fact that the relatively few researchers who have studied marital rape were looking at a crime of violence that is just as serious and life threatening as rapes committed by men not the victims' husbands. Samples were selected by a variety of techniques, but all researchers took care to screen out any cases that would not fit the legal definition of sexual intimacy by force or threat of force. Their reports make it abundantly clear that their cases of marital rape were not simple bedroom arguments or lovers' quarrels.

Although undoubtedly an underreport, the largest study to date, using a random sample of adult women, found that 14% of ever-married wives had been raped by husbands or former husbands. In another study, 10% of a large sample of women reported that force or threatened force was used. Other studies using samples of battered women found that between 23% and 50% were sexually assaulted by spouses. All studies showed that most raped wives had been repeatedly victimized. Obviously, rape is neither rare nor infrequent in marital relations.

Factors that promote marital rape are historical, legal, economic, and social. The patriarchal family of British common law established the rights of husbands' ownership of their wives and wives' lack of legal protection from rape by husbands. Common law was adopted in the United States, and until recently, husbands in this country were protected from prosecution for wife rape by a marital exemption clause in rape laws. Abused wives frequently endure repeated rapes and lives of pain and terror because of economic dependence on husbands, and data presented showed the reality of entrapment for many. The acceptance of violence in the American culture and the association made between male sexuality and violence has created a distorted image of masculinity for many men. The rape myth featured so often in the media and pornography teaches men that rape is rewarded and not punished.

Next, research findings reveal that most marital rape victims suffer extreme and long-lasting trauma. Helping professionals can learn about the dynamics of marital rape and become sensitized to the possibility that clients presenting certain symptoms are victims. Skilled professionals will be most effective when they deal with the problem rather than the symptoms.

The obvious solution to ethical issues in marital rape has been the object of much effort over the past years: legal reform to criminalize marital rape. The arguments against it have not been supported by the evidence in this country and others.

Looking to future direction requires examining the contributions of research to date, and the need for more and larger studies, not only of raped wives but of their rapist husbands. In the area of reform legislation, there have been some successes and a few losses, but the efforts for progress are certain to continue and eventually prevail. Research to date has provided enough information to educate many persons in positions to help victims of marital rape or wives vulnerable to attack. On the individual level, young women may marry on a stronger economic level and thus be less vulnerable to marital rape and dependency. At the same time, a new model of masculinity may be promoted by a society that refuses to accept images of aggressive and brutal male sexuality, as now portrayed in the media and pornography.

If these things occur, rape will be reduced and marital rape will become merely a historical fact.

REFERENCES

Adamo, Monsignor, S. J. (December 7, 1984). Time for a new definition of wifely obedience. *Philadelphia Daily News.*

Bard, M., & Ellison, K. (1974). Crisis intervention and investigation of forcible rape. In L. Brodyaga, M. Gates, S. Singer, M. Tucker, and R. White (Eds.), *Rape and its victims: A report for citizens, health facilities, and criminal justice agencies* (pp. 165–167). Washington, DC: Department of Justice.

Bart, P. B. (1981). A study of women who both were raped and avoided rape. *Journal of Social Issues, 4,* 123–137.

Bart, P. B., & Jozsa, M. (1980). Dirty books, dirty films, and dirty data. In L. Lederer (Ed.), *Take back the night: Women on pornography* (pp. 204–217). New York: William Morrow.

Black, C. (1979). Children of alcoholics. *Alcohol Health and Research World, 1,* 23–27.

Bowker, L. H. (1983a). Marital rape: A distinct syndrome? *Social Casework: The Journal of Contemporary Social Work,* Vol. 64, *June,* 347–352.

Bowker, L. H. (1983b). *Beating wife-beating.* Lexington, MA: Lexington Books.

Brown, D. (May 19, 1981). Man on trial again on wife rape count. *Los Angeles Times,* p. II-6.

Brownmiller, S. (1976). *Against our will: Men, women and rape.* New York: Bantam.

Calkins, R. (April 5, 1981). Wife in spousal-rape case slain. *Fresno Bee* (pp. B1–B7).

Calvert, R. (1974). Criminal and civil liability in husband-wife assaults. In S. Steinmetz & M. Straus (Eds.), *Violence in the family* (pp. 88–91). New York: Harper & Row.

Carter, N. A. (December, 1982). Distortion of scripture supports domestic violence. *Response,* pp. 34–35, 45.

Chase, S. (1982). Outlawing marital rape: How we did it and why. *Aegis,* Vol. 35, *Summer,* 21–26.

Davidson, T. (November, 1977). Wife beating: It happens in the best of families. *Family Circle,* pp. 62, 68, 70, 72.

Diamond, I. (1980). Pornography and repression: A reconsideration of "who" and "what." In L. Lederer (Ed.), *Take back the night: Women on pornography* (pp. 187–203). New York: William Morrow.

Dobash, R. E., & Dobash, R. P. (1979). *Violence against wives: A case against the patriarchy.* New York: Free Press.

Donovan, J. (January 14, 1985). When a husband rapes his wife. *San Francisco Chronicle* (pp. 1–4).

Doron, J. B. (August, 1980). *Conflict and violence in intimate relations: Focus on marital rape.* Paper presented at the annual meeting of the American Sociological Association, New York.

Egner, D. (July 18, 1980). Killer gets no-parole life term. *San Jose Mercury.*

Eisenberg, S. E., & Micklow, P. L. (1977). The assaulted wife: Catch-22 revisited. *Women's Rights Law Reporter,* Vol. 3, March, 138–161.

Feshbach, S., & Malamuth, N. (November, 1978). Sex and aggression: Proving the link. *Psychology Today, 7,* 111–117, 122.

Finkelhor, D. (May, 1984). *Marital rape: The misunderstood crime.* Address to the New York County Lawyer's Association.

Finkelhor, D., & Yllo, K. (1983). Rape in marriage: A sociological view. In D. Finkelhor, R. J. Gelles, G. T. Hotaling, & M. A. Straus (Eds.), *The dark side of families* (pp. 119–130). Beverly Hills, CA: Sage.

Finkelhor, D., & Yllo, K. (1985). *License to rape.* New York: Holt, Rinehart & Winston.

Fleming, J. B. (1979). *Stopping wife abuse: A guide to the emotional, psychological, and legal implications for the abused woman and those helping her.* Garden City, NY: Anchor Press.

Footlick, J. K. (May 8, 1979). Beating the rape rap. *Newsweek,* p. 41.

Fox, R. (1968). Treating the alcoholic's family. In R. J. Catanzaro (Ed.), *Alcoholism* (pp. 105–115). Springfield, IL: Charles C Thomas.

Freeman, M. D. A. (1981). But if you can't rape your wife who(m) can you rape? The marital rape re-examined. *Family Law Quarterly, 1,* 1–29.

Frieze, I. H., (September, 1980). *Causes and consequences of marital rape.* Paper presented at the annual meeting of the American Psychological Association, Montreal, Canada.

Geis, G. (1978). Rape-and-marriage: Law and law reform in England, the United States, and Sweden. *Adelaide Law Review, 2,* 284–303.

Geis, G. (August, 1980). *Rape and marriage: Historical and cross-cultural considerations.* Paper presented at the annual meeting of the American Sociological Association, New York.

Groth, A. N., with Birnbaum, H. J. (1979). *Men who rape: Psychology of the offender.* New York: Plenum Press.

Hanneke, C. R., & Shields, N. M. (1981). *Patterns of family and non-family violence: An approach to the study of violent husbands.* Paper presented at the National Conference for Family Violence Researchers, Durham, NH.

Hanneke, C. R., Shields, N. M., & McCall, G. J. (November, 1985). *Assessing the prevalence of marital rape.* Paper presented at the annual meeting of the American Criminological Association, San Diego.

Hilberman, E., & Munson, K. (1978). Sixty battered women. *Victimology, ¾,* 460–470.

Kanowitz, L. (1969). *Women and the law: The unfinished revolution.* Albuquerque, NM: University of New Mexico Press.

Kurman, W. (1980). *Marital rape: A comparative study—Great Britain and California.* Unpublished paper.

Landau, S. F. (September, 1976). *The rape offender's perception of his victim: Some cross-cultural findings.* Paper presented at the Second International Symposium on Victimology, Boston, MA.

LeGrand, C. (1973). Rape and rape laws: Sexism in society and law. *California Law Revew, 61,* 919.

Malamuth, N. M. (1981). Rape proclivity among males. *Journal of Social Issues, 4,* 138–157.

Martin, D. (1976). *Battered wives.* San Francisco: Glide.

Martin, D. (1979). Presentation before the State of California Assembly Criminal Justice Committee Hearing on AB-546, April 23.

May, M. (1978). Violence in the family: An historical perspective. In J. P. Martin (Ed.), *Violence and the family* (pp. 135–168). New York: Wiley.

MacFarlane, K., L. L. Jenstrom, & B. M. Jones (1980). Conclusion: Aspects of prevention and protection. In B. M. Jones, L. L. Jenstrom, & K. MacFarlane, (Eds.), *Sexual abuse of children: Selected readings,* (pp. 123–126). U. S. Department of Health and Human Services, Office of Human Development Services. Washington, DC: U. S. Government Printing Office.

Mettger, Z. (1982). A case of rape: Forced sex in marriage. *Response, 2,* 1–2, 13–16.

Mitra, C. (1979). . . . for she has no right or power to refuse her consent. *Criminal Law Review,* September, 558–565.

Ms. Magazine (1982). When a wife says no. . . . Beyond the Rideout case. April 23.

O'Donnell, W. J. (1980). *Consensual marital sodomy and marital rape—The role of the law and the role of the victim.* Paper presented at the annual meeting of the Academy of Criminal Justice Sciences.

Pagelow, M. D. (September, 1977). *Blaming the victim: Parallels in crimes against women—rape and battering.* Paper presented at the annual meeting of the Society for the Study of Social Problems, Chicago, IL.

Pagelow, M. D. (June, 1980). *Does the law protect the rights of battered women? Some research notes.* Paper presented at the annual meeting of the Law and Society Association and the ISA Research Committee on the Sociology of Law, Madison, WI.

Pagelow, M. D. (1981). *Woman-Battering: Victims and their experiences.* Beverly Hills, CA: Sage.

Pagelow, M. D. (1982). Children in violent families: Direct and indirect victims. In S. Hill & B. J. Barnes (Eds.), *Young children and their families* (pp. 47–72). Lexington, MA: D. C. Heath.

Pagelow, M. D. (1984). *Family/violence.* New York: Praeger.

Queen's Bench Foundation. (1976). *Rape: Prevention and resistance.* San Francisco: Queen's Bench Foundation.

Rawlings, S. W. (1980). Families maintained by female householders, 1970–79. *Current Population Reports, Special Studies,* Series P-23, No. 107. Department of Commerce, Bureau of the Census. Washington, DC: U. S. Government Printing Office.

Response (November, 1979). Husband convicted of raping wife. Vol. 3(3), p. 4.

Russell, D. E. H. (1975). *The politics of rape: The victim's perspective.* Briarcliff Manor, NY: Stein & Day.

Russell, D. E. H. (1980a). *The prevalence and impact of marital rape in San Francisco*. Paper presented at the annual meeting of the American Sociological Association, New York.

Russell, D. E. H. (1980b). Pornography and violence: What does the new research say? In L. Lederer (Ed.), *Take back the night: Women on Pornography* (pp. 218–238). New York: William Morrow.

Russell, D. E. H. (1982). *Rape in marriage*. New York: Macmillan.

Russell, D. E. H. (1984). *Sexual exploitation: Rape, child sexual abuse, and workplace harassment*. Beverly Hills, CA: Sage.

Sachs, A., & Wilson, J. H. (1978). *Sexism and the Law: Male beliefs and legal bias*. New York: Free Press.

Schulder, D. B. (1970). Does the law oppress women? In R. Morgan (Ed.), *Sisterhood is powerful* (pp. 153–175). New York: Vintage.

Schulman, J. (1980). The marital rape exemption in the criminal law. *Clearinghouse Review,* p. 136.

Shields, N. M., & Hanneke, C. R. (1983). Battered wives' reactions to marital rape. Rape in marriage: A sociological view. In D. Finkelhor, R. J. Gelles, G. T. Hotaling, & M. A. Straus (Eds.), *The dark side of families* (pp. 119–130). Beverly Hills, CA: Sage.

Siller, S. (1982, April). ''Wife rape''—who really gets screwed. *Penthouse,* pp. 104–105.

Smart, C. (1977). *Women, crime and criminology: A feminist critique*. London: Routledge & Kegan Paul.

Stannard, U. (1977). *Mrs. Man*. San Francisco: Germain.

Stoller, R. (1975). *Perversion: The erotic form of hatred*. New York: Pantheon.

Time Magazine (1979). Wife rape: The first conviction. October 8, p. 80.

U. S. Bureau of the Census, (1980). Current Population Reports, Series P-60, No. 125. *Characteristics of the population below the poverty level: 1979*. Department of Commerce. Washington, D.C.: Government Printing Office.

U. S. Bureau of the Census, (1981). Current Population Reports, Series P-23, No. 112. *Child support and alimony: 1978*. Department of Commerce. Washington, DC: U. S. Government Printing Office.

U. S. Bureau of the Census, (1983a). Current Population Reports, Series P-60, No. 137. *Consumer income*. Department of Commerce. Washington, DC: U. S. Government Printing Office.

U. S. Bureau of the Census, (1983b). Current Population Reports, Series P-60, No. 138. *Characteristics of the population below the poverty level: 1981*. Department of Commerce. Washington, DC: U. S. Government Printing Office.

Walker, L. E. (1979). *The battered woman*. New York: Harper Colophon.

Weitzman, L. (1981). *The marriage contract: Spouses, lovers, and the law*. New York: Free Press.

Weitzman, L. (1985). *The divorce revolution*. New York: Free Press.

Weingourt, R. (1985). Wife rape: Barriers to identification and treatment. *American Journal of Psychotherapy, 2,* 187–192.

10

Husband Battering

SUZANNE K. STEINMETZ and JOSEPH S. LUCCA

INTRODUCTION

My wife started out hitting me and when I restrained her she started kicking and that's when
she did the damage . . . what I remember was her kicking the bottom of my foot, kicking my
legs, it did hurt . . . I have always felt more powerful than her and knowing that if I started
hitting her I could hurt her, I made a conscious effort . . . to rule out physical violence.
(Brown, 1982)

Research on victimization resulting from discrimination has focused on racial minorities
(e.g., Blacks, Hispanics, and Indians, and on women). Thus, it is not surprising that
research on spouse violence has tended to focus almost exclusively on wife abuse.
Although studies of infanticide (Radbill, 1974) and homicide (Wolfgang, 1958) clearly
indicate that women have the potential to be violent, their use of physical violence on their
husbands has carefully been avoided.

Unfortunately, to ignore the phenomena of the battered husband not only denies the
existence of this type of violence, but assumes that the consequences in terms of the
physical injury to the victim and the psychological damage to both the victim and the
children that witness these attacks are inconsequential. Considerable data on the power of
social modeling and social learning suggest that this behavior will have profound effects
on the children.

With more women employed in the labor force, often with two jobs, the stress
resulting from these multiple roles heightens the likelihood of abuse occurring. It is
critical that we understand all forms of family violence if we hope to remove the cloak of
secrecy and break the cycle of violence. Some historical and current issues may provide
insights to help understand why this dearth of information on the battered husband exists.

Historical Overview

Historically, men have been given the right to control women and children, through
abusive means if necessary. Women and children were often seen as chattel along with

SUZANNE K. STEINMETZ and JOSEPH S. LUCCA • Department of Individual and Family Studies,
Life and Health Sciences, University of Delaware, Newark, DE 19716.

farm animals and property. However, if a women were to use physical force against her husband, society would perceive this to be a threat to the established social order.

The post-Renaissance charivari, a noisy demonstration intended to shame and humiliate wayward individuals in public, targeted persons whose behavior was considered to be a threat to the patriarchal community social order. Thus, a husband who allowed his wife to beat him in 18th-century France was made to wear an outlandish outfit and ride backwards around the village on a donkey.

The fate of these men in Paris was to kiss a large set of ribboned horns (Shorter, 1975). Beaten husbands among the Britons were strapped to carts and ''paraded ignominiously through the booing populace.'' The assaultive wife was also punished by being forced to ride backwards on a donkey, drink wine, and wipe her mouth with the animals tail.

In Colonial America, communities tended to punish the wife that was abusive toward her husband, rather than ridicule and humiliating him. Perhaps this reflected the precarious circumstances of the colonies and requirement to have all couples live peacefully. For example, Joan Miller was charged by the elder because of ''Beating and reviling her husband and egging her children on to help her, bidding them to knock him in the head and wishing his victuals might choke him'' (Demos, 1970, p. 73).

The Battered Husband as a Humorous Topic

The subject matter of comic strips, specifically those revolving around a domestic theme, is also revealing. The caricature of husbands is one in which he is shown to deviate from the strong, self-assertive, intelligent, ideal image and assumes the character traits culturally defined as feminine. The wife in these comics is justified in playing the dominant role and in chastising her erring husband, because he has not fulfilled his culturally prescribed roles.

Barcus (1963), in a survey of every comic strip appearing in March for the years 1943, 1953, 1958 in the bound files of Puck: The Comic Weekly and three Boston newspapers, a sample representing most of the major nationally syndicated Sunday papers, found that domestic relations was a theme in 41% of the comics examined. These domestic relations are presented as caricatures reflecting a stereotype of husbands as fatter, bald, less virile, and of wives as taller and bigger than their husbands.

This is most poignantly exhibited in the domestic comic strip ''Bringing up Father.'' Making its debut in 1913, this comic strip revolves around a newly rich Irish immigrant (Jiggs) who prefers his former life-style of corn beef, cabbage, and billiards, and who endures the physically violent attacks by his wife (Maggie), who is unsuccessfully attempting to emulate upper-class life-styles.

Saenger's (1963) study of 20 consecutive editions of all comic strips appearing in the nine leading New York City newspapers during October, 1950, provides additional insights. He found that females were more likely than males to be shown as having a greater mastery over their environment (48% vs. 10%) and that 19% of the males but only 4% of the females were pictured as helpless. He also noted that whereas husbands were the victims of hostility and attack in 63% of all conflicts, wives were victims in only 39% (see Table 1).

Furthermore, males were more likely to initiate physically aggressive acts then were females (10% vs. 7%). However, only 1% of the females, but 14% of the males were recipients of domestic physical aggression. Additional analysis revealed that in 73% of the comic strips the wives were more aggressive; in 10% husband and wife were equal; and in only 17% of the strips were the husbands portrayed as being more aggressive than their wives.

The popularity of these domestic relations comics was most likely sustained because they approximate, in comic, nonserious manner, common family situations, allowing men and women to carry out in fantasy actions that they have not been able to carry out in reality (Steinmetz, 1977–78). The wife in the comics, although justified in playing the dominant, chastising, physical violent role, because her husband did not fulfill his culturally prescribed roles, is simultaneously described in undesirable, nonfeminine terms.

The impact of comics is impressive. In one study covering a 12-year period, over 56% of both male and female readers ranked the category *comic strips* as ''most frequently'' read (Swanson, as cited in Robinson & White, 1963). The second ranking category, *war,* was listed by 35% of the respondents. Because a large portion of this 12-year survey occurred during World War II, it is surprising that the category *war* was a poor second to the comics. The portrayal of family life in comics therefore not only reflects life-styles but also is in a position to influence or reinforce family-related behavior.

It is true that comics tend to be based on a distortion of reality. However, the consistent appearance of battered husbands in early court and community records both in Europe and the United States, the persistence of battered husbands as dominant theme in comics, and the stability of the finding that husbands equal wives as victims of marital homicide—the most severe form of violence—reinforce our belief that husband battering is not a new phenomenon.

Although it is not possible to ascertain the effect that comics have on contemporary domestic relations, continued representation of these models in the media desensitizes us to negative effects of this form of interaction, making it more acceptable. A contemporary example of this phenomenon is provided by Gelles' (1974) interview of a wife who explained how she retaliated against a drunken husband who slapped her for no apparent reason:

> I know I was stronger than he was, drunk that is, so I gave him a good shove and kick—whatever I could kick—I didn't aim. And then he'd end up on the floor and I'd beat the daylights out of him. (pp. 78–79)

Female versus Male Violence

An examination of street crime suggests that although rates for female perpetrators of criminal violence are increasing dramatically, they are still considerably lower than comparable crimes for men. As the data in Table 2 indicate, men are more likely than women

Table 1. Marital Violence in Comics

	Perpetrator of aggression	Victims of attack	Initiate violence	Recipients of violence
Husbands	10	63	10	14
Wives	73	39	7	1

Note. Data adapted from Saenger (1963).

to be perpetrators or victims of a wide range of violent activities (U. S. Bureau of Census, 1977, 1978; U.S. Department of Justice, 1978).

With one notable exception, rape, in which women constitute over 99% of the victims, men are more likely to be victims of street crime. Men constitute about 80% of the homicide victims; nearly 70% of the robbery victims and about 70% of the victims of aggravated assault (U. S. Bureau of Census, 1979).

There has been considerable speculation about the causes and implications of the dramatic increase in crime rates among women. However, the greatest increase in female criminal activity parallels the increasing number of women who hold positions of trust in the business world.

One explanation for these trends is expansion of the opportunity structure (Simon, 1976). If women are not part of the mafia, there will be no women involved in "contract" activities. Furthermore, if women do not hold high administrative positions with considerable power, then women are not able to participate in white-collar crime. As women gain access to areas traditionally reserved for men, we may expect a wider range of criminal behavior to be exhibited.

Although the documentation on husband beating is not as extensive as that on wife beating, we do know that over 3% of 600 husbands in mandatory conciliation interviews listed physical abuse by their wives as a reason for the divorce action (Levinger, 1966). Although this is far lower than the nearly 37% of wives who mentioned physical abuse, it is consistent with some other data that suggest that there is about a 1:12 or 1:13 ratio of abused husbands to abused wives (see Table 3).

Based on police records and a random sample of New Castle County, Delaware families during 1975, it was estimated that 7% of the wives and just over one half percent (.6) of husbands would be victims of severe physical abuse by their spouse (Steinmetz, 1977a). Statewide data collected between January 1, 30, 1981, revealed that there were 423 reported incidents of wife abuse and 33 reported incidents of husband abuse. Thus, whereas the actual number of reported abuse grew considerably, possibly due to increased

Table 2. Victims and Offenders of Street Crime[a]

	Victims of violent crimes[b] (rates/100,000)		Offenders of violent crimes[c] (rates/100,000)	
	Males	Females	Males	Females
Murder[d]	9.3	2.5	7.8	1.2
Forcible rape	3.9	84.6	14.9	0.5
Robbery	438.0	252.0	64.7	4.9
Aggravated assault	1614.8	897.1	112.7	17.6

[a] Data for offenders is for 1983 for victims in 1981. Data is converted to rates/100,000 for comparability.

[b] Data from U.S. Department of Justice, Washington, D.C., Federal Bureau of Investigation, *Crime in the United States, 1983*, (pp. 182–183). Tables 32 and 33.

[c] Data from U.S. Department of Justice, *Source Book of Criminal Justice Statistics* (pp. 341–342. Table 3.21.)

[d] Data from U.S. Department of Commerce, Bureau of the Census, *Statistical Abstract of the United States*, 1985 (p. 170). Table 284.

services and wide advertising of their existence, the ratio of 12 or 13 abused women to 1 abused man remained constant in police records.

It should be noted, however, that this ratio was based on police statistics and reflects only those abusive situations that were reported by the victim, or were sufficiently visible to others (e.g., neighbors) that the police were called. Data gathered from sources that are more representative of the general population suggest that for less violent forms of spouse abuse husbands and wives are nearly equal in most respects (see Table 4).

The data from a nationally representative study of family violence (Straus, Gelles, & Steinmetz, 1980), reported that although the total violence scores for spouse abuse were very similar, wives tended to be slightly higher in almost all categories except pushing and shoving. Steinmetz (1977–78) reported similar findings for several other studies (see Table 4).

Only one study, Gelles (1974), found husbands exceeding wives in the use of all types of violence except "hitting with something," a mode which deemphasized physical strength. In this study, 47% of husbands had used physical violence on their wives, whereas only 33% of the wives had used violence on their husbands.

The differences may have resulted from the samples. Half of the respondents in Gelles' study were selected from the police blotter because of reported domestic violence or were identified by the social service agency. Wives are more likely to seek agency-related help or call the police.

Although the previously cited data represent the percentages of husbands and wives who have used physical violence against a spouse, they do not tell us the frequency with which these acts occur. The data indicate that not only do the percentages of wives that have used physical violence often exceed that of the husbands, but wives' average violence score tended to be higher (Steinmetz, 1977–78). For example, data from the

Table 3. Comparisons of Husband and Wife Abuse over Time

Study	Date	Husband abuse	Wife abuse	Ratio
Levinger: Divorce petitions	1966	19	222	1:11.7
Police statistics: New Castle County 1-year period	1975	2	24	1:12.0
Police statistics: New Castle County 6-month period	1981	18	262	1:14.5
Straus et al.: National survey* severe violence	1975	4.6	3.8	0.83:1**
Straus & Gelles: National survey* severe violence	1985	4.4	3.0	0.68:1**

*Numbers are reported as rate per 100 couples.

**It is unlikely that severly battered women who were still living with the batterer participated in these studies because of the high risk that being caught talking with an outsider represented. The ratios for the national survey data indicate higher rates for wife-to-husband violence than for husband-to-wife violence. Furthermore, the differential between the two increased over a period of 10 years.

national study revealed that wives committed an average of 10.3 acts of violence against their husbands during 1975, whereas their husbands averaged only 8.8 acts against their wives.

Only Gelles (1974) found husbands to exceed their wives in use of physically violent modes. He found that 11% of the husbands and 5% of the wives engaged in marital violence between two and six times a year, and 14% of the husbands and 6% of the wives used violence between once a month and daily. Wives exceed husbands in one category, however: 11% of the husbands but 14% of the wives noted that they "seldom" (defined as between two and five times during the marriage) used physical violence against their spouse.

Oswald (1980) examined the histories of patients at the Royal Infirmary of Edinburgh because of parasuicide. During 1977 and 1978, 592 admissions of women who were married (or living with a man) and between 20 and 40 years of age, answered 30 items that contained questions on victim and perpetrator of violence. They found 299 reported domestic violence; and 263 were victims of violence. Of this number 124 (46%) reported that they themselves were excessively violent and 36 (12%) had been perpetrators of violence but were not the victim of violence.

IGNORING THE BATTERED HUSBAND PHENOMENON

Abuse of men, as a topic of investigation, has received very little attention. There are two possible reasons for this. Men will go to great lengths to avoid reporting that they are abused, because such an admission would stigmatize them in the eyes of others. As a result, men tend to report only the most extreme abuse, and would not dream of reporting lesser abuse—such as slapping or kicking—which women routinely report. In other words, a greater percentage of women are likely to report less severe injuries, and as a result, the highly visible evidence would suggest that women are abused more often than men, whereas this actually is not the case. A second factor is that men often have greater resources (money, credit, status, power) that allows them to utilize private sources of help and avoid reporting their victimization.

Table 4. Women as Victims and Perpetrators of Spousal Violence

Study	N	Throw things		Push shove		Hit slap		Hit with object		Threaten with knife/gun		Use knife or gun		Use of any violence		Mean freq.	
		H	W	H	W	H	W	H	W	H	W	H	W	H	W	H	W
Gelles (1974)	80	22	11	18	1	32	20	3	5	5	0	—	—	47	33	—	—
Steinmetz (1977a)	54	39	37	31	32	20	20	10	10	—	—	2	0	47	43	3.5	4.0
Steinmetz (1977b)	52	21	21	17	13	13	13	10	12	—	—	—	—	23	21	6.0	7.8
Steinmetz (1977c)	94	31	25	22	18	17	12	12	14	—	—	—	—	32	28	6.6	7.0

Note. Table numbers are percentages (%).

There also are a relative lack of empirical data on the topic. The selective inattention by the media and researchers, the greater severity of physical damage to women, which makes their victimization more visible, and the reluctance of men to acknowledge abuse at the hand of women, makes it more apparent why the battered husband has received so little attention.

The discussion of the husband-abuse data cited earlier suggests that husband beating constitutes a sizable proportion of marital violence. As discussed earlier 3% of the husbands in Levinger's study considered their wife's physically abusive treatment of them to be grounds for divorce. This percentage might have been larger had the following factors not been present.

First, Levinger's study, conducted before no-fault divorce, showed that women had nearly twice the number of total complaints as men. Therefore, unless one assumes that it is always the husband's fault when a marriage fails, it appears that women might be more comfortable voicing their complaints.

A second factor to be examined is the time frame during which Levinger's study was conducted. At that time, considerable fault had to be established in order for a divorce to be granted. The traditional role of a husband in a divorce action at that time was to take the blame for the failure. Thus, even if the husband desired the divorce, etiquette demanded that he allow his wife to initiate the action. During a conciliatory interview it is reasonable, then, to expect the husband to be less ready to expose his wife's faults. Some support is provided for this position by examining the types of complaints commonly made by husbands (i.e., sexual incompatibility, and in-laws, both traditionally accepted male-oriented complaints).

Finally, the male in our society is under pressure to maintain a dominant position over a female (Balswick & Peek, 1971; Steinmetz, 1974). The psychological stress of recognizing the wife's physical dominance makes it unlikely that many men would be willing to admit their physical weakness to a third party.

The stigma attached to this topic, which is embarrassing for beaten wives, is doubly so for beaten husbands. The patriarchal concept of the husbands's right to chastise his wife with a whip or rattan no bigger than his thumb is embedded in ancient law and was upheld by a Mississippi court in 1824, "in case of great emergency and with salutary restraints" (*Bradley v. State*, Walker, 158, Miss., 182-184). This idea has provided some legal and social understanding for the woman who has suffered because her husband has gone beyond permissible bounds. Because there is no recognition of the woman's right to chastise her husband, there is little likelihood that society will recognize that the wife may go beyond that which is permissible.

As one respondent who had been terrorized by a knife-wielding spouse and has gone to work with deep fingernail gashes on his face related: "I never took the fights outside, I didn't want anyone to know. I told the guys at work that the kids did it with a toy."

This fear of stigma also affects the official statistics collected on husband–wife violence. Curtis (1974) reported that whereas violence by men against women was responsible for about 27% of the assaults and 17.5% of the homicides, violence by women against men accounted for 9% of the assaults and 16.4% of the homicides in his study. Thus, although women commit only about one third as many assaults against men as men commit against women, the number of cross-sex homicides committed by the two groups are nearly identical.

Wilt and Bannon (1976) warned that caution should be applied when interpreting the Curtis finding. They note that

nonfatal violence committed by women against men is less likely to be reported to the police than
is violence by men against women; thus, women assaulters who come to the attention of the
police are likely to be those who have produced a fatal result. (p. 20)

Also helping to camouflage the existence of husband beating is the terminology used
to describe it. This can be illustrated by referring to Gelles' monograph *The Violent Home*
(1974). An examination of the entries in the subject index shows that, although there is
one page each devoted to "wife-to-husband" and "husband-to-wife" violence, seven
pages under the heading "wife beating," two under "battered wife," yet no corresponding listing can be found for "husband beating." However, Gelles's data provide ample
evidence that many wives do in fact beat their husbands. In addition to the data from
Gelles's study summarized in Table 1, many quotas from his respondents support this. For
example, one respondent noted, "He would just yell and yell—not really yell, just talk
loudly, and I couldn't say anything because he kept talking, so I'd swing" (Gelles, 1974,
p. 80).

Even though Gelles reports that one respondent, a retired cook, was often verbally
and physically attacked by his jealous wife, and quotes another as saying, "My wife is
very violent. It's a miracle that I didn't go out because she really put a hell of a dent in my
head," these are not labeled as husband beatings. Thus, although Gelles readily acknowledges that men are physically victimized by their wives, he does not provide a discussion
of this phenomenon as a distinct parallel to wife beating. Because Gelles's study was the
first study ever systematically to examine spouse abuse, and the term *wife-abuse* was
fairly new, it is easy to understand his choice of terms. What is even more puzzling,
however, is the denial of this phenomenon in Walker's (1984) book on wife battering.

This cyclical aspect of family violence is demonstrated by her study of over 400
battered women. She reported that 67% of the women were battered as children (41% by
their mothers, 44% by their fathers); about 20% had brothers and sisters who were also
battered; 44% of their fathers battered their mothers; and 29% of their mothers battered
their fathers. Furthermore, 28% of these battered women reported that they battered their
own children and 5% attributed this behavior to being angry at their husband.

She further reported that 15% of these battered women used violence against their
spouse (either in retaliation or self-defense) when in a battering relationship, and five %
continued this violent behavior after they left the first relationship and had entered into a
nonbattering relationship. Her conclusion that these data "refute the 'mutual combat' or
'battered man' problem as being a large one" (1984, p. 150) is indeed puzzling.

Even if one were willing to assume that 5% of the these new relationships characterized by husband battering were relatively inconsequential, the nondirect, next-genera-
tion effects noted by Walker (the 41% of children battered by their mothers, the 29% of
mothers who battered the father, the 5% of women who batter the child because they are
angry at the husband) surely must be considered significant. Given the data from nationally representative samples, these women may differ only in the degree of violence
experienced and perpetrated from non-shelter-based samples.

These findings are especially disturbing in light of three factors, which popular
culture has suggested should mitigate against women using violence against their husbands. First, as a result of their socialization, women are taught better impulse control—
they stop aggressive behavior before any danger occurs. Second, women are more verbal
than men, and therefore men resort more readily to physical means to support their
dominant position. A third explanation focuses on the superior physical strength of men

and their greater capability of causing more physical damage to their spouses than wives are capable of doing to their husbands.

In reality, the contention that women are socialized for greater impulse controls appears to have little support, at least as far as marital fights are concerted. The data provided in Table 4, plus insights gained from the in-depth interviews, suggest that women are as likely to select physical violence to resolve marital conflicts as are men.

Furthermore, child abusers are more likely to be women. Throughout history women have been the prime perpetrators of infanticide (Straus, Gelles, & Steinmetz, 1973). Although it is recognized that women spend more time with children and are usually the parent in a single-parent home (which makes them prone to stress and strains resulting in child abuse) and that fathers in similar situations might abuse their children more severely, these findings do indicate that women have the potential to commit acts of violence and that under certain circumstances they do carry out these acts.

Wolfgang (1958), in an investigation of homicides occurring between 1948 and 1952, found that spouses accounted for 18% of the incidents and that there were virtually no differences between the percentage of husbands or wives who were offenders. According to FBI statistics, 15% of the homicides in 1975 were between husband and wife. In 7.8% of the cases the husbands were victims, whereas in 8% of the cases the victims were wives (U.S. Bureau of the Census, *Vital Statistics Reports,* 1976). In 1984 there were about 1700 spousal homicides 43% of the victims were husbands (*Uniform Crime Reports,* 1984).

The second point is also questionable. Although the myth of the verbally abusing, nagging woman is perpetuated in the media, mainly in comic form, the data do not support this myth. There appeared to be small random differences in the use of verbal violence in the families studied. Furthermore, Levinger (1966), in his study of divorce applicants, found that wives were three times more likely to complain of verbal abuse than their husbands.

It appears that the last reason is more plausible. The data reported suggest that at least the intention of men and women to use physical violence in marital conflicts is equal. Identical percentages of men and women reported hitting or hitting with an object. Furthermore, data on homicide between spouses suggest that an almost equal number of wives kill their husbands as husbands kill their wives (Wolfgang, 1958). Thus it appears that men and women might have equal potential for violent marital interaction; initiate similar acts of violence; and when differences of physical strength are equalized by weapons, commit similar amounts of spousal homicide.

The major difference appears to be the males ability to do more physical damage during nonhomicidal marital physical fights. When the wife slaps her husband, her lack of physical strength plus his ability to restrain her reduce the physical damage to a minimum. When the husband slaps his wife, however, his strength plus her inability to restrain him result in considerably more damage.

An apt illustration is provided by a newspaper article describing the beating a physically weaker husband had received from this wife. This article noted that a wealthy, elderly New York banker had won a separation from his second wife who was 31 years his junior. During the 14-year marriage the husband had been bullied, according to the judge, by hysteria, screaming tantrums, and . . . various physical violence practiced on the man . . . ill-equipped for fist fights with a shrieking woman.'' The judge noted that the husband wore constant scars and bruises. Once his wife shredded his ear with her teeth;

another time she blackened his eyes; and on another occasion injured one of his eyes so badly that doctors feared it might be lost (Wilmington Evening Journal, April, 21, 1976, p. 2).

Why Do Husbands Stay?

In answer to the question,'' Why would a woman who has been physically abused by her husband remain with him?'' Gelles (1974, p. 650) suggested that there are three major factors influencing wives' decision to leave. The less severe and the less frequent the violence, the more the wife experienced violence as a child, and the fewer the resources and power the wife has, the more likely she is to stay with their husband.

These three factors were also found to influence the husbands' decision to stay. Lower levels of violence were not likely to be considered a major concern. Only when the violence appeared to be affecting the children, rather than affecting the husband's physical safety, did the husband consider leaving. The background of violent wives is often characterized by violence and trauma. One violent wife, as a child, witnessed her own father force her mother, who was in the last stages of pregnancy, to walk home in a the snow carrying bags of groceries. The father drove behind his wife in a car bumping her with the car to keep her moving and beating her when she stopped or stumbled. Another wife felt responsible for her father's suicide, which occurred when she was 10. Still another wife as a teenager slept with weapons under her pillows and lived in constant fear of brutal beatings from her alcoholic father (Steinmetz, 1977–78).

The perceived availability of resources also affects the man's decision to leave. According to most studies (as well as popular knowledge), women remain because they feel that the children will be worse off if they leave. Not only does the wife often lack the economic resources to provide adequately for the children, but she feels that separation will have a more harmful effect on the children than would remaining with her abusive husband. It is always assumed that the husband's greater economic resources could allow him to leave more easily a disruptive marital situation. Not only do men tend to have jobs that provide them with an adequate income, but they have greater access to credit and are not tied to the home because of the children. This perspective rests on erroneous sexist assumptions.

Although males, as a group, have considerably more economic security, if the husband leaves the family, he is still responsible for a certain amount of economic support of the family in addition to the cost of a separate residence for himself. Thus, the loss in standard of living is certainly a consideration for any husband who is considering a separation. Furthermore, it is assumed that because wives are "tied to their homes,'' they would be the ones who would most likely regret it if they moved. Until recently, custody was almost always awarded to mothers, thus the mother remained in the family home while father sought a new residence. Interviews with abused men suggest that leaving the family means leaving many hours of home improvements, family rooms, dens, workshops, in other words the comfortable and familiar, that which is not likely to be reconstructed in a small apartment.

Probably the most erroneous assumption, however, is that the husband's decisions to leave would not be influenced by concern over the children. Often the husband becomes the victim when he steps in to protect the children and becomes the target of abuse. These men are afraid to leave for fear that further violence would be directed toward the children. Recognizing that men are not likely to receive custody of the children, even in a era of increased recognition of their ability to care for them, men feel that by staying they are providing some protection for their children. These men also express the idea that keeping the family together at all costs is best for the children. Another man, who lived in terror for 2 years and did not know when his wife would attack him with knives and other objects, an almost daily occurrence, remained because as an orphan, he knew what it was like to be without a father. Also, he considered his wife to be attractive, personable, a good housekeeper and mother and, except for her violent attacks, a good wife. The wife, however, was insecure, dissatisfied with herself, had low self-esteem, and was uncomfortable with her low position as a secretary, and with a paycheck that was smaller than her husband's. She wanted a career and to be the economically dominant partner (Steinmetz, 1977–78).

Why, then do these husbands not protect themselves? Several reasons evolve. The first, based on chivalry, considers any man who would stoop to hit a woman to be a bully. The second, usually based on experience, is a recognition of the severe damage that a man could do to a woman. In fact, several men expressed the fear that if they ever lost control, they could easily kill their wives. One husband noted that he hit his wife only once, "in retaliation with hands and fist, and smacked her in the mouth. She went flying across the room." Because he realized how badly he could hurt his wife, he continued to take the physical abuse. He noted, with hindsight, that probably she continued her abuse because she knew she should get away with it.

A final reason expressed by the beaten men is perhaps a self-serving one. The combination of crying out in pain during the beating and having the wife see the injuries, which often take several weeks to heal, raises the wife's level of guilt, which the husbands consider to be a form of punishment (Steinmetz, 1977–78).

A Cross-Cultural Examination of Husband Abuse

Aggressive family interaction in the United States appears to be quite different from that found in a country such as Sweden where physical punishment is prohibited, and child abuse seems to be relatively uncommon (Zeigert, 1983). If there are social/cultural factors that influence levels of aggression, then it would appear that one could reduce aggression by changing these factors. For example, a change in ideology could effect such a change. In preliberation China, physical abuse between husband and wife, mother-in-law and daughter, parents and child, and the landlord and peasant was common. Oppression of the weak and less powerful had a long tradition in Chinese culture, and this oppression fostered physical abuse. However, the equalitarian ideology of the People's Republic of China does not support the use of physical force to resolve interpersonal conflict; as a result, physical punishment is rare and child abuse and wife beating are unheard of (Sidel, 1972).

However, things have recently changed in China with the end of Mao's reign. Individuals are allowed more independent decision-making opportunities, and reports of acts of aggression are surfacing. Under the current one-child policy incidents of wife abuse and child abuse, specifically infanticide or wife killings when the single child is a female, have also become a problem (Beck, Rohter, & Friday, 1984).

Although caution must be taken in the linking of societal levels of aggression to interpersonal and familial levels of aggression, there is both theoretical and empirical support for this relationship. Studies based on the data in the Human Relations Areas files found that the incidence of wife beating in 71 primitive societies was positively correlated with invidious displays of wealth, pursuit of military glory, bellicosity, institutionalized boasting, exhibitionistic dancing, and sensitivity to insults (Slater & Slater, 1965). These descriptions sound curiously similar to the macho male's attempts to dominate that are often linked to wife abuse in the United States.

Lester (1980), also studying primitive cultures, found that wife beating was more common in societies characterized by high divorce rates and societies in which women were rated as inferior. Societies that experienced not only high rates of drunkenness, but also high rates of alcohol-related aggression, also had higher rates of wife beating.

In another study, data on marital violence from six societies, the United States, Canada, Finland, Israel—with city and Kibbutz subsamples)—Puerto Rico, and Belize (British Honduras)—with subsamples of Spanish-speaking Creoles and Caribs—were compared (Steinmetz, 1981). Although analysis of these data must be considered preliminary, it appears that the percentage of husbands and wives who use violence apparently did not predict the severity and frequency of the violent acts (see Table 5). Finland, in which over 60% of husbands and wives were reported to have used violence, had the lowest mean frequency scores of actual violent acts. On the other hand, the Kibbutz sample from the Israeli data had the fewest number of husbands and wives using violence, but those who did use violence were extremely violent. In each society, the percentage of husbands who used violence was similar to the percentage of violent wives. The major exception was Puerto Rico, in which twice as many husbands used physical violence to resolve marital conflicts as did the wives.

Wives who used violence, however, tended to use greater amounts. For example, although twice as many husbands in Puerto Rico used violence than did the wives, the frequency scores of wives were greater ($X = 5.8$ versus 6.60). In the Kibbutz sample, almost equal percentages of husbands and wives used each type of violence. However, those wives who resorted to violence used considerably more than did the husbands ($X = 12.56$ versus 9.91).

Table 5. Cross-Cultural Comparisons of Marital Violence

Country		Throwing things %		Pushing shoving %		Hitting slapping %		Hit with something %		Use of any violence %		Mean frequency %	
		H	W	H	W	H	W	H	W	H	W	H	W
Finland	44	20	23	18	14	16	14	9	9	61	64	2.19	2.18
Puerto Rico	82	28	16	22	11	25	11	22	11	49	25	5.78	6.60
British Honduras	231*	24	21	25	23	23	22	19	18	39	38	6.83	6.38
Spanish speaking	103	23	22	27	26	25	20	20	19	40	39	5.85	5.73
Creole	79	24	21	19	17	22	18	15	15	34	29	7.78	7.17
Carib	37	31	30	30	27	24	27	22	19	51	54	7.37	6.20
U.S.A.	94	31	25	22	18	17	12	12	14	32	28	6.60	7.00
Canada	52	21	21	17	13	13	13	10	12	23	21	6.00	7.80
Israel	127	14	14	13	12	15	14	13	13	22	20	8.42	8.65
Kibbutz	63	16	14	16	14	17	16	14	14	21	16	9.91	12.56
City	64	13	13	11	9	13	13	13	11	22	20	7.59	7.38

Note. From "A Cross-Cultural Comparison of Marital Abuse" by S.K. Steinmetz, 1981, *Journal of Sociology and Social Welfare, 8* (2), p. 411. Reprinted by permission.
*Contains 12 additional cases that were mixed families.

The data suggest other interesting questions. Whiting and Child (1953) found less wife beating in societies that lived in extended family forms; thus, the levels of violence in the Kibbutz sample as compared with nuclear family (city) sample were surprising. However, Demos (1970) noted that to survive the cramped living quarters, early colonists went to great length to avoid family conflict. It appears that they vented their hostilities on neighbors, and conflicts between neighbors were extremely high. Is it possible that preserving community tranquility is of extreme importance, and therefore the Kibbutz family keeps conflict within the family to preserve more important communal tranquility.

Summary

The critics of research on battered husbands have labeled women's violence against their husbands as ''usually insignificant physical attacks'' (Field & Kirchner, 1978). However, we contend that physical violence between spouses is never insignificant. Although an initial attack may be mild, it is often a precursor to more violent attacks, and may serve as a later justification for a husband's violence toward his wife.

In an earlier article, ''The Battered Husband Syndrome,'' it was concluded:

> Although the data discussed do not represent, for the most part, a systematic investigation of representative samples of battered husbands, it is important to understand husband beating because of the implications for social policies to help resolve the more global problem of family violence. (Steinmetz, 1977–78, p. 507)

When the focus remains on the battered wife, the remedies often suggested revolve around support groups, crisis lines, and shelters for the woman and her child. This stance overlooks a basic condition of violence between spouses—a society that glorifies violence if done for the ''right reasons,'' the good of society, or that of one's own family. It is critical to shift at least some of the blame from individual family members to basic sociocultural conditions so that more resources will become available to help families and a greater emphasis will be placed on changing the attitudes and values of society (Steinmetz, 1977–78).

Almost 10 years have passed since the first article on battered husbands appeared. Knowledge in this area has expanded and professionals in the field realize more than ever the importance of reducing all forms of domestic violence.

References

Balswick, J. O., & C. Peek (1971). The inexpressive male: A tragedy of American society. *Family Coordinator, 20* (4), 363–368.

Barcus, F. E. (1963). The world of Sunday comics. In D. M. White & R. H. Abel (Eds.), *The Funnies, an American Idiom* (pp. 190–218). Glencoe: The Free Press.

Beck, M., Rohter, L., & Friday, C. (1984, April 30). An unwanted baby boom. *Newsweek.*

Brown, R. (1982, October). Battered husbands need help. *Sunday News Journal,* pp. 1–4.

Curtis, L. A. (1974). *Criminal violence: National patterns and behavior.* Lexington, MA: Lexington Books.

Demos, J. (1970). *A little commonwealth.* New York: Oxford University Press.

Field, M., & Kirchner, R. M. (1978). Services to battered women. *Victimology, 3*(1–2), 216–222.

Gelles, R. J. (1974). *The violent home: A study of physical aggression between husbands and wives.* Beverly Hills, CA: Sage.

Lester, D. (1981). A cross-cultural study of wife abuse. *Aggressive Behavior, 6,* 361–364.

Levinger, C. (1976). Sources of marital dissatisfaction among applicants for divorce. *American Journal of Orthopsychiatry, 36* (5), 803–807.

Oswald, I. (1980, December). Domestic violence by women. *The Lancet,* p. 1253.

Radbill, S. X. (1968). A history of child abuse and infanticide. In R. E. Helfer & C. H. Rempe (Eds.), *The battered child* (1st ed., pp. 3–21). Chicago, IL: University of Chicago Press.

Robinson, E. J., & White, D. M. (1963). Who Reads the Funnies—and Why? In D. M. White & R. H. Abel (Eds.) *The funnies, an American idiom* (pp. 179–232). Glencoe: The Free Press.

Saenger, G. (1963). Male and female relation in the American comic strips. In D. M. White & R. H. Abel (Eds.), *The funnies: An American idiom* (pp. 219–223). Glencoe, IL: The Free Press.

Shorter, E. (1975). *The making of the modern family.* New York: Basic Books.

Sidel, R. (1972). *Women and child care in China.* New York, NY: Hill & Wang.

Simon, R. J. (1976). American women and crime. *The Annals of the American Academy of Political and Social Science, 423,* 31–46.

Slater, P., & Slater, D. (1965). Maternal ambivalence and narcissism. *Merrill Palmer Quarterly, 11,* 241–259.

Steinmetz, S. K. (1977a). *The cycle of violence: Assertive, aggressive and abusive family interaction.* New York, NY: Praeger Press.

Steinmetz, S. K. (1974). Male Liberation—Destroying the stereotypes. In E. Powers & M. Lee (Eds.), *The Process of Relationships* (pp. 55–67). Minneapolis: West Publishing Co.

Steinmetz, S. K. (1977b). Secondary Analysis of data from ''The use of force for resolving family conflict: The training ground for abuse.'' *Family Coordinator,* Vol. 33(4), 19–26.

Steinmetz, S. K. (1981). Cross cultural marital abuse. *Journal of Sociology and Social Welfare, 8,* 404–414.

Steinmetz, S. K. (1987). Family violence: Past, present, and future. In M. B. Sussman & S. K. Steinmetz (Eds.), *Handbook of marriage and the family.* New York: Plenum Press.

Straus, M. A., Gelles, R. J., & Steinmetz, S. K. (1980). *Behind closed doors: Violence in American families.* New York, NY: Doubleday.

Straus, M. A., & Gelles, R. J. (1986). Societal change and change in family violence from 1975 to 1985 as revealed by two national surveys. *Journal of Marriage and the Family 48:* 465–479.

Tiger, L. (1969). *Men in groups.* New York, NY: Random House.

U. S. Bureau of the Census (1976). *Vital statistics reports: Annual summary for the United States,* Vol. 24, no. 13. Washington, DC: National Center for Health Statistics.

U. S. Department of Commerce, Bureau of the Census (1977). *Statistical abstract of the United States* (p. 177).

U. S. Department of Commerce, Bureau of the Census (1978). *Statistical Abstract of the United States* (pp. 180–183).

U. S. Department of Justice (1978). *Sourcebook of criminal justice statistics* (p. 401).

U. S. Department of Justice (1985). *F.B.I. uniform crime reports.* Washington, DC: U.S. Government Printing Office.

Walker, L. (1984). *The battered women syndrome.* New York: Springer.

Whiting, J. W. M., & Child, T. L. (1953). *Child training and personality: A cross-cultural study.* New Haven, CT: Yale University Press.

Wilt, G. M., & Bannon, J. D. (1976). *Violence and the police: Homicides assaults and disturbances.* Washington, DC: The Police Foundation.

Wolfgang, M. (1958). *Patterns in criminal homicide.* New York, NY: Wiley.

Zeigert, K. A. (1983). The Swedish prohibition of corporal punishment: A preliminary report. *Journal of Marriage and the Family,* Vol. 45, 917–926.

11

Elder Abuse

KARL PILLEMER and J. JILL SUITOR

INTRODUCTION

Although difficulties exist in the study of all forms of family violence, it may be that nowhere have so many obstacles to understanding been encountered as with the abuse of the elderly. The problem of battered elders came to the public's attention almost a decade ago, and the ensuing years have seen the development of intervention programs at the state and local level, and the expression of major concern at the federal level (Salend, Kane, & Satz, 1984). Reports on elder abuse have appeared in such mass media publications as *Newsweek* and *Parade Magazine,* and the problem has been addressed on national television. However, in spite of such wide interest in domestic mistreatment of the elderly, we know surprisingly little about this phenomenon.

A number of exploratory studies of elder abuse have been conducted; however, the methodological weaknesses of this research have been so pronounced that reliable results have rarely been obtained. Perhaps for this reason, only a few of the most frequently cited studies have ever been published in academic journals. The authors of review articles on the topic agree that there is no reliable estimate of the prevalence of elder abuse, and that the causes of maltreatment remain unidentified (Hudson & Johnson, 1987; Pedrick-Cornell & Gelles, 1982; Yin, 1985). Thus, we are in a curious situation in which major intervention programs are being implemented all over the country for a phenomenon (a) that we do not know how to define; (b) for which we have no reliable estimate of the number of persons affected; and (c) about which we know little regarding risk factors.

In this chapter, we hope to shed new light on the problem of elder abuse by going beyond previous attempts to review the literature on the topic. In particular, our theoretical perspective incorporates two bodies of research whose relevance to elder abuse has thus far not been systematically explored: the gerontological literature on relations between adult children and their elderly parents; and research on the quality of marital relationships. It is our belief that elder abuse need not only be examined as a separate and distinct phenomenon, but can also be understood in part as an outgrowth of family conflict in later life. This perspective allows us to draw on more general findings regarding the

KARL PILLEMER and J. JILL SUITOR • Family Research Laboratory, University of New Hampshire, Durham, NH 03824.

quality of relationships between the aged and their families. We attempt to integrate this literature with research on other forms of family violence to provide a theoretical framework for understanding elder abuse.

The chapter begins with the presentation of three case studies, followed by a discussion of the definition of elder abuse. Next, we review the evidence regarding the extent of maltreatment of the elderly, and provide new data on spousal violence among the aged. Then, in a more theoretical discussion, we present the framework for the study of elder abuse just mentioned. The chapter concludes with a review of intervention strategies and suggestions for future research.

CASE STUDIES

The notion of physical abuse of the elderly is a disquieting one to most people, and, as we know with child and spouse abuse, disturbing phenomena are frequently denied. Even those who are familiar with the literature on family violence may have difficulty conceptualizing the circumstances under which elder abuse occurs. Because of the relative strangeness of the phenomenon, we present the following case studies to give graphic evidence of the forms that domestic violence against the elderly can take. We have also chosen cases to show the wide range of situations that can fall under the term *elder abuse*. These case studies are drawn from an interview study of physically abused elderly persons (Pillemer, 1985a).

Case I

Mr. A. was a 64-year-old man who lived with his wife and 22-year-old son in the second floor apartment of an old three-decker building. Mr. A. had multiple sclerosis, and had recently experienced a substantial decline in health; nevertheless, he was still ambulatory and was able to drive a car. When the interviewer arrived, Mr. A. was tidying up as best he could around the small apartment. However, he was often quite weak and unsteady on his feet.

At the time of the interview, Mr. A. had been the victim of physical abuse by his son, Edward, for about 3 years.[1] Edward had been discharged from the Marine Corps after having what his father termed a nervous breakdown. He became very violent during his breakdown and, his father attested, "had to be held down by five Marines." Although Edward was never an easy person to get along with, the breakdown and discharge made him much worse. Since that time, he had been repeatedly hospitalized for psychiatric reasons. He had been married to and divorced from another former mental patient, and at the time of the interview was living with a prostitute and her children, which bothered Mr. A. tremendously.

Mr. A. reported that Edward came by the house almost every day, in spite of the fact that Mr. A. had obtained a restraining order to prevent such visits. Mr. A. found these visits almost uniformly unpleasant. They generally involved requests for financial assistance. Mr. A. complained about his son's unwillingness to help him in any way, which he felt "is not the way a son should act." When asked why he didn't bar Edward from the house and totally break off contact with him, Mr. A. responded that he was afraid of his son:

> He starts kicking stuff around . . . he has also assaulted me three times. He hit me
> in the head, and on my body, and knocked me down. He takes off when we call

---

[1]All of the names used in the case studies are pseudonyms.

the police, but always comes back. He comes in here banging at the door, going to knock my door down. I don't want him disturbing the peace. I've got tenants upstairs and downstairs, and so not to make a scene I let him in. It's just a case of where I'm handicapped and if I ever start fighting with him, I'd probably be hurt bad . . . in other words, I can't defend myself . . . I don't go looking to fight with him because it's like a hornet's nest. If he goes off, off his faculty, he could really hurt me bad. Which I don't want; I'm hurting enough.

Mr. A. did not see any solution to his situation. He was unwilling to abandon his son entirely or have him arrested, and he did not wish to leave his home and move to elderly housing, where he would be more protected. To exacerbate the situation, Mr. A.'s friends and relatives had become less likely to visit, due to their fear of Edward's outbursts. Thus, Mr. A. had become rather isolated during the period prior to the interview.

I just hope to God that, like I say, there's peace in the house. That's what I want, and I'm looking forward every day that things will be corrected. That's the size of it, and I just hope nobody has to go through what we are going through, my wife and my family. It's something—it's your own flesh and blood. I'm looking for an answer, and I just hope to God that there's an answer someplace in the near future.

Case II

Mrs. Y. and her husband lived in a small house in a working class neighborhood. The interview took place in what had once been the dining room, and was now serving as her bedroom. She lay in a hospital-style bed, with her hands lying limply on her chest. She was almost entirely paralyzed, and could only move her head and neck. She had been bedridden for 3 years, and was assisted by the visits of home health aides, a woman she hired for weekends, and a neighbor. Her husband was a victim of Alzheimer's disease; his condition had become severe 5 years earlier, at which time he had ceased working.

Mrs. Y. asserted that before the onset of Alzheimer's disease, her husband was "a saint." She reported, "He was quiet, fussy about his clothes, modest, shy. We had a good relationship. He was never violent." She said that more recently, he had become argumentative and angry. She still tried to talk with him, but generally received little response. At times, he would become extremely agitated and hit her. One incident was particularly terrifying for her:

I was saying something to him, and he got angry. He put his hands around my throat and started to choke me. There was nothing I could do. I started to cry and then he stopped. He saw the tears in my eyes, and stopped.

Mrs. Y. attributed the abusive behavior to her husband's illness, which she said had transformed him. She was extremely reluctant to institutionalize him, however. She asserted that nursing homes are "bad," and that it would be a betrayal to place him in one. She reported a sense of obligation to him for his past kindness to her. Again, this was a situation without any clear prospect for resolution until the deteriorating physical condition of the two partners necessitated a change in living situation.

Case III

Mrs. D. lived in a moderately sized, attractive house in a pleasant suburban neighborhood. She was 70 years old, and lived with her son, Alan, and grandson; until their separation shortly before the interview, her daughter-in-law and two more grandchildren had resided with her. The daughter-in-law, Edna, had been repeatedly abusive to Mrs. D.

Although Mrs. D. acknowledged that her daughter-in-law sometimes was pleasant to her, the conflicts were many. Mrs. D. was heavily involved in caring for her grandchildren, especially in the past few years, when both parents were employed. She was extremely attached to her grandchildren, and referred to them frequently in conversation. Edna was dependent on Mrs. D. for child care, but also argued violently with her about the children. They also fought about the house; Edna wanted Mrs. D. to turn it over to her. Toward the end of the relationship with her husband, Edna began to drink more heavily, and to have affairs with other men.

During that period, a series of violent events occurred between Mrs. D. and Edna. During one argument, Mrs. D. recounted:

> She grabbed me. She scratched me all over my arms. All scratches, and she pulled me off of the chair where I was sitting near the sewing machine. She pulled me off. Well, when she did that, I grabbed her hair. I said, "You're not going to do that to me." Well, when I grabbed her hair, she slapped me and threw me across my kitchen there, and I went against the refrigerator and I lost my balance. When I regained my balance I said to her, "How can you do this to me when I was so good to you?" I said, "I was even better to you than my own daughter," which is true. And she leaned across the counter and she spit right in my face. Then she went downstairs.

Mrs. D. then called her sister-in-law, who urged her to contact the police. Mrs. D. obtained a restraining order against the daughter-in-law, who left shortly after the incident. Divorce proceedings began, and Mrs. D.'s life became more settled. However, she worried almost constantly about the grandchildren, who lived with her daughter-in-law, and tried to see them as often as she could.

We have presented three cases of domestic violence in which an elderly person was the victim. The perpetrators were a son, a husband, and a daughter-in-law. The connection among these cases may not be immediately obvious; superficially, the common thread is the violent act. However, the evidence discussed below does point to certain commonalities in families in which elder abuse occurs. In a later section, our goal will be to identify elements in abusive relationships that may distinguish them from nonabusive ones, and thus to uncover factors specifically associated with violence toward elders. Before turning to these concerns, we will discuss definitional issues in the study of elder abuse, and present information on the extent of the problem.

DEFINITIONAL ISSUES

There is, at present, no consensus regarding the definition of elder abuse, and efforts to define this term accurately have met with little success. As Callahan (1981) noted, "With some of these definitions there seems to be a drive to include all forms of troubled interpersonal relationships under the rubric of violence and abuse" (p. 2). T. F. Johnson (1986), in a comprehensive review of definitions of elder abuse, provides an example of this problem. She noted that definitions often include psychological mistreatment of the elderly. This type of abuse has been seen as including such behaviors as making the old person feel ashamed of his or her behavior, ridiculing the elder, shouting at him or her, or interfering with the old person's decision making regarding his or her own activities. In contrast, in the study of other forms of family maltreatment, the term *abuse* has generally been limited to actions that are much further beyond the range of normal human relationships, such as physical violence that results in injury, or is intended to result in injury (Crystal, 1986).

A second issue is the inability to compare findings among studies, due to the lack of consistency in defining abuse. An example can be provided by examining two of the most cited studies. Lau and Kosberg (1979) included four categories in their study: physical abuse, psychological abuse, material abuse, and violation of rights. Block and Sinnott (1979) included the first three categories, omit violation of rights, and add poor residential environment. The apparent overlap is deceptive, however, because similarly labeled categories contain different types of injuries and abuse. Lau and Kosberg divided physical abuse into classes that may or may not involve injuries (direct beatings, lack of personal care, lack of food, lack of medical care, and lack of supervision), whereas Block and Sinnott included only a list of various injuries (bruises and welts, sprains and dislocations, malnutrition and freezing, abrasions, lacerations, cuts and punctures).

As another example, Hudson and Johnson (1987) note that Lau and Kosberg (1979) categorized withholding personal care as physical abuse, whereas Douglass, Hickey, and Noel (1980) placed it under active neglect, and Sengstock and Liang (1982) subsumed it under the category of psychological neglect. To be sure, in each of these studies, the authors carefully attempted to create clear definitions. It is the inconsistency among definitions that makes it difficult to synthesize the outcomes of various studies.

Rather than attempting to resolve the debate over the definition of elder abuse, we will respond to the theme of this book by focusing on domestic violence against the elderly (persons 65 or older). We employ the simple and clear definition of violence used by Straus, Gelles, and Steinmetz (1980): ''an act carried out with the intention or perceived intention of causing physical pain or injury to another person'' (p. 20). In this chapter, we use the terms *domestic violence against the elderly* and *elder abuse* interchangeably.

PREVALENCE OF ELDER ABUSE

There have been two attempts to determine the prevalence of elder abuse using population surveys. Although both of these studies suffer from methodological weaknesses, they provide valuable information. Block and Sinnott (1979) surveyed three groups by mail: community agencies, a random sample of elderly persons living in the community, and health and human service professionals. Respondents drawn from these sources were questioned about a range of types of maltreatment, including physical, financial, and emotional abuse and neglect. The response rate was very low: only 1 agency in 24 responded, as did only 16% of the elderly and 31% of professionals. The elderly sample yielded a total of 26 reports of some form of abuse or neglect, or a 4% rate of abuse.

Block and Sinnott's (1979) findings have been extrapolated to the total elderly population of the United States, resulting in a figure of nearly one million cases nationwide. However, as Block and Sinnott noted, this estimate may not be reliable because of the low response rate. Additionally, this study was confined to the District of Columbia, further reducing the generalizability of the findings. In spite of these methodological limitations, the 4% figure frequently appears in reports on elder abuse. Such reports often go on to describe this abused 4% as the ''tip of the iceberg,'' and intimate that a much higher proportion (up to 10%) of the elderly may be abused (cf. House Select Committee on Aging, 1985).

In contrast, a very low estimate comes from a survey conducted by Gioglio and

Blakemore (1983). This study is unusual, in that it is the only survey of elder abuse and neglect based on a random probability sample of a state population (New Jersey) for which information is currently available.[2] Of the 324 persons in the sample, only five reported some form of maltreatment. Projecting this figure to the entire noninstitutionalized population of New Jersey, Gioglio estimated that approximately one percent of the elderly, or 8,000 persons, would report having been victimized. Interestingly, only one of the five cases involved physical maltreatment; thus, the incidence of physical abuse measured by this study appears to be extremely low.

A recent national study of family violence (Straus & Gelles, 1986) provides additional data on the incidence of physical abuse among the elderly, although it is restricted to violence between spouses. These data also allow us to compare the rate of spouse abuse among the elderly to that found among couples of younger ages. The data were collected during telephone interviews with a national probability sample of 5,168 currently married adults, 520 of whom were 65 years of age or older.[3]

Marital violence was measured by use of the Conflict Tactics Scale (CTS) developed by Straus (1979). The CTS is administered by reading respondents a list of behaviors in which they might have engaged when they had a dispute with their spouse/partner, and asking them to tell the interviewer how often they had engaged in each of the behaviors during the previous year. The 18-item scale begins by inquiring about the frequency with which the respondent had "discussed the issues calmly," and proceeds gradually to more aggressive behaviors, such as "did or said something to spite the other one" and "threw or smashed or hit or kicked something," and ultimately to eight items about the use of physical violence: threw something at the other one; pushed, grabbed or shoved the other one; slapped the other one; kicked, bit, or hit with a fist; hit or tried to hit with something; beat up the other one; threatened with a knife or gun; or used a knife or gun.

After the respondents describe their own behaviors, they are asked how frequently their spouses engaged in each of the behaviors during the previous year. Each item is coded on a scale from 0 (never) to 6 (more than 20 times). For the present analysis, the responses were dichotomized into "never" and "one or more times." Data on wife-to-husband and husband-to-wife violence were examined separately.

As shown in the top row of Table 1, 3.3% of the elderly respondents reported that husband-to-wife violence had occurred in their marriages within the previous year. These data also show that there was a very strong negative relationship between age and rate of husband-to-wife violence; in fact, the rate of husband-to-wife violence within the previous year was almost seven times greater among couples in which the respondent was 30 or younger than among couples in which the respondent was 65 years of age or older. A similar pattern was found when examining the rate of wife-to-husband violence within the previous year, as shown in the bottom row of Table 1.

It is important to point out, however, that the rates of spousal violence among the elderly just presented should not be taken as an indication of the overall incidence of elder abuse; they represent only the rate of violence among elderly individuals who are currently married. Only 55% of the elderly are married—40% of the women and 86% of the men—(U. S. Bureau of the Census, 1985, p. 36), and are therefore at risk for this type of

[2]A random-sample prevalence survey of elder abuse in the Boston metropolitan area has recently been completed by David Finkelhor and Karl Pillemer; however, incidence figures from this survey are not yet available.
[3]Married and cohabiting individuals were included in the sample; we will use the term *spouse* to refer to individuals who are cohabiting as well individuals who are married.

violence. At present, similar data for abuse of the elderly by their children and other relatives are not available.

The relatively low rates of spousal abuse just presented should not be used to suggest that elder abuse is not a social problem worthy of further attention. As the case studies presented earlier demonstrate, domestic abuse of the elderly is a source of a substantial amount of human suffering among those families in which it occurs. In order to reduce the incidence of elder abuse, we believe that we must understand the factors that may precipitate it. In particular, our knowledge of risk factors must be improved before prevention programs that allow for early intervention with potentially abusive families can be developed. Therefore, we will now turn to a discussion in which we develop a framework for understanding factors that may lead to elder abuse.

A Framework for Understanding Elder Abuse: Combining Two Literatures

In order to place the framework proposed here in proper context, it is necessary to begin with a brief discussion of the difficulties in utilizing existing research findings on elder abuse. One major problem in interpreting results from previous studies is the conceptual problem already noted: poor definition of the term *elder abuse*. The remaining four difficulties are methodological in nature. First, different criteria have been used to determine the population at risk for elder abuse. For example, some researchers have included persons under 60 years of age in their samples, whereas most others have limited their studies to persons 60 or over. Other investigations have included only persons sharing a residence with the abusers (Block & Sinnott, 1979), or caretakers of the elderly (Steinmetz & Amsden, 1983), whereas O'Malley, Segars, Perez, Mitchell, and Knuepfel (1979), Gioglio & Blakemore (1983), and Wolf, Godkin, and Pillemer (1984) included all abused or neglected elders.

Second, studies have employed widely differing methods for obtaining data, ranging from Gioglio and Blakemore's (1983) statewide random sample survey to Lau and Kosberg's review of patients' records. Third, many studies rely on professional reports of cases of abuse, rather than on direct interviews with victims or abusers. Fourth, few of the studies have included comparison groups, thus reducing their generalizability. For example, some investigators have asserted that the abused and neglected elderly are likely to be physically and/or mentally impaired. However, without a comparison group, it is impossible to know if they are more or less impaired than other persons.

Table 1. Rate of Husband-to-Wife and Wife-to-Husband Physical Violence per 100 Couples by Respondent's Age

	Respondent's age			
	30 or Younger	31–50	51–64	65 or Older
Husband-to-wife physical violence	22.0	11.6	5.3	3.3
Total N	(1246)	(2421)	(981)	(520)
Wife-to-husband physical violence	24.4	12.1	5.1	4.2
Total N	(1246)	(2420)	(982)	(520)

KARL PILLEMER and
J. JILL SUITOR

Taken together, these problems suggest that a thoretical framework for understanding domestic violence against the aged cannot be derived from previous research. In this section, we consider two sets of factors that may have the ability to help predict the occurrence of abuse. We first consider factors that have been found to be precipitants of other forms of family violence. In so doing, we mirror earlier attempts to identify risk factors for elder abuse: the extension of concepts relating to spouse abuse and child abuse to maltreatment of the aged. However, in order to construct a more exhaustive model to explain elder abuse, we have included a second body of research as well: the more general literature on relations between spouses and between parents and their adult children.

In the framework proposed here, the family-violence-related variables are treated as being directly related to elder abuse; we have termed them *direct precipitants*. The variables relating to the more global pattern of relations among family members are considered to be *predisposing factors* for elder abuse. They provide the context in which domestic violence against the aged is likely to occur.

Direct Precipitants: Findings from the Family Violence Literature

Our review of the literature on family violence suggests that there are five major factors related to domestic violence in general which may also be related to elder abuse. These are:

1. Intra-individual dynamics
2. Intergenerational transmission of violent behavior (''cycle of violence'')
3. Inequitable levels of dependency between abuser and abused
4. Social isolation
5. External stress

There is greater evidence that the first three factors may be related to elder abuse; we have therefore discussed these in somewhat more detail. Our discussions of stress and social isolation are more brief.

Intra-individual Dynamics. Intra-individual theories blame abuse on some pathological characteristic of the abuser, usually mental illness of some kind. This approach has been widely employed to explain spouse and child abuse, although it has been criticized by some experts (cf. Gelles, 1974). However, there is evidence that intra-individual factors may play a part in elder abuse.

Douglass *et al.* (1980) included the ''flawed development'' of the abuser as one cause of abuse, which results from problems in the childhood of the abuser. Similarly, Lau and Kosberg (1979) referred to the problem of the non-normal child (e.g., mentally ill or retarded, or alcoholic) who has always been cared for by parents, yet may be expected to care for them if the parents become impaired. Further, research by Wolf, Strungnell, and Godkin (1982) found a considerable degree of mental illness among elder abusers; 31% were reported to have a history of psychiatric illness. Pillemer (1985a) also found abusers to be much more likely to have a history of psychiatric hospitalization than a nonabuse control group.

One other intra-individual characteristic that has gained acceptance as a partial explanation of why child and spouse abuse occur is alcohol and drug abuse (cf. Coleman & Straus, 1983; Kantor & Straus, 1986; Sedge, 1979). Preliminary evidence has indicated that a similar relationship between substance abuse and domestic violence may exist among the elderly (Pillemer, 1985b; Wolf *et al.*, 1984).

Intergenerational Transmission of Violent Behavior. Social learning theory holds that a child learns to be violent in the family setting in which a violent parent has been taken as a role model. When frustrated or angry as an adult, the individual relies on this learned behavior and lashes out violently. This theory has led to the concept of a cycle of violence that suggests, for example, that abused children grow up to become child abusers.

Findings from the Straus, Gelles, and Steinmetz (1980) national survey support this notion. Their study revealed that a greater degree of physical punishment at the hands of either parent was positively associated with a higher rate of abusive violence toward that person's own children. Children who observed their fathers striking their mothers also had a higher rate of violence toward their children. Consistent with this, an extensive review of the literature (Hotaling & Sugarman, 1986) identified witnessing parental violence during childhood or adolescence as one of the strongest risk factors for the abuse of wives in adulthood.

No evidence exists at present to determine whether elder abusers have experienced violent upbringings. Such a connection would indeed seem likely, based on the strength of this finding in other forms of abuse. It is important to note, however, that a difference may exist between elder abuse and child and spouse abuse regarding the transmission of violent behavior. Obviously, children who abuse the elderly were not themselves abused as elderly parents; the cycle of violence must therefore take one of two different forms. In one case, the formerly abused child strikes out at his or her own abuser. This pattern involves a psychological process with elements of retaliation as well as imitation. In the other case, the adult child models a pattern of abusive behaviors that he or she has seen his or her parents exhibit toward their own elderly parents (i.e., the child's grandparents).

Dependency and Exchange Relations. Another commonly cited factor in the elder abuse literature is the resentment generated by the dependency of an older person on a caretaker. In fact, the belief that the dependency of elderly individuals is a major cause of abuse is probably the most widely held in the literature (cf. Steinmetz & Amsden, 1983). This view has developed in large part from gerontological research on the strains of family caregiving to elderly relatives. Thus, Davidson (1979) tied abuse directly to the "crises" created by the needs of an elderly parent for care. Steinmetz (1983) argued that families undergo "generational inversion," in which the elderly person becomes dependent on his or her children for financial, physical, and/or emotional support, leading to severe stress on the part of the caregiver. As the costs of the relationship grow for the caregiver, and the rewards diminish, the exchange becomes perceived as unfair. If the caretaker feels unable to escape the situation, he or she may then become abusive.

However, because many elderly persons are quite dependent on their relatives (cf. Brody, 1985; Cantor, 1983; Kulys & Tobin, 1980), the question therefore arises: Why are some of these dependent individuals abused and others not? Because abuse occurs in only a small proportion of families, no direct correlation between dependency of an older person and abuse can be assumed. In fact, Phillips (1983) failed to find any difference in level of impairment between a group of abused elderly and a control group.

Although it may seem contradictory, preliminary research suggests that another cause of abuse may be the continued dependency of abuser or abused. Wolf, Strugnell, and Godkin (1982) found that in two thirds of their cases, the perpetrator was reported to be financially dependent on his or her victim. Hwalek, Sengstock, and Lawrence (1984), in a case-control study, also found that the financial dependency of the abuser on the elderly victim was an important risk factor in elder abuse.

KARL PILLEMER and
J. JILL SUITOR

Pillemer's (1985a,b) results support this argument even more strongly. He found that 64% of the abusers in his sample were dependent on their victims financially, and 55% were dependent on the victims for housing. In the nonabuse control group, financial dependency of a comparison relative was reported by only 38% of the elderly, and housing dependence by relatives was reported by only 30%. Both differences were statistically significant ($p < .05$). In general, Pillemer found the abusers to be heavily dependent individuals, including disabled or cognitively impaired spouses and children who were unable to separate from their parents.

Why should the dependency of an adult child or spouse on an elderly person result in physical abuse? A theoretical explanation of this phenomenon can be based on a concept from social exchange theory: that of power. Finkelhor (1983), in his attempt to identify common features of family abuse, noted that abuse can occur as a resonse to perceived powerlessness. Acts of abuse, he noted, "seem to be acts carried out by abusers to compensate for their perceived lack or loss of power" (p. 19). Thus, spouse abuse in younger populations has been found to be related to a sense of powerlessness, and the physical abuse of children "tends to start with a feeling of parental impotence" (p. 19). For example, it may be that the feeling of powerlessness experienced by an adult child who is still dependent on an elderly parent is especially acute, because it goes so strongly against society's expectations for normal adult behavior. This perceived power deficit appears to have more explanatory power than the notion that the abuser holds much power in the relationship (for a more complete discussion of this explanation, see Pillemer, 1985b).

In summary, dependency seems to play a critical role in elder abuse, but it is not yet clear who is depending on whom in these abusive relationships. Does an elderly person come to make excessive demands on caregivers? Are abusers persons who have remained dependent on the abused into later life, with unrealistic expectations of what the abused might provide? Or is the critical issue an imbalance in dependency, regardless of the direction it takes? Future research must examine such factors as the need for assistance of the abused, feelings of caregiving burden on the part of the abuser, and the dependency of the abuser.

Social Isolation. Social isolation has also been found to be characteristic of families in which other forms of domestic violence occurs (Gelles, 1972; Gil, 1971; Hennessey, 1979; Justice & Justice, 1976; Stark, Flitcraft, & Frazier, 1979). This is probably because behaviors that are considered to be illegitimate tend to be hidden. Detection of family violence can result in informal sanctions from friends, kin, and neighbors, and formal sanctions from police and the courts. Thus, all forms of family violence are likely to be less frequent in families that have friends or relatives who live nearby (Nye, 1979). The presence of an active social network may be a particularly strong deterrent to elder abuse, because it is viewed as a highly illegitimate behavior. Support for this argument has been provided by case-control studies by Phillips (1983) and Pillemer (1985c), which found abused elderly persons to have less social contact.

External Stress. A number of investigators have found a positive relationship between external stress (as differentiated from the stress that results from interpersonal relationships in the family) and child and wife abuse (Gil, 1971; Justice & Justice, 1976; Straus *et al.*, 1980). A stress perspective on abuse can be seen as an alternative to the theories previously discussed. In Gelles and Straus' (1979) terms, it is a sociocultural theory, rather than a social-psychological or intra-individual one, in that it emphasizes social structural and macrolevel variables, such as unemployment and economic conditions. However, the social stress model alone cannot explain elder abuse, as it does not account for why some families respond to stress with abuse and others do not. To date, no systematic exploration has been conducted of the relationship between stress and elder abuse, although Sengstock and Liang (1982) provided preliminary support for such a relationship.

To summarize, the family violence literature points to five factors that could lead to elder abuse: intra-individual dynamics, intergenerational transmission of violent behavior, dependency of abuser and/or abused, social isolation, and external stress. In the framework proposed here, these factors may directly precipitate domestic violence against the elderly. That is, families that have one of these characteristics may be at greater risk of elder abuse. To the extent that a family has more of these characteristics, it will be more at risk.

However, as noted earlier in this chapter, we do not believe that these factors alone provide an adequate framework in which to understand elder abuse. In order to understand more fully this phenomenon, we will review findings from the more general literature on family relationships.

Predisposing Factors: The Family Relations Literature

The literature on elder abuse has developed largely apart from the large body of research that exists on family relations among the elderly. We view this as a limitation of research on elder abuse, in particular because it removes this problem from the broader study of family relationships. In this section, we will include a discussion of more global relations between adult children and their elderly parents and those between spouses. We will attempt to demonstrate that findings on the determinants of the quality of family relations of the elderly can provide important insights into the factors that lead to abuse.

Adult Child–Parent Relations. Most of the literature on intergenerational relations has focused on patterns of interaction and instrumental support between adult children and their parents; however, in recent years, there has been increasing interest in examining the affectional aspects of adult child–parent relations. In this section, we will review the studies that have attempted to explain the factors affecting the quality of relations between adult children and their elderly parents.[4]

It is important to note two limitations of this literature for our purposes. First, the large majority of these studies focus on the relationship between adult children and their mothers, as opposed to fathers; and second, many of the investigations examine the relationship between mothers and their adult daughters, rather than children of both genders. We do not see the first characteristic as particularly problematic for our purposes. By 1984, 60% of the American population over 64 years of age was female, and their proportion is expected to continue to increase until at least the end of this century (U. S. Bureau of the Census, 1985, pp. 24–25). Consistent with this demographic trend, virtually every study has shown that women are most often the targets of abuse by their younger family members (cf. T. Johnson *et al.*, 1985, for a comprehensive review). Additionally, the studies we reviewed that included fathers and mothers did not report consistent gender differences in the factors affecting parent–child relations. Similarly, an examination of the studies that included sons and daughters did not reveal consistent gender differences in the factors affecting adult

---

[4]This review excludes factors about which there is substantial disagreement in the literature (for example, the effects of changes in parents' or children's marital status).

KARL PILLEMER and
J. JILL SUITOR

child–parent relations. Thus, in the absence of evidence to the contrary, we believe that it is reasonable to assume that the factors we will discuss similarly affect the relations of elderly parents with their sons and daughters.

First, the most consistent finding among the studies we reviewed is that parents' health is positively associated with feelings of closeness and attachment between them and their adult children (Baruch & Barnett, 1983; Cicirelli, 1981; Johnson & Bursk, 1977; Mindel & Wright, 1982). One reason for this may be the effects of parents' health on the previously established flow of support between the generations. That is, adult children may have to increase substantially their level of support to previously independent parents, as well as to accept a lessening or termination of the parents' provision of support to the children.

A second, related factor comes from the literature on the effects of disruption of the established flow of support between generations. These studies suggest that this change may reduce positive feelings. Cicirelli (1983a,b) found that high levels of parental dependency and of children's helping behaviors could lead to negative feelings on the part of adult children. Thompson and Walker's (1984) study revealed that middle-aged daughters and their mothers who reported high reciprocal aid patterns had the highest levels of attachment, and those who reported the lowest levels of reciprocal aid scored lowest on attachment. Similarly, Adams (1968) found that affectional ties were weaker when adult children's provision of help to their widowed parents was unreciprocated. In summary, it appears that perceived equity of support plays an important part in the quality of adult child–parent relations.

Third, parents' and adult children's satisfaction with one another's performance of family roles may also affect their relationship. Johnson's (1978) findings indicated that mothers' and daughters' satisfaction with one another's family role performance contributed to the quality of their relationship. Houser and Berkman (1984) reported that the quality of the mother–child relationship was not related to either partner's actual role performance; however, mothers' satisfaction with their relationship with their children was related to what they believed their children's behaviors would be if they were called upon. Thus, it appears that mothers' satisfaction with their children's commitment to family role performance may affect parent–adult child relations.

Last in this discussion, changes in the degree of status similarity between adult children and their parents may affect their relationship. The effects of increased status similarity on the mother–daughter relationship were illustrated by Fischer's (1981) finding that this relationship assumed greater importance from the daughters' perspective when they themselves became mothers. Fischer's findings are similar to those presented more than two decades ago by Young and Willmott (1957) and Komarovsky (1962), suggesting a consistent pattern of increased closeness in mother–daughter relations when daughters begin to share a larger number of social statuses with their mothers.

Decreases in status similarity also appear to have the potential to affect relations between adult children and their parents. Although Adams' (1968) original findings did not show a consistent relationship between adult children's upward or downward mobility and affectional closeness to either parent, a later analysis provided evidence that upward mobility could affect daughters' relations with their parents. Specifically, working-class daughters who had married into middle-class families were closer to their parents-in-law than to their own parents.[5] Further, several studies have suggested that the status dis-

[5]Personal communication with Bert Adams, April, 1986.

similarity that develops when adult children surpass their parents educationally may have particular potential for creating difficulties between the generations (Billson & Terry, 1982; Bruce, 1970; Piorkowski, 1983; Suitor, 1987).

To summarize, four factors emerge from this literature as contributing to the quality of adult child–parent relations: (a) parents' health; (b) parents' degree of dependency on their adult children and ability to reciprocate support; (c) parents' and children's satisfaction with one anothers' performance of family roles; and (d) changes in the degree of status similarity between parents and their children.

Marital Relations in the Later Years. Marital relations among the elderly have received surprisingly little attention, considering the dramatic increase in research on older persons in recent years. Consequently, we will need to draw on the more general literature on marital satisfaction and adjustment as well (i.e., those studies that included younger respondents) in our attempt to understand the factors that may affect the quality of marriage in the later years. This literature has grown to several hundred articles and books during the past few decades; thus, we will not attempt to review it in its entirely. Instead, we will restrict our attention to those studies whose findings appear to be relevant to older couples.[6]

Various measures of psychological well-being have consistently been found to be associated with marital satisfaction both among the general population and specifically among the elderly. Andrews and Withey (1976) found respondents' evaluations of their marital relationships to be positively associated with measures of global well-being; Glenn and Weaver (1981) reported that marital happiness was strongly related to global happiness; and Lee (1978) found marital satisfaction was correlated with older persons' morale. Although these cross-sectional studies cannot determine the causal direction in these correlational findings, it is reasonable to assume that marital satisfaction and psychological well-being act on one another reciprocally.

Spouses' satisfaction with one another's family role performance has also been found to be associated with marital adjustment. Bahr, Chappell, and Leigh (1983), Chadwick, Albrecht, and Kunz (1976), and Nye and McLaughlin (1976) all reported that both husbands' and wives' evaluations of one another's performance of the therapeutic role contributed to marital satisfaction. Two of these studies (Bahr *et al.*, 1983; Chadwick *et al.*, 1976) also found spouses' evaluations of one anothers' performance of the household role to be important to marital satisfaction.

Several studies have provided evidence that status transitions precipitated by negative life events are often associated with lower levels of marital adjustment. For example, Larson (1984) found lower levels of marital adjustment among blue-collar men following the loss of their jobs. Similarly, Simmons and Ball (1984) reported lower levels of marital adjustment among couples in which husbands had experienced spinal cord injuries during the marriage than among couples in which the injury had preceded the marriage.

Suitor's (1984) panel study of married mothers' return to school suggests that status transitions may lead to declines in partners' satisfaction with one another's family role

---

[6]We will not include the discussion of several variables that have been shown to affect marital relations at other stages of the life cycle, but either have been investigated only with younger populations, or do not appear to be relevant to the elderly, such as age at time of marriage. As with our review of the literature on adult child–parent relations, the present review excludes factors about which there is substantial disagreement in the literature. In this case, the most important of these issues include the effects of wives' employment, spouses' physical health, and the presence of either younger or adult children.

performance, perhaps helping to explain why status transitions often result in lowered marital adjustment. Suitor found that marital happiness declined over the women's first year of university study among couples in which wives were enrolled full time, and changed little among couples in which wives were enrolled part time. An analysis of her qualitative data revealed that the decline in marital happiness among full-time students and their husbands was due to a decrement in those wives' performance of the household and therapeutic aspects of their family roles, and a subsequent decrement in their husbands' performance of the therapeutic role, in response to the changes in their wives' role performance.

Similarity of attitudes and values also appears to be important to marital adjustment and satisfaction, particularly in the later years. Levinger and Breedlove (1966), Barry (1970), Hicks and Platt (1970), and Bowen and Orthner (1983) reported a positive relationship between marital satisfaction and actual and perceived value similarity. However, none of the analyses they presented examined whether the importance of value similarity differed by age or stage in the family life cycle. Medling and McCarrey's (1981) investigation revealed that value similarity was only weakly related to marital satisfaction across earlier stages of the family life cycle, but assumed greater importance in explaining marital satisfaction among older spouses.

Two recent studies conducted on very different substantive issues suggest that equity may also play a part in marital satisfaction and adjustment. Davidson, Balswick, & Halverson (1983) found that husbands and wives were least satisfied with their marriages when they felt that they received more expressions of love and affection than they gave. For wives, receiving less than they gave was also associated with lower levels of marital adjustment, whereas for husbands, underbenefitting was unrelated.

Yogev and Brett's (1985) study of the division of household labor and marital satisfaction also suggests that equity is important in marital relations. Their investigation revealed that patterns of contributions to household labor were differentially associated with marital satisfaction, depending on the respondents' gender and their spouses' employment status. However, across all of these categories, perceiving oneself as contributing more than one's share of the household labor was associated with lower levels of marital satisfaction.

Recent work by Filsinger and Wilson (Filsinger & Wilson, 1984; Wilson & Filsinger, 1986) has shown that higher levels of religiosity are positively related to marital adjustment. A detailed analysis of the importance of various aspects of religiosity (Wilson & Filsinger, 1986) revealed that couples' marital adjustment was positively related to a high levels of ritualistic involvement in religion, high levels of personal religious experience, and conservative religious beliefs. These studies of religion and marital satisfaction have not examined the effects of age. However, given the greater importance of religion to the elderly (Ward, 1984), it is possible that religiosity may play a larger role in marital adjustment among older couples.

To summarize, this literature indicates that there are six factors that affect marital adjustment and satisfaction and are relevant for couples in the later years: (a) psychological well-being; (b) status transitions, particularly if precipitated by negative life events; (c) satisfaction with one another's performance of family roles; (d) value similarity; (e) equity; and (f) religiosity.

In conclusion, we have been able to identify four factors that appear to be related to the quality of adult parent–child relations, and six factors that appear to be related to spousal relations in later life. Our review also indicates that the dynamics of relations between spouses differ somewhat from those that involve adult children; thus, it is reasonable to assume that the factors precipitating marital violence among the elderly will differ, at least in part, from those precipitating adult children's abuse of their elderly parents. Based on our view that elder abuse can be viewed in the context of troubled family relationships, we anticipate that these variables will have some ability to help to identify the circumstances under which abuse is likely to occur.

The Two Literatures: What Can They Tell Us?

In Table 2 we have provided a summary of the factors discussed in the preceding sections. In order to illustrate how this framework could be applied to an individual case, we will now refer back to the case studies section. As noted, Mr. A. (Case I) was abused by his adult son Edward. Of the four factors that contribute to the quality of adult child–parent relations, three appear to be helpful in explaining Mr. A.'s situation. First, his health had recently declined; second, he was highly dissatisfied with his son's performance of family roles; and third, Edward's downward mobility had created a substantial degree of status dissimilarity between the father and son. Further, of the five immediate precipitants from the family violence literature, three clearly apply to this situation. Edward was severely psychologically disturbed; he was heavily dependent on Mr. A. financially and emotionally; and the family was socially isolated.

Although this framework may be fruitfully applied to such individual cases of elder abuse, we believe that it is better suited for use as a guide for future research. Thus, we encourage researchers to take into consideration the predisposing and precipitating factors that we have outlined earlier when developing research designs. The relationship between the two sets of factors can be conceived as a theoretical path diagram. We have shown an example of this in the top half of Figure 1. In this example, the predisposing factor—in this model, decline in parent's health—forms the context in which the abusive acts are more likely to occur; and the family-violence-related factors—parent's dependency and social isolation—are the direct precipitants. To give an example involving spousal elder

---

Table 2. Predisposing Factors and Direct Precipitants of Elder Abuse

Predisposing factors	Direct precipitants
Adult child–parent relations:	
1. Parents' health	1. Intra-individual dynamics
2. Parents' dependency	2. Intergenerational transmission of violent behavior
3. Parents' and children's satisfaction with one anothers' performance of family roles	3. Inequitable levels of dependency between abuser and abused
4. Changes in degree of status similarity between parents and children	4. Social isolation
Spousal relations:	5. External stress
1. Psychological well-being	
2. Status transitions (particularly when precipitated by a negative life event)	
3. Satisfaction with one anothers' performance of family roles	
4. Value similarity	
5. Equity	
6. Religiosity	

abuse, experiencing a status transition precipitated by a negative life event may increase the occurrence of social isolation and decrease marital adjustment, thus increasing the likelihood of abuse, as shown in the bottom half of Figure 1.

It is important to point out that many of the relationships among the factors in the theoretical framework we have developed have not yet been explored. We believe that research is critically needed on these variables, because it will lead to the development of more powerful explanatory models of elder abuse and family relations in later life.

INTERVENTIONS

Our lack of knowledge regarding the extent, nature, and dynamics of elder abuse makes the rational planning of social remedies very difficult. In the absence of a comprehensive national policy toward this problem, states and local communities have designed programs to help abused elderly persons. The intervention strategies that have been employed thus far can be categorized into three basic types: mandatory reporting laws, protective services programs, and direct services. The first two intervention strategies—

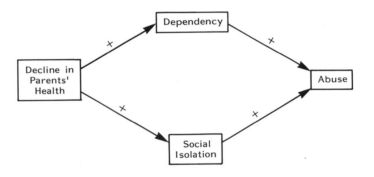

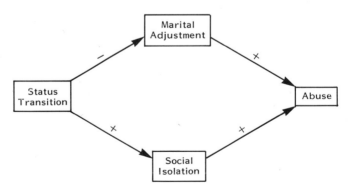

Figure 1. Theoretical path diagrams of the relationship between predisposing factors and direct precipitants of elder abuse.

mandatory reporting and protective services—are highly controversial. In the absence of data on elder abuse, the arguments over these interventions have involved primarily anecdotal evidence and speculation. In practice, the opposition to these initiatives has not been strong; at least 42 states and the District of Columbia now have mandatory reporting laws (House Select Committee on Aging, 1985). In this section, we will briefly review mandatory reporting and protective services, and then discuss service options.

Mandatory Reporting Laws

Mandatory reporting laws require certain groups of people (usually health and social service professionals) to report suspected cases of abuse to designated authorities. The goal of these laws is to facilitate the identification of abused older people, and thereby allow the state to intervene in their situation. There is, however, tremendous variation from state to state in the laws. Definitions vary as to whom should be classified as abused. Some states, for example, only intervene in cases in which the abuse is caused by another person, whereas others include the categories of self-neglect and self-abuse. States also differ as to whether there is a central registry for complaints. Further, penalties for failure to report differ greatly, ranging from no sanctions whatsoever to substantial fines in some states (Salend *et al.,* 1984).

Proponents of mandatory reporting argue that such laws are the best method for bringing cases to light. Without these statutes, they hold, few persons would report cases of suspected abuse. In contrast, opponents such as Faulkner (1982) claim that mandatory reporting laws will not lead to the identification of new cases, but instead to the reporting of ones that are already known to other service providers. Further, the opponents note that funding is rarely sufficient to allow for effective follow-up on suspected cases and for services to treat the abused. In 1984, for example, states spent only about $2.90 per older resident for elder protective services, compared to $22.00 per child resident for child protective services (House Select Committee on Aging, 1985). In the absence of such services, some observers fear that older persons will be inappropriately institutionalized (Crystal, 1986).

Protective Services

Protective services programs for the elderly are equally controversial. Most public protective services programs assign a legal intervention role to social workers. Such programs generally also involve the use of legal surrogate options, such as guardianship or conservatorship, when the elderly person is judged to be incompetent (Callendar, 1982, p. 3). Members of the legal community have been the strongest critics of protective services. They see such programs as an intrusion on the civil liberties of the elderly and as a way of infantilizing them. They argue that most states define abuse so broadly that they allow for a potentially stigmatizing intrusion into families with merely the normal range of human problems (Callahan, 1981). Further, critics hold that guardianship, which takes away many of the rights of an old person, is frequently used when it is not warranted.

Service Options

There is an enormous range of services that could be used by abused elderly persons and their families. These service options can be categorized into three general groups:

services for the victim, services for the abuser, and linkage services that bring together service providers and persons in need.

Services to Victims. Most discussions of service needs of abused elders list health and social services that are not specific to abuse. Such services are generally most appropriate for cases in which the victim is impaired and dependent, and in which the abuse is related to strain on the caregivers. As noted earlier, the research evidence indicates that this pattern of physical abuse occurs only in a minority of cases. However, in such situations, the following types of services may be helpful in reducing the strain families experience:

- Housing services: respite care to allow relatives a break from caregiving, and permanent alternative housing such as rest homes, congregate housing, and in extreme cases, nursing homes
- Health services: home health aides, home nursing, personal care attendants, adult day health centers, and in-home occupational, speech, and physical therapy
- Home maintenance services: assistance in housekeeping, heavy chores, shopping, and meal preparation
- Supportive services: friendly visitor programs, senior centers, and recreation programs
- Guardianship and financial management: protective services, voluntary conservatorship or guardianship, counsel for elderly persons in guardianship hearings

In other cases, the victim is a relatively independent person who is abused by a dependent relative. Such situations require a different set of interventions. As has been argued elsewhere (Finkelhor & Pillemer, 1984), many cases of elder abuse involve spouse abuse, and even child-to-parent cases have close parallels with the situation of abused spouses: legally independent adults who live together out of choice for a variety of material and emotional reasons. Thus, several interventions that have been effective with victims of spouse abuse may be fruitful when used with abused elders as well.

One such service option is self-help groups, in which victims come together to provide one other with support, to allay the sense of stigma and self-blame, and to help each other cope with the abusers (Breckman, 1985). Another service for battered elders is the emergency shelter or safe house. This mode differs radically from placing the victim in a nursing home, which occurs in some cases of elder abuse. The shelter is temporary, and presumes that after a chance to escape the abuser, the victim can move to a new living situation, or return to the relative who is now aware that no more abuse will be tolerated.

Finally, although not precisely a service, the parallel to spouse abuse also suggests that criminal justice sanctions could be more widely used in cases of elder abuse. In general, police and prosecutors have been reluctant to intervene in family violence. However, recent research suggests that police involvement may reduce revictimization (Sherman & Berk, 1984). Thus, arrest may be a deterrent in elder abuse.

Services to Abusers. Many services could be offered to the abusers themselves. Children who have remained unhealthily dependent on elderly parents may be helped by psychological counseling and by concrete assistance in establishing a separate residence and finding employment. Similarly, abusive spouses or children who are caring for the victim might benefit from caregiver support groups and the range of supportive long-term care services listed above. Self-help groups for elder abusers analogous to those for younger wife abusers would probably also be beneficial.

Linkage Services. For services to reach those in need, mechanisms are needed that link providers of services to potential consumers. Such services include the following:

- Case management services: assignment of an individual to an abusive family who arranges services for those involved and monitors their progress.
- Transportation: special needs vans and subsidized taxi fares
- Information and referral: a central clearinghouse and "hotline" for persons in need of services

Although it seems likely that all of these services would be of some help to abused elders and their families, the effectiveness of these interventions has not been systematically evaluated. As we discuss in the following section, experimental demonstration projects are needed to examine the relative success of each of the service options described in this section.

SUMMARY AND CONCLUSIONS: RECOMMENDATIONS FOR FUTURE RESEARCH

Rather than merely summarizing the information we have presented in earlier sections of this chapter, we will conclude with a set of recommendations for improving knowledge of elder abuse. Given the lack of firm research findings on elder abuse, we believe that it is more appropriate to make proposals for future research, rather than for practice and policy. The most critical need at present appears to be for information about the incidence and causes of elder abuse; without this, plans for intervention into the problem of elder abuse are, at best, educated guesses and at worst, opportunistic political compromises. In light of this observation, we propose eight recommendations for consideration in future investigations.[7] It should be noted that most of these recommendations are applicable to other forms of maltreatment besides physical abuse (e.g., psychological and material abuse, and neglect).

1. Researchers, policy makers, and practitioners should work intensively to develop more precise definitions of elder abuse and neglect. Much work needs to be done to develop clear and comprehensive definitions of elder abuse. In the absence of a uniform definition, it is of critical importance that researchers strive for clarity in the definitions they employ. In particular, simultaneous treatment of a variety of types of maltreatment under the term *elder abuse* has been a major flaw in previous research efforts. Abuse and neglect should be considered as separate phenomena, in that abuse is a conscious action toward another individual, whereas neglect is the failure to perform a caregiving activity or to provide for basic needs. Existing research indicates that differences exist between these two categories (Giordano, 1982; Wolf *et al.*, 1984).

Given the lack of consensus, it is possible that the question of how to define elder abuse could be treated as an empirical issue. One promising approach is to conduct vignette studies to determine the way in which professionals and the general public view elder abuse. Such studies present synopses (or vignettes) of maltreatment situations and ask respondents whether they consider each situation abusive (Rossi & Nock, 1982). Samples could be drawn from health professionals, social workers, and the elderly them-

[7]The following recommendations were developed in the context of the Research Conference on Elder Abuse and Neglect, held at the University of New Hampshire in October, 1985.

KARL PILLEMER and
J. JILL SUITOR

selves. Similar approaches have been used with considerable success to study other forms of abuse (Finkelhor, 1984). Although the results of these studies would not resolve the definitional problem, they would provide a basis for eventual agreement on a definition.

2. Studies should be conducted that involve direct interviews with victims rather than with professionals. The majority of previous studies have involved reviews of agency records or interviews with professionals who encounter elder abuse cases. Although this approach has provided valuable preliminary information, there is little justification for continuing to focus on professionals for information about elder abuse. Instead, studies should attempt whenever possible to interview victims directly. Professionals often have very different perceptions about an elder abuse situation than do the elderly persons themselves.

3. Perpetrators of elder abuse should be studied. To date, there have been no studies of persons who abuse elderly relatives. Evidence from research on other forms of family violence has shown that perpetrators may actually be somewhat more willing to discuss the abuse situation than the victims. Conducting research on victims alone provides only one part of the total picture. The perspectives of both parties are necessary to achieve a more complete understanding of elder maltreatment. In particular, studies in which the victim and the perpetrator are interviewed would allow for a much better understanding of the dynamics of elder abuse.

4. Studies should be designed to include comparison groups. Case-comparison studies are needed to identify possible causes of elder abuse. Such studies compare a group of abuse victims with a group of nonabused persons. Most existing studies have collected data on small samples of elder abuse victims drawn from intervention programs, after which attempts have been made to generalize from those samples to the larger elderly population. However, without a comparison group, it is impossible to determine the extent to which abuse victims differ from the elderly in general. For example, some studies have argued that poor health or functional impairment leads to elder abuse. Yet, many elderly people who are not abused have chronic conditions: we need to know whether abused elders are more often or more severely impaired than are nonabused elders.

5. A national incidence and prevalence survey of elder abuse and neglect should be conducted. As noted earlier, there is at present no reliable estimate of the extent of elder abuse. Without incidence or prevalence estimates, policymakers do not know how high a priority to give the problem. Although there are methodological difficulties in conducting such surveys, they have been carried out successfully with other forms of family violence (Finkelhor, 1984; Straus *et al.*, 1980). A nationwide survey is necessary, as there may be regional differences in the incidence of elder abuse.

6. Questions on elder abuse and neglect should be included in existing national surveys. In addition to conducting a national incidence survey, questions relating to elder abuse could be included in existing data collection. The most promising option in this area is the Health Interview Survey (HIS), in which a sample of the United States population is interviewed each year. The core elements of this survey cover various health problems and the utilization of health resources. However, each year there is a supplement to the HIS that varies according to current information needs. A series of items on elder abuse could be included in a future supplement. The precise nature of questions to be included would need to be carefully determined. As an example, the HIS routinely asks about any injuries respondents have sustained. For elderly respondents, it would be possible to ask, as a follow-up question, whether such injuries are abuse-related.

7. Existing intervention programs should be systematically evaluated. At present, we know very little regarding the effectiveness of various types of intervention into elder abuse cases. Virtually no research has been conducted on whether programs currently in operation actually benefit those they serve, or whether they may in fact have negative effects on clients. A high priority for researchers must be to use sophisticated evaluation research techniques to determine the impact of treatment programs. Without such careful evaluation, funds may be wasted on inappropriate services which fail to help—and may even harm—elder abuse victims and their families.

Most important, mandatory reporting laws are being passed in many states in the absence of any evidence of their effectiveness. The impact of these laws must be explored. Research possibilities include making comparisons between states with and without mandatory reporting and initiating demonstration projects within a state in which mandatory reporting would be introduced in selected regions. Results could then be compared to areas without such statutes. Further, existing state Adult Protective Services programs should be subjected to rigorous evaluation. New programs should include funds for such evaluations in their budgets, in order to minimize the risks of intervention to elderly persons.

8. Finally, it is essential to bring more sophisticated theoretical approaches to the study of elder abuse. We hope that this chapter demonstrates the importance of building on broader existing bodies of literature in the study of family relations and family violence. By conceiving of elder abuse as an extreme point on a continuum of family relations of older persons, which ranges from harmonious and supportive to highly conflictual and abusive, it will be possible to develop more powerful models to explain domestic violence against the elderly.

REFERENCES

Adams, B. (1968). *Kinship in an urban setting*. Chicago, IL: Markum.

Andrews, F. M., & Withey, S. B. (1976). *Social indicators of well-being: American perceptions of life quality.* New York: Plenum Press.

Bahr, S. J., Chappell, C. B., & Leigh, G. K. (1983). Age at marriage, role enactment, role consensus, and marital satisfaction. *Journal of Marriage and the Family, 45*, 795–804.

Barry, W. (1970). Marriage research and conflict: An integrative view. *Psychological Bulletin, 73*, 41–54.

Baruch, G., & Barnett, R. C. (1983). Adult daughters' relationships with their mothers. *Journal of Marriage and the Family, 45*, 601–606.

Billson, M., & Terry, M. B. (1982). In search of the silken purse: Factors in attrition among first-generation students. *College and University, 58*, 57–75.

Block, M., & Sinnott, J. (1979). *The battered elder syndrome study*. College Park, MD: Center on Aging.

Bowen, G. L., & Orthner, D. K. (1983). Sex-role congruency and marital quality. *Journal of Marriage and the Family, 45*, 795–804.

Breckman, R. (November, 1985). *Elder abuse intervention: The staircase model.* Paper presented at Annual Meeting of the Gerontological Society of America, New Orleans, LA.

Brody, M. (1985). Parent care as a normative family stress. *The Gerontologist, 25*, 19–29.

Bruce, J. M. (1970). Intragenerational occupational mobility and visiting with kin and friends. *Social Forces, 49*, 117–127.

Callahan, J. J. (March, 1981). Elder abuse programming: Will it help the elderly? Paper presented at the National Conference on the Abuse of Older Persons, Boston, MA.

Callender, W. (1982). *Improving protective services for older Americans: A national guide series*. Portland, ME: Center for Research and Advanced Study: University of Southern Maine.

Cantor, M. H. (1983). Strain among caregivers: A study of experience in the United States. *The Gerontologist, 23*, 597–604.

Chadwick, B. A., Albrecht, S. L., & Kunz, P. R. (1976). Marital and family role satisfaction. *Journal of Marriage and the Family, 38,* 431–440.

Cicirelli, V. (1981). *Helping elderly parents: Role of adult children.* Dover, MA: Auburn House.

Cicirelli, V. (1983a). Adult children and their elderly parents. In T. H. Brubaker (Ed.), *Family relationships in later life* (pp. 31–46). Beverly Hills, CA: Sage.

Cicirelli, V. (1983b). Adult children's attachment and helping behavior to elderly parents: A path model. *Journal of Marriage and the Family, 45,* 815–826.

Coleman, D., & Straus, M. (1983). Alcohol abuse and family violence. In E. Gottheil, K. A. Druley, T. E., Skolada, & H. M. Waxman (Eds.), *Alcohol, drug abuse and aggression* (pp. 104–121). Springfield, IL: Charles C. Thomas.

Crystal, S. (1986). Social policy and elder abuse. In K. Pillemer & R. S. Wolf (Eds.), *Elder abuse: Conflict in the family* (pp. 331–340). Dover, MA: Auburn House.

Davidson, B., Balswick, J., & Halverson, C. (1983). Affective self-disclosure and marital adjustment: A test of equity theory. *Journal of Marriage and the Family, 45,* 93–102.

Davidson, J. (1979). Elder abuse. In M. R. Block and J. D. Sinnott (Eds.), *The battered elder syndrome: An exploratory study* (pp. 49–55). College Park, MD: Center on Aging.

Douglass, R., Hickey, T., & Noel, C. (1980). *A study of maltreatment of the elderly and other vulnerable adults.* Ann Arbor, MI: University of Michigan Institute of Gerontology.

Faulkner, L. (1982). Mandating the reporting of suspected cases of elder abuse: An inappropriate, ineffective, and ageist response to the abuse of older adults. *Family Law Quarterly, 16,* 69–91.

Filsinger, E. E., & Wilson, M. R. (1984). Religiosity, socioeconomic rewards, and family development: Predictors of marital adjustment. *Journal of Marriage and the Family, 46,* 663–670.

Finkelhor, D. (1983). Common features of family abuse. In D. Finkelhor, R. J. Gelles, G. T. Hotaling, & M. Straus (Eds.), *The dark side of families: Current family violence research.* Beverly Hills, CA: Sage.

Finkelhor, D. (1984). *Child sexual abuse: New theory and research.* New York: Free Press.

Finkelhor, D., & Pillemer, K. (August, 1984). *Elder abuse: Its relationship to other forms of domestic violence.* Paper presented at the Second National Conference on Family Violence Research, Durham, NH.

Fischer, L. R. (1981). Transitions in the mother–daughter relationship. *Journal of Marriage and the Family, 43,* 613–622.

Gelles, R. (1972). *The violent home.* Beverly Hills, CA: Sage.

Gelles, R. (1974). Child abuse as psychopathology: A sociological critique and reformulation. In S. Steinmetz & M. Straus (Eds.), *Violence in the family* (pp. 190–204). New York: Dodd, Mead.

Gelles, R., & Straus, M. (1979). Determinants of violence in the family: Toward a theoretical integration. In W. R. Burr, R. Hill, F. I. Nye, & I. L. Reiss (Eds.), *Contemporary theories about the family* (Vol. 1, pp. 549–581). New York: Free Press.

Gil, D. (1971). *Violence against children: Physical child abuse in the United States.* Cambridge, MA: Harvard University Press.

Gioglio, G., & Blakemore, P. (1983). *Elder abuse in New Jersey: The knowledge and experience of abuse among older New Jerseyans.* Trenton, NJ: New Jersey Department of Human Services.

Giordano, N. H. (1982). *Individual and family correlates of elder abuse.* Unpublished doctoral dissertation, University of Georgia.

Glenn, N. D., & Weaver, C. N. (1981). The contribution of marital happiness to global happiness. *Journal of Marriage and the Family, 43,* 161–168.

Hennesey, S. (1979). Child abuse. In M. R. Block & J. D. Sinnott (Eds.), *The battered elder syndrome: An exploratory study* (pp. 19–32). College Park, MD: Center on Aging.

Hicks, M., & Platt, M. (1970). Marital happiness and stability: A review of the research in the 60s. *Journal of Marriage and the Family, 32,* 553–574.

Hotaling, G. T., & Sugarman, D. (1986). An analysis of risk markers in husband to wife violence: The current state of knowledge. *Violence and Victims, 1,* 101–124.

Houser, B. B., & Berkman, S. L. (1984). Aging parent/mature child relationships. *Journal of Marriage and the Family, 46,* 295–299.

House Select Committee on Aging (1981). *Elder abuse: An examination of a hidden problem.* Washington, DC: Government Printing Office.

House Select Committee on Aging (May 10, 1985). *Elder abuse: A national disgrace.* (Executive Summary). Washington, DC: Government Printing Office.

Hudson, M., & Johnson, T. (1987). Elder neglect and abuse: A review of the literature. In C. Eisdorfer (Ed.), *Annual review of gerontology.* New York: Springer.

Hwalek, M., Sengstock, M., & Lawrence, R. (November, 1984). *Assessing the probability of abuse of the elderly.* Paper presented at the Annual Meeting of the Gerontological Society of America, San Antonio, TX.

Johnson, E. S. (1978). "Good" relationships between older mothers and their daughters: A causal model. *The Gerontologist, 18,* 301–306.

Johnson, E. S., & Bursk, B. J. (1977). Relationships between the elderly and their children. *The Gerontologist, 17,* 90–96.

Johnson, T., Hudson, M., & O'Brien, J. (1985). *Elder neglect and abuse: An annotated bibliography.* Westport, CT: Greenwood Press.

Johnson, T. F. (1986). Critical issues in the definition of elder mistreatment. In K. Pillemer & R. S. Wolf (Eds.), *Elder abuse: Conflict in the family* (pp. 167–196). Dover, MA: Auburn House.

Justice, B., & Justice, R. (1976). *The abusing family.* New York: Human Sciences Press.

Kantor, G., & Straus, M. (April, 1986). *Alcohol and family violence.* Paper presented at the National Alcoholism Conference on Alcohol and the Family, San Francisco, CA.

Komarovsky, M. (1962). *Blue-collar marriage.* New York: Random House.

Kosberg, J. I. (Ed.). (1983). *Abuse and maltreatment of the elderly: Causes and Interventions.* Littleton, MA: John Wright, PSG.

Kulys, R., & Tobin, S. (1980). Older people and their "responsible others." *Social Work, 25,* 138–145.

Larson, J. H. (1984). The effect of husband's unemployment on marital and family relations in blue-collar families. *Family Relations, 33,* 503–511.

Lau, E., & Kosberg, J. (1979). Abuse of the elderly by informal care providers. *Aging,* September/October, 10–15.

Lee, G. R. (1978). Marriage and morale in later life. *Journal of Marriage and the Family, 40,* 131–139.

Levinger, G., & Breedlove, I. (1966). Interpersonal attitude and agreement: A study of marriage partners. *Journal of Personality and Social Psychology, 3,* 367–372.

Medling, J. M., & McCarrey, M. (1981). Marital adjustment over segments of the family life cycle: The issue of spouses' value similarity. *Journal of Marriage and the Family, 43,* 195–203.

Mindel, C. H., & Wright, R. (1982). Satisfaction in multigenerational households. *Journal of Gerontology, 37,* 483–489.

Nye, F. I., & McLaughlin, S. (1976). Role competence and marital satisfaction. In F. I. Nye (Ed.), *Role structure and analysis of the family* (pp. 191–205). Beverly Hills, CA: Sage.

Nye, F. I. (1979). Choice, exchange, and the family. In W. R. Burr, P. Hill, F. I. Nye, & I. L. Reiss (Eds.), *Contemporary theories about the family* (Vol. 2, pp. 1–41). New York: The Free Press.

O'Malley, H., Segars, H., Perez, R., Mitchell, V., & Knuepfel, G. (1979). *Elder abuse in Massachusetts: A survey of professionals and paraprofessionals.* Boston, MA: Legal Research and Services for the Elderly, Unpublished manuscript.

Pedrick-Cornell, C., & Gelles, R. (1982). Elderly abuse: The status of current knowledge. *Family Relations, 31,* 457–465.

Phillips, L. (1983). Abuse and neglect of the frail elderly at home: An exploration of theoretical relationships. *Journal of Advanced Nursing, 8,* 379–392.

Pillemer, K. (1985a). *Domestic violence against the elderly: A case-control study.* Unpublished doctoral dissertation, Department of Sociology, Brandeis University.

Pillemer, K. (1985b). The dangers of dependency: New findings on domestic violence against the elderly. *Social Problems, 33,* 146–158.

Pillemer, K. (1985c). Social isolation and elder abuse. *Response to the victimization of women and children,* Fall, 1–4.

Piorkowski, G. K. (1983). Survival guilt in the university setting. *Personnel and Guidance Journal, 61,* 620–622.

Rossi, P. H., & Nock, S. L. (1982). *Measuring social judgements: The factorial survey approach.* Beverly Hills, CA: Sage.

Sager, A. (1974). *Learning the home care needs of the elderly.* Brandeis University, Florence Heller School.

Salend, E., Kane, R. A., & Satz, M. (1984). Elder abuse reporting: Limitations of statutes. *Gerontologist, 24,* 61–69.

Sedge, S. (1979). Spouse abuse. In M. Block & J. Sinnott (Eds.), *The battered elder syndrome* (pp. 33–48). College Park, MD: Center on Aging.

Sengstock, M., & Liang, J. (1982). *Identifying and characterizing elder abuse.* Detroit, MI: Wayne State University, Institute of Gerontology, unpublished manuscript.

Sherman, L. W., & Berk, R. A. (April, 1984). *The Minneapolis domestic violence experiment*. Police Foundation Reports, 1.

Simmons, S., & Ball, S. E. (1984). Marital adjustment in couples married before and after spinal cord injury. *Journal of Marriage and the Family, 46*, 943–945.

Stark, E., Flitcraft, A., & Frazier, W. (1979). Medicine and patriarchal violence: The social construction of a "private" event. *International Journal of Health Services, 9*, 461–493.

Steinmetz, S. (1983). Dependency, stress, and violence between middle-aged caregivers and their elderly parents. In J. I. Kosberg (Ed.), *Abuse and maltreatment of the elderly* (pp. 134–139). Littleton, MA: John Wright PSG.

Steinmetz, S., & Amsden, D. J. (1983). Dependent elders, family stress, and abuse. In T. H. Brubaker (Ed.), *Family relationships in later life* (pp. 173–192). Beverly Hills, CA: Sage Publications, Inc.

Straus, M. (1979). Measuring intrafamily conflict and violence: The Conflict Tactics (CT) Scales. *Journal of Marriage and the Family, 41*, 75–88.

Straus, M., Gelles, R., & Steinmetz, S. (1980). *Behind closed doors: Violence in the American family*. New York: Doubleday.

Straus, M. A., & Gelles, R. J. (1986). Societal change and change in family violence from 1975 to 1985 as revealed by two national surveys. *Journal of Marriage and the Family, 48*, 1–15.

Suitor, J. J. (August, 1984). *Marital happiness among returning women students and their husbands: Differential effects of part-time and full-time enrollment*. Paper presented at the Annual Meeting of the American Sociological Association, San Antonio, TX.

Suitor, J. J. (1987). Mother-daughter relations when married daughters return to school: Effects of status similarity. *Journal of Marriage and the Family, 49*, 435–444.

Thompson, L., & Walker, A. J. (1984). Mothers and daughters: Aid patterns and attachment. *Journal of Marriage and the Family, 46*, 313–322.

U. S. Bureau of the Census (1985). *Statistical abstract of the United States, 1984*. Washington, DC: U.S. Government Printing Office.

Walker, L. (1978). Battered women and learned helplessness. *Victimology, 2*, 525–534.

Ward, R. A. (1984). *The aging experience*. New York: Harper and Row.

Wilson, M. R., & Filsinger, R. E. (1986). Religiosity and marital adjustment: Multidimensional relationships. *Journal of Marriage and the Family, 48*, 147–152.

Wolf, R., Godkin, M., & Pillemer, K. (1984). *Elder abuse and neglect: Findings from three model projects*. Worcester, MA: University of Massachusetts Medical Center, University Center on Aging.

Wolf, R., Strugnell, C., & Godkin, M. (1982). *Preliminary findings from three model projects on elderly abuse*. Worcester, MA: University of Massachusetts Medical Center.

Yin, P. (1985). *Victimization and the Aged*. Springfield, IL: Charles C. Thomas.

Yogev, S., & Brett, J. (1985). Perceptions of the division of housework and child care and marital satisfaction. *Journal of Marriage and the Family, 47*, 609–618.

Young, M., & Willmott, P. (1957). *Family and kinship in East London*. Baltimore, MD: Penguin.

12

Family Homicide

When Victimized Women Kill

ANGELA BROWNE

INTRODUCTION

A woman calls the police emergency number, begging for help. She says she just shot her husband. Officers who arrive at the scene note that she is bruised and there is some evidence of an altercation. While ambulance attendants work on the dying man, police locate the weapon and test the woman's hands for traces of gunpowder. They wrap her hands in plastic and lead her to a squad car, threading their way around neighbors gathered on the sidewalk. The woman is taken to jail, where she is interrogated about what happened. She attempts to reply to the officers' questioning, although her responses are disoriented and confused and she will later remember little of what she said. At some point, she is informed that her husband is dead. She is asked to strip to the waist so that pictures can be taken of her injuries and is booked on suspicion of first degree murder. Later testimony reveals that she had been beaten and sexually assaulted by her mate for several years, and that he threatened to kill her shortly before the shooting took place. In recent months, she made several attempts to get help. She has no prior criminal record; she has a family, and has held a steady job.

Neighbors are shocked by the killing. Such things do not happen in their part of town. Relatives are grieved and defensive. They struggle with what they will say when questioned; what to say in court, when the private lives of their family become front page news. His family, who knew the most about his abusiveness, are in the worst position: Will they aid in this woman's defense, when she has just killed their son or brother? Could they have prevented it? Should they have done something more? Was his drinking to blame? Or was it her fault, for staying with him? They knew he sometimes hit her, but no one ever dreamed she would kill him.

Portions of this chapter have also appeared in *Advances in Applied Social Psychology* (Vol. 3). M. Sakes & L. Saxe (Eds.), Hillsdale, NJ: Erlbaum, 1986.

ANGELA BROWNE • Family Violence Laboratory, Horton Social Science Center, University of New Hampshire, Durham, NH 03824.

What leads a woman who has occupied the role of victim and who usually has no history of violent, or even illegal, behavior to use deadly force against her mate? What factors in an abusive relationship precipitate a homicide committed by the woman? And what factors—in the woman's perceptions, in the relationship, and in our society—contribute to her remaining with a man who assaults her or threatens to take her life?

This chapter presents a picture of battered women who kill, the violence they live with, and the pattern of events that leads them to homicide. Data are based on information drawn from the author's study of 42 women who were facing charges for murder or attempted murder in the death or serious injury of their mates. Dynamics in the relationships of these women are compared to those of a group of women who had been involved in abusive relationships in which no lethal incident had occurred, resulting in the identification of factors that indicate high risk for a lethal incident perpetrated by the victim. A theoretical framework is suggested for how the women's perceptions lead them to such a drastic alternative. Further, parallels between responses of abused women to their situation and those of other types of victims are noted. The chapter also includes a discussion of the contributions that social exchange and social judgment theories can make to our understanding of victimized women's choices and their evolution from predominantly passive responses to the suddenly active one of homicide.

Research on Violence between Partners

Little is known about those cases in which an abusive relationship culminates in the death of a spouse. The study of physical violence among family members is still in its infancy. It was not until the 1960s that researchers even began to talk about child abuse in families (Kempe, Silverman, Steele, Drogemueller, & Silver, 1962). At that time, there were almost no reports on abused wives, and those that existed attributed the abuse to personality disorders in both the perpetrator and the victim (e.g., Schultz, 1960; Snell, Rosenwald, & Robey, 1964). In the early 1970s, Murray Straus, Richard Gelles, and others began extensive research on family violence from a sociological point of view (Gelles, 1974, 1979; Straus, 1971, 1973; Straus, Gelles, & Steinmetz, 1980), and the prevalence of spouse abuse began to receive serious attention. (For a more complete review of the research on family violence during this period, see Gelles, 1980.) The first significant publications on the topic of wife abuse were Erin Pizzey's *Scream Quietly or the Neighbors Will Hear* (published in England in 1974), and Del Martin's *Battered Wives* (published in the United States in 1976).

Much of the early writing on battered women was theoretical, based on impressions gained from working with women in shelters or clinical practice, or on sociological theories relating wife abuse to society's general discrimination against women (Chapman & Gates, 1978; Hilberman & Munson, 1978; Roy, 1977). In 1979, Lenore Walker's *The Battered Woman* was published, based on her clinical experience and using social learning theory as a basis for understanding abused women's reactions to violence. Irene Frieze and her colleagues began to apply attribution theory to women's perceptions of their abusive relationships and to study types of battered women (Frieze, 1979; Washburn & Frieze, 1980). Walker also undertook an intensive survey study, interviewing over 400 respondents from six states (Walker, 1981, 1984). Still, these investigations did not attempt to explore the nature of severe violence or to inquire into those relationships that ended in death; although data on murder cases in the United States indicate that many spousal homicides are preceded by a history of abuse and that women jailed for slaying their mates often have been assaulted by them (Bourdouris, 1971; Chimbos, 1978; Lindsey, 1978; Stephens, 1977; Totman, 1978). Despite their importance, the dynamics in abusive relationships that result in such extreme denouements were still unknown.

Widows by Their Own Hand

In May of 1980, I began work as a consultant to defense attorneys on legal cases in which abused women were charged with the death or serious injury of their abusive mates.[1] I remember some of what I was thinking the morning of my first interview with one of those women. What would it be like to spend the day with someone who had killed another person? What would she say? How would she act? She turned out to be a lot like other women I knew—like friends or family, like women in general, except that she had lived through an experience that, even to her, seemed unimaginable. I began looking for books to read about women who kill partners, or even about partners who kill partners. I found only two (Chimbos, 1978; Totman, 1978). It seemed that the place to learn was from the women themselves. For the next 3 years, I conducted interviews with accused women, read corroborating documents, worked with their attorneys, and followed the outcome of their trials. Their stories were unusual and little known. However, given the incidence of homicides between partners and the frequency with which a history of abuse is a factor, they can not be called unique.

Stacey and Shupe (1983) contend that "no society of any consequence can survive if its family institution crumbles from within" (p. 203). Research on relationships that include severe battering between adult intimates constitutes only part of the picture of violence within the family. The fear and devastation in these homes spawns wider and wider rings of impact in our society—from the children whose relationships are affected (and who, in turn, affect the lives of their families), to the taxpayer whose dollars support the prosecution of offenders and pay for intervention needed by the victims and other troubled family members. The cost, in terms of resources, human life, and suffering, is far too high.

Assault and Homicide at Home

Early studies on criminal victimization focused primarily on violent incidents occurring outside of the home. Most of these studies were conducted with incarcerated offenders, and there was a strong tendency to label these individuals as comfortably different than the rest of society. Their problems were seen as coming from an unusual home background, "unique" in violence or disorder; or as attributable to a medical or psychological condition, which then provided a pathological explanation for their behavior. Newspapers and other media emphasized the more sensational crimes and criminals, and a common impression was formed that the risk of personal injury lay in individuals outside one's circle of intimates. Assault was believed to occur primarily on the streets of cities or in barroom brawls, murders and rapes were committed by deranged strangers on the unsuspecting, and a discussion of child molestation called up the image of a "dirty old man" lurking near a park or gradeschool playground. Crimes that did occur within the family were rarely reported, and those that became known were seen as oddities. The average family, it was assumed, afforded nurturance and protection to its members. Those

[1]This work was done as part of a consulting team at Walker & Associates in Denver, Colorado.

individuals who left their homes and families were sometimes stigmatized, forcibly returned, or punished.

Yet, current evidence forces us to suspect that a hidden reservoir of criminal victimization has existed almost unnoticed, and in fact has been given permission to thrive within our culture. The 1980 National Crime Survey compared violent crimes involving intimates with crimes involving strangers and noted that, whereas the victim was injured 54% of the time when the attacker was a stranger, three fourths of the victims sustained injuries when their attacker was related. Three fifths of the attacks by relatives occurred at night, so most of these victims were "safe at home" at the time of the assault. Estimates on the number of children that are physically abused by parents range from 3.5% to 14% (e.g., National Study of the Incidence and Severity of Child Abuse and Neglect, 1981; Straus *et al.*, 1980). Even if one used the 3.5% estimate, that would still be 1.7 million physically battered children per year.

Estimates of the incidence of violence between adult partners are just as alarming. In a national survey of over 2,000 homes, conducted in 1975 and published in 1980, more than one-quarter of married couples reported at least one instance of physical abuse between them (Straus *et al.*, 1980); 16% reported violence in the year prior to the study. Over one third of these incidents were serious assaults involving acts such as punching, kicking, hitting with an object, and assaults with a knife or a gun. A follow-up survey, conducted in 1985, found the exact same percentage reporting violent incidents in the twelve months prior to that study (Straus & Gelles, 1986). These results are supported by a Harris (1979) poll conducted in Kentucky, using similar questions, which found that 21% of the 1,793 women respondents reported at least one physical attack by a male partner. (This would project to 169,000 women in that state alone.) Over two thirds of women who had been separated or divorced during the previous year reported violence occurring in that relationship. Although the majority of respondents in these studies did not report violence, these estimates still mean that *over a million-and-a-half women in the United States are physically assaulted by a male partner each year.* Of course, such figures are prone to substantial underreporting. Still, they refute the image of the family as the predictably safe haven it was once thought to be.

Although threatening or attacking another person is illegal, when it happens within a family, the episodes rarely come to the attention of authorities. Even if the assaults are reported, they are often not accorded the serious treatment given to similar attacks by strangers. Harris (1979) found that 43% of the women who had been abused told no one, and only 4% of the reported assaults resulted in court action. Studies show that the rate of prosecution and conviction in criminal cases drops sharply when there is a current or prior relationship between the victim and assailant (Field & Field, 1973; U. S. Commission on Civil Rights, 1982). It is often only when someone is seriously injured or killed that strict action is taken; battered women reporting attacks on threats by spouses are familiar with being referred for personal mental health treatment, or asked why they do not leave home, rather than being assisted with effective and case-appropriate alternatives. Left without adequate recourse, some family altercations continue to escalate in severity until they result in death.

Homicides between Partners

The rate of homicide among families in the United States is quite high when compared to that of many other countries; higher, for instance, than the rate for all homicides in countries such as England, Denmark, and Germany (Straus, 1985). Nearly one fourth of the nation's homicide victims in 1984 were related to their assailants: 4,408 murders in that one year were committed by family members. Of homicides occurring within the family, by far the largest category is that of a spouse killing a spouse. In 1984, nearly half (48%) of intrafamilial homicides, or the deaths of over 2,000 people, were between partners. Of these, the majority of the victims were women: Two thirds (1,310) were wives killed by husbands, and one third (806) were husbands killed by wives.

Women do not usually kill other people; they perpetrate less than 15% of the homicides in the United States (Jones, 1980; Uniform Crime Reports, 1983). When women do kill, it is often in their own defense. A report by a government commission on violence estimated that homicides committed by women were seven times as likely to be in self-defense as homicides committed by men (Crimes of Violence, 1969).

In his classic study of criminal homicide, Wolfgang (1967) noted that 60% of the husbands who were killed by wives "precipitated" their own deaths (i.e., were the first to use physical force, strike blows, or threaten with a weapon), whereas victim precipitation was involved in only 9% of the deaths of wives. A review of police records on spousal homicides in Canada found that almost all of the wives who had killed their mates had previously been beaten by them (Chimbos, 1978). In such cases, it is the abusive mate who becomes the final victim.

Women charged in the death of a mate have the least extensive criminal records of any female offenders. However, they often face harsher penalties than men who kill their partners. FBI statistics indicate that fewer men are charged with first or second degree murder for killing a woman they have known than are women who kill a man they have known. And women convicted of these murders are frequently sentenced to longer prison terms than are men (Schneider & Jordan, 1981). The following case serves to illustrate the discrepancies in attitudes that may lead to this uneven sentencing:

> In 1978, an Indiana prosecutor, James Kizer, refused to prosecute for murder a man who beat and kicked his ex-wife to death in the presence of a witness and raped her as she lay dying. Filing a manslaughter charge instead, Kizer commented, "He didn't mean to kill her. He just meant to give her a good thumping." (Jones, 1980, p. 308)

In contrast, each of the women in the present investigation had a documented history of physical abuse by the man she slayed. In many cases, the files contained police photographs of the woman's injuries at the time of her arrest, and in some instances the woman was taken to a hospital for x-rays or treatment, prior to being transported to jail. All of the women reported that they had been threatened by the abuser and that the incident occurred in an attempt to protect themselves or a child from further harm.

Yet, of the 36 women whose husbands died, all but nine were charged with first degree murder; none was charged with manslaughter. Results of the study give some insight into the seriousness of domestic violence, and highlight how a lack of adequate responsiveness to early contacts with these cases exacerbates the dangers already existent in the situation.

APPROACH TO A STUDY OF HOMICIDE

The purpose of the investigation was to learn more about severely abusive relationships and the perspectives of women involved in them and to see if particular factors discriminated between abusive relationships in which no lethal incident occurred and those that culminated in homicide by a woman victim. The study focused on the women's actions (e.g., the killing of a mate) in the context of their perceptions based on prior physical assaults by that partner, and the impact that the abuse and situational or societal variables had on their assessment of the danger and of alternatives available to them. This effort is exploratory and results should not be treated as representative of all spousal homicides in which a woman kills her mate.[2] It may have general relevance, however, for cases in which a woman kills a man who has been abusing her over a period of time. (See Browne, 1987, for a more complete discussion of the homicide study, as well as quantitative and qualitative findings).

The Sample

The 42 women in the homicide group had been charged with a crime in the death or serious injury of their mates. Initial contact with them was made when their attorneys requested an evaluation based on some evidence that the woman had been battered by the deceased. These women came from 15 different states, and seven were incarcerated awaiting trial at the time of the interview. Thirty-three were charged with murder, three with conspiracy to commit murder, and six with attempted murder. (In reporting the results of this study, no distinction is made between women who were charged with murder and those charged with attempted murder or conspiracy, because the same dynamics seemed to apply to both types of cases; see also Chimbos, 1978.) Of the women who went to trial after the interview, 20 (about half) received jail terms, 12 were given probation or a suspended sentence, and 9 (less than one quarter) were acquitted. In one case, the district attorney's office determined that the killing was justified on the grounds of self-defense and dropped the charges. Jail sentences ranged from 6 months to 25 years, and one woman was sentenced to 50 years.

It is difficult to find an appropriate comparison group for abused women who were not identified as battered until they committed a homicide in response to the violence. In the present study, the nonhomicide group was drawn from data collected on a subset ($n = 205$) of women interviewed in a previous research study.[3] The sample was generated using referral sources (e.g., mental health centers, shelters, private practitioners, emergency rooms) and direct advertising, including public service announcements on radio and television, newspaper ads, and posted notices. Subjects were self-identified and self-referred, and were considered eligible to participate if they reported being physically abused at least twice by a man with whom they had an ongoing intimate relationship or to whom they had been married. These women came from a six-state region of the United States and were from both urban and rural areas.[4] They were either still in the abusive relationship (e.g., living with their partner) at the time of the interview, or had been out of the relationship less than one year.

Physical abuse was defined as any assaultive or coercive physical act by one person against another, with or without evident resultant injury. Psychological abuse included factors such as excessive possessiveness or jealousy, restriction of normal activity, sur-

[2]Random sampling procedures are not feasible when studying battered women who have killed their abusers, because the general incidence in the population is so low. Thus, statistical significance must be interpreted cautiously. Significant findings do indicate, however, a relatively large difference or relationship in the data.
[3]NIMH grant #R01MH30147, Lenore E. Walker, Principal Investigator.
[4]Health and Human Services Region VIII.

veillance, enforced sleep deprivation, extreme verbal harassment, threats of future physical abuse, and threats to kill. Actions such as Russian roulette or forcing the women to watch while a pet animal was killed were also included under psychological abuse. All subjects had experienced at least two physically abusive incidents; most of the women in both groups reported at least four. Nearly all of the women in the homicide sample were living with their partners at the time of the incident, although a few had been separated from their mates for up to 2 years prior to the homicide.

The Questionnaire

A semistructured questionnaire was used to gather data on the homicide and nonhomicide cases. This allowed for the systematic collection of information, while also giving an opportunity for the interviewee to fill in details and background that might not otherwise have been obtained. The questionnaire included a section on the woman's family of origin, her relationship with her parents, and any previous physical or sexual abuse she may have experienced. General questions were asked about the background of the abusive mate and about typical interactions in her relationship with him. In addition, women were asked to give a narrative account of four specific battering incidents: the first occurrence of violence in the relationship, a "typical" violent incident, a subsequent incident that was one of the most frightening to the woman, and the last violent incident prior to our interview. (These incidents are referred to as first, second, third, and fourth; but although they occurred in that order, the time lapse between them—and the number of other abusive episodes that may have occurred in the interim—varied by case.) By asking about these four incidents, it was possible to assess more accurately the severity and escalation of the violence, and to look for patterns in abusive relationships over time. The interview was quite extensive and took 8 to 10 hours to complete. Although this was a taxing process for both subject and interviewer, it yielded a wealth of data about a little-known area. Also, the opportunity to place the events in context seemed to be therapeutic for most women.

Self-Report Issues

The reliability of self-report data is often questioned, although all research done on victims is, by nature, retrospective self-report. This is of special concern in homicide cases, however, when one can no longer learn the deceased's version of the story and the survivor is facing criminal charges in relation to the incident. In the present study, extensive use was made of police reports, hospital records, and witness statements to verify the women's accounts. Interestingly, it was actually easier to document women's stories in the homicide cases than in the nonhomicide group, because private records became available and witnesses came forward to testify when they were no longer afraid of retaliation by the abuser. When discrepancies were found, it was usually in the direction of understatement. Women who had been battered over a period of time forgot some incidents (which were uncovered through hospital records, witness reports, and other sources) and were often reluctant to report the mate's sexual abuse of a child or their own physical or sexual abuse in childhood, for fear of doing damage to other family members. Some women also were reluctant to describe severe physical and sexual abuse out of a sense of shame, or for fear others would think they were crazy.

Contributions of the Study

In previous investigations of homicide between partners, information was gathered on survivors who were convicted of a crime in the death of their mates (Chimbos, 1978; Totman, 1978; Wolfgang, 1958, 1967). Most of these subjects were incarcerated or had previously served time in jail for the offense. However, studying only those adjudicated guilty often produces biases in the data. Cases that result in acquittals are not included, nor are cases in which the charges are dropped. In the present study, half of the cases would not have been tapped in a survey conducted only with incarcerated populations. In addition, previous samples were drawn from a particular geographical area, which also may contribute to bias. In the current study, further diversity was added by drawing subjects from different areas of the country. Results of this study indicate that certain factors are strongly associated with abusive relationships that culminate in homicide. Knowledge of these factors may aid in identification of cases at particularly high risk, and could be used as a guide to intervention and a basis for social policy recommendations.

RESULTS OF A COMPARATIVE STUDY

Few demographic differences were found between women in the two groups. Women in the homicide group were a few years older on the average (36 vs. 31 years of age), and had slightly larger families (2.3 vs. 1.97 children) and more relationships with men (2.5 vs. 1.3). They also had slightly more battering relationships with men: 1.5 versus 1.3 for the nonhomicide group, including the one on which they were reporting. There were no significant differences in the length of the relationships, however: 80% of the women in both groups were married to the abuser, with the average length of the marriage being 6.9 years for the homicide group and 7.7 years for the nonhomicide group. Over half (66%) of the women in the homicide group and 76% of women in the nonhomicide group were white, with Spanish Americans, Chicanos, blacks, and Native Americans also represented. (There were no Native Americans in the homicide sample.) Women in the homicide group came from slightly higher class backgrounds, but the nonhomicide group had somewhat more formal education (12.2 vs. 11.8 years of schooling—not a significant difference). Nearly half of the homicide group and 33% of the nonhomicide group were employed most or all of the time during their relationship with the batterer.

Comparisons Involving the Women's Mates

There were no significant differences in the men's class of origin, with 87% of men in the homicide group and 93% of men in the nonhomicide group coming from lower- or working-class families. Women in the homicide group tended to come from a higher class background than their mates, but there were no significant differences between women and men in the nonhomicide group. Men in the nonhomicide group were significantly more educated (averaging 11.7 years of schooling vs. 10.6 years for men in the homicide group). In both groups, the women were better educated than their mates. Employment patterns were not significantly different between the men, with 48% of men in the homicide group and 53% of men in the nonhomicide group employed during most of the relationship. There were no significant differences between time employed for couples in the homicide group, with less than half of both women and men being employed most or all of the time. However, in the nonhomicide group significantly more men than women were fully employed.

Childhood Experiences with Violence

Nearly 71% of women in the homicide group and 65% in the nonhomicide group reported that they had been the victims of and/or witnessed physical abuse in their family of origin. This included seeing their mother physically abused by a father or father surrogate, witnessing parental abuse of siblings, abuse of themselves by parents, and abuse from other relatives. Sexual assault during childhood was also frequently reported: 57% of women in the homicide group and 54% in the nonhomicide group reported at least one completed or attempted sexual assault as a child. Most of these were intrafamilial, perpetrated by a father, stepfather, mother's boyfriend, brother, or other male relative. Threats and beatings also sometimes accompanied these incidents. Although the reported incidence of these occurrences is high, these experiences did not differentiate between the two groups of women. Women also reported that their mates had come from abusive homes. Eighty-four percent of the men in the nonhomicide group had reportedly witnessed or been the victims of abuse during childhood. In the homicide group, 18% of the women did not know that information about the childhood of their mates, but of those who did, 91% reported abuse occurring in the man's childhood home.

Significant Differences in Behavior of the Men

Differences between the men in the homicide and nonhomicide groups emerged on four variables: drug use, alcohol use, arrest records, and child abuse. The use of both prescription and street drugs was much higher for men in the homicide group. For example, it was reported that 29% of the men used street drugs every or almost every day by the end of the relationship, whereas only 7.5% of men in the nonhomicide group were reported to use street drugs that often. Even stronger differences were found in the men's drinking patterns. Eighty percent of the men in the homicide group reportedly became intoxicated every day or almost every day, compared to 40% in the nonhomicide group. There were also significant differences in the percentage of men who had been arrested. Over three quarters (77%) of men in the nonhomicide group had been arrested (for offenses ranging from drunk driving to murder), whereas 92% of the men in the homicide group had a past history of arrest. The incidence of child abuse was also significantly higher for men in the homicide group: 71% reportedly abused the children as well as their partner, compared to 51% in the nonhomicide group. Some of this abuse also involved the sexual assault of a child.

Comparison of Abusive Acts, Resultant Injuries, and Threats

Women were asked about: (a) specific violent acts that occurred during each of the four battering incidents for which information was gathered, (b) the outcome, in terms of injuries, and (c) the frequency with which these incidents occurred. Typical battering episodes involved a combination of violent acts, verbal attacks, and threats. Types of physical abuse ranged from being slapped, punched, kicked, or hurled bodily, to being choked, smothered, or bitten. Women reported attacks in which they were beaten with an object, injured with a weapon, scalded with hot liquid, or held underwater. Although slightly more violent acts were reported by women in the homicide group, the difference was not significant. There were, however, major differences in the severity of resultant injuries. Women in the homicide group were significantly more injured in both the second (a typical) and third (one of the worst) incidents, and overall sustained more, and more severe, injuries than did women in the nonhomicide group. Types of injuries ranged from bruises, cuts, and black eyes to concussions, broken bones, and miscarriages caused by beatings. Permanent injuries included damage to joints, partial loss of hearing or vision, and scarring from burns, bites, or knife wounds. The frequency with which abusive incidents occurred also proved to be quite different for the two groups: nearly 40% of women in the homicide group reported that abusive incidents occurred more than once a week by the end of the relationship, whereas only 13% of women in the nonhomicide group reported that frequency.

Another important difference between the groups was in threats to kill. Eighty-three percent of men in the homicide group reportedly threatened to kill someone other than themselves, compared to 59% of men in the nonhomicide group. Over 61% of women in the homicide group, and 51% in the nonhomicide group, also reported that their mates had threatened to commit suicide (this difference was not significant). There were also significant differences in threats made by the women. Nine percent of women in the nonhomicide group said that they had threatened to kill their abuser, whereas 22% of the homicide group said that they had made that threat, usually as a warning about him hurting them or a child any further. Almost half of the women in the homicide group had threatened to commit suicide, compared to 31% of the nonhomicide group.

Sexual Assault by the Partner

Sexual assault by a partner was another area in which highly significant differences emerged. Over 75% of the women in the homicide group reported that they were forced to have sexual intercourse on at least one occasion, compared with 59% of the nonhomicide group. In the homicide group, if it happened at all, it usually happened more than just once or twice: 14% said it occurred one to three times, 22% said more than three times, and 39% said they were raped "often." Only 13% of the nonhomicide group said that rape occurred often, whereas 27% said it occurred from one to three times. Nearly 62% of the homicide group also reported that their mates had forced or urged them to perform other sexual acts against their will, compared to 37% of the nonhomicide group. These acts included the insertion of objects in the woman's vagina, forced anal or oral sex, bondage, forced sex with others, and sex with animals. One woman reported being raped with her husband's service revolver, a broom handle, and a wire brush. Some sexual assaults were quite severe and involved a combination of sexual and other physical abuse and threats. Often they lasted for hours and resulted in the woman being severely injured and psychologically devastated.

Comparison of Relationships over Time

The majority of men showed remorse or sorrow after abusive incidents, although these percentages declined over time. This decline was especially precipitous for men in the homicide group: over 87% reportedly showed sorrow after the first incident, 73% after the second incident, and only 58% after the third—or one of the worst—incidents. In contrast to the decline in contrition, it was found that, for both groups, the abuse tended to become more severe as the relationship progressed. Again, there were significant differences between the homicide and nonhomicide groups. Nearly 80% of women in the homicide group reported that the abuse worsened over time, compared to 58% of women who reported this pattern in the nonhomicide group.

Summary of Findings

To summarize the significant differences, then, men in the homicide group used drugs and alcohol more often than men in the nonhomicide group, and were arrested more often. The incidence of child abuse by men in the homicide group was also significantly higher. Battering of women partners was more frequent in the homicide group, and the resulting injuries more severe. More men in the homicide group than the nonhomicide group threatened to kill someone other than themselves, whereas more women in the homicide group threatened to kill themselves or their mate. The incidence of rape and other forced or threatened sexual activities was also much higher in the homicide than the nonhomicide group. Comparing abusive relationships over time, the physical abuse tended to become more severe in both the homicide and nonhomicide groups, but such increases were much more common in the homicide group, while the decline in reported contrition was more precipitous.

In order to place the major variables in a single picture, a discriminant function analysis was conducted using all of the abuse-related variables for which between-group differences reached the .001 significance level. This analysis identified seven variables that, in linear combination, best discriminated between women who had a history of abuse by their partners and finally seriously injured or killed them, and women who were abused by their mates but did not take lethal action against them. Variables that best predicted membership in the homicide group included severity of the woman's injuries, the man's drug use and frequency of intoxication, the frequency with which abusive incidents occurred, forced or threatened sexual acts by the man, the woman's suicide threats, and the man's threats to kill.

In talking about their relationships with their partners, women in the homicide group reported that they had felt hopelessly trapped in a desperate situation, in which staying meant the possibility of being killed, but attempting to leave also carried with it the threat of reprisal or death. In her book on marital rape, Russell (1982) suggested that

> The statistics on the murder of husbands, along with the statistics on the murder of wives, are both indicators of the desperate plight of some women, not a sign that in this one area, males and females are equally violent. (p. 299)

A QUESTION OF SURVIVAL

It would be comforting to think that women in the homicide group—and indeed, the abusive couples we have discussed—are quite different from the rest of us. Some theorists have attempted to look for pathology in the women victims, contending that personality disorders are responsible for the precipitation, or at least the continuation, of their abuse (Blum, 1982; Shainess, 1979). Although living in constant fear and experiencing physical attacks obviously creates sufficient stress to affect women's behaviors in significant ways, data from the majority of empirical studies conducted during the last decade does not support an assumption of personal pathology (see Finkelhor, Gelles, Hotaling, & Straus, 1983, for examples of recent research). Few differences have been found between abused and nonabused women that are not primarily related to having experienced assault or intimidation (e.g., Rosenbaum & O'Leary, 1981). Indeed, Hotaling and Sugarman (1986), in reviewing findings from the last 15 years of empirical investigations on husband-to-wife violence, note that the strongest precipitant of victimization in women is simply being female. Characteristics of the man with whom a woman is involved are actually better predictors of a woman's chances of being victimized than are characteristics of the woman herself. The behaviors of abused women in these relationships are predominantly in reaction to the level of threat and violence perpetrated by the abuser: women chose the responses that seem most likely to minimize the danger and to facilitate their survival.

Although preliminary studies on homicides between partners have clarified some of the dynamics of these relationships, the research raises many more questions than it answers. The next section offers a theoretical framework for the evolution of an abusive relationship into a lethal incident perpetrated by the woman and discusses the basis for the woman's perceptions of threat and danger, the correspondence of her reactions to those known to be typical of victims, and the factors that contribute to her sense of entrapment in a deadly situation. The potential contribution of social exchange theory to understanding the choices a woman makes in these situations, and the possible application of social judgment theory to a woman's adaption to, and then rejection of, the violent relationship, are also mentioned. Although this model is highly speculative, it is hoped that it will provide a springboard for further hypothesis testing on abusive relationships that result in homicide.

The Spiral of Violence

As evidenced by results of the comparative study, women in the homicide group were the victims of increasingly frequent and severe attacks by their partners. Qualitative data from the interviews indicated that this resulted in a sense of desperation in the victimized woman (Browne, 1987). This desperation was based on the woman's experience with violence at the hands of the abuser, the escalation in the frequency and severity of violent acts, and the severity of the outcome in terms of injuries. The man's threats of future violence or threats to kill were taken very seriously, as threats had become realities so often in the past. A woman's belief in her partner's ability to do her harm was exacerbated by the perception—often based on a decline in contrition or remorse—that the man no longer cared what he did to her, and that his inhibitions against hurting her would be even further reduced by this lack of concern.

In addition to the extremity of the violence perpetrated against them and the lack of empathy with their suffering, women in the homicide group also had a sense that the men's behavior in general was out of control, based on the increasing frequency of intoxication, accelerated drug use, and violence and threats against others. All of the partner's actions began to seem unpredictable, and potentially deadly.

Shock Reactions of Victims to Abuse

Faced with this extreme situation, it is interesting to note that the reactions of the women corresponded quite closely with the reactions of other types of victims to trauma. In contrast to theories that would interpret their behaviors as indicative of personality disorder, their responses to violence is what we would expect from an individual who is confronted with a life-threatening situation. For example, research on both disaster and war victims indicates that, during the impact phase when the threat of danger becomes a reality, an individual's primary focus is on self-protection and survival. Victims experience feelings of shock, denial, disbelief, and fear, and reactions of withdrawal and confusion (Chapman, 1962; Mileti, Drabek, & Haas, 1975). They may deny the threat, leading to a lag in accurately defining the situation, or respond with dazed or apathetic behavior (Bahnson, 1964; Miller, 1964; Powell, 1954). A battle reaction in war situations includes a response of severe passivity in the face of danger, and a lack of escape behaviors even when those are possible. Observers noted that, as the level of danger became overwhelming, defensive strategies were employed and the individual became increasingly involved with internal defense mechanisms, causing external activity to diminish and giving the appearance of extreme apathy (Kardiner, 1959; Spiegel, 1955; Withey, 1962). Studies of crime victims also indicate that during a personal offense, the victim may offer little or no resistance, in an attempt to minimize the threat of injury or death (Bard & Sangrey, 1979).

Probably the type of victimization that most closely approximates the experiences of battered women is abuse related to captivity, such as that experienced by prisoners of war. In these situations, the captor or assailant has a major influence on the victim's assessment of the danger and of the alternatives available. Studies show that victims tend to select coping strategies based on their evaluation of alternatives and their appraisal of whether a particular method of coping will further endanger them and to what degree (Arnold, 1967; Lazarus, 1967). A crucial variable in this decision is the perceived balance of power between the captor and the victim. The coping strategy selected is weighed against the aggressor's perceived ability to control or to harm. For example, in situations of extreme helplessness such as concentration camps, surprisingly little anger is shown toward the captors, and this may be a measure of the captors' power to retaliate. "Fight or flight" responses are inhibited by this perception, and depression often results, based on the perceived helplessness of the situation. Victim's perceptions of their alternatives become increasingly limited, and those that exist often seem to constitute too great a threat to survival (Lazarus, 1967).

Like other victims of trauma, battered women's affective, cognitive, and behavioral responses often become distorted by their single focus on survival (Walker & Browne, 1985). They may develop a whole range of responses that seem to mitigate the severity of abuse during violent episodes, such as controlling their breathing or not crying out when in pain. However, they may not have developed any plans for escaping the abusive situation. Consistent with findings in the literature on victims, women in the homicide group experienced reactions of shock, denial, depression, anxiety, and fear. They also showed a marked tendency to withdraw immediately after abusive incidents, rather than to seek help. As the relationship progressed, the women's perceptions of viable alternatives became increasingly limited. They seemed to develop survival, rather than escape, skills; that is, they attempted to cope with the immediate threat by appeasing the violent partner and avoiding actions that might further anger him, but saw most other alternatives as too dangerous to pursue.

Weighing the Alternatives

The way in which abused women weigh the alternatives available to them is similar to the process described in Thibaut and Kelley's (1959) exchange model as characteristic of nonvoluntary relationships. Their theory focuses on the balance of costs and rewards realized by each participant in a relationship, with the conclusion that a negative balance will eventually cause that individual to terminate the interaction. They acknowledge, however, that some relationships exist in which an individual is forced to remain, even though the individual would prefer not to. In these interactions, the fate of one participant is in the hands of the other, and the restraining participant has the power to impose heavy costs on the captive participant. This power is further enhanced when ''agents outside the dyad . . . place social or physical barriers' against the victim's leaving (p. 170).

According to Thibaut and Kelley (1959), interactions in nonvoluntary relationships focus primarily on costs, rather than on rewards, and—similar to the theories of Arnold (1967) and Lazarus (1967)—the captive participant weighs alternatives based on the other's perceived power to control and to harm. Thibaut and Kelly note that, ''the greater the penalties for escape (or attempted escape), the poorer the outcomes that a prisoner can be forced to endure,'' and that the captor's power becomes ''more a matter of the punishments he can apply or withhold rather than, as in voluntary relationships, a question of . . . rewards'' (p. 170–171). At this point, the constraining member's power is limited only by ''the instruments [the captor] has for inflicting pain and by his scruples about making [the prisoner] suffer'' (p. 171).

Consistent with this theory, women in the homicide group deemed most alternatives too costly when weighed against the known abilities of the abuser to impose penalties. As mentioned earlier, the abuser's scruples against inflicting pain seemed to be weak or nonexistent, and the women's focus had often narrowed to immediate attempts to cope with the violence. They were frequently in terror, yet were constrained in the situation by the man's threats of harm or death if they left or attempted to leave. They were further persuaded of the risk in this alternative if they had tried to leave and were beaten for it. Their fears were justified: a study in Michigan showed that up to 50% of wives who left their abusive husbands were sought out and further terrorized or abused by them (Moore, 1979). In situations where the abuser has warned the victim not to leave, chosing to do so may escalate the very danger from which she is trying to escape.

As suggested by Thibaut and Kelley (1959), the abuser's power to constrain and punish is supported by strong societal barriers against obtaining effective protection from an assaultive mate (Blair, 1979; Field & Field, 1973; U.S. Commission on Civil Rights, 1982). A battered woman sometimes risks reprisal or death to seek out legal remedies, only to find the legal system unable or unwilling to help her. Lack of adequate provision for safe shelter, relocation, or protection from further aggression also contributes to an abused women's sense of entrapment in a violent relationship. This realization contributes to their conclusion that they must attempt to survive within the situation. As Thibaut and Kelley contend, when the probability of escape appears to be extremely low, ''the least costly adjustment'' for a victim may involve a ''complex of adaptions'' and ''dramatically shortening one's time perspective to a moment-to-moment or day-to-day focus'' (p. 180).

The Application of Social Judgment Theory

How does a battered woman go from this seemingly passive response pattern to the highly active one of homicide? Although individuals have the legal right to defend themselves against the threat of imminent serious bodily harm or death, based on a reasonable perception of the danger (LaFave & Scott, 1972; Thyfault, 1984), the process by which a woman makes a transition to this mode of reacting is still largely unknown. Although the experimental testing of the social judgment theory proposed by Sherif and Hovland (1961) has produced some contradictory results (Wrightsman, 1972), their concept of a latitude of acceptance for stimuli, and of assimilation and contrast effects, may make a contribution to our understanding of the evolution in a violent relationship toward a homicide committed by the woman.

Sherif and Hovland's (1961) theory involves the concept of a continuum on which incoming stimuli are ordered. This becomes a reference scale by which the individual judges a given stimulus as acceptable or unacceptable. The latitude of acceptance is that range of possibilities that the individual is willing to agree with or adapt to. Stimuli that fall outside that range are either in the latitude of rejection, or the latitude of noncommitment (neither acceptable nor unacceptable). According to Sherif and Hovland, these latitudes are defined by endpoints, or anchors, that determine the extremes of the scale. Internal anchors are those originating within the individual, whereas external anchors are provided by outside factors or social consensus. In the absence of outside referrents, internal anchors play an especially important role in an individual's evaluation of a situation. Past learning experiences, such as prior experience with similar stimuli, also effect the placement of stimuli on the scale. An important part of Sherif and Hovland's theory is the the concept of assimilation and contrast: an external anchor that falls at the end of a series, or even slightly above the series, will produce a shift of the range—or assimilation—toward that anchor. However, if an anchor is placed too far from a series, a contrast effect will ensue, and the anchor will be perceived as being even more extreme than it really is.

If one views the escalation of violent acts by the abuser as ordered along a continuum, then the latitude of acceptance for a battered woman would be that range of activities to which she can adapt. This latitude would be greatly determined by her prior socialization experiences as a woman, and by prior learning experiences with similar stimuli, such as violence in her childhood home. Because society's standards on violence against wives are ambiguous, and because abused women rarely discuss their victimization with others, it can be assumed that, apart from their prior learning history, battered women are quite dependent on their internal anchors to determine the latitude of behaviors they will accept. As abusive acts continue to fall near the endpoints of the range, Sherif and Hovland's (1961) model would predict that assimilation of those actions would occur, and that the woman's latitude of acceptance would shift to accomodate them. This is consistent with findings in the literature on victims. In extreme environments, human beings alter their behavior quite dramatically if it is necessary to survive. Thus, when the situational demands created by the abuser are extreme, an abused woman may respond with extreme behavior in order to coexist.

Early in the relationship, this adaptation may consist of minimalization or extreme appeasment. In discussing the reactions of persons in captivity, Biderman (1967) suggested that a normal human being might be incapable of sustaining a totally hostile or antagonistic interaction over a long period of time. Further, periods of acquiescence might be necessary for psychological and emotional survival. A certain level of abuse and tension becomes the status quo: women progress from being horrified by each successive incident, to being thankful they survived the last one. The criterion is survival. Their latitude of acceptance is determined by what they believe they can live through. Judging from reports of women in the homicide group, battered women do adapt to the violence they live with to a great extent. By the end of their relationships, women in the homicide group were living with abuse they would not have thought endurable at an earlier stage. They were involved in a constant process of assimilation and readjustment.

If we follow the conceptualization of Sherif and Hovland (1961), the contrast phenomena would come into effect when an act occurs that the woman perceives as significantly above the normal range of violence. In investigating events immediately prior to a lethal incident, we noted that women often told us, "He had never done that before." Often there was a sudden change in the pattern of violence that indicated to them that their death was imminent. One attack would be so much more violent or degrading than all the rest that, even with their highly developed survival skills, the women believed it would be impossible to survive the next one. Or an act would suddenly be beyond the range of what the women were willing to assimilate. Frequently this involved the onset of abuse of a child. Women would state "He had never threatened the baby before," or "I could stand him beating me, but then he hurt my daughter."

Contrast theory would predict that, once the woman had defined the act as significantly outside her latitude of acceptance, she would judge it as being more extreme than it really was. Actually, given the amount of minimalization and assimilation engaged in by victims, and the tendency of the abused women in our study to understate the levels of violence in their relationships, it is more likely that the women were at last simply making a realistic appraisal of the danger. Their final hope had been removed. They did not believe they could escape the abusive situation and live, and now they could no longer survive within it.

CONCLUSIONS

The current study focused on the perceptions of women victims and their reactions to abuse by a male partner. These perceptions are crucial, both from a legal and a psychological standpoint, if we are to understand the dynamics that lead an abused woman to take lethal action against her abuser.

Tacit social support exists for the abuse of family members in our society. This is reflected in and reinforced by our traditions of noninvolvement in family matters, a man's "rights" in dealing with his wife and children, and the gender stereotyping that favors a male's expression of dominance and aggression. Lack of effective legal system response to assaults in which the victim is a wife, and the lack of social support for adequate and established alternatives to assure the victim's protection from further aggression, allow the violence in abusive relationships to escalate. An abused woman is left in a potentially deadly situation from which she sees no practical avenue of escape. As is typical of victims, women react with responses of fear and adaption, weighing their alternatives in accordance with their perceptions of the threat, and attempting to choose those options that will mitigate the danger and facilitate their survival.

Yet in some cases, the violence escalates beyond the level a victim can assimilate. By the end of their relationships, women in the homicide group were subjected to frequent and injurious attacks from partners who were likely to be drinking heavily, using drugs, sexually assaulting them, and threatening murder. Most of these women had no history of violent behavior. However, in these relationships, the women's attempts to survive with an increasingly violent and unpredictable mate eventually resulted in an act of violence on their part as well.

I am grateful to Tim Collins and Steve Ipsen at the University of Colorado for their invaluable assistance in analysis of these data, to Phil Shaver for his detailed comments on an earlier draft of the results, and to the psychology department at the University of Colorado at Denver for its research facilities during the 3 years I worked on this project. I also wish to thank David Sugarman for his contributions to my thinking on the application of social judgment theory.

REFERENCES

Arnold, M. B. (1967). Stress and emotion. In M. H. Appley & R. Trumball (Eds.), *Psychological stress*. New York: Appleton-Century-Crofts.

Bahnson, C. B. (1964). Emotional reactions to internally and externally derived threats of annihilation. In G. H. Grosser, H. Wechsler, & M. Greenblatt (Eds.), *The threat of impending disaster*. Cambridge, MA: The M.I.T. Press.

Bard, M., & Sangrey, D. (1979). *The crime victim's book*. New York: Basic Books.

Biderman, A. D. (1967). Captivity lore and behavior in captivity. In G. H. Grosser, H. Wechsler, & M. Greenblatt (Eds.), *The threat of impending disaster*. Cambridge, MA: The M.I.T. Press.

Blair, S. (1979). Making the legal system work for battered women. In D. M. Moore (Ed.), *Battered women* (pp. 101–118). Beverly Hllls, CA: Sage.

Blum, H. P. (1982). Psychoanalytic reflections on "The beaten wife syndrome." In M. Kirkpatrick (Ed.), *Women's sexual experiences: Explorations of the continent*. New York: Plenum Press.

Bourdouris, J. (1971). Homicide in the family. *Journal of Marriage and the Family, 33,* 667–676.

Browne, A. (1987). *When battered women kill*. MacMillan/Free Press.

Chapman, D. W. (1962). A brief introduction to contemporary disaster research. In G. W. Baker & D. W. Chapman (Eds.), *Man and society in disaster*. New York: Basic Books.

Chapman, M. R., & Gates, M. (Eds.). (1978). *The victimization of women*. Beverly Hills, CA: Sage.

Chimbos, P. D. (1978). *Marital violence: A study of interspousal homicide*. San Francisco: R & E Research Associates.

Coleman, K. H., Weinman, M. L., & Hsi, B. P. (1980). Factors affecting conjugal violence. *Journal of Psychology, 105,* 197–202.

Crimes of violence. (1969). A staff report to the National Commission on the Causes and Prevention of Violence. Washington, DC: U.S. Government Printing Office.

Field, M. H., & Field, H. F. (1973). Marital violence and the criminal process: Neither justice nor peace. *Social Service Review, 47,* 221–240.

Finkelhor, D., Gelles, R., Hotaling, G., & Straus, M. (1983). *The dark side of families*. Beverly Hills, CA: Sage.

Frieze, I. H. (1979). Perceptions of battered wives. In I. Frieze, D. Bar Tal, & J. Carroll (Eds.), *New approaches to social problems* (pp. 79–108). San Francisco: Jossey-Bass.

Gelles, R. J. (1974). *The violent home: A study of physical aggression between husbands and wives*. Beverly Hills, CA: Sage.

Gelles, R. J. (1979). *Family violence*. Beverly Hills, CA: Sage.

Gelles, R. J. (1980). Violence in the family: A review of research in the seventies. *Journal of Marriage and the Family, 42,* 873–885.

Harris & Associates. (1979). *Survey of spousal violence against women in Kentucky*. (Report No. 792701) Louis Harris & Assoc.

Hilberman, E., & Munson, L. (1978). Sixty battered women. *Victimology: An International Journal, 2,* 460–471.

Hotaling, G. T., & Sugarman, D. B. (1986). An analysis of risk markers in husband to wife violence: The current state of knowledge. *Violence and Victims, 1*(2), 101–124.

Jones, A. (1980). *Women who kill*. New York: Fawcett Columbine Books.

Kardiner, A. (1959). Traumatic neuroses of war. In S. Arieti (Ed.), *American handbook of psychiatry* (Vol. 1). New York: Basic Books.

Kempe, C. H., Silverman, F. N., Steele, B. F., Droegemueeler, W., Silver, H. (1962). The battered child syndrome. *Journal of the American Medical Association, 181,* 107–112.

LaFave, W. R., & Scott, Jr., A. W. (1972). *Handbook on criminal law.* St. Paul, MN: West.

Lazarus, R. S. (1967). Cognitive and personality factors underlying threat and coping. In M. H. Appley & R. Trumbull (Eds.), *Psychological stress.* New York: Appleton-Century-Crofts.

Lindsey, K. (1978, September). When battered women strike back: Murder or self-defense. *Viva,* 58–59; 66–74.

Martin, D. (1976). *Battered wives.* San Francisco: Glide.

Mileti, D. S., Drabek, T. E., & Haas, J. E. (1975). *Human systems in extreme environments.* Institute of Behavioral Science, University of Colorado.

Miller, J. G. (1964). A theoretical review of individual and group psychological reactions to stress. In G. H. Grosser, H. Wechsler, & M. Greenblatt (Eds.), *The threat of impending disaster.* Cambridge, MA: The M.I.T. Press.

Moore, D. M. (1979). Editor's introduction: An overview of the problem. In D. M. Moore (Ed.), *Battered women* (pp. 7–9). Beverly Hills, CA: Sage.

National Study of the Incidence and Severity of Child Abuse and Neglect. (1981, September). *Study findings.* (DHHS Publication No. PHDS 81-30320). U.S. Department of Health & Human Services. Washington, DC: U.S. Government Printing Office.

Pizzey, E. (1974). *Scream quietly or the neighbors will hear.* London: Penguin Books.

Powell, J. W. (1954). *An introduction to the natural history of disaster* (Vol. 2). Final contract report, Disaster Research Project, Psychiatric Insitute, University of Maryland.

Rosenbaum, A., & O'Leary, K. D. (1981). Marital violence: Characteristics of abusive couples. *Journal of Consulting and Clinical Psychology, 49,* 63–71.

Roy, M. (1977). Research project probing a cross-section of battered women. In M. Roy (Ed.), *Battered women: A psychosocial study of domestic violence* (pp. 24–44). New York: Van Nostrand Reinhold Company.

Russell, D. E. H. (1982). *Rape in marriage.* New York: MacMillian.

Schneider, E. M., & Jordan, S. B. (1981). Representation of women who defend themselves in response to physical or sexual assault. In E. Bochnak (Ed.), *Women's self-defense cases: Theory and practice* (pp. 1–39). Charlottesville, VA: The Michie Company Law Publishers.

Schultz, L. G. (1960). The wife assaulter. *Journal of Social Therapy, 6,* 103–111.

Shainess, N. (1979). Vulnerability to violence: Masochism as a process. *American Journal of Psychotherapy, 33,* 174–189.

Sherif, M., & Hovland, C. (1961). *Social judgment.* New Haven, CT: Yale University Press.

Snell, J. E., Rosenwald, R. J., & Robey, A. (1964). The wifebeaters wife: A study of family interaction. *Archives of General Psychiatry, 11,* 107–113.

Spiegel, J. P. (1955). Emotional reactions to catastrophe. In S. Liebman (Ed.), *Stress situations.* Philadelphia & Montreal: J. B. Lippincott.

Stacey, W., & Shupe, A. (1983). *The family secret.* Boston, MA: Beacon Press.

Stephens, D. W. (1977). Domestic assault: The police response. In M. Roy (Ed.), *Battered women: A psychosocial study of domestic violence* (pp. 164–172). New York: Van Nostrand Reinhold.

Straus, M. A. (1971). Some social antecedents of physical punishment: A linkage theory interpretation. *Journal of Marriage and the Family, 33,* 658–663.

Straus, M. A. (1973). A general systems theory approach to a theory of violence between family members. *Social Science Information, 12,* 105–125.

Straus, M. A., & Gelles, R. J. (1986). Societal change and change in family violence from 1975 to 1985. *Journal of Marriage and the Family, 48.*

Straus, M., Gelles, R., & Steinmetz, S. (1980). *Behind closed doors: Violence in the American family.* Garden City, NY: Anchor Press.

Thibaut, J. W., & Kelley, H. H. (1959). *The social psychology of groups.* New York: Wiley.

Thyfault, R. (1984). Self-defense: Battered woman syndrome on trial. *California Western Law Review, 20,* 485–510.

Totman, J. (1978). *The murderess: A psychosocial study of criminal homicide.* San Francisco: R & E Research Associates.

Uniform Crime Reports. (1983, September). *Crime in the United States.* Federal Bureau of Investigation. U.S. Department of Justice, Washington, DC.

United States Commission on Civil Rights. (1982). *Under the rule of thumb: Battered women and the administration of justice*. Washington, DC: U.S. Government Printing Office.

Walker, L. E. (1979). *The battered woman*. New York: Harper & Row.

Walker, L. E. (1981). *The battered woman syndrome: Final report*. NIMH Grant #R0130147.

Walker, L. E. (1984). *The battered woman syndrome*. New York: Springer.

Walker, L. E., & Browne, A. (1985). Gender and victimization by intimates. *Journal of Personality, 53*(2), 179–195.

Washburn, C., & Frieze, I. H. (1980, March). *Methodological issues in studying battered women*. Paper presented at the meeting of the Association for Women in Psychology, Santa Monica, CA.

Withey, S. B. (1962). Reaction to uncertain threat. In G. W. Baker & D. W. Chapman (Eds.), *Man and society in disaster*. New York: Basic Books.

Wolfgang, M. E. (1958). *Patterns in criminal homicide*. New York: Wiley.

Wolfgang, M. E. (1967). A sociological analysis of criminal homicide. In M. E. Wolfgang (Ed.), *Studies in homicide*. New York: Harper & Row.

Wrightsman, L. S. (1972). *Social psychology in the seventies*. Belmont, CA: Wadsworth.

IV
SPECIAL ISSUES

13

Violence among Intimates

An Epidemiological Review

EVAN STARK and ANNE FLITCRAFT

THE EPIDEMIOLOGICAL APPROACH TO DOMESTIC VIOLENCE

This chapter will describe how domestic violence is distributed in various populations, identify its demographic features, and distinguish its etiology, insofar as this is possible, by comparing violent with nonviolent groups. Within certain limits, we identify the clinical components and sequelae of the problem, set them in a social context that makes them intelligible, and ask if there are antecedent problems or risk factors that community interventions should target.

The epidemiologist's ideal is a well-defined disease, a suspected agent, and a host or carrier population that is distinguished by clear symptoms or risk factors. As a branch of medicine close to public health, epidemiology emphasizes etiological factors, such as physical agents or individual behaviors and problems, that can be easily defined and measured. Cause and effect should occur with sufficient temporal contiguity to make onset clear, and the carrier population should be large and accessible enough to sample reliably.

Domestic violence only fulfills this last condition: the victim population is large and relatively accessible. Depending on the criteria, victims may comprise from 5% to 20% of the United States population. The problem lies in wide disagreement about how to define and measure the dependent variable.

Case identification requires answering two questions, how should violence (or abuse) in domestic life be defined and which relations should be included as domestic? Without agreement on case identification, it is impossible to determine incidence (the new cases in a population during a given period) or prevalence (the total number of cases).

Definitions of violence used by researchers range from any use of force in the family setting, including sibling fights as well as spousal homicide, (Straus, Gelles, & Steinmetz, 1980), through physical assault on wives only (Berk, Berk, Loseke, & Ranma, 1983). Stark, Flitcraft *et al.*, (1981), meanwhile, identified abuse with any clinical

EVAN STARK • Department of Public Administration and Sociology, Rutgers University, Newark, NJ 07102. **ANNE FLITCRAFT** • Department of Medicine, University of Connecticut, Farmington, CT 06032.

presentation (regardless of severity) for which assault by a social partner is mentioned or indicated.

Legal definitions of what types of violence are domestic differ from state to state. Whereas awareness of these differences will help clinicians allocate resources appropriately, what distinguishes a problem epidemiologically is that its manifestations are differentiated by well-recognized principles, as in a disease, or, in the absence of a well-understood logic, by clinical experience, as in a syndrome. To resolve the controversy about definition, therefore, we need to weigh the clinical evidence supporting competing claims.

Feminists argue that male violence against women and children is different than other forms of domestic violence because it converges with broader patterns of discrimination. This combination of assault and discrimination against women leads to entrapment and is manifested in a distinct clinical profile—"the battering syndrome"—which evokes a range of psychosocial problems alongside injury. However, the majority of nonfeminist clinicians and researchers approach various forms of domestic violence—including wife–husband assault and elder abuse—as symptomatic of distinct family dynamics, psychopathology, and stress. Here, what is distinctive is not so much the outcome—the abuse of one family member or another—but its source in a family history of abuse, behavioral problems such as alcoholism, personality deficits, or psychopathology.

These competing claims have political significance for the expenditure of clinical and other public resources. To the women's movement, domestic violence is the expression of unequal power and the appropriate response is to "empower" abused women—who are termed survivors—through some combination of community support and advocacy. By contrast, the huge therapeutic and child abuse establishment approach the abused family member as a victim requiring the sort of rescue institutionalized in child protective services. So the question of definition bears on whether public monies generally will go to community-based groups or to established professionals, and whether the aim of intervention is supporting the autonomy of women and children or strengthening the family unit. By fixing attention on certain aspects of the problem rather than others, epidemiology enters this political debate. It is obligated to map its way carefully through the controversy in a way that at least makes the terms of disagreement clear.

The Research Universe

To determine whether male violence against women or family violence is the more appropriate clinical concern, we report findings that bear on acts of physical force among adult social partners regardless of their marital or domiciliary status. The focus on acts of assault or abuse—the smallest unit of force—allows us to investigate the relation between acts, outcomes, and patterns. By including spouse abuse, violence against children emanating from spousal violence, and violence against single, divorced, and separated women, we take a perspective that is broader than the large body of research concerned only with battered women (Stark, Flitcraft, & Frazier, 1979; Schulman, 1979; Walker, 1979), but narrower than one including any aggressive act in the family context (Straus *et al.*, 1980). Use of the generic term *spouse* to describe abuse indicates concern for males assaulted in the family context as well as females, and for relationships in which both partners are equally abusive (intraspousal violence). The vast body of evidence concerns woman abuse. However, wife–husband assault and abuse between same sex lovers are realities to which clinicians must be sensitive.

In particular, whereas we include evidence on violence among dating couples—usually ignored in domestic violence research—we exclude evidence on mental abuse, abuse of the elderly, sibling violence, children's violence against parents, and evidence on child abuse that has no bearing on adult–adult violence.

However great the suffering that may result from mental abuse, its definition and link to violence are too vague to warrant its inclusion here (cf. Walker, 1979). Meanwhile, although Straus *et al.* (1980) conclude that 53% of children in the United States use severe force against their siblings and that two thirds of families use physical punishment as a form of parental discipline, we find no hard evidence to link these acts to adult–adult violence.

According to a U.S. House Committee on Aging Report, elderly abuse may affect as many as 4% of all persons over 65 in the U.S. each year. However, there has been no representative population survey of the problem and nonprobability interview surveys report rates of physical abuse that range from a high of 55% (O'Malley, 1979) to less than 3% (Lau & Kosberg, 1979). The population at highest risk appears to be very elderly low-income women who suffer some impairment. But, when Gratton (1982) randomly sampled 317 cases from this high-risk group, he was able to confirm only one case of physical abuse, an incidence rate of .003%. The seriousness of the problem is suggested by a 6-month review of *Uniform Crime Report* statistics in New Jersey (1984) indicating that 3% of police calls involve physical abuse of the elderly. To date, husbands and sons appear to be primarily responsible for elderly abuse, economic stress and alcohol are important situational components, and women comprise the majority of victims regardless of how abuse is defined. This apparent similarity to the abuse of women should be explored.[1] We can make only these limited observations about elderly abuse because nothing definitive is known about its incidence, prevalence, or etiology.

Child abuse is excluded, finally, because in few areas has so much been alleged with so little clinical or empirical support, particularly about the abusive propensities and deficits of mothers. We present evidence on child abuse only if it bears directly on the controversy about whether violent men or an inheritance of pathology are at the root of domestic violence.

Methodological Criteria

Our working definition allows us to assess which model of domestic violence is the more appropriate by comparing and contrasting woman abuse generally, spouse abuse, and violence against wives. We report only those studies whose design conforms to strict epidemiological criteria.

The most popular causal theories in the domestic violence field have not been adequately tested. Violence may be transmitted across generations, as many clinicians and social scientists contend. But believing the evidence for this view requires a prodigious faith in memory and veracity and accepting definitions of childhood abuse that range from inappropriate mothering (Steele, 1976) to physical battering (Straus *et al.*, 1980). And the

---

[1]Ironically, while female independence appears to be a key motive for violence against women by their husbands and boyfriends, it is the dependence of elderly women that apparently excites the ire of husbands and sons. At the same time, a growing feminist literature emphasizes that home care almost always means care of women by women, placing virtually the entire responsibility for an infirm parent on the daughter or sister. Not surprisingly, therefore, among the minority of female abusers of the elderly, daughters feature prominently (Lau & Kosberg, 1978).

corollary that stress triggers violence given a lack of coping resources or an inherited predisposition to violence is even more difficult to operationalize. Allegations in this work about onset and causal direction hopelessly disregard Susser's caution (1973) about temporal contiguity. For instance, the poor coping skills of some abused women are more likely to be the product of violence (Walker, 1979) or of frustrating helping encounters (Stark & Flitcraft, 1983) than the source of a violence-prone personality. There is as little empirical basis for opposing arguments that proceed as if violence were intrinsic to male character (Brownmiller, 1975) or passivity to female socialization (Martin, 1977).

The material summarized here was selected on the basis of its *internal* and *external validity:* the degree to which a study design identifies characteristics specific to domestic violence in a given population and/or permits generalization to the total universe of battered women. The first criterion is met by client-based case control comparisons between violent and nonviolent groups; the second, by representative (or probability) samples from the larger population.

Case-Control Studies involve institutionalized, client or "normal" populations in which the group identified with domestic violence is systematically compared and/or matched with at least one group of persons not identified with domestic violence. The control design helps ensure that differences identified will be real distinguishing characteristics of violent and nonviolent groups. But, generalizability from client-based control studies is limited by "sample selection bias," i.e., by the unrepresentativeness of any given client group.

Representative Studies typically use random survey designs to tap responses to standard measures and devise comparison groups on the basis of these responses through statistical manipulation. Assuming a minimum level of sample selection bias, representative studies based on random survey designs have a high degree of generalizability. But, standardized questions may not accurately "operationalize" domestic violence or respondents may refuse to answer or distort information ("response bias").

A good study design is no guarantee of important findings. These depend on the prior generation of plausible hypotheses, usually from descriptive studies of client populations and clinical observational studies that look at a few cases in depth.

The bulk of domestic violence research describes the experience of women victims. However indispensible, much of this work, because it fails to identify what is distinctive about battering, can give rise to seriously misleading generalizations. For instance, on the basis of questioning only battered women, British psychiatrist J. J. Gayford (1975a, b) concluded that the various problems they had showed such women "need protection against their own stimulus-seeking activities. Though they flinch from violence like other people, they have the ability to . . . provoke attack from the opposite sex." But, a group of nonbattered women with a similar background might have an identical profile. Disregarding this possibility, a Select Committee on Violence in Marriage in Britain used Gayford's testimony to justify its finding that battered women "had been inadequately prepared for adult life."

Clinical observation, meanwhile, permits rich detail and an exploration of etiological pathways. Again, however, the absence of standardized measures or comparison groups limits the utility of such work for our present purposes.

Different methods answer certain questions better than others. Surveys are best suited to measuring environmental factors and aggregate behaviors whereas case-control studies highlight what is distinctive about specific client populations. The selection of methods—like the hypotheses they test—reflects very different professional and/or political orientations and a singular lack of communication between survey researchers and clinicians is one result. For instance, although surveys emphasizing social factors show that men are the assailants in from 25% to 50% of all child abuse (Gil, 1973), partially because men are difficult to access in treatment settings, there are no client-based studies of male abusers and no programs targeting child-abusing men. The exclusion of descriptive and clinical assessments from this review reveals our personal bias that battering is a social rather than a private event in which interpersonal dynamics are less important than social and institutional factors.

Explanations of Domestic Violence: Pathology or Politics?

Ever since the debate about domestic violence began a century ago, with Francis Power Cobbe's "Wife Torture in England" (1878), the field has been dominated by the women's movement and various charitable groups. Attention was once again drawn to the issue in the early 1970s, this time by a growing social movement that had opened more than 700 community-based shelters for battered women by 1980 (Schecter, 1982). These shelters emphasize peer support, female empowerment, and systems advocacy. But as researchers and health and protective service providers have become increasingly involved, the emphasis has begun to shift from male violence to family violence more generally, from the politics of gender to pathology and victimization, and from community-based advocacy and support to professional therapy and rescue.

The stress/pathology model promoted by service professionals highlights evidence, to quote Straus and Steinmetz (1975), that "the family is the most physically violent group or institution that a typical citizen is likely to encounter." In this view, woman abuse is a point on a continuum extending from sibling rivalry through spousal homicide and abuse of elderly parents. (Gelles, 1974; Straus *et al.*, 1980). Psychopathology allegedly originating in the family of origin is transmitted across generations and triggered in parents or children by some combination of relational deficits, lack of coping skills, behavioral problems (such as alcohol abuse), and environmental stressors (such as poverty). Following child abuse research, this model also emphasizes the importance of identifying and targeting risk factors.

A number of problematic assumptions in this approach can be assessed through the research literature. One involves abused husbands. The violent family model relies heavily on claims that whereas women are more easily injured in family fights—allegedly because they are weaker—they are no less abusive than men. However, the status of this claim remains unclear, in part because the survey methods employed to support it fail to establish the intention (e.g., assault or self-defense), consequence (e.g., injury), duration, or context of violent acts. Another problematic assumption involves the thesis that violent men have themselves been beaten or witness to violence as children and that when they beat their wives, their wives, in turn, beat the children. Still another is the alleged causal role of alcohol and other psychiatric problems in violence and victimization. We will want to know, for example, whether battered women (or their assailants) are more likely to abuse alcohol—or evidence other behavior disorders—than nonbattered women (or nonviolent men) and whether such a disproportionate risk proceeds or follows the onset of abuse. Meanwhile, the alleged importance of environmental stress should be reflected in vastly higher rates of abuse among vulnerable groups, such as blacks or the unemployed. A final key to the pathology/stress model involves how we explain widely noted discrepancies between survey data on acts of force and the paucity of data in clinical records.

According to Walker (1979), this may reflect a helplessness syndrome evoked by violence that undermines self-esteem and prevents victims from seeking or taking advantage of help. In a more sophisticated interpretation of clinical evidence, Hilberman (1980) described a stress-response syndrome to violence evident among abused mental patients and characterized by agitation, anxiety, depression, and extreme passivity.

The political model advanced by the battered women's movement emphasizes that violence against women is the most common and serious expression of a pattern of forceable subordination that includes the physical and sexual abuse of children. Violence or victimization may sometimes be learned. But, the political view holds abuse is typically motivated by situational conflicts over authority and resources and by threats to male privilege posed by women struggling for personal independence. As Finn (1985) and Dobash and Dobash (1974) have shown, fights over ''who's the boss?,'' money, sex and child care are at the heart of abuse. Women stay in such relationships—and so are battered—less because of pathology, self-blame, or helplessness than because the helping system implicitly collaborates with violent men by supporting traditional family roles and treating victims as if they were the problem. As a result of the combination of sex discrimination, an inappropriate helping response, and male violence, women's options are cut off, they become entrapped in violent homes, and may develop many of the behavioral and personality problems said to cause abuse.

The evidence will be used to evaluate several of these assumptions. If male violence against women rather than family dynamics is the problem, then we should find woman abuse among nonmarried as well as married women and the typical batterer should be no different than the nonbattering male. In addition, we should find that batterers, rather than abused women, are the typical child abusers. As important, if woman battering is different in kind (not simply in degree) from the problems suffered by siblings, men, or the elderly, then battered women should reveal a distinct clinical profile that emerges only after the onset of abuse. Although a reluctance on the part of victims to report their problem is consistent with the pathology model, a finding of professional neglect and inappropriate treatment would support the political contention that discrimination combines with violence in woman battering.

Analysis will also suggest the most appropriate approach to intervention. If clinical cases are only the tip of the iceberg, as the pathology model implies, then identifying hidden cases through early risk factors is important. Moreover, family treatment models—including parent education and couples' therapy—should be emphasized if violent families or inadequate personalities are the root of the problem. But, if gender inequality supported by institutional maltreatment shapes male–female relations into abusive violence and battering, then the shelter's emphasis on female empowerment, systems advocacy, and closing what Reiker and Carmen (1984) call the gender gap in psychotherapy is more appropriate.

RESEARCH FINDINGS

Data Sources

There are no preexisting data bases from which to derive reliable estimates of domestic violence, no widely recognized identification procedures have been adopted, and reporting is sporadic even in those states where it is mandatory. Although woman battering may be associated with the psychiatric diagnosis of posttraumatic stress disorder, spouse abuse and battering are not recognized diagnoses in the health or mental health systems. Until some form of national surveillance is implemented, estimates of incidence and prevalence must be based on representative surveys and sparse institutional data.

One source of information on the most severe forms of domestic violence—homicide and aggravated assault—are the FBI's *Uniform Crime Reports* (UCR). Based on monthly information from over 15,000 law enforcement agencies, the UCR contain a Supplementary Homicide Report (SHR) with information on the age, race, and sex of the victim as well as the relationship to the offender. From the UCR (1980), for example, we learn that 844 husbands were killed by wives in 1979 and 1009 wives by husbands. In 1982, fully 17% of the 21,012 reported homicides in the country involved family members. Depending on whether we count extended family members, close acquaintances, and dating couples, so-called primary homicides account for between 20% and 66% of all reported homicides (Boudouris, 1971; Stephens, 1977). Other surveys, meanwhile, report that intraspousal violence accounts for anywhere from 11% to 52% of all assaults (Boudouris, 1971; Pittman & Handy, 1964).

The UCR data do not indicate whether or not the victim and perpetrator live together—a common criterion for domestic violence—and only include those serious instances of criminal assault/murder that have been reported to the police and then, by the police, to the FBI. Without knowing what percentage of all domestic violence cases are reported to police, it is impossible to determine prevalence with UCR data.

A more accurate source of prevalence data is the National Crime Survey taken each year by the U.S. Department of Justice from a stratified, multistage cluster sample of approximately 62,000 households. Information bearing on domestic violence comes from questions on rape and assault victimization and accompanying data on medical treatment, property loss, characteristics of the victim–offender relationship, and whether or not police were notified. The NCS includes many crimes not reported to police, but if a criminal incident includes several different acts, only the most serious is counted (e.g., robbery over assault). This may account for an estimate, based on NCS figures, that only 1% of the ever married were assaulted by a spouse or ex-spouse in 1977 (Gaquin, 1977–78).

Accurate epidemiological data on domestic assault are difficult to gather in clinical settings. Because physicians rarely record abuse or list it as a diagnosis in medical records, case finding based on physician reporting or discharge diagnoses seriously and consistently underestimate the magnitude of the problem (Stark *et al.*, 1979). However, Appleton (1980) and Hilberman and Munson (1977–78) have shown that sensitive probing evokes accurate patient accounts. And Stark *et al.* (1981) showed that a critical record review or interview process designed to elicit a trauma history can identify abuse victims and persons whose histories suggest abuse.

Incidence, Prevalence, Frequency, Severity, and Sequelae of Abuse

Survey Results. To date, only one representative United States survey has specifically measured violent acts among cohabitants. Sampling 3,300 families, Straus *et al.*, (1980) estimate there are 3.9 million instances of spouse abuse annually, 3.8% or 1.8 million wives are abused by husbands and 4.6% or 2.2 million husbands are abused. An estimated 12.6% have ever experienced a ''severe'' violent episode (6 million couples), and 28% report some use of force. Two other surveys also report alarming results. An estimated 20% of the adult residents of Suffolk County, Long Island, have hit or been hit by their spouse (Nisonoff & Bitman, 1979). Meanwhile, Szinovacz (1983) found that 26% of the women but 30% of the men had been abused in a sample of 103 couples from Pennsylvania towns. However, in a random survey of couples in Delaware, Steinmetz (1977–78) found no cases of husband abuse.[2]

Three state surveys have focused exclusively on violence against women. A Harris Poll of Kentucky housewives (Schulman, 1979) found that 10% had been abused during the year (80,000 women) and 21% had ever been abused. A North Carolina sample revealed that 21% had ever been beaten as adults by "a person they knew" (Genteman, 1980). Finally, a probability sample of 1,210 female residents of Texas, age 18 or older found that 8.5% had been abused during the year and 29.7% had been abused "ever" (Teske & Parker, 1983).

Despite their appeal, annual rates of violent acts do not establish incidence because there is no way to determine a new case. Nor are the various prevalence estimates strictly comparable. Though many men are clearly hit by their wives, figures on husband abuse vary too widely to determine the extent or seriousness of the problem. More consistent figures on intraspousal violence suggest a prevalence of from 12% to 20%, but again without establishing a firm basis for clinical concern. Only the data on violence against women are consistent across county, state, and national surveys. We can safely estimate that between 20% to 25% of the adult women in the United States have been physically abused at least once by a male intimate: that is between 12 and 15 million women.

By contrast with the paucity of information on spousal violence in the general population, survey data consistently show that violence is an isolated incident for less than a third of the abused women: 47% of husbands who beat their wives do so three or more times a year (Straus et al., 1980). And NCS data (Klaus & Rand, 1984) and the Texas survey (Teske & Parker, 1983) indicate that between 25% and 30% of all abused women suffer "serial victimization," many beaten as frequently as once a week! Findings bearing on the probability that intraspousal violence will result in injury vary widely. Thus, whereas 49% of the victims of "family assaults" reported to the NCS suffered some injury, 24% of the abused women in the Texas sample had been injured seriously enough to require medical treatment. By contrast, only 9% of the incidents reported by the Kentucky housewives to the Harris survey resulted in injury requiring medical treatment (Schulman, 1979). Knives and guns are not used in the majority of abusive incidents, but their use is not uncommon (Straus et al., 1980). Finally, sexual assault frequently accompanies physical abuse. According to a survey of ever-married women in San Francisco, 14% have been raped by their current or former husbands. (Russell, 1980, 1982).

Dating Couples. Woman battering has been considered primarily a family problem, even by survey researchers. The Texas survey included nonmarried women, but asked about abuse only by "a husband or live-in partner." Despite this, at least one representative survey and a number of client studies indicate that the majority of abuse victims are single, separated, or divorced and that the risk of battering actually increases with separation or divorce (Gentemann, 1980; Stark et al., 1979, 1981). Therefore, we cannot assume that women are protected from ongoing violence if they are living alone.

---

[2]Steinmetz sampled 57 intact couples with two children in New Castle, Delaware, and identified four wives as assault victims, but no husbands. She then compared her data to police files where she found 26 spouse assault cases, 24 involving women and 2 involving men. From this, she drew the astounding conclusion that "husband abuse is the most unreported crime in America," estimating that 250,000 husbands are "battered" in the U.S. each year. This "finding" was widely publicized. (For a full discussion of Steinmetz's work see Pagelow, 1985.)

By contrast with studies focusing on domestic violence, studies about violence among nonmarried persons target college students exclusively, choosing to term reported abuse premarital or courtship violence as if a difference between violence against married and unmarried women had been established. Among the many studies in this genre, the two using randomized samples found that 19% and 31.5% respectively were victims of physical aggression or threats (Bogal-Allbritten & Allbritten, 1983; Murphy, 1984). Large nonrandom surveys reflect similar findings, ranging from 13.5% of 2,338 students from seven United States schools (Makepeace, 1984) to 42% of 354 female college students at a large Southeastern University (Comins, 1984). Moreover, in the seven college survey, 46% of those with a violent experience reported an injury, with 5% receiving an injury serious enough to warrant medical care. These figures are comparable to or higher than the injury rates reported by domestic assault victims to the NCS and support the view that dating violence is a subset of violence against women.

Medical Consequences

Injury. Battering may be the single most common source of serious injury to women, accounting for more injury than auto accidents, muggings, and rape combined. Stark (1984) and Stark *et al.* (1981) reviewed the complete medical records of 3,676 women randomly selected from among female patients presenting with injury to a major metropolitan emergency room during a single year. Although a mere 1% ($n = 73$) of the 5,040 injury episodes ever presented by these women were identified by clinical staff as due to abuse or battering, a review of the adult trauma history revealed that fully 40% of the episodes were either identified by victims as resulting from a deliberate assault by an intimate other, or that this could be surmised from the circumstances. Also using the trauma history, the authors concluded that 19% of the women presenting to the emergency service with injury had a history of abuse. This compares to 11% presenting with injuries resulting from auto accidents, usually thought to be the most common source of serious injury. Clinicians identified only one battered woman in 35, and even these few diagnoses had little therapeutic relevance. By contrast with the institutional prevalence of 19%, the number of old and new cases, just 4% of the women presented during the year with their first at-risk episode, what might be termed the institutional incidence. In other words, 75% to 80% of the battering cases seen by medicine are ongoing. These figures have been independently confirmed by Anwar (1976), Appleton (1980), and McClear and Anwar (1986).

The Battering Syndrome. Although battering and abuse are sometimes used interchangeably, battering can be used epidemiologically to refer to a syndrome attendant upon spouse abuse and characterized by a history of injury (often including sexual assault), general medical complaints, psychosocial problems, and unsuccessful help seeking. In reviews of hospital records, Stark (1984), Stark *et al.* (1979) and Stark *et al.* (1981) and Rosenberg, Stark, and Zahn (1985) have identified a *battering syndrome* among abused women in which a history of trauma is accompanied by a disproportionate risk of rape, miscarriages, and abortion, alcohol and drug abuse, attempted suicide, child abuse, and mental illness. Paralleling this multiproblem profile is a history of help seeking marked by neglect and by inappropriate and punitive responses. According to Stark and Flitcraft (1987), the dual trauma of personal assault and institutional victimization lead to an increasing sense of isolation, entrapment, self-destructive behaviors, and even homicidal rage. Although abuse may involve either partner or both, to date battering has been identified only among women and is therefore synonymous with woman battering.

Using a stratified sampling procedure to compare battered women and nonbattered women, Stark *et al.* (1981) concluded that abusive injury is distinguished by its sexual nature, not its severity. Battered women are 13 times more likely than nonbattered women to be injured in the breast, chest, and abdomen, and three times as likely to be injured while pregnant. Frequent medical visits, particularly with vague complaints, and an extended medical history are direct functions of ongoing abuse. Almost one battered woman in five has presented at least 11 times with trauma, and another 23% have brought 6 to 10 abusive injuries to the attention of clinicians.

Medical Utilization. The greatest proportion of medical visits by battered women do not involve trauma but general medical, behavioral, and psychiatric presentations. Battered women are more likely to present depression, anxiety, family/marital/sexual problems (19% vs. 8%) and vague medical complaints (12% vs. 3%). As a result of these presentations, nontrauma medicine provides most of their care. For example, Stark (1984) and Stark and Flitcraft (1981) report that 25% of all obstetrical patients are abused women; this has been independently confirmed by Helton (1985). Meanwhile, 25% of all female patients seen by emergency psychiatry are abused. These percentages are even higher than in the emergency surgical service.

Alcohol and Drug Abuse. Battering appears to be the single most important context yet identified for female alcoholism. Since the association of alcohol abuse in women with adverse life events was reported, numerous writers have argued that alcoholism in women is more likely to arise from psychological stress and a specific precipitating circumstance than heavy drinking in men. The association of female alcoholism and violence is rarely made, however, although Hilberman and Munson (1977–78) made the intriguing observation that "the woman patients in a nearby alcohol rehabilitation program were almost all victims of parental and marital violence." Allan and Cooke (1985) cautioned that the structured interviews and life-stress scales used in much alcohol research rely on recall to distinguish onset, leaving it unclear whether alcohol is the context or consequence of stress.

Stark and Flitcraft (1981) reported that the rate of alcoholism among battered women is significantly greater than among nonbattered women (16% vs. 1%). A comparison of the recorded onset of alcoholism and of abusive injury among battered and nonbattered women indicates that 74% of the alcohol cases emerge only after the onset of abuse, suggesting abuse is the context for alcoholism among this population, not the reverse. Indeed, battered women who are also alcoholic have a higher rate of emergency medical utilization than any other population, an indication of the complex nature of woman battering as it evolves. Extrapolating to the medical population as a whole, approximately 50% of all female alcoholism may be precipitated by abuse.

Whereas battered women evidence no more drug abuse than nonbattered women prior to the onset of abuse, afterwards their corrected relative risk is 9, indicating that battering is associated with an increased risk of drug abuse that is 9 times greater than expected (Stark, 1984; Stark & Flitcraft, 1981).

Rape. Battering may be the single most important context for rape.

Descriptive studies frequently mention sexual assault as a factor in abusive relationships. Although battered women are more likely than nonbattered women to present as raped, rape is a relatively rare event in the medical setting. Reviewing the medical records of rape victims who used the surgical service over 2 years ($n = 174$), Roper, Flitcraft, and Frazier (1979) concluded that one third had a documented history of rape. Among victims over age 30, 58% were battered.

The Medical Response. Descriptive studies frequently report inadequate professional care, including neglect and the treatment of abused women with secondary problems such as alcoholism as "deliberate deviants" (Kurz & Stark, 1987; Stark & Flitcraft, in press). Despite their failure to identify abuse, physicians are more likely to refer battered women to emergency psychiatry (37% to 7%) and to label them as hysterics, neurotic, hypochondriacal, and as having psychosomatic disorders. Battered women are also more likely to be prescribed tranquilizers or pain medication and eventually to be institutionalized at the state mental hospital. At advanced stages of abuse, clinicians interpret secondary consequences, such as female alcoholism, as the cause of the violence and intervene to stop these secondary problems with a variety of punitive and/or family maintenance strategies that entrap women in violent relationships (Stark, 1984; Stark *et al.*, 1979). Battered women who attempt suicide are more likely than nonbattered attempters to receive no follow-up. Finally, battered mothers of abused children are more likely to have their children placed in foster care than nonbattered mothers (Stark & Flitcraft, 1985). Interestingly, child protective services rarely interview the potential foster father, a possible reason for high rates of child abuse in foster homes.

Mental Health Consequences

Nonrandom samples in mental health settings have included outpatient as well as inpatient populations, used interview as well as record review techniques, and focused on men as well as women. Although these studies provide important insight into the mental health correlates and sequelae of domestic violence, in lieu of survey data identifying which battered women utilize mental health facilities, the external validity of this work is limited.

Psychiatric Problems. Fully 20% of the abused population evidence mental health problems in addition to physical injury. More than a third (37%) carry a diagnosis of depression or another situational disorder, and 1 abused woman in 10 suffers a psychotic break. That psychiatric problems may be the context of abuse among some women is suggested by their slightly higher use of psychiatric services before the first recorded abusive episode. Still, 78% of the abused women using psychiatric services after the onset of abuse have not done so previously and differences in psychoses emerge only after the onset of abuse. At the same time, battered women are also far more likely than nonbattered women to be given a pseudopsychiatric label such as hysteric, hypochondriac, crock, etc. in the absence of evidence of mental illness. Indeed, 86% of all labels appear in the medical histories of abused women (Stark, 1984; Stark & Flitcraft, 1981; Rosenberg *et al.*, 1985).

Abuse appears to be one of the most important single background factors for patients in mental health settings. Hilberman and Munson (1977–78) found that half of 60 women referred for psychiatric consultation in a rural medical clinic were in battering relationships, but only four had been previously identified. Approximately half of all female inpatients have been physically and/or sexually abused, about twice the number of males who report abuse. But where adult abuse characterizes the women's experience, the majority of males report abuse as teenagers, primarily by their fathers (Carmen, Reiker, & Mills, 1984; Post *et al.*, 1980). Compared with an age-matched group of nonbattered patients, battered women are more likely to carry a diagnosis of personality disorder according to DSM-II (Back, Post, & D'arcy, 1980). Interestingly, in this highly disturbed population, there are no differences between battered and nonbattered groups on clinical scales of the MMPI or in the incidence of suicide attempts. Abused female inpatients exhibit markedly impaired self-esteem, direct their anger inward (often in self-destructive acts), and believe "that the abuse can be explained only by their essential 'badness.' " By contrast, abused males (mainly adolescents) are more likely to channel feelings of self-hatred into aggression toward others (Carmen *et al.*, 1984).

Stark (1984) reported that fully 25% of the women utilizing a psychiatric emergency service have a history of domestic violence. Although abuse was recorded as a specific problem in 25 of 429 visits made by the battered group, it never appeared as a final diagnosis. Battered women using this service are less likely than nonbattered women to manifest psychotic illness, but more likely to present situational and personality disorders. Even among this population of multiproblem individuals, alcoholism is twice as common among battered than nonbattered women (20% vs. 10%). Despite a marked absence of psychiatric disease, battered alcoholics have a mean rate of psychiatric emergency service utilization three times greater than nonbattered alcoholics and a trauma history 10 times as great.

Suicide Attempts. Battering appears to be the single most important context yet identified for female suicide attempts.

In *Suicide,* Durkheim associated "fatalistic suicide" with "excessive regulation," futures that were "pitilessly blocked," "violently choked" passions and with "physical or moral despotism" (Johnson, 1979). Where psychiatric research has linked female suicide attempts to family conflict, the explanation offered is underlying psychiatric disease, general hostility, depression, or a rigid personality (Neuringer, 1964; Vinoda, 1966; Weisman, Fox, & Klarman, 1973). Descriptive studies by Gayford (1975a), Pagelow (1976) and Walker (1979) report 35% to 40% of abused women attempt suicide, but these samples are nonrepresentative.

Though there are no differences between battered and nonbattered women prior to the first reported episode of abuse, subsequently, battered women evidence a relative risk of attempted suicide that is 4.8 times as high. Of the 10% who attempt suicide, almost 50% do so more than once (Stark, 1984; Stark & Flitcraft, 1981). Twenty-six percent of all female suicide attempts presented to the hospital in a year are associated with battering, whereas fully 50% of the black women who attempt suicide are abused. The battered women (26% of the population) account for 42% of all traumatic attempts and are significantly more likely to attempt more than once (20% vs. 8%). Eighty-five percent of these women are seen in the hospital for at least one abusive injury prior to their first suicide attempt, again highlighting the importance of abuse as a precipitant. Furthermore, 44% (vs. 11%) mention marital conflict as the precipitating factor, an interesting finding because 70% of the abused women are single, divorced, or separated (Stark, 1984; Stark & Flitcraft, 1981).

Child Abuse. Woman battering appears to be the single most important context for child abuse. In these cases, the majority of the assailants are the male batterers.

A range of psychological and behavioral problems in children result from violence among parents, including internalizing behavior, nervousness, and sadness (Cohn & Christopoulos, 1984); anxiety disorders (Levine, 1975), depression (Brown, Pelcovitz, & Kaplan, 1983) nightmares, violence toward siblings and pets, respiratory distress and a range of somatic complaints (Hilberman & Munson, 1977–78). And correlational evidence links the physical abuse of children with battering. Straus *et al.* (1980) reported that the risk of child abuse is 12% higher where the husband hits his wife, Stewart and deBlois

(1981) found child abuse was two times as common among battered than nonbattered women, and Stark and Flitcraft (1985) reported that battered women evidence an excess risk of 5. But estimates of the exact association vary widely. Thus, whereas Levine (1975) uncovered physical abuse among only 1.7% of the children of battered mothers in his private practice, Hilberman and Munson (1977–78) found fully a third of the children in the rural population of battered women had been physically or sexually abused.

If the frequency of child abuse in battering relationships remains unclear, the impact of battering on child abuse is well documented. In a review of a year's sample of mothers whose children had been ''darted'' for suspected physical abuse or neglect (n = 116), Stark and Flitcraft (1985) reported 45% are battered women, the highest percentage thus far identified in any client population. Compared to the nonbattered mothers, the battered mothers are less likely to come from a multiproblem background including incest and/or alcoholism and no more likely to have a background that includes violence. Still, physical abuse (as opposed to neglect) is more than twice as likely among the children of the battered mothers.

The propensity for batterers to abuse their children is widely mentioned (Coleman, 1980; Washburn & Frieze, 1981). And although there are no case studies of or programs specifically directed toward male child abusers (Martin, 1983), surveys estimate that fathers or father substitutes comprise from 40% to 55% of all assailants (American Humane Society, 1978; Baher, 1976; Gil, 1973). Stark and Flitcraft (1985) reported that fathers or father substitutes are three times as likely to be the abusing parent in families where the mother is also battered, accounting for 50% of all child abuse in these families.

Personality, Demographic, and Vulnerability Factors

Battered Women. Apart from the increased incidence of mental health problems following abuse reported by Stark (1984) and Stark and Flitcraft (1981), studies correlating personality traits with physical abuse fail to establish cause and effect. Several studies report greater personality disturbance among battered women than among comparison groups. But studies with the most reliable designs report few if any differences in personality. Battered women appear more aggressive (or hostile) than comparison groups and may suffer a loss of self-esteem. But, outside the psychiatric hospital, little support is found for the view that battered women blame themselves for the violence or otherwise evidence a helplessness syndrome. No consistent personality profile has been identified for battered women. Where some turn anger inward in classic psychoanalytic fashion, a substantial number are aggressive, independent, and overtly hostile to their assailants. These behaviors, as well as excessive fear evident in frequent changes in address or phone numbers, are often appropriate given the real dangers in abusive relationships.

Early psychiatric reports of abused women reflected the stereotyped view that they ''ask for it'' by exhibiting behavior that is inappropriately aggressive, masculine, frigid, and masochistic (Ball, 1977; Scott, 1974; Snell, Rosenwald, & Robey, 1964). Feldman (1980) described the abused woman as overly emotional, aggressive, concrete in her mode of thinking, with weakened ties to reality when under stress. Similarly, Contoni (1981) emphasized role reversal, inappropriate sexual expression, lack of trust, conflict over dependency, and either a lack or excess of control.

These findings have not been supported in comparison studies, however. Thus, when Graff (1980) matched samples of battered and nonbattered women, he found they were generally alike. Though the abused women were more hostile and dominant, they were also more social, sympathetic, and skeptical. When Telch and Lindquist (1984) compared violent, nonviolent but distressed, and nonviolent nontherapy couples, they found that aggressiveness was the only factor distinguishing battered women. Finally, Star (1978) reported that battered women exhibit more independence and ego strength than controls, whereas Finn (1985), in a study of issues provoking violence, emphasized the importance of power balances in the relationship and suggested the abuse victim has a better sense of reality than her assailant, particularly with respect to sexual relations.

Another portrayed stereotype emphasizes low self-esteem and passivity (Shainess, 1977). Battered women are pictured as shy and reserved (Weitzman & Dreen, 1981), more likely than controls to submit to rules (Star, 1978), and as suffering from a help-lessness syndrome (Walker, 1979) that leads them to blame themselves for violence, avoid helping services altogether, or delay using medical care (Petro, 1978).

Evidence on how abuse affects self-esteem is mixed. Hartik (1979) administered the Tennessee Self-Concept Scale and the 16 Personality Factor Questionnaire to abused and nonabused married women. The abused women showed less ego strength, lower self-esteem, and were generally less satisfied with themselves. Similarly, Hofeller (1980) reported battered women evidence lower self-esteem (but no other differences) in a matched sample. But, researchers have generally failed to find low self-esteem among abused client populations (cf. Carmen *et al.*, 1984). Thus, in Telch and Lindquist's careful comparison of violent couples in therapy with two comparison groups, battered women showed no differences in self-esteem and the authors concluded this was not a reliable discriminator. Stewart and deBlois (1981) found no differences between battered and nonbattered women, Back, Post, and D'Arcy (1980) found no differences on MMPI clinical scales among the battered and nonbattered inpatient populations they studied, and Coleman (1980) reported no differences between battered and nonbattered women on the Bem Sex Role Inventory when gender type was controlled. When Walker (1983) used a semantic differential scale to examine the self-perceptions of battered women, she found they were stronger, more independent, and more sensitive than other women, contradicting her earlier predictions of learned helplessness. Meanwhile, contrary to earlier allegations, abused patients actually seek medical help even more promptly than auto accident victims (Stark, 1984). Feelings of helplessness may as often result from a history of institutional victimization as from violence, and the view of abused women as helpless victims (rather than survivors) may actually prompt interventions that reduce a woman's ability to cope. Two important descriptive studies of shelter populations fail to find any evidence that women feel responsible for the pattern of violence (Frieze, 1979; Pagelow, 1976). In all probability, hospitalization is a source of low self-esteem among abused mental patients, whereas the more positive self-perceptions of women in shelters reflect their emphasis on support and advocacy.

Male Batterers. Apart from the association of abusive behavior and alcohol, no personality factors have been identified that consistently distinguish batters from nonbatterers.

Descriptive studies emphasizing the psychopathological roots of battering trace male violence to a vulnerable self-concept (or low self-esteem); a complex of helplessness, powerlessness, or inadequacy; conflicts over being dependent; traditional attitudes, particularly about sex; pathological jealousy; fear of abandonment, alternating with a desire for control over women and children; an inability to communicate feelings or to identify feelings in others (empathy); and a lack of assertiveness (Ball, 1977; Makmon, 1978; Saunders, 1982; Weitzman & Dreen, 1982). But comparison studies fail to substantiate that these features are distinctive.

Although batterers evidence low self-esteem, are less assertive than their spouses, and lack communication skills, they share these traits with nonviolent males in distressed relationships (Rosenbaum & O'Leary, 1981; Telsch & Linquist, 1984). Furthermore, control studies report no differences in their expressiveness or empathy, in authoritarianism and dogmatism, in *N*power (the need for power or control), in expectations of others, in attitudes toward violence, or in adversarial sexual beliefs (Browning, 1983; Dvoskin, 1981). Thus, although the negative traits identified by descriptive studies are linked to marital difficulties, they appear to be general attributes of American males rather than of violent men specifically.

Vulnerability Factors. Research on domestic violence has focused more closely on acts and their consequences than on background or etiological factors. Efforts to operationalize major causal theories lack consistency in how the problem is defined and measured and fail to establish a clear temporal sequence that demonstrates that an alleged characteristic, such as low self-esteem, is a cause or risk factor rather than an outcome of violence. Even where certain factors are shown to correlate with and precede domestic violence, the lack of longitudinal research, a failure to differentiate samples along the dimension in question or to demonstrate statistically that a given factor(s) can predict violent outcomes either alone or in combination, make it difficult to specify causal pathways with any certainty (Hotaling & Sugarman, 1985).

Researchers following the child abuse model emphasize risk factors, personal or group characteristics, and behaviors or environmental conditions whose presence increases the probability that an individual or group will suffer a certain problem. A factor may increase risk without causing a disorder. But a number of questionable assumptions about causality are nevertheless implied in most risk factor analysis. Moreover, a factor, such as a childhood history of violence, may contribute to a disorder among some sufferers, but have so small an impact on overall prevalence that its use in an early warning or identification system is nil. Meanwhile, the simple possession of a risk factor is often equated with responsibility for the problem. Finally, without establishing a clear temporal sequence, the alleged risk may really be a product of abuse. As yet, there is no evidence that changing certain characteristics of victims will be 'protective' in the way that stopping smoking protects against lung cancer.

No factor other than male violence appears to precipitate any substantial degree of woman battering. Conversely, apart from age, no factors have been consistently found to increase a woman's risk of abuse. Race, income, occupation, alcohol, an inheritance of violence, isolation and status inconsistency are frequently cited risk factors, but their importance remains ambiguous (Hotaling & Sugarman, 1984). Given these caveats, we discuss the demographic, behavioral, and relational features of domestic violence as what Brown and Harris (1978) term *vulnerability factors*. Such factors appear to interact with the situational dynamics of domestic conflict to increase the likelihood that violence will result and that the woman exposed to these factors will be battered.

Race. Black women are more likely to be abused than white women. It is unclear, however, whether this excess risk is a function of race, income, or other factors. Straus *et al.* (1980) and Schulman (1979) have reported a prevalence among blacks that is two to three times greater than among whites. But black women are twice as likely as whites to report their problem (Schulman, 1979). And Casawave and Straus (1979) found that among groups with similar income, blacks were less likely than whites to experience spousal violence.

Income, Occupation, and Status. Studies consistently report an inverse relation between income and domestic violence. Certain white-collar occupations (or occupational environments) may be associated with elevated risk. And status inconsistency may increase a woman's chance of being victimized.

Despite early reports that domestic violence is common in upper- and middle-class communities, numerous studies, including the national representative survey, find substantially higher rates of domestic violence among the poor and working class (Gelles, 1974; Peterson, 1980; Stark, 1984; Steinmetz, 1974; Straus *et al.*, 1980). The extent to which reporting bias explains these differences is unclear. Still, the most exacting statistics demonstrate only a 3% difference between the spousal violence reported by low-income women (11%) and women with family incomes of $25,000 or above (8%), with 10% of middle-income women reporting abuse (Schulman, 1979). Indeed, couples with the lowest educational levels (school dropouts), a frequent indicator of low income, are less prone to violence than those who had attended high school.

Similarly, although unemployment of males and their victims has been linked to woman battering. (Stark *et al.*, 1981; Straus *et al.*, 1980) without factoring out race, income, and education, it is impossible to tell whether being without a job in itself increases risk. And, one representative sample found housewives had a lower risk of violence than employed women (Horning, McCullough, & Sugimoto, 1981).

In an early paper, Steinmetz (1977) argued that occupational environment (rather than employment status *per se*) was an important stimulus to violence and survey data points alternately to clerical and service workers or managers and professionals as at highest risk (Gaguin, 1977; Schulman, 1979). There is some evidence that women's risk of victimization increases if their occupational and educational status are inconsistent (e.g., if education is high and job status low) or if their status is higher than their male partner's (Hotaling & Sugarman, 1984). By contrast, status inconsistency among men does not differentiate abusive males (Horning *et al.*, 1981; Hotaling & Sugerman, 1984; O'Brien, 1971).

Age. Although acts of domestic violence are more common among couples under 30 than among 31- to 50-year-olds (Dvoskin, 1981; Straus *et al.*, 1980), age does not differentiate battered from nonbattered women in clinical populations (Post *et al.*, Stark & Flitcraft, 1981), possibly because women may remain in battering relationships even after abusive acts are infrequent.

Marital Status. Married women are the least likely and single, separated, and divorced women the most likely to experience assault by a male intimate.

Early surveys assessed domestic violence only among intact couples, reinforcing a widespread belief that wives were the exclusive targets of battering (Schulman, 1979; Straus *et al.*, 1980). The NCS data, however, indicate that separated women are the most vulnerable group with divorced women next and married women last. Further, 75% of the clinical population of battered women are single, separated, or divorced, and a woman's risk of abuse increases with separation (Stark & Flitcraft, 1981). Conversely, whereas only 15.6% of all assaults among married women are domestic, fully 55% of assaults among separated women are by a male intimate.

Social Isolation/Mobility. Violent couples and battered women are consistently reported to be more socially isolated than controls (Garbarino & Sherman, 1980; Stark,

1984), a particular problem among military families (Bowen, 1984). Because isolation is a frequent consequence of ongoing abuse, however, we cannot say whether isolation is a significant vulnerability factor.

Pregnancy. Among abused women, pregnancy is a high-risk period.

Although family pressures, including number of children, are frequently cited risk factors for battering, battered women in the medical complex average no more children than nonbattered women (Stark, 1984). Still, they are pregnant nearly twice as often, significantly more likely to have a miscarriage or abortion, and more likely to be pregnant at the time of their injury (Stark & Flitcraft, 1981), again highlighting the importance of sexual assault. The Texas survey found that 28% of the abused women in their population were beaten while pregnant (Teske & Parker, 1983). And between 20% and 25% of all obstetrical patients are abused women (Helton, 1985; Stark *et al.*, 1981).

Alcohol. Although alcohol abuse among battered women is a common sequelae of deliberate injury, alcohol abuse has been consistently associated with violence by men.

Although alcohol abuse distinguishes battered women from control groups (Stark *et al.*, 1981; Telch & Lindquist, 1984), the largest proportion of battered women who abuse alcohol do so only after the onset of assaultive violence.

The correlation of alcohol use and abusive behavior has been frequently demonstrated for men (Telch & Lindquist, 1984), but cause and effect are unclear. Coleman and Straus (1983) reported that men who drink often are more than 15 times as likely to abuse their wives as nondrinkers. And alcoholism is a frequently mentioned precursor to child abuse. Still, Byles (1979) and Orne and Rimmer (1980), in a comprehensive literature review, concluded that a causal role for alcohol cannot be supported. Alcohol is a factor in fewer than 8% of the domestic abuse cases where police are called (McClintock, 1978). In sum, although alcohol probably increases the risk of abusive violence, in lieu of conclusive evidence it should be considered a contextual factor to be treated separately from the violence.

Violence in the Family of Origin. Violence in the family of origin increases both a woman's vulnerability and a man's propensity to abuse his wife and/or children. But, the vast majority of abused women and male abusers have not been beaten as children and the vast majority of persons who have been beaten as children are not involved in violent realtionships.

Straus *et al.* (1980) claimed that "the majority of today's violent couples are those who were brought up by parents who were violent to each other" and, further, that "children who are abused grow up to be abusing parents." But this widespread belief is unfounded.

The first question is whether a childhood experience of abuse or parental violence separates partners in currently violent relationships from nonviolent partners. A second question is whether such a childhood experience is a sensitive or a specific indicator of adult violence/victimization? Is there, in other words, a high probability that a child with such an experience will become a batterer or victim or, conversely, that a batterer or his victim will have experienced childhood violence?

Survey and case-control studies report significant correlations between current victimization and a woman's experience of abuse or parental violence as a child (Dvoskin, 1981; Schulman, 1979; Straus *et al.*, 1980). Stark and Flitcraft (1985) compared the actual pediatric records of battered and nonbattered women and found that the abuse victims had an excess risk of childhood abuse 14 times higher than expected (15% to 1%). However, two well-designed studies using multiple comparison groups and collecting data from men and women found no significant effect of childhood violence on later victimization (Rosenbaum & O'Leary, 1981; Telch & Lindquist, 1984). All of these studies, including the two with negative findings about physical abuse as a child, report that witnessing parental violence as a child effects subsequent victimization. Unfortunately, definitions of the dependent and independent variables in this research run the gamut from physical punishment to serious abuse. Another problem is reporter bias. For instance, a current victim of violence will be more likely than a nonvictim to report violence in her childhood.

Evaulating evidence on the childhood experience of current batterers is even more problematic. Psychiatric researchers have supported the thesis that violence is transmitted intergenerationally—the so-called cycle of violence theory—primarily by examining small and highly unrepresentative groups of prominent law-breakers, such as Charles Manson, presidential assassins, delinquents, and convicted murderers (Button, 1973; Solnit, Goldstein, & Freud, 1977). Meanwhile, the basis for the claim by Straus *et al.* (1980) that the transmission thesis has been proved "beyond a doubt" is the support garnered by B. F. Steele (1976). But to Steele, childhood abuse or neglect is a "lack of empathetic mothering," a definition that falls far outside the criteria of domestic violence employed here.

Most studies linking childhood violence to adult victimization also report a significant effect of exposure to violence as a child on current assaultive behavior (Straus *et al.*, 1980; Telch & Lindquist, 1984), with Coleman (1980) reporting that witnessing childhood violence is the best predictor of violence by men. Although some association probably exists, caution is appropriate given the array of definitions employed and the probability that current victims and assailants will rationalize their current predicament by overreporting childhood victimization.

Even if a link between childhood violence and adult victimization and/or abuse is accepted, how sensitive and specific is childhood violence as an indicator? Extrapolating from their sample, Stark and Flitcraft (*et al.,* 1981; 1985) have suggested that fully 79% of women with a history of documented child abuse may be battered women, a very high degree of sensitivity, and one battered woman in four may have a childhood history that includes child abuse, making child abuse relatively specific as well. This also means that 75% of currently battered women do not have a childhood history of violence. In lieu of longitudinal and prospective data, generalizations should not be made based on these findings.

Straus *et al.* (1980) presented extensive data on the sensitivity and specificity of childhood violence as an indicator of current battering behavior, demonstrating that men from violent childhoods (5% of the total population) are three times as likely to hit their wives and 10 times more likely to abuse them as men from nonviolent childhoods. However, the currently nonviolent group is far larger than the group in their sample that is currently abusive in our terms. As a result, extrapolating to the population as a whole, this data indicates that 90% of the children from violent homes and even 80% of the children from the homes that are most violent do not become batterers. Moreover, although a boy who witnessed wife abuse is three times as likely to abuse his wife as a boy who did not witness parental abuse, given the relative proportions of children from violent and nonviolent homes, (5% to 37%), a current batterer is more than twice as likely to have had a nonviolent childhood (7:3) and seven times more likely to come from nonviolent than from the most violent homes. In sum, childhood exposure to violence appears to be neither a sensitive nor a specific indicator of battering by men.

Conclusions

As the battered women's movement has grown, it has evoked interest from and become increasingly dependent on the assistance of researchers and a range of helping professionals. In this process, the feminist identification of battering with gender inequality has been challenged by a model that emphasizes the psychological roots and dynamics of family violence, the stress/pathology model. In this view, violent behavior and victimization are learned in childhood, culturally supported, and provoked by current stressors, such as poverty and unemployment, and transmitted from one family member to another. Assailants and victims are distinguished by a common profile: they are dependent, hostile, unable to communicate or empathize with the feelings of others and have low self-esteem. Victims in particular suffer from self-blame, helplessness, and other personality deficits. The logical extension of this analysis is the identification of risk factors (such as alcoholism, unemployment, or social isolation), treatment of injured and impaired family members and counseling designed to strengthen family coping.

The political model views violence in the home as the extension into private life of the social control exercised by men over women and children in virtually every institution. The basis for this control is men's privileged access to resources and the occasion for violence the threat to this privilege, both real or perceived, posed by women's growing independence. Far more important than an inheritance of violence or psychopathology in this approach are situational dynamics involving power balance in areas ranging from sexuality through work. In the family model, woman battering is distinguished by the physical consequences of the fact that men hit harder. By contrast, the political model views woman battering as different in kind from other family fights and as holding the key to domestic violence overall, including child abuse. Institutional maltreatment plays a crucial role in battering as well. As help is either denied or actually turned against the abused woman, her options are closed, she feels entrapped, and may become alternately passive or hostile. In the stress/pathology model, these are predisposing personality deficits. Moreover, woman battering is a danger in all intimate relations among adults, not merely among cohabitants.

By contrast with the professional approach, the battered women's shelters define the abused woman as a survivor whose incredible coping skills provide the basis for individual empowerment and system advocacy (Schecter, 1982). Violence is the key issue for treatment (though secondary pathology should be cared for as well) and separating women in treatment and invoking legal sanctions to stop the violence are powerful ethical and therapeutic statements about responsibility for the violence. Although some women may chose to return to previously violent relationships, the therapeutic imperative is protection and autonomy, not family functioning (Stark & Flitcraft, 1987).

The epidemiological evidence supports some aspects of the stress/pathology paradigm. For instance, homicide and assault data indicate that women hit and kill husbands almost as often as they are attacked and killed and sometimes even more frequently. A significant subgroup of abused males has been identified as well among mental hospital inpatients, although they are primarily adolescents. In addition, abused psychiatric patients exhibit a posttraumatic stress syndrome whose hallmarks are the same self-blame and impaired self-esteem found among rape victims (Burgess & Holstrom, 1974) and Vietnam veterans (Rosenheck, 1985–86). The family background and demographic characteristics of abused women indicate that for perhaps as many as one in four, current violence reflects some combination of inherited pathology, including a childhood experience of abuse or parental violence, and environmental stress. Moreover, male children who experience or witness violence are far more likely than children from nonviolent families to become batterers as adults. Environmental stressors that appear to increase a couple's vulnerability to violence include low income, minority status, unemployment and status inconsistency. Alcohol may also be a risk factor for men and, to a lesser degree, for female victims as well.

The most important tenets of the stress/pathology model find little support, however, including the importance of husband abuse; the predisposing role of psychopathology, personality deficits, and family problems; and the utility of identifying risk factors.

Husband and wife abuse appear similar only so long as all acts of force are equated irrespective of their social, historical, and political context and consequence. Police and crime data indicate that complaints of wife–husband assault are almost nonexistent (Dobash & Dobash, 1979; Steinmetz, 1977–78). Most important, there are no clinical reports of a battering syndrome among men similar to the profile identified among women. Still, limited claims about wife–husband assault would appear incontrovertible. Although a certain amount of wife–husband violence is undoubtedly defensive, it seems implausible that women are violent only in response to men, as some feminists claim. Moreover, the notion that women are only reactive can reinforce institutional biases that deprive aggressive women of equal protection and undermine a woman's capacity to act effectively on her own behalf. This does not change the fact that even if a woman wins a particular fight, because of the social support given to male authority she ends up "battered," not the male.

Outside the psychiatric facility, there is no consistent evidence that battered women share a common personality profile either as context or consequence of their abuse. In response to psychological tests, abused women have as frequently appeared to be aggressive as passive, to be independent and dominant as dependent, and to evidence ego strength as well as impaired self-concepts. Meanwhile, the disproportionate incidence of alcoholism, drug abuse, attempted suicide, child abuse, and mental illness among abused women arises only after the onset of abuse, and so cannot be its cause. Where early claims that women delayed seeking help supported the image of pathology and helplessness, it now appears that professional neglect explains the paucity of institutional statistics on the problem. By contrast, mental health clients appear open about abuse when sensitively questioned (Hilberman & Munson, 1977–78), and fully 50% of the abused women in the medical setting positively identify a male intimate as a source of their problem (Stark, 1984). Finally, the Texas survey documents that fully 25% of the women abused during the previous year and 63% of those ever abused have divorced or permanently left their husband or live-in partner, discounting the image of abused women as helpless.

Evidence that batterers have a distinguishing personality profile is equally weak. Battering males are generally unassertive, evidence impaired self-esteem, and lack communication skills. But they share these deficits with men in distressed but nonviolent marriages. Moreover, batterers appear identical to controls in their attitudes toward violence and sexuality, their authoritarianism, and in their empathy and expressiveness.

The data on intergenerational transmission does not support the cycle of violence theory as an explanation of woman battering or child abuse. A childhood experience with parental violence is neither a sensitive nor specific indicator of violence among males. The vast majority of batterers and battered women have not experienced violence in their families of origin and the vast majority of persons who experience violence in their childhood do not become batterers or battering victims. Further, men (not abused women) are the typical child abusers in violent homes, and the battered mothers of abused children are actually less likely than their nonbattered counterparts to have had a childhood that includes violence, incest, or alcoholism. As Kaufman and Zigler (1986) argued, rather than persist in the false belief that "violence begets violence," future researchers should investigate the mechanisms and factors that affect the transmission of abuse among a minority and that inhibit such transmission among the vast majority. Although data linking a childhood experience of abuse to current battering appears sensitive and specific, prospective studies developed around a variety of hypotheses are called for to substantiate this connection.

There is some evidence that blacks are more prone to violence (and to abuse) than whites, but this may reflect overreporting by blacks. There are slightly more abusive relationships as one moves down the income ladder. Abuse is more common among younger adults and unemployment or status inconsistency may also increase a woman's vulnerability. For men, alcohol abuse is highly associated with battering, though whether as cause or context remains unclear. A risk profile of violent couples based on a combination of low-income, minority status, unemployment, status inconsistency, alcoholism, and an inheritance of violence might prove to be a sensitive indicator of abuse. But its lack of specificity prevents such a profile from aiding identification, particularly in police, medical, mental health or other multiproblem case-loads. It should prove far more useful to base identification protocols on site-specific assessments of how abuse is typically presented.

The political model is widely accepted by the battered women's movement. But because funds required for carefully designed case-control or survey research have been garnered primarily by proponents of the stress/pathology paradigm, evidence for the political model is sketchy and anecdotal. Even so, support for its basic tenets has been consistent, suggesting that future research should follow this paradigm more closely.

The prevalence, frequency, the accumulated severity of abuse, and the psychosocial pattern it evokes, in combination with an inappropriate helping response, distinguish woman battering from other forms of domestic violence and suggest a distinct response. Changing the behavior and attitudes of service professionals and removing the structural incentives for them to neglect abuse are important first steps to early identification and prevention. Professional education and the development of appropriate protocols should extend to the tertiary sites where the multiple sequelae of abuse are now treated as primary problems, particularly to alcohol rehabilitation, suicide prevention, and child abuse programs. With respect to child abuse especially, liaison with battered women's shelters should be combined with aggressive management of the male violence responsible for 45% or more of all such abuse.

To date, there have been no clinical, descriptive or case-observation studies of abused males. For this reason, it is impossible to affirm unhesitatingly the major claim of the feminists, namely that its political dynamic makes woman battering clinically distinct. In lieu of persuasive evidence to the contrary, however, it seems warranted to conclude that woman battering results from the dual trauma of male violence and institutional victimization, and that its consequence is to further subordinate the personal power of women to the already greater authority of men.

REFERENCES

Allan, C. A., & Cooke, D. J. (1985). Stressful life events and alcohol misuse in women: A critical review. *Journal of Studies on Alcohol, 46,* 147–152.

American Humane Society. (1978). *National analysis of official child neglect and abuse reporting.* Denver, CO: Author.

Anwar, R. (1976). *Woman abuse: retrospective review of all female trauma presenting to the emergency room.* Philadelphia, PA: Medical College of Pennsylvania.

Appleton, W. (1980). The battered woman syndrome, *Annals of Emergency Medicine, 9,* 84–91.

Back, S. M., Post, R. D., & D'Arcy, H. (September, 1980). *A comparison of battered and nonbattered female psychiatric patients.* Paper presented at the meeting of the American Psychological Association, Montreal, Canada.

Baher, E. (1976). *At risk: an account of the work of the battered child research department,* NSPCC, Boston, MA: Routledge & Kegan Paul.

Ball, M. (1977). Issues of violence in family casework. *Social Casework, 58,* 3–12.

Berk, R. A., Berk, S. F., Loseke, D. R., & Rauma, D. (1983). Mutual combat and other family violence myths. In D. Finkelhor, R. Gelles, G. Hotaling, & M. Straus (Eds.), *The dark side of families: Current family violence research.* Beverly Hills, CA: Sage.

Bogal-Allbritten, R. B., & Allbritten, B. (1983, August). *The hidden victims: Premarital abuse among college students,* Paper presented at the meeting of the American Psychological Association: Anaheim, CA.

Boudouris, J. (1971). Homicide and the family, *Journal of Marriage and the Family, 33,* 667–676.

Bowen, G. (1984). Spouse abuse: Incidence and dynamics, *Military Family, 33,* 667–682.

Brown, A. J., Pelcovitz, D., & Kaplan, S. (1983, August), *Child witnesses of family violence: A study of psychological correlates.* Paper presented at the meeting of the American Psychological Association, Anaheim, CA.

Brown, G. W., & Harris, T. (1978). *Social origins of depression—A study of psychiatric disorder in women.* London: Tavistock.

Browning, J. J. (1983). *Violence against intimates: Toward a profile on the wife assaultor.* Unpublished Ph.D Dissertation, Department of Psychology, University of British Columbia.

Brownmiller, S. (1975). *Against our will: Men, women and rape.* New York: Simon & Schuster.

Burgess, A., & Holmstrom, L. (1974). Rape trauma syndrome, *American Journal of Psychiatry, 131,* 981–986.

Button, A. (1973). Some antecedents of felonious and delinquent behavior. *Journal of Clinical Child Psychology, 2,* 35–38.

Byles, J. A. (1979). Violence, alcohol problems and other problems in disintegrating families, *Journal of Studies on Alcohol, 39,* (3).

Carmen (Hilberman), E., Rieker, P., & Mills, T. (1984). Victims of violence and psychiatric illness. *American Journal of Psychiatry, 141,* 378–383.

Casanave, N. A., & Straus, M. A. (1979). Race, class, network embeddedness and family violence: A search for potent support systems. *Journal of Comparative Family Studies, 10,* 281–299.

Cobbe, F. P. (1878). Wife-torture in England. *The Contemporary Review, XXXII,* 55–87.

Cohn, D. A., Christopoulos, Kraft,C., & Emery, R. (August, 1984). *The psychological adjustment of school-aged children of battered women: A preliminary look,* Paper presented at the Second National Conference for Family Violence Researchers, Durham, NH.

Coleman, K. H. (1980). Conjugal violence: What 33 men report. *Journal of Marital and Family Therapy, 6,* 207–213.

Coleman, D. H., & Straus, D. H. (1983). Alcohol abuse and family violence. In E. Gottheil, A. Druley, I. E. Skolada and H. Waxman (Eds.), *Alcohol, drug abuse, and aggression.* Springfield, IL: Charles C Thomas.

Comins, C. A. (August, 1984). *Courtship violence: A recent study and its implications for future research.* Paper presented at the Second National Conference for Family Violence Researchers, Durham, NH.

Contoni, L. (1981). Clinical issues in domestic violence. *Social Casework, 62,* 3–12.

Dobash, R., & Dobash, R. E. (August, 1974). *Violence between men and women within the family setting.* Paper presented at the VIII World Congress of Sociology, Toronto, Canada.

Dobash, R. E., & Dobash, R. (1977–78). Wives: The appropriate victims of marital violence. *Victimology, 2,* 426–442.

Dvoskin, J. A. (1981). *Battered women—An epidemiological study of spousal violence.* Unpublished Ph.D Dissertation, Department of Psychology, University of Arizona.

Feldman, L. S. (1980). *Conjugal violence: A psychological and symbolic interactionist analysis.* Dissertation Abstracts International, *40*(7) 3390–B, No. 79-28687.

Finn, J. (1985). The stresses and coping behavior of battered women. *Social Casework,* 341–349.

Flaherty, E. W. (1985). *Identification and intervention with battered women in hospital emergency departments,* Final Report (Grant # R01 MH37180), National Institute of Mental Health.

Frieze, I. R. (1979). Percpetions of battered wives. In I. R. Frieze, D. Bar-Tal, & V. S. Carroll (Eds.), *New approaches to social problems* (pp. 79–108). San Francisco: Jossey-Bass.

Gaquin, D. A. (1977–78). Spouse abuse: Data from the National Crime Survey, *Victimology, 2,* 632–643.

Garbarino, J., & Sherman, D. (1980). High-risk families and high-risk neighborhoods. *Child Development, 51,* 188–198.

Gayford, J. J. (1975a). Wife battering: A preliminary survey of 100 cases. *British Medical Journal, 1,* 194–197.

Gayford, J. J. (1975b). Battered wives. *Medicine Science and the Law, 15,* 237.

Gelles, R. (1974). *The violent home.* Beverly Hills, CA: Sage.

Genteman, K. M. (1980, March). *Attitudes of North Carolina women toward the acceptance and causes of wife beating.* Paper presented at the meeting of the Southeastern Women's Studies Association, Nashville, TN.

Gerson, L. W. (1978). Alcohol related acts of violence: Who was drinking and where the acts occurred. *Journal of Studies on Alcohol, 39,* 1294–1296.

Gil, D. (1973). *Violence against children: Physical child abuse in the United States.* Cambridge, MA: Harvard University Press.

Graft, T. T. (1980). *Personality characteristics of battered women.* Dissertation Abstracts International, *40* (7-B), 3395.

Gratton, R. T. (1982). *An empirical study of abuse of the elderly.* Unpublished MSW Thesis, Smith College School of Social Work.

Hartik, L. M. (1979). *Identification of personality characteristics and self-concept factors of battered women,* Dissertation Abstracts International, *40,* (2-B), 893.

Helton, A. S. (1985). *Battering during pregnancy: A prevalence study in a metropolitan area,* Unpublished M.S. Thesis, College of Nursing, Texas Woman's University, Denton, TX.

Hilberman, E. (1980). Overview: The "wife-beater's wife" reconsidered. *American Journal of Psychiatry, 137,* 1336–1347.

Hilberman, E., & Munson, K. (1977–78). Sixty battered women. *Victimology, 2,* 460–470.

Hofeller, K. H. (1980). *Social, psychological and situational factors in spouse abuse.* Dissertation Abstracts International, *41,* (1-B), 408.

Horning, C. A., McCullough, B. C., & Sugimoto, T. (1981). Status relationships in marriage: risk factors in spouse abuse. *Journal of Marriage and the Family, 43,* 675–692.

Hotaling, G. T., & Sugerman, D. B. (1984). An identification of risk factors in *Domestic violence surveillance system feasibility study. phase I report,* Rockville, MD: Westat.

Johnson, K. (1979). Why do women kill themselves? *Suicide and Life Threatening Behavior, 9*(3), 145–153.

Johnston, M. E. (1984). *Correlates of early violence experience among men who are abusive toward female mates.* Paper presented to the Second National Conference for Domestic Violence Researchers, Durham, NH.

Kaufman, J., & Zigler, E. (1987). Do abused children become abusive parents? *American Journal of Orthopsychiatry, 57*(2), 186–193.

Klaus, P. A., & Rand, M. R. (1984). *Family violence.* Special report by the Bureau of Justice Statistics. Department of Justice: Washington, DC.

Kurz, D., & Stark, E. (1987). Health education and feminist strategy: The case of woman abuse. In M. Bograd & K. Yllo (Eds.), *Feminist perspectives in wife abuse.* Beverly Hills, CA: Sage.

Lau, E. A., & Kosberg, V. I. (1979). Abuse of the elderly by informal care providers. *Aging, Sept./Oct.,* 10–15.

Levine, M. (1975). Interparental violence and its effect on the children: A study of 50 families in general practice. *Medicine science and the law, 15* (3), 172.

Makepeace, J. M. (August, 1984). *The severity of courtship violence injuries and individual precautionary measures.* Paper presented at the Second National Conference for Family violence Researchers, Durham, NH.

Makmon, R. S. (1978). Some clinical aspects of inter-spousal violence. In J. M. Eekelaar & S. N. Katz (Eds.), *Family violence: An international and interdisciplinary study.* Toronto: Butterworths.

Martin, D. (1977). *Battered wives.* New York: Pocket Books.

Martin, J. (1983). Maternal and paternal abuse of children: Theoretical and research perspectives. In D. Finkelhor et al. (Eds.). *The dark side of families: Current family violence research.* (pp. 293–305). Beverly Hills, CA: Sage.

McClear, S. V., & Anwar, R. (1986). *A study of women presenting in an emergency medical department.* Unpublished paper, Medical College of Pennsylvania.

McClintock, F. H. (1978). Criminological aspects of family violence. In J. P. Martin (Ed.), *Violence and the family* (pp. 146–172). New York: Wiley.

Murphy, J. E. (August, 1984). *Date abuse and forced intercourse among college students,* Paper presented at the Second National Family Violence Research Conference, Durham, NH.

Neuringer, C. (1964). Rigid thinking in suicidal individuals, *Journal Consulting Psychology, 28,* 54–56.

Nisonoff, L., & Bitman, I. (1979). Spouse abuse: Incidence and relationship to selected demographic variables. *Victimology, 4,* 131–140.

O'Brien, J. E. (1971). Violence in divorce prone families. *Journal of Marriage and the Family, 33,* 692–698.

O'Malley, H. (1979). *Elderly abuse: A review of the recent literature,* Boston, MA: Legal research and Services for the Elderly.

Orne, T. C., & Rimmer, J. (1980). Alcoholism and child abuse: A review. *Journal of Studies on Alcohol, 42* (3).

Pagelow, M. D. (1976). *Preliminary report on battered women.* Paper presented at the Second International Symposium on Victimology, Boston, MA.

Pagelow, M. D. (1985). The 'battered husband syndrome?' Social problem or much ado about nothing? In N. Johnson (Ed.), *Marital violence* (172–195). London: Routledge & Kegan Paul.

Peterson, R. (1980). Social class, social learning and wife abuse. *Social Service Review, 54,* 390–406.

Petro, J. (1978). Wife abuse. *Journal of the American Medical Association, 240,* 240–241.

Pittman, D. J., & Handy, W. (1964). Patterns in criminal aggravated assault, *Journal of Criminal Law, Criminology and Police Science, 55,* 462–470.

Post, R. D., Willett, A. B., Franks, R. D., House, R. M., Beck, S., & Weissberg, M. P. (1980). A preliminary report on the prevalence of domestic violence among psychiatric inpatients, *American Journal of Psychiatry, 137,* 974–975.

Reiker, P. P., & Carmen (Hilberman), E., (1984). *The gender gap in psychotherapy: Social realities and psychological processes.* New York: Plenum Press.

Roper, M., Flitcraft, A., & Frazier, W. (1979). *Rape and battering: A pilot study,* Department of Surgery, Yale Medical School.

Rosenbaum, A., & O'Leary (1981). Marital violence: Characteristics of abusive couples. *Journal of Consulting and Clinical Psychology, 41,* 63–71.

Rosenberg, M. L., Stark, E., & Zahn, M. A. (1985). Interpersonal violence: Homicide and spouse abuse. In J. M. Last (Ed.), *Maxcyroseneau: Public health and preventive medicine,* (12th ed., New York: Appleton-Century Crofts.

Rosenheck, R. (1985–86). Malignant post-Vietnam syndrome. *American Journal of Orthopsychiatry, 55,* 166–177.

Russell, D. (1980). *The prevalence & impact of marital rape in San Francisco,* Paper presented at the meeting of the American Scoiological Association.

Russell, D. (1982). *Rape in marriage.* New York: Macmillan.

Saunders, D. G. (1982). Counselling the violent husband. In P. A. Keller, & L. G. Ritt (Eds.), *Innovations in clinical practice, Vol. I.* Sarasota: Professional Resource Exchange.

Schulman, M. A. (1979). *Survey of spousal violence against women in Kentucky,* Harris Study #792701. Conducted for Kentucky Commission on Women. Washington, DC: U.S. Government Printing Office.

Schechter, S. (1982). *Women and male violence.* Boston, MA: South End.

Scott, P. D. (1974). Battered wives. *British Journal of Psychiatry, 125,* 433–441.

Shainess, N. (1977). Psychological aspects of wife battering. In M. Roy (Ed.), *Battered women* (pp. 174–189). New York: Van Nostrand Reinhold.

Snell, J. E., Rosenwald, R. J., & Robey, A. (1974). The wifebeater's wife: A study of family interaction. *Archives of General Psychiatry, 11,* 107–112.

Solnit, A., Goldstein, J., & Freud, A. (1977). *Beyond the best interest of the child.* New Haven, CT: Yale University Press.

Star, B. (1978). Comparing battered and nonbattered women, *Victimology, 3,* 32–44.

Stark, E. (1984). *The battering syndrome: Social knowledge, social therapy and the abuse of women,* Unpublished Ph.D Dissertation, Dept. of Sociology, SUNY-Binghamton.

Stark, E., & Flitcraft, A. (1983). Social knowledge, social policy and the abuse of women. In D. Finkelhor (Eds.), *The dark side of families,* Beverly Hills, CA: Sage.

Stark, E., & Flitcraft, A. (1985). Woman-battering, child abuse and social heredity: What is the relationship? In N. Johnson (Ed.), *Marital violence.* Sociological Review Monograph # 31. London: Routledge & Kegan Paul.

Stark, E., & Flitcraft, A. (1987). Personal power and institutional victimization: Treating the dual trauma of woman battering. In F. Ochberg (Ed.). *Post traumatic therapy.* New York: Bruner/Mazel.

Stark, E., Flitcraft, A., & Frazier, W. (1979). Medicine and patriarchal violence: The social construction of a ''private'' event, *Internalional Journal of Health Services, 9,* 461–493.

Stark, E., Flitcraft, A., Zuckerman, D., Grey, A., Robison, J., & Frazier, W. (1981). *Wife Abuse in the medical setting: An introduction for health personnel,* Monograph # 7, Office of Domestic Violence: Washington, DC.

Steele, B. F. (1976). Violence within the family. In R. E. Helfer & C. H. Kempe (Eds.). *Child abuse and neglect: The family and the community.* Cambridge: Ballinger.

Steinmetz, S. K. (1974). Occupational environment in relation to physical punishment and dogmatism. In M. Straus & Steinmetz (Eds.). *Violence in the family.* New York: Harper & Row.

Steinmetz, S. K. (1977–78). The battered husband syndrome, *Victimology, 2,* 499–509.

Stephens, D. W. (1977). Domestic assault: The police response. In M. Roy (Ed.). *Battered women: A psycho-sociological study of domestic violence.* New York: Van Nortrand Reinhold.

Stewart, M. A., & deBlois, C. S. (1981). Wife abuse among families attending a child psychiatry clinic. *Journal of the American Academy of Child Psychiatry, 20,* 845.

Straus, M., & Steinmetz, S. K. (1975). The family as a cradle of violence. In M. Straus & S. K. Steinmetz (Eds.), *Violence in the family.* New York: Dodd Mead.

Straus, M., Gelles, R., & Steinmetz, S. K. (1980). *Behind closed doors: A survey of family violence in america.* New York: Doubleday.

Susser, M. (1973). *Causal thinking in the health sciences.* New York: Oxford University Press.

Szinovacz, M. E. (1983). Using couple data as a methodological tool: The case of marital violence, *Journal of Marriage and the Family, 45,* 633–644.

Telch, C. F., & Lindquist, C. U. (1984). Violent versus nonviolent couples: A comparison of patterns. *Psychotherapy, 21,* 242–248.

Teske, R. H. C., & Parker, M. L. (1983). *Spouse abuse in Texas: A study of women's attitudes and experiences,* Criminal Justice Center, Sam Huston State University: Huntsville, TX.

Vinoda, K. S. (1966). Personality characteristics of attempted suicides, *British Journal of Psychiatry, 112,* 1143–1150.

Walker, L. (1979). *The battered woman.* New York: Harper & Row.

Walker, L. (1983). The battered woman syndrome study. In D. Finkelhor, R. Gelles, G. Hotaling, & M. Straus (Eds.), *The dark side of families.* Beverly Hills, CA: Sage.

Washburn, C. (1983). A feminist analysis of child abuse and neglect. In D. Finkelhor, R. Gelles, G. Hotaling, & M. Straus (Eds.), *The dark side of families* (pp. 289–293). Beverly Hills, CA: Sage.

Weissman, M., Fox, K., & Klarman, G. (1973). Hostility and depression associated with suicide attempts. *American Journal of Psychiatry, 130,* 450–455.

Weitzman, J., & Dreen, K. (1982). Wife beating: A view of the marital dyad. *Social Casework, 63,* 259–265.

14

Prevention of Wife Abuse

ANDREA J. SEDLAK

Violence in the family takes many forms and has many victims. As treated in this volume, it includes physical violence and sexual abuse and is directed against children, adolescents, wives, husbands, elderly relatives, and siblings. Because there is no reason at present to assume that these various phenomena follow identical, or even substantially similar dynamics, the task of evaluating the current knowledge on prevention for all categories of family violence will be formidable, requiring a separate monograph or textbook in its own right. This chapter will not attempt to cover the full gamut of family violence but, like others in this volume, will instead focus on a single category of family violence—physical violence by men against women in cohabiting and/or conjugal relationships.

Although the literatures of the various helping professions have given considerable discussion to the general issue of prevention, very little attention has been directed toward specifically preventing family violence. The relative neglect of this problem is especially disturbing in light of its evident prevalence and serious consequences. This chapter will summarize current knowledge concerning family violence prevention, emphasizing conceptual distinctions that can lend coherency to what has been achieved in this area, integrating the existing empirical evidence concerning risk factors and intervention outcomes, and delineating some of the particularly troublesome ethical and legal issues that are inherent in attempts to address the problem of family violence.

Description of the Problem

In colloquial terms, to *prevent* a problem simply means to do something to keep it from happening. The term has a more elaborate meaning, however, as it is currently used in public health, social services, and mental health. Prevention can occur at any of three levels, depending on the stage at which one applies preventive measures.

Primary prevention refers to activity that stops the problem before it occurs (e.g., immunization, sanitation in public health; stress management skills, training in effective communication in mental health). Primary prevention has been further subdivided into

---

ANDREA J. SEDLAK • Westat, Inc., 1650 Research Blvd., Rockville, MD 20850.

proactive services, which prevent the initial occurrence of factors that increase the likelihood of the problem, and *reactive* services, which are undertaken in the face of existing risk factors in order to prevent the problem itself from occurring (Catalano & Dooley, 1980).

Secondary prevention involves activity designed to eradicate the problem at a very early stage. At this level of prevention, the problem has already manifested itself in some way, and the measures which are taken aim to both eliminate the problem and to avoid its more severe stages (e.g., early detection and treatment of correctable conditions in public health; therapy during early, nondebilitating stages of dysfunction in mental health).

Tertiary prevention aims to ameliorate a serious problem once it has developed, reducing the duration and/or severity of its consequences and preventing its recurrence (e.g., treatment of established diseases in public health; crisis intervention in mental health; cf. Gilbert, 1982).

It is important to recognize that this three-level scheme originated in connection with simple, clearly circumscribed disease entities in the public health arena and that there are nontrivial problems in translating it to other types of phenomena, such as family violence. The scheme applies imperfectly at best where (a) there is little agreement about the exact definition of the phenomenon (cf. Chap. 13 in this volume), (b) the problem is not easily delineated in time (what precisely marks its onset and how does one define a cure?), or (c) its etiology is poorly understood and causal factors appear multiple and interactive. Not surprisingly then, when the scheme is applied to family violence or to any problem in family processes or interactions, the three levels do not have fixed or obvious referents (cf. Giovannoni, 1982; Mace, 1983).[1] Despite these ambiguities, however, researchers and service providers in the area of family violence have continued to apply these terms. As a result, future confusions in the literature will only be avoided if all authors make a concerted effort to be clear about their intended meanings. In any event, the three-level scheme is helpful in emphasizing that prevention always consists of intervention efforts of some type and in conceptualizing interventions in relation to the problem's evolution, with primary prevention considered to be ideal.

Attempts to avoid a given problem altogether (primary prevention) or to detect it in the early stages (secondary prevention) rely heavily on knowledge concerning risk factors or risk markers. In relation to wife abuse, *risk factors* are attributes or characteristics that are associated with an increased likelihood of husband-to-wife violence, but that are not outcomes or consequences of this violence. Nor are risk factors necessarily causes or determinants (Last, 1983). Risk factors can be distinguished on the basis of whether they are related to the occurrence of wife abuse in a given couple, to its level of severity once it has occurred, or to both its occurrence and severity. Risk factors can also be distinguished according to whether they can conceivably be modified by intervention and whether they are causally related to the problem.

---

[1]For example, depending on how one defines violence and on what one regards as its onset, a given intervention may be regarded as primary, secondary, or tertiary prevention. Working with a couple in which the husband pushes and slaps the wife may be
- *primary prevention* if pushing and slapping are not regarded as forms of violence *per se* but only as interaction patterns that are associated an increased likelihood of future violence;
- *secondary prevention* if these behaviors are seen as manifestations of early stages in a violence problem which, left unchecked, is likely to progress toward more serious violence in the future; or
- *tertiary prevention* if pushing and slapping are considered to be serious manifestations of family violence in themselves.

Table 1. Goals at Each Level of Prevention with Respect to Four Possible Targets

Prevention level	Risk factors for problem's occurrence	Actual occurrence of problem	Risk factors for problem's severity	Actual development of high severity
Primary/proactive	Avoid	*	*	*
Primary/reactive	Remove	Avoid	*	*
Secondary/proactive	Remove	Remove	Avoid	*
Secondary/reactive	Remove	Remove	Remove	Avoid
Tertiary	Remove	Remove	Remove	Remove

*Not relevant if targeted prevention is effective.

Table 1 depicts the aims of each level of prevention in relation to these different categories of risk factors, to the occurrence of the problem itself, and to its degree of severity. As this table suggests, interventions occur increasingly after the fact as one approaches the level of tertiary prevention. Note that this table extends the terminology introduced by Catalano and Dooley (1980) by applying the distinction between proactive and reactive interventions to the secondary level of prevention as well, where it pertains to those risk factors associated with the severity of the problem.

With respect to wife abuse, effective prevention efforts avert or remove modifiable risk factors that are causally related to the problem. Some risk factors are modifiable for the specific individuals or couples who manifest them (e.g., low assertiveness, high marital discord), and reactive and proactive services can be applied to these. Others may only be modifiable proactively, for future individuals (e.g., childhood exposure to family violence). The known risk factors for wife abuse are identified in the next section of this chapter.

Secondary prevention efforts can be aided by screening devices that use knowledge of risk factors for the occurrence of family violence (even those risk factors that are not modifiable or causal) to narrow the search for early stage cases of the problem. Sensitive diagnostic tests can then be used to determine which of the cases screened-in as likely to be violent actually are. The issues involved in identification of wife abuse cases are discussed immediately following the risk factor review.

Finally, it is important to evaluate the effectiveness of any intervention strategy applied at any of the levels of prevention and to apply the knowledge gained through this evaluation to developing future strategies. The remaining sections of this chapter focus on the existing approaches to prevention, their evaluation, and the ethical and legal issues they raise.

EPIDEMIOLOGICAL FINDINGS[2]

Because the incidence and prevalence of family violence are treated elsewhere in this volume, the evidence pertaining to those questions will not be reiterated here. This section

[2]The work underlying the review in this section was supported by Contract No. 200-84-0755 from the Violence Epidemiology Branch at the Centers for Disease Control (CDC), Atlanta, GA, and reflects the efforts of several people. The author would like to acknowledge considerable contributions by Gerald Hotaling (University of

reports the results of a review of the existing literature on risk factors for husband-to-wife violence.[3] Given the wealth of studies that have appeared on the subject in the past decade, a critical synthesis of the evidence concerning the correlates of wife abuse should be generally useful to both researchers and service providers. This assessment may help to dispel myths and misconceptions, to identify the ways in which the existing knowledge base is flawed, and to direct future work on the question.

Data Sources and Standards of Evidence

For this review, a comprehensive search of published and unpublished works in psychology and sociology was undertaken. Relevant studies were located through (a) a search of *Psychological Abstracts* and *Sociological Abstracts* from 1970 through June of 1986; (b) a review of *Dissertation Abstracts International,* Section B, from 1978 through June 1986; (c) an examination of an extensive bibliography compiled by the Spouse Abuse Clearinghouse at the Family Violence Research Program, University of Texas at Tyler; (d) a direct search of the contents of key journals for 1984 through June 1986 to identify more recent relevant articles not yet abstracted; and (e) an overview of un-published papers from five conferences: two National Conferences for Family Violence Researchers at the University of New Hampshire (1981 and 1984), and the last three annual meetings of the American Psychological Association.

These sources were searched for studies that met four criteria: first, the study had to provide unambiguous evidence concerning husband-to-wife violence. Studies were ex-cluded if they used a combined or global measure of family violence that reflected violence in other family relationships or if they focused on dating couples rather than on couples who were married or cohabiting. Second, studies had to have as their focus the measurement of acts of physical violence. Not included were those studies that did not limit the definition of wife abuse to physical violence against wives, but that also focused on psychological abuse and/or verbal aggression. Third, studies had to offer sufficient information to allow a reader to determine whether a given relationship was statistically significant. Some reports that did not indicate the results of statistical analyses were included if they gave the reader enough data to allow calculation of appropriate statistical tests. Fourth, the study design and methodology had to provide adequate evidence con-cerning the covariation or correlation of a given characteristic or feature with the occur-rence and/or severity of wife abuse.

Risk Factor Findings

Studies were divided into those offering evidence about the risk factors for the occurrence of wife abuse at the societal or community level, those focusing on occurrence risk factors at the individual level, and those giving evidence concerning individual risk factors for the severity and/or frequency of wife abuse.

Societal and Community-Level Risk Factors. Many writers have emphasized that wife abuse receives considerable support from patriarchal structures and norms and

New Hampshire) and David Sugarman (Rhode Island College), as well as the comments of Mark Rosenberg, James Mercy, and Linda Saltzman (Violence Epidemiology Branch, CDC), Gary Bowen (University of North Carolina), Evan Stark (Rutgers University), and Murray Straus (University of New Hampshire).

[3]Throughout this chapter, the phrases *wife abuse* and *husband-to-wife violence* include physical violence by men against women who currently are or who have ever been married or cohabiting in a conjugal relationship.

from pervasive societal attitudes tolerating violence. In contrast to the frequency of comment about these factors, efforts to establish empirical support following traditional research methodologies have been almost nonexistent. Only two studies dealing with societal risk factors were located through the literature search.

Masumura (1979) conducted a cross-cultural survey, examining a worldwide sample of 86 primitive societies. Cross-cultural codes were established for a number of societal characteristics, including the incidence of wife abuse, on the basis of ethnographic descriptions of the societies. The incidence of wife abuse (absent, infrequent, or common) was found to covary with theft, personal crime, homicide, feuding, and an index that indicates the overall level of societal violence. Patrilineal inheritance and patrilocal residence were also positively related to wife abuse, but the correlations were not significant. Overall, the findings of this study supported a relationship between the incidence of wife abuse and societal levels of other forms of violence.

Yllo (1980, 1983; Yllo & Straus, 1981) obtained support for the idea that the incidence of wife abuse is related to the status of women by using states as the unit of measurement, and relating state-level rates of serious violence against women to measures reflecting women's status on four dimensions: economic, educational, political, and legal. State-level measures of wife abuse incidence were derived from Straus' national survey data (Straus, Gelles, & Steinmetz, 1980) and aggregate measures were based on the interviews with respondents in 30 states. The correlation between serious wife abuse and the overall status of women was not significant, but the correlation with women's legal status approached significance. A more detailed examination of the data revealed a curvilinear relationship between women's overall status and wife-beating. Serious wife abuse was most common in states where women's status was low, but wives in those states where women had achieved their highest status were also subjected to a great deal of abuse. Yllo and Straus (1981) concluded that wife abuse tends to be common where there is an inconsistency between women's status in economic, educational, political, and legal institutions and the social norms that dictate that their status in the family should be subordinate. Although this investigation provides encouraging preliminary evidence in support of women's status as a community-level risk factor, its results should be interpreted cautiously, because they were based on a data set that was not designed to provide reliable state-level measures of the incidence of wife abuse.

Individual Risk Factors for Occurrence. Seventy-two reports concerning 63 independent investigations met the requirements for evidence concerning risk factors for occurrence at the individual level. For thirty-six characteristics, the research evidence was relatively clear concerning whether any relationship with the simple occurrence of wife abuse existed, and if so, whether this relationship was positive (wife abuse increasing with the characteristic) or negative (wife abuse decreasing with the characteristic). The research evidence was considered relatively clear when there were a minimum of three studies which examined the characteristic in question and when at least two out of three studies reported the same pattern of findings. An additional criterion was applied to take account of the widely varying quality of research evidence in the literature—even if two-thirds of the relevant studies showed a consistent finding, the research evidence was *not* defined as clear if any representative survey of the general population reported findings contrary to this predominant pattern.

According to these standards, six characteristics were clearly *disconfirmed* as having any relationship with the occurrence of wife abuse, and thirty characteristics were confirmed to correlate with the occurrence of wife abuse.

Risk Factors for Severity/Frequency. In contrast to risk factors for the simple occurrence of wife abuse, there is a notable lack of research focusing on the correlates of severity or frequency. This review uncovered only 10 studies that offered information about the statistical significance of the relationship between severity or frequency and victim, abuser, or couple characteristics. Across these studies, only four characteristics had been examined by a minimum of three studies. A predominant pattern of findings emerged for only two of these characteristics,[4] with one characteristic (the couple's marital status) shown to be unrelated to wife abuse.[5]

The only characteristic that has been consistently related to the severity and/or frequency of wife abuse to date is the *abuser's own experiences of abuse as a child.* Fagan, Stewart, and Hansen (1983) found that this characteristic predicted the severity of the victim's injuries, and both Brown (1986) and Hofeller (1980) found that it related to the severity of the abuse itself.

Summary

From this review, a number of conclusions can be drawn. First, numerous studies implicate the abuser's exposure to parental violence in childhood. Second, there has been substantial support for the finding that being an abused child tends to be associated with being a victim of wife abuse. Third, there are a number of studies that link the occurrence of wife abuse with the occurrence of child abuse in the household. Fourth, the abuser's experiences of being abused as a child predict the severity of the injuries he inflicts. Taken together, these findings indicate the interdependence of prevention for these different categories of family violence. Preventing child abuse in a household may not only relate to the occurrence of wife abuse in that particular household, but may also reduce the likelihood that the female children will grow up to enter into and/or remain in conjugal relationships where they are abused and the severity of the abuse inflicted by those male children who grow up to become abusive husbands. Preventing spouse abuse in a household will reduce the likelihood that the male children will be abusive toward their own partners as adults. This last point implies, as many researchers have long argued, that intervention in current wife abuse circumstances (tertiary prevention) will reduce the incidence of this problem in future generations (primary prevention). Contrary to the opinions of many writers, however, the pattern relating wife abuse victims to exposure to parental violence is not so clear-cut, as fewer than two-thirds of the relevant studies supported such a relationship.

Most of the other victim-related risk factors with substantial support have been shown to be products of the abuse rather than precursors (cf. drug use, notable psychopathological symptomatology, and apprehension/tension/anxiety). Only one characteristic with more than three studies supporting its association remains as a possible antecedent of wife abuse for the victim: the victim's degree of self-sentiment/self-acceptance. In view of the fact that it is the victim's characteristics that have been most extensively studied, the lack of an extensive set of victim-related risk factors emphasizes

[4]Evidence was contradictory concerning remaining two characteristics: abuser's age and abuser's use of alcohol.
[5]The couple's marital status was found to be unrelated to the severity of wife abuse in two of three studies (Gaquin, 1977–78; Tauchen, Witte, & Long, 1985), with only Berk, Berk, Loseke, and Rauma (1983) reporting a finding that divorce or separation was associated with less serious injuries to the wife.

the essential similarity between women who become victims of wife abuse and those who do not.

Abuser characteristics have been studied far less frequently than victim characteristics, yet there is considerable evidence in support of connections between the occurrence of wife abuse and the husband's abuse of alcohol. A man who abuses alcohol is also likely to abuse his wife, independent of whether or not he is inebriated at the time of the abusive incidents *per se*. Thus, programs aimed at reducing the incidence of alcohol abuse among men may well have a preventive influence on the incidence of husband-to-wife violence.

The couple's marital status also relates to the occurrence of wife abuse. Wife abuse is less likely to occur among persons who are married in comparison to those who are separated, divorced, cohabitating, or remarried. To some degree, this couple characteristic is ambiguous in that it may be because of the fact that wife abuse may cause a couple to separate and/or divorce. However, the fact that cohabiting couples also show higher rates of wife abuse indicates that marital status may well be an antecedent risk factor for wife abuse as well. Although many studies have found that abusive couples generally have much poorer marital adjustment/satisfaction than nonabusive couples, there is evidence that this complaint distinguishes battered women from nonbattered women after the first abusive incident but not beforehand (cf. Stark *et al.*, 1981). This may mean that marital adjustment is actually poorer after the onset of wife abuse, that abuse increases the women's willingness to complain about poor marital adjustment, or both dynamics may operate simultaneously. The prevention implications of these findings are similarly unclear, but they would seem to suggest that the couple's definition of their relationship and its general level of quality have important linkages to the occurrence of wife abuse.

Research is lacking in several important areas:

- Few of the studies have used multiple control groups, and risk factor analyses of survey data generally fail to control for confounding factors. As a result, it is rarely possible to determine whether a given characteristic is associated with wife abuse *per se* or instead with an accompanying feature, such as marital distress.
- Most of the available information concerns victim, abuser, or couple risk factors for the occurrence of wife abuse, whereas extremely few studies provide information about community-level risk factors or about couple- and individual-level risk factors associated with the frequency or severity of wife abuse.
- Researchers have generally neglected to examine the temporal relationship(s) between wife abuse and characteristics found to be correlated with it, which has left many of the known correlates in the ambiguous correlate category—unclear as to whether they are risk factors for or consequences of wife abuse.
- Little attention has been given to the possible interactive effects of wife abuse risk factors, so it is not known whether and to what extent one risk factor may mitigate or accentuate the influence of another.

This review indicates that there is very little solid evidence on which to base secondary and tertiary prevention efforts, because few studies have been informative about the factors that distinguish different levels of the severity or frequency of wife abuse. At the same time, service providers cannot ignore the needs of currently violent couples while awaiting further research findings. The subsequent sections of this chapter focus on the issues involved in identifying wife abuse and on the existing intervention strategies, their effectiveness, and the legal and ethical dilemmas they engender.

IDENTIFICATION OF WIFE ABUSE

It is necessary to identify or diagnose cases of wife abuse in order to study associated risk factors or to intervene in the problem. The studies reviewed in the preceding section identified existing cases of wife abuse and examined the factors associated with its occurrence and/or severity. Interventions at different points in the evolution of the problem must also target appropriate recipients of the intervention services—whether these be couples currently at risk, persons involved in the early stages of wife abuse, or cases of serious and ongoing husband-to-wife violence. Thus, for research or for services, it is necessary to classify persons or couples according to whether or not they represent cases that fit the criterion of interest. This section discusses a number of issues surrounding the classification or measurement of wife abuse cases.

Accuracy

Although many writers have emphasized the prevalence of wife abuse (e.g., Langley & Levy, 1977), they have generally been referring to any use of physical force by husbands against wives. In contrast, the more serious forms of violence are far less common—occurring at a rate of about 4 per 100 couples (cf. 3.8%, Straus, 1977–78). Thus, wife abuse, at least in its more serious forms, would be considered a relatively rare event in measurement terms. There are unique measurement problems associated with rare events, and any efforts to develop tools to identify wife abuse must take account of these problems—whether these devices are designed to identify high-risk cases prior to any overt abuse, to detect cases in their early stages, or to diagnose serious cases.

The difficulty posed by the fact that wife abuse is a relatively rare event can be understood by considering the ability of any measuring instrument to classify wife abuse cases in the way desired. Regardless of whether one wants to identify at-risk couples or actual ongoing cases of wife abuse, no identification or screening device is entirely perfect. No risk factor is perfectly associated with the occurrence of wife abuse or with its different levels of severity. Even direct questions about abusive experiences or behaviors often rely on self-reports (cf. the Conflict Tactics Scale, Straus, 1979), which may be seriously distorted by respondents' efforts to present themselves in a socially desirable way. The degree to which any screening or diagnostic method succeeds in its purpose can be viewed from two different perspectives: (a) *sensitivity*—the proportion of true cases of wife abuse that are correctly identified as such, and (b) *specificity*—the proportion of cases that are not wife abuse cases that are correctly recognized as nonviolent cases.

These two features, sensitivity and specificity, are interdependent. The more stringent one's measuring device (the more careful one is to avoid labeling a person or couple as abusive), the greater its specificity and the lower its sensitivity. On the other hand, the more relaxed one makes the criteria for what will be screened-in, the more sensitive and the less specific the device is. In assessing the sensitivity or specificity of a test or measure, one compares a classification of cases based on the test scores with their classification based on some independent criterion. For example, cases of wife abuse may be identified by therapists and nonviolent cases obtained from another source, as for a case-control study. One can then assess the sensitivity and specificity of the instrument by examining the ability of test scores to reconstruct these two groups. Note that any assessment of specificity or sensitivity can only be approximate, because no independent classification of cases can be regarded as a perfect indicator of true cases. Also note that two kinds of misclassifications will occur: (a) *false positives*—some cases that should not be screened-in will be (more numerous when specificity is low), and (b) *false negatives*—some cases which should be screened-in will be missed (more numerous when sensitivity is low).

The predictive value of a method for screening or identifying cases is defined as:

$$\text{Predictive value} = \frac{\text{True cases screened-in}}{\text{Total cases screened-in}} \tag{1}$$

The total cases that are screened-in include both the true positives and the false positives. The percent of true positives can be calculated as:

$$\text{True positives screened-in} = \text{Prevalence}^6 \times \text{Sensitivity} \tag{2}$$

The percent of false positives is given by:

$$\text{False positives screened-in} = (1-\text{Prevalence}) \times (1-\text{Specificity}) \tag{3}$$

Thus, the predictive value of a measure, or the proportion of true cases that are screened by a test, is a function of three factors: (a) its sensitivity, (b) its specificity, and (c) the true prevalence of wife abuse:

$$\text{Predictive value} = \frac{\text{Prevalence} \times \text{Sensitivity}}{(\text{Prevalence} \times \text{Sensitivity}) + (1-\text{Prevalence})(1-\text{Specificity})} \tag{4}$$

According to this formula, the predictive value of any measuring device will be low whenever prevalence itself is low, *even for high levels of specificity and sensitivity* (cf. Ahlbom & Norell, 1984). Quantitatively, even if one were to develop a device that achieved 95% sensitivity and 95% specificity, then assuming that the true prevalence of serious wife abuse is about 4%, the predictive value of classifying cases with the device would only be 44.2%. This means that of those cases screened-in by the device only 44.2% would be true cases, accurately screened-in, and there would be more false positives (55.8%) than true positives. This problem is graphically illustrated in Figure 1, which includes examples of common and rare phenomena. The distributions in the upper half of the figure depict a situation where the phenomenon of interest is common, affecting about half the total population. There, only a small proportion of the individuals who are defined to be cases by the identification tool are not true cases (i.e., are false positives). The lower half of the figure differs in that true cases comprise a much smaller subset of the total population. There, false positives make up a far greater proportion of the defined cases.

This problem of screening accuracy has been a central concern in the literature on child abuse (cf. Daniel, Newberger, Reed, & Kotelchuck, 1978; Garbarino, 1980; Kotelchuck, 1982; Light, 1974; McMurtry, 1985), where error rates lead to very inefficient allocation of services. In connection with spouse abuse, the problem of low predictive value of identification devices can be expected to interfere with the study of risk factors and to intrude in the process of screening for services. On the one hand, a high rate

---

[6]Measured as a percentage.

of false positives will reduce detectable group differences between identified violent and nonviolent comparison cases, obscuring real differences between true representatives of these groups. The extent to which this has distorted the findings reported in the previous section cannot be directly determined, but its influence should be recognized. On the other hand, a high rate of false positives may inconvenience the process of screening for services—but in itself will not render a device useless for this purpose. This view is contrary to that expressed by Gelles (1984), who concluded that, because the relatively low prevalence of spouse abuse would lead to a high rate of false positives, "screening for prediction will *never be feasible.*" Even in the earlier example, the use of the instrument can focus service efforts on a subgroup where the prevalence of wife abuse is more than 10 times that of the population at large (i.e., 44.2% vs. 4%). The most important consideration in the use of any screening device is what one actually does with the cases that are screened-in by the measure. Using it to identify persons and couples who warrant further careful questioning, follow-up, and to whom various supportive and educational

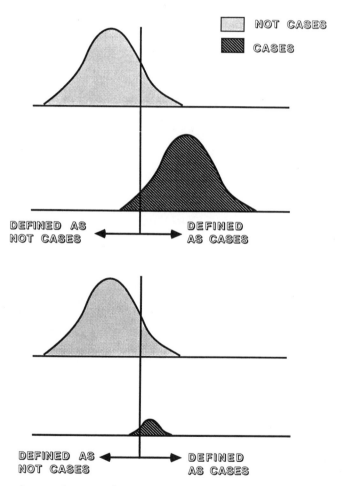

Figure 1. Distributions of cases and noncases for common events (in upper half) and rare events (lower half of figure), showing the higher proportion of false positives (noncases defined as cases) when the event is rare.

services can be offered is very different from using such a test to apply a stigmatizing diagnostic label or to justify intrusive interventions.

Identification Measures

Two structured tests have been developed for use in identifying cases of ongoing wife abuse. The Conflict Tactics Scale (CTS) (Straus, 1979) is perhaps the most well-known of these, and is the more general of the two instruments, providing for questions about violence among all members of the household. The more recently developed Index of Spouse Abuse (ISA) (Hudson & McIntosh, 1981) was designed to specifically measure spouse abuse. Both instruments assess the occurrence of husband-to-wife violence and its relative severity.

The Conflict Tactics Scale (Straus, 1979) includes a violence component that inquires about the use of physical violence in resolving disagreements and conflicts in the family. The violence component includes less serious force (e.g., slapping, pushing, grabbing), and what Straus has termed an abusive violence subset that includes acts assumed to carry a risk of serious injury. As noted earlier, the complete CTS inquires about all possible combinations of family roles and directionalities (i.e., wife-to-husband, husband-to-wife, parent-to-child, child-to-child). The reliability and validity of the 9-item husband-to-wife violence component have been documented.[7] Reliability measured by item-total correlation was found to be .87 (Straus, 1979), and coefficient alpha has been calculated as .83 (Straus, 1979) and .86 (Lockhart, 1985). Efforts to document the validity of the CTS have focused on the total scale and on the husband-to-wife component. In support of its construct validity, Straus (1979) has cited a number of findings generated by the scale that are in keeping with theoretical predictions concerning marital and intra-familial violence. The initial assessment of the concurrent validity of the husband-to-wife items was based on reports by different family members on the occurrence of husband-to-wife violence during the previous year. The intercorrelations of these reports ranged from .33 to .64 (Bulcroft & Straus, 1975).

Szinovacz (1983) argued that the use of overall percent agreement scores or correlations (even nonparametric correlations) is inappropriate in connection with wife abuse. Because of its relatively low frequency, such correlations will primarily reflect relatively high agreement about the nonoccurrence of violence. Using a nonrepresentative general population sample of 103 couples, Szinovacz (1983) privately interviewed each spouse using the CTS while the other completed a questionnaire. Whereas 82% of the couples agreed overall (about either the occurrence or nonoccurrence of husband-to-wife violence), agreement was considerably lower (27%) when only occurrence was considered. That is, among couples where one spouse reported the occurrence of violence, only a minority of the partners' reports were in agreement. Based on these data, one can generate estimates of the incidence of husband-to-wife violence ranging from a low of 7% (considering only those reports in which both spouses agree) to a high of 26% (considering any report of wife abuse by either spouse). In addition, there was little agreement between

---

[7]There have been two forms of the CTS, differing slightly in their format (proportion of items unrelated to physical violence), their intended method of administration (self-administered vs. face-to-face interview administration), and in the wording of some of the questions. The reliability and validity findings reported in the text represent the union of the results for both forms.

spouses on the occurrence of specific violence behaviors, with wives reporting more husband-to-wife violence than their husbands acknowledge.[8]

In conclusion, Szinovacz suggested that although direct questions concerning marital violence are likely to result in considerable underreporting of wife abuse, it may be possible to minimize this type of distortion by having both spouses respond to these questions and defining the occurrence of wife abuse on the basis of an admission by either spouse. Using this strategy, it may be possible to reduce the incidence of underreporting by using sequential or simultaneous private interviews with each spouse. This approach may raise respondents' concerns about providing answers which are consistent with those of their partners.

Recently, Jouriles and O'Leary (1984) also reported findings that indicated low to moderate agreement between spouses on the occurrence of marital violence, suggesting that the occurrence-agreement rate is not notably different in couples from clinic samples compared with couples from the general community—despite sample differences in the reported frequency of wife abuse. Using a self-administered version of the CTS, they examined responses from 65 couples attending a marital therapy clinic and 37 happily married couples from the community. In the maritally discordant sample, 36% of the women reported experiencing wife abuse at some point in their marriages, compared to only 9% in the happily married sample. Raw percentage occurrence-agreement on the husband's use of violence was 50% in the clinic sample, and 38% in the community sample, but when corrected for the base frequencies in these two groups by using Cohen's Kappa (a statistic that controls for chance agreements), the two samples were found to be remarkably similar: 43% agreement in the clinic sample, and 40% in the community sample. There was a slight tendency for clinic husbands to underreport their own violent behavior (and/or for their wives to overreport their partner's violence). Similar results concerning occurrence-agreement were reported by O'Leary and Arias (1984) for a sample of 400 couples about to be married who were recruited through newspaper and radio ads, where percentage occurrence-agreement was 55% for the husband's violence. These authors pointed out that the general levels of these reliabilities are very similar to those found for spouse reports of daily relationship events in general (e.g., Elwood & Jacobsen, 1983).

Overall, O'Leary and Arias concluded that the Conflict Tactics Scale is psychometrically adequate for detecting sample differences in incidence rates. Note, however, that its utility for identifying specific couples in need of service is a separate question. At present, even with appropriate item modifications, it would appear to be far less than ideal for specific diagnostic purposes. Moreover, it ignores many important contextual aspects of the violence, such as motives (e.g., self-defense), prior and subsequent interactions, and resultant injuries (Pleck, Pleck, Grossman, & Bart, 1978). Because it is one of the few standardized measures available, it is probably inevitable that it will be used to help identify couples in need of service. Given the substantial discrepancies in reports between spouses, however, a cautious approach would seem advisable, with ample supplementary information obtained through other methods.

---

[8]Similar patterns were observed by Okun (1983), who reported that there were dramatic divergences between batterers' reports and those of their battered wives—the men reported committing far less frequent and less serious violence than reported by their spouses. The findings in both of these studies may at least partly derive from a more general tendency of females, even as third party observers, to report more family violence than males (cf. Gully, Pepping, & Dengerink, 1982).

Hudson and McIntosh (1981) reported the development of a 30-item scale, the Index of Spouse Abuse (ISA), for use as a diagnostic aid as well as to monitor and evaluate progress in clinical treatment programs for wife abuse. The ISA was designed to assess the severity of physical and nonphysical abuse by spouses in separate subscales. The physical abuse subscale (ISA-P) is of interest here. Like the CTS, the ISA is comprised largely of direct inquiries concerning experiences of violence, but unlike the CTS it is limited to violence occurring within conjugal relationships.

The reliability of the ISA-P as measured by coefficient alpha was shown to be quite good (.90 with a sample of 398 female university students and .94 with 64 abused shelter residents and 43 nonabused comparison women). Concurrent validity and construct validity were also supported—the former by demonstrating a point-biserial correlation of .73 between the clinical status of the abused and nonabused women and the ISA-P scores; the latter by low average correlations (.11) with measures concerning problems unrelated to the marital relationship, slightly higher average correlations (.29) with personal and social problems expected to relate to or reflect the quality of the marital relationship, and a relatively high correlation with clinical status (.75).

Based on the data from the abused and nonabused samples, the optimal clinical cutting score for identifying respondents as likely victims of physical spouse abuse was calculated as a ISA-P score of 10 (given a potential range of 0 to 100). This score classified the women with a 9.3% false positives rate and a 7.8% false negatives rate (using the women's shelter status as the criterion).

Several limitations of the ISA have been noted by its authors. The clinical cutting score and the associated statistics concerning false positives and false negatives may have been biased by the use of a relatively severely abused criterion group (from battered women's shelters). Future revisions of this cutting score may, therefore, be necessary. Also, the distinction between the subscale for physical abuse and that for nonphysical abuse was not supported by the data. In fact, the two subscales intercorrelated strongly (.86), which suggests a lack of specificity (although this, too, may have derived from the severely abused character of the criterion sample).

Like the CTS, the ISA is a self-report measure and subject to distortions from respondents' efforts to present themselves in a socially desirable manner. This would mean that a large proportion of persons involved in wife abuse should tend to deny or minimize the abuse they receive or inflict. Moreover, retrospective self-report measures are likely to suffer from memory-related distortions as well. As a result, the identification of specific cases of wife abuse would be facilitated by developing rapport and trust with respondents and by supplementing scores on tests such as the CTS and ISA with information from other sources.

Screening Aids

The need for screening arises primarily in medical, mental health, and general-purpose shelters, where clientele may seek services without referring to the problem of wife abuse. The Wife Abuse Inventory (WAI) was developed by Lewis (1983) for use as a screening device with women who seek social and/or economic services to aid in identifying those who are at risk of physical abuse by their male partners. The inventory consists of 34 scale items, which Lewis (1985) conceptually classified into rating questions concerning the husband's self-image, the family's degree of social isolation, and the couple's style of conflict resolution. The internal consistency of the instrument is acceptably high

(.90 for split half reliability, .90 for coefficient alpha). To date, there have been two studies of the instrument's validity and its ability to correctly discriminate between abused and nonabused women has been reported as 78% (Lewis, 1984), and 96% (Lewis, 1985), depending on the samples used. A discriminant analysis (Lewis, 1985) showed that among the three categories of items, those pertaining to the couple's styles of conflict management accounted for the greatest portion of abused versus nonabused between-group variance.

Although these findings suggest that the WAI may be a useful preliminary tool to include in a screening protocol, there are several reasons to be cautious about its use. First, the validity studies have been very limited, based on small and nonrepresentative samples of women, so it is not clear how well the WAI will generally discriminate abused from nonabused women among the client populations Lewis has targeted for its use. Second, the specificity of the WAI appears to be relatively low. Scores on the WAI also discriminate women who have been emotionally abused from those who have not, and women who report having been raped by their male partners from those who do not. It is not, however, clear that the scale is able to differentiate among physical abuse, emotional abuse, and marital rape. In fact, the data so far would suggest that the WAI measures general abuse and is not specific to physical husband-to-wife violence.

A third reason for caution in using the WAI is that the suggested applications for its use have outdistanced its empirical foundations. There is some danger that uninformed practitioners will apply it in ways that are not warranted. Because the WAI was not systematically designed to assess empirically documented risk markers for wife abuse, it should not be used to determine whether prevention efforts aimed at altering these risk markers are effective (or to assess the effectiveness of intervention programs). Nor, as Lewis (1985) acknowledged, is it useable for diagnosis *per se* in detecting existing wife abuse cases. In its present state of development, the WAI would appear to be best applied in concert with other identification and assessment methods. Those women whose WAI scores identify them as at risk for wife abuse can be questioned about their experiences at greater length and advised of or offered available services.

Stark *et al.* (1981) conducted an extensive study of wife abuse among 2,676 women presenting with injuries to the Emergency Surgical Service of a large city hospital during a one-year period. On the basis of their findings, they have offered a set of guidelines for an index of suspicion concerning wife abuse among such clientele. They suggest that various aspects of the trauma event itself trigger supportive and frank discussion regarding possible wife abuse, including the following:

- *Multiple injuries.* Cases of multiple injuries often derive from abuse, and bilateral injuries are even more likely to be abuse-related.
- *Body map.* Accidents generally injure extremities, especially hands and feet, but deliberate assault involves a high incidence of injuries to the face, neck, chest, breasts, and abdomen.
- *Rape.* Given that abusive men are also likely to sexually assault their partners, rape crisis teams should be sensitive to the possibility that a presenting victim was raped by her conjugal partner.
- *Pregnancy.* The conjunction of traumatic injury and pregnancy is a high-risk presentation. Stark *et al.* (1981) found that abused women were more likely to be beaten during pregnancy and to have higher rates of miscarriage than nonabused women.

In addition, counter to popular impressions, severity of injury was noted to be a rather poor indicator of wife abuse. Instead, Stark *et al.* suggested that clinicians inquire as to the patient's trauma history as a routine component of treating traumatic injuries. One obstacle to effectively identifying wife abuse in medical and mental health contexts is resistance on the part of clinicians and physicians—the protocol differs considerably from the histories typically taken in these contexts. Considerable effort may be necessary to educate these professionals concerning the need for an adjusted protocol to identify these cases, but there is evidence that interventions in the form of lectures to emergency room physicians can substantially alter patterns of diagnoses (Mascia, 1983). Also, as a general strategy, Stark *et al.* (1981) recommended that clinic staff be involved in developing the screening protocols by helping to identify the types of high-risk presentations likely to appear at different service sites, which will vary with the services, triage, and referral patterns of a given facility (Stark *et al.*, 1981).

The logic underlying this last recommendation applies beyond the medical service context. The specific screening techniques and guidelines that will prove most effective will vary with the nature of the facility, the reasons for its use, and the risk factors for wife abuse in the particular client population in question. Additional research on client population risk factors would greatly facilitate further development of effective screening approaches and strategies.

INTERVENTION AND TREATMENT METHODS

A variety of intervention programs have been developed to combat wife abuse. The earliest wife abuse programs were developed to provide services to the women who are its direct victims. Subsequent programs targeted their efforts more broadly, toward prevention and early detection in the community at large and/or to ameliorating the effects of wife abuse on the children in these families. The most recently developed services deal with the actual source of the problem and work to stop the violent behavior of men who batter. This section overviews current knowledge in each of these program areas. In addition, special attention is given to the controversy concerning the use of couples' counseling for husband-to-wife violence and to recent developments in the legal system's approach to the problem.

Programs for Battered Women

Initial intervention programs aimed at combatting wife abuse focused on the women who were its victims and included shelters, hotlines, crisis intervention programs, and counseling services for abused wives. Despite being the most long-standing services for wife abuse, however, they are historically a very recent development. Programs for battered wives essentially began in the early 1970s and experienced considerable growth throughout the following decade. The first known shelter was founded in England in 1971 by Erin Pizzey (1974). In 1972, Women's Advocates in St. Paul, Minnesota, began offering shelter to battered women in the United States (Davidson, 1978; Vaughan, 1979). Since then, shelters, safe houses, or refuges as they are variously called, have mushroomed throughout the United States, Britain, and Europe. In mid-1976, there were only 11 known shelters in the United States (Pagelow, 1977), but by early 1980 this number had risen to over 500 (Hart, 1980).

Although battered women programs are located in all states, they vary considerably in per capita representation. Kalmuss and Straus (1983) found the strongest predictor of their availability to be the level of feminist organization in a state, as indexed by the number of members of the National Organization for Women (NOW) and of local NOW groups. This factor proved to be a more effective predictor of the availability of wife abuse programs than was per capita income, political culture, legislation allocating funding for domestic violence, or individual feminist sentiment (as indicated by sales of *Ms.* magazine).

Shelters. Generally, shelters are grassroots efforts, beginning at the community level with little money and little government assistance. Shelters reflect the character of the groups that administer them, and these can be divided into three categories on this basis: feminist groups, traditional social service providers, and Al-Anon and religious organizations (Ferraro, 1981). The latter two categories of groups often adopt a family-dynamic orientation to the problem of spouse abuse (cf. Peltoniemi, 1981). Although much existing literature on shelters stresses feminist approaches and an organized feminist constituency appears instrumental in determining their availability, the majority of shelters are operated by professionals who do not define themselves as feminists (Ferraro, 1981).

Most shelters are filled on a virtually constant basis, many reporting that they must often turn women away. Their primary goal is to secure the woman's safety and provide an environment in which she can make practical plans for a safe future. Shelters usually have established criteria for accepting women into residency[9] and they typically provide only short-term residence, between 4 and 6 weeks. Most shelters in the United States follow what Ferraro (1981) has termed the self-sufficiency ethos, in which their superordinate goal is to "empower" the women clients. Their services usually focus on establishing alternative living arrangements to the battering situation and on connecting the women with social services in the community that will allow them to live independently of their batterers. Some shelters include family-oriented programs and/or programs for the batterer as well (Colorado Association for Aid to Battered Women, 1979; Ferraro, 1981; Gentry & Eaddy, 1980; Lynch & Norris, 1977–78; Miller, 1980; Vaughan, 1979; Walker, 1978d).

One of the primary measures of shelter effectiveness has been the proportion of clients who do not return to their abusers, which has generally comprised a majority of shelter clients. Some researchers claim that 45% to 50% do not return to their abuser after their shelter stay (Colorado Association for Aid to Battered Women, 1979; Snyder & Scheer, 1980; Walker, 1978d). Others have reported estimates ranging from two-thirds to more than four-fifths not returning (Aguirre, 1985; Doherty, 1981). Even assuming that the observed percentages overestimate return rates, shelters do appear to be successful in helping a substantial proportion of their clients to break their ties with their abusive partners.

Gauging shelter effectiveness by the proportion of women returning to their relationships obscures other benefits that may derive from the shelter experience. To avoid

[9]For example, they may require that the woman have experienced real or threatened physical abuse and exclude women whose experiences have not involved actual physical violence. Ferraro (1981) reported that, in the shelter she studied, deciding which clients were "appropriate for residency" was a very subjective process, which depended on current space availability and on counselors' "gut feelings" about each client. As Loseke and Berk (1981) have emphasized, identifying how initial shelter contact is related to shelter entry is critical to understanding how helpseeking relates to service delivery in this area.

becoming a mere "crash pad" that battered women might use as a "safety valve" on a periodic bais without trying to substantially change their situations, many shelters make concerted efforts not only to provide a physical alternative to the relationship, but also to have a significant impact on the woman's psychological and emotional states. To the extent that a shelter adopts such goals, it may be quite similar to a variety of other wife abuse counseling and crisis intervention programs and share the goals of such programs, as outlined later. Several of the more recent studies of shelter effectiveness have gone beyond simply documenting return rates and begun to identify changes that occur during shelter residence in the woman's psychological and emotional states and in her subsequent relationship with her abuser.

Women who reside longer in a shelter are less likely to return to their abusers. In addition, after staying some weeks in a shelter, women are found to be significantly less depressed (Sedlak, 1983; Zuckerman & Piaget, 1982), to have higher scores on internal locus of control, and to have more friendships with people unconnected with their abusers (Sedlak, 1983). Also, women who form close relationships with other shelter residents or who identify with a shelter role model are less likely to return to their abusers (Dalto, 1983).[10]

Women who return to abusive partners may cognitively and emotionally progress toward a permanent solution as a result of their shelter residency. Walker (1978d) argued that a woman may need to leave and return three or four times before she is ready to leave permanently. She claimed that the percentage of women who do not return to their batterers rises dramatically if the shelter will readmit women who return home and then change their minds. Findings reported by Okun (1983), Porter (1983), and Snyder and Scheer (1980) also attest to the influence of past separations, showing that battered women who terminate their relationships after shelter residence have experienced significantly more previous conjugal separations than had those who return to their partners.

A shelter stay may substantially alter, even paradoxically actually improve, a woman's relationship with her abuser. Ridington (1977–78) believes that a woman who returns home is often better able to deal with her situation as a result of her shelter stay. Seward (1980) and Vaughan (1979) have claimed that the shelter stay signified to the abuser that the woman will not tolerate the abuse and this may motivate him to seek treatment. In this connection, it is notable that those women whose husbands were in counseling at the time they left the shelter (Aguirre, 1985), or who sought conjoint marital counseling after their shelter residency (Snyder & Scheer, 1980) tended to return to their partners. Shelter programs generally report that nearly 19% of their clients achieve a successful resolution in the relationship (Colorado Association for Aid to Battered Women, 1979). Snyder and Scheer (1980) found further support for these claims, observing that of those who returned home, only 12% reported having been abused in a 6-week follow-up contact.

Unfortunately, evaluation of shelter programs is still relatively elementary. Although there have been numerous assessments of return rates, there have been few efforts to document the cognitive-emotional changes that occur during shelter stays. Moreover, next to nothing is known about the processes by which shelters affect women's decisions, about how to improve a shelter's effectiveness, or about the specific effects shelters have on those women who return to their abusers. If, however, shelter programs are to be

---

[10]Evidence is contradictory, however, concerning whether there are changes in the women's self-esteem (Sedlak, 1983; Zuckerman & Piaget, 1982) and about whether the women's use of services during their shelter stay relates to their ultimate outcomes (Aguirre, 1985; Zuckerman & Piaget, 1982).

effective in benefiting all women, including those who return, these questions must be addressed.

Counseling/Therapy with Abused Wives. Whereas shelters are oriented to the abused woman who wishes to leave the relationship (at least temporarily), many abused women who seek social services intervention do so while remaining with their abusers (Carlson, 1977; Dobash & Dobash, 1979; Loseke & Berk, 1981, 1982).[11] Service providers typically report that the majority of abused women who come for counseling want to remain in their marriages, but without the violence (e.g., Geller & Walsh, 1977–78).

The literature abounds with recommendations concerning techniques for counseling battered women. Many authors agree that the traditional mental health system has hurt more than helped many battered women by promoting the use of tranquilizers, by focusing on internal and intrapsychic causes that tend to blame the victims, and by inappropriate referrals and diagnoses that actually stabilize abusive relationship patterns (cf. King, 1981; Stark & Flitcraft, 1981).

Whether counseling is provided within a shelter or some other service context, typical goals in counseling a battered woman include decreasing her psychological dependence on the abuser, helping her to realize that she is not a helpless victim but does have power over her own life, reestablishing her self-esteem, combatting traditional sex-role concepts and any concomitant tendency to blame herself or to rationalize her abuse, dissuading her of beliefs that she can control the abuse, and decreasing her acceptance or tolerance of the use of physical force in interpersonal disputes (Carlson, 1977; Colorado Association for Aid to Battered Women, 1979; Gregory, 1976; Pagelow 1978; Ridington, 1977–78; Straus *et al.*, 1980; Vaughan 1979; Walker, 1978a, c, d, 1984). An abused woman may sometimes seek a counselor's or therapist's help for the violence itself, but at other times she may present with a different reason (cf. Walker, 1984). Directors at one large New York agency (Geller & Walsh, 1977–78) classify their battered women clients into three categories: (a) those who want to separate from or divorce their husband—to whom they offer individual counseling and referral assistance, (b) those who want to end the violence in their current relationship—for whom attempts are made to involve the abusive partner in couple therapy; and (c) those whose perceive their options as restricted to remaining in the relationship under the current circumstances—for whom the preferred approach is group therapy with other women in similar situations. Thus, counselors or therapists variously use crisis intervention, individual psychotherapy, or group therapy with battered women.

There is an ongoing debate among service providers as to whether it is best to use a staff of professionally trained counselors and therapists or whether peer counselors, many of whom are themselves former battered women, can be equally effective. In the absence of data on the subject, opinions abound. As Roberts (1984) pointed out, neither advanced training nor a battering history should be simplistically regarded as automatic predictors of success, as a configuration of skills and attitudes are probably necessary.

Unfortunately, there is remarkably little research evidence concerning the relative effectiveness of different counseling approaches or strategies. Some practitioners believe that the group therapy approach is the most effective in promoting battered women's

---

[11]According to one representative survey of the general population, less than 1% of women who reported experiencing abuse by a partner at some point in their lives said that they had used the services of a shelter (Teske & Parker, 1983). In contrast, nearly 12% of the nonrepresentative sample of women studied by Pagelow (1981) reported having gone to a battered women's shelter.

emotional independence and in reducing their feelings of isolation (Fleming, 1979). Subjective evaluations by battered women themselves show that the women consider women's groups and battered women's shelters to be the most effective formal help sources (Bowker, 1984; Bowker & MacCallum, 1981). However, Huston (1986), who has recently reviewed the objective evidence supporting claims for the unique therapeutic effectiveness of women's groups, concluded that there is only suggestive support for these assumptions.[12] Overall, research on the relative effectiveness of different types of interventions with battered women would be of great benefit in guiding future service programs for these clients.

Community Outreach and Interventions with the Children

Many shelters and advocacy groups systematically attempt to educate the community about wife abuse and to alter the societal attitudes which support it. They may, for example, provide speakers to schools and to community social organizations, distribute literature, offer public service announcements in different media, and provide informational referrals as well as crisis intervention on a wife abuse hotline (cf. Colorado Association for Aid to Battered Women, 1979; Miller, 1980; Roberts, 1981). Such programs constitute primary as well as secondary prevention efforts in that they aim to reduce factors that are considered to increase the risk of wife abuse and to stimulate help seeking at the early stages of a wife abuse problem. Unfortunately, no published accounts of evaluation studies of these programs could be located, and existing information appears to consist entirely of subjective impressions of their perceived impact.

A number of agencies and shelters have, in recent years, established programs for children of battered women (cf. Alessi & Hearn, 1984; Gentry & Eaddy, 1980; Hughes, 1981, 1982, 1986) in an effort to help remedy some of the many problems they experience as a result of being exposed to the violence. These children have had their lives disrupted by the violence and are in crisis together with their mothers. Moreover, as has already been discussed, one of the most serious consequences of their experiences is the likelihood that they will repeat the pattern of wife abuse in their own adult lives. Such primary prevention programs vary considerably in scope, ranging from simple biweekly meetings involving the children or the addition of play therapy to shelter services (e.g., Rhodes & Zelman, 1986) to multifaceted programs with several coordinated components and linkages to other community agencies. In general, however, services to children are in their infancy, with large gaps even in the most developed programs. Jaffe, Wilson, and Wolfe (1986) reported an evaluation of an intervention program for children in which children were assigned to two age groups (8–10 or 11–13 years) and met for 10 sessions to discuss aspects of their experiences and explore coping and safety skills. The evaluation demonstrated that the children showed significant improvement over wait-list controls in measures of self- and mother-rated overall adjustment and in school performance and behavior.

An innovative multifaceted approach was adopted in a model program in Arkansas (Hughes, 1981, 1982, 1986) that involved peer, sibling, and family group meetings and

---

[12]Rounsaville, Lifton, and Bieber (1979) did not use objective measures, but claimed successful outcomes for those women who remained in treatment (6 of an original group of 31). Apart from this report, the literature offers only one case study (Meyers-Abell & Jansen, 1980) showing a reduction in depression and increase in assertiveness by an individual in group treatment.

targeted four major areas of intervention: the children, their mothers, the schools, and shelter staff members. Interventions with the children were conducted individually and in groups—peer, sibling, or family. The most important issues dealt with in these meetings included the rationale for the shelter's prohibition against physical force, the problems associated with the use of violence, and alternative methods of interpersonal problem solving. Interventions with the mothers were primarily child focused and directed toward improving parenting awareness and skills. Shelter residence typically meant that the children attended a new school. The school liaison component of the program included efforts to improve communications with these new teachers, educating them about the children's experiences, and offering assistance as future needs arose. Finally, the shelter staff themselves were trained in interacting with the children and serving as models of appropriate parenting behaviors. Preliminary data (Hughes & Barad, 1982) concerning the effectiveness of this intervention after an average of 21 days of residence showed significant improvements on only one measure. The children were significantly less anxious at the second testing. The findings did not confirm expectations concerning decreases in behavior problems and increases in self-esteem and preferences for non-violent disciplinary methods. More recently, an informal evaluation of this program showed that 69% of the mothers perceived their children's behavior to have improved either a little or a lot, and 81% reported an improved relationship with their children (Hughes, 1986).

Although Emery, Kraft, Joyce, and Shaw (1984) did not provide specialized services to the children, they did evaluate changes in the children's adjustment following shelter residence. Assessments were completed during residence at the shelter and again 4 months later, and comparisons were made with children in a matched control group of families. Mothers rated the children on a standardized measure, the Child Behavior Checklist (CBCL), which yields scores on two broad dimensions: internalizing behaviors (e.g., sad, nervous, anxious, cries too much), and externalizing behaviors (e.g., hyperactive, aggressive, impulsive, loud, demands attention). At the 4-month follow-up, the children had significantly fewer internalizing problems, but their scores were still a full standard deviation above the norm on this index. Although the children's level of internalizing problems on follow-up proved to be related to parental conflict patterns 4 months earlier, there was no attempt to relate follow-up adjustment to in-shelter experiences, so little is known about how children-oriented programs might affect their outcomes.

Overall, current knowledge concerning the effectiveness of interventions with children and with surrounding communities is rudimentary. Although individual programs sometimes conduct informal evaluations of their efforts, the results of these are not generally available in the literature. Moreover, systematic comparisons with alternative approaches or with control groups are almost nonexistent, so little can be said concerning the absolute or relative merits of different child or community intervention programs.

Programs for Men Who Batter

In sharp contrast to the rapid growth of services for battered women, interventions for the abusers have developed more slowly. In 1975 there were only two known services for abusive men. This number had increased to an estimated 80 programs by 1981 (Roberts, 1984) and in 1982 was placed at about 150 (Mettger, 1982). The last 3 years have seen a remarkable increase in such services, with the majority now in existence established since 1983 (Sonkin, Martin, & Walker, 1985). Several recent surveys of programs for abusers have been published (Feazell, Mayers & Deschner, 1984; Finn, 1985; Roberts, 1982, 1984; Star, 1983), providing an overview of their diversity in orientation, agency affiliation, and treatment modality and content.

Some programs offer services exclusively to abusive males, whereas others see spouse abusers as part of a broader clientele (Feazell *et al.*, 1984). Programs exclusively for men who batter can be further differentiated according to the nature of the offering agency. Some are organizations comprised of former batterers and/or grassroots organizations of men committed to ending violence against women. Others are associated with battered women's programs. Still others are specialized services within established agencies that offer a broad spectrum of counseling and therapy services to the community (Mettger, 1982; Roberts, 1984).

Traditional theories of psychotherapy have not offered clear-cut direction for designing programs to treat abusive men. Moreover, programs that train counselors and therapists do not explicitly prepare their graduates to contend with this problem and none of the states have licensure requirements specifying such preparation (Searle, 1985). As a result, most service providers have developed their approaches from direct experience with clients and from networking with other service providers in the field (Sonkin *et al.*, 1985). Not surprisingly, there is considerable diversity of opinion concerning what services should be offered and which treatment approaches are optimal (Davis, 1984; Weidman, 1986).

Treatment modalities cover a wide spectrum (individual counseling for the abuser, abuser group therapy, marital/couples therapy, and couples group therapy) and some programs offer combinations of these modalities (Star, 1983; Weidman, 1986). Roberts (1984) found that the group approach was the most popular format, with 60% of a national sample of 44 programs using group counseling either alone or in conjunction with other modes of treatment. At the same time, slightly more than one third preferred a combined approach incorporating individual, group, and couples counseling. There is an ongoing controversy as to the efficacy (and advisability) of couples therapy for spouse abuse, as detailed in the next section.

Proponents of group treatment argue that it breaks down social isolation and reduces extreme dependency on the partner, affords the men increased opportunities to recognize their general problem with anger control, provides role models for change, offers a safe and supportive context in which to practice new behaviors and skills, expands their options in times of crisis, and increases their self-esteem as they support others (cf. Searle, 1985).[13] The benefits of the group format may be extended by the additional use of a buddy system, wherein buddies check up on each other during the week and/or call each other if they need help in problem situations (cf. Mott-McDonald Associates, 1979).

Concerning the content of treatment, there has been some argument as to whether attitude change is a necessary priority or whether behavioral skills should receive emphasis (cf. Adams & McCormick, 1982; Finn, 1985; Martin, 1985; Neidig, 1985). As a result, some treatment approaches give more emphasis to behavioral skills development and changes, whereas others emphasize changes in attitudes and cognitions. Despite these differences, however, treatment programs often share remarkably similar goals and content, and many incorporate both attitudinal and behavioral change components. All share the

---

[13]Assumptions about the characteristics of abusive men have guided choices of treatment format and content, despite the fact that these have been based on clinical impressions, rather than on systematic risk factor analyses.

treatment goal of stopping the violence, and most insist that the abuser be accountable for the violence and explicitly acknowledge his responsibility for his own behavior (Roberts, 1984). Although a few programs do adopt a more traditional psychotherapeutic approach, the absence of aggressive ventilation therapy (the cathartic release school of thought[14]) is noteworthy. This approach has come under considerable criticism and is even deemed to be dangerous in relation to spouse abuse treatment (Bagarozzi & Giddings, 1983; Mott-McDonald Associates, 1979; Myers & Gilbert, 1983; Walker, 1978b).

Treatments focusing on skills development and behavioral changes include methods designed to improve the men's ability to recognize their stressors and react to them differently, to manage their anger more effectively, and to increase their abilities to accomplish interpersonal goals in other ways as by greater assertiveness, an expanded repertoire of interpersonal problem-solving strategies, and better communication skills (Feazell et al., 1984; Mott-McDonald Associates, 1979; Waldo, 1986; Weidman, 1986). These treatment approaches may employ various behavior therapy techniques, such as the use of an anger diary to help identify cues to violence, systematic desensitization using relaxation training to reduce the anger response to such cues, interruption of behavioral sequences that lead to violence by the use of a time out strategy, explicit search for and reinforcement of nonviolent responses to frustration and anger, and concrete arrangements for avoiding any reinforcement of violence (Bagarozzi & Giddings, 1983; Edelson, 1984; Edelson, Miller, Stone, & Chapman, 1985; Mott-McDonald Associates, 1979; Myers & Gilbert, 1983; Saunders, 1984a; Sonkin et al., 1985). Behavior change approaches are characteristically highly structured and typically include goal setting, leader modelling, rehearsal/role-playing, and feedback.

Treatment approaches emphasizing changes in attitudes and cognitions include consciousness-raising as well as cognitive restructuring approaches. Consciousness-raising is designed to alter rigid sex role expectations, increase insight into the personal and social roots of spouse abuse, heighten awareness of emotions, and foster supportive relationships with other men (Adams & McCormick, 1982; Finn, 1985; Saunders, 1984a; Weidman, 1986). Additional efforts to alter emotional/cognitive patterns may focus on developing greater individuation of the spouses (Grayson, Mathie, Wampler, Dennis, & Lynch, 1984), on enhancing responses empathic to the partner (Sonkin et al., 1985), and on the use of cognitive restructuring/reality therapy to reduce irrational beliefs that precipitate anger (cf. Bagarozzi & Giddings, 1983; Edelson, 1984; Edelson et al., 1985; Faezell et al., 1984; Mott-McDonald Associates, 1979; Saunders, 1984a). In contrast to behavior change strategies, these more cognitive approaches typically use a relatively unstructured and nondirective therapeutic context and rely heavily on constructive confrontation to effect cognitive/attitudinal changes.

In general, most treatment programs target both behavioral and attitudinal changes, and thus share a number of treatment strategies. Different programs offer different combinations of some or all of the earlier mentioned treatment approaches, and may emphasize some treatment components over others. The diversity of treatment programs in this respect may insure against oversimplifying the problem of spouse abuse by expecting a single treatment model to be effective with all abusers, a concern expressed by Roy (1982). At present, however, approaches for tailoring treatment programs to the needs of specific abusers are relatively undeveloped and, rather than being empirically grounded

---

[14]This approach, represented by Bach and Wyden (1968) maintains that periodic release of "pent up" aggressive impulses is necessary and constructive.

on systematic evidence, reflect primarily theoretical speculation and clinical judgments. For example, Schlesinger, Benson, and Zornitzer (1982) suggested classifying abusive men according to the etiology (organic/psychotic vs. not) and generality of their violence (both in and out of the home vs. in the home only) and recommended that different treatment approaches be employed with clients in different categories. Walker (1984) also recommended that treatment be geared to the offender, differentiating first from chronic offenders and also identifying men who require incarceration during treatment. Professionals treating abusive men have also stressed that clients be screened for their lethality potential prior to deciding on a treatment program, and that they be appropriately referred to other agencies or services for problems such as alcohol and/or drug abuse (cf. Feazell *et al.*, 1984; Sonkin *et al.*, 1985; Walker, 1984).

Consistent with the diversity of approaches in this arena, there appears to be little consensus concerning the advisable length of therapy with batterers (cf. Grayson *et al.*, 1984), with some practitioners advocating relatively short-term programs (e.g., Waldo, Firestone, Anderson, & Guerney, 1983) and others advising longer-term treatment (e.g., Sonkin *et al.*, 1985). To some degree, these discrepancies may reflect differences in the treatment component(s) considered to be crucial. For example, Sonkin *et al.* (1985) reported that whereas they have found that anger management skills can be developed adequately in a period of 6 to 12 months, improving self-esteem and resolving issues and attitudes concerning power in relationship may take considerably longer. Another arena of controversy concerns whether group facilitators must necessarily be male. Those programs that have women as co-leaders maintain that although the group may require an initial period of adjustment, this passes relatively quickly and a woman facilitator may in fact be a beneficial presence, helping the men to unlearn stereotypic sex role attitudes (cf. Mettger, 1982).

Programs for abusers share a pervasive problem of high attrition and low client motivation. The vast majority (70%) report that their greatest problem is the lack of motivation and commitment by the men (Roberts, 1984). Programs report that between one third and one half of the batterers drop out of treatment after the first session (Feazell *et al.*, 1984; Saunders, 1984a), and even higher attrition rates have been reported (Roberts, 1984). Thus, there is general agreement that batterers need a strong incentive to come to and remain in treatment (Feazell *et al.*, 1984). The strongest motivator appears to be the men's fear of losing their partner. They tend not to recognize wifebeating as a problem until the women have left them, or have threatened to do so (Myers & Gilbert, 1983; Saunders, 1984a). Once the immediate crisis is past and their partner returns, it is not uncommon for the men's motivation for treatment to end (Roberts, 1984).

Despite agreement that incentive for treatment is needed, there is little agreement concerning what the optimal incentive should be (Feazell *et al.*, 1984). Although the criminal justice system can serve as an important motivator (Mott-McDonald Associates, 1979; Roberts, 1984), the advisability of counseling men who have entered a program nonvoluntarily (through court mandate) is a point of strong disagreement. Some programs discourage or refuse to accept court-mandated clients, arguing that counseling is ineffective under such circumstances because mandated clients resist change and sabotage the counseling process (cf. Roberts, 1984).[15] Proponents of court-mandated counseling argue

---

[15]Other complications in the use of court-mandated counseling also arise. For example, such programs need to be implemented very soon after a battering incident rather than postponing arraignment until weeks after the arrest, as is typical, because such delay presents too much opportunity for the victim to drop the charges and

that getting the abuser to attend a treatment program at all is the greater part of the battle, and that the court can provide the external motivation needed for some men to enter and stay in treatment (Martin, 1985; Walker, 1984). They claim that although a period of initial resistance may occur among such clients, the court-mandated versus self-referred clients evidence little difference after this period (cf. Mettger, 1982; Star, 1983). Some also favor court-mandated counseling on the basis that it frees the victim from the responsibility of motivating the abuser via threats to leave or divorce him.

It is important to recognize that courts vary in the ways in which they mandate counseling. Some actually convict the offender, sentence him to imprisonment, and then stay this sentence pending completion of the counseling program. Others offer pretrial diversion programs, deferring ruling on the charges and dismissing the case upon successful completion of the counseling program (Finn, 1985; Waldo, 1987). Some pretrial diversion programs may additionally offer to purge the record of the arrest upon successful completion of treatment. Finally, some courts offer offenders the choice of entering the treatment program, whereas others simply mandate the treatment without providing offenders any option. As reiterated in the following, there is currently no information concerning the relative effectiveness of these different approaches.

Although there are a number of published papers describing the format of specific treatment programs and reporting clinical impressions of their effectiveness, many fail to provide systematic evaluation studies. In fact, studies of treatment effectiveness and follow-up data on clients have generally received little attention. To some extent this is attributable to limited program funds and staff time, but to some degree it may also derive from a lack of knowledge concerning evaluation methods and procedures (Finn, 1985). Although Star (1983) reported that most agencies and organizations do use simple, informal evaluation methods such as client feedback (e.g., Saunders, 1984a; Waldo, 1987), very few of even these informal evaluations have emerged in a published or readily accessible forum. More systematic assessments of effectiveness rely on recidivism rates (e.g., Waldo et al., 1983). Estimates of nonrecidivism during the period of treatment are said to range as high as 90% during the course of treatment itself, and to 67% to 75% after one year of follow-up (Feazell et al., 1984). Finally, the better-designed studies of treatment effectiveness have found significant differences in recidivism between treated and untreated men or between pre- and posttreatment rates of violence (Waldo, 1986). Sonkin et al. (1985) suggested that the degree to which a client is motivated to change may be the primary predictor of success in any given case. Nevertheless, the relative scarcity of publicly accessible results of outcome evaluations makes it difficult to generate informed hypotheses concerning the factors affecting differential success rates.

Couples Counseling

The advisability of treating the abuser and spouse together in conjoint couples counseling has been a subject of ongoing debate (Mott-McDonald Associates, 1979).

---

diminishes the effectiveness of any treatment that does occur (Roberts, 1984). Service providers must work closely with the court to coordinate court mandates with the treatment periods and regimes considered necessary for successful intervention (Mott-McDonald Associates, 1979). Finally, inequities in treatment policies, such as sanctions for nonattendance and/or reoffenses, may divide a group when both court-mandated and self-referred clients are included in the same group (Sonkin, 1985; Star, 1983).

Despite the fact that some authors have characterized conjoint couples therapy as infrequently used or as generally unaccepted (Neidig, 1985; Sonkin, 1984), nearly one third (32%) of battered women's shelters responding to one survey (Lindegren, no date) reported the use of conjoint therapy of some type. There is considerable variation in the way couples therapy is implemented as well as in the content and techniques used in this context. Some approaches use male and female co-therapists (Walker, 1978b), whereas others use couples groups (e.g., Deschner, 1984; Deschner, McNeil, & Moore, 1986; Guerney, Waldo, & Firestone, 1987; Myers, 1984). Some implement couples therapy only after the violence has been controlled following individual sessions with the abuser (and victim) (e.g., Walker, 1978b), and others implement couples therapy concurrently with individual or group therapy for the abuser (e.g., Edelson et al., 1985; Weidman, 1986).

Clinicians who adopt a family systems approach to spouse abuse assume (a) that wife battering occurs in specific types of relational structures, (b) that it results from an interactional system in which behavior transactions follow predictable and repetitive sequences, and (c) that it may itself serve a functional role in maintaining the marital system (Bograd, 1984). Many of those who approach spouse abuse from this theoretical perspective consider conjoint couples counseling or therapy to be the treatment of choice for this problem (e.g., Geller, 1982; Geller & Walsh, 1977–78; Geller & Wasserstrom, 1984; Schlesinger et al., 1982). They argue that this approach makes it easier for the therapist to assess the interaction patterns that lead to and/or maintain the violence (Mott-McDonald Associates, 1979). Another advantage of conjoint treatment is that it provides a context within which one can simultaneously deal with the husband's violent behavior and with the effects of his violence on his partner (Geller, 1982). Third, it precludes any secrets with the therapist and thereby avoids the suspicion and distrust engendered when the partners are seen separately in concurrent therapy approaches (Geller & Wasserstrom, 1984). Finally, it allows the therapist to address directly a partner's resistance to (or misunderstanding of) positive changes in the abuser (Saunders, 1984a).

Those opposing conjoint approaches argue that violence is an individually learned behavior and that the abuser must assume responsibility for the violence. First, opponents doubt the safety and efficacy of a joint approach in the absence of a strict no-violence contract. There is real concern that conjoint therapy may compromise the victim's safety and exacerbate the violence if used before the man has achieved control over his violence (cf. Adams & Penn, 1981; Mott-McDonald Associates, 1979; Purdy & Nickle, 1981). Moreover, the battered woman may well be reticent to disclose anything negative in front of her abuser if she risks violent retaliation. Second, critics argue that the violence must be the first and central issue in any treatment program. Conjoint therapy is seen as minimizing the importance of the violence by focusing equally or even predominantly on other issues (Bograd, 1984; Edelson, 1985). Third, the conjoint approach is said to cloud (if not distort) the issues of responsibility for the violence (Bograd, 1984). It can give the impression that the violence is caused to some degree by the woman and can lead the abuser to feel it is not really his problem (Adams & Penn, 1981; Martin, 1985). At one extreme are those family therapists who are even unwilling to label the battered woman as a victim (Goodstein & Page, 1981; Neidig, 1985). More moderate clinicians may acknowledge the woman's victimization, but imply that she can (and hence should) control her husband's feelings and actions, which thereby attenuates his responsibility for the violence (Bograd, 1984). Fourth, traditional couples therapy is oriented toward improving the relationship, and it subordinates individual needs to this goal. Critics emphasize that intervention with battering couples must focus on strengthening the individuals first, and relegate the survival of the relationship to a lesser priority (Walker, 1978b).

Less extreme viewpoints on both sides of this controversy have recently emerged. On the one hand, Bograd (1984) has noted that adopting a systemic framework in thinking about the problem does not require that one use conjoint therapy. In line with this stance, some family systems practitioners have also taken the somewhat unorthodox view that a systemic approach does not preclude holding the husband to be solely accountable for the violence (cf. Bograd, 1984; Cook & Frantz-Cook, 1984; Geller, 1982). On the other hand, those who oppose the general use of conjoint therapy do acknowledge that it might be a useful follow-up to individual work with the man in those cases where the couple chooses to stay together (Mott-McDonald Associates, 1979) and where the violence has stopped (Purdy & Nickle, 1981). As a result, no-violence contracts are becoming a commonly imposed precondition to the use of conjoint couples therapy and a number of those who offer conjoint couples counseling have established ending the violence as their highest priority goal (cf. Saunders, 1984a).

Again, evaluation studies are sadly lacking. Although informal reports concerning the general effectiveness of specific programs have been published (cf. Geller, 1982; Geller & Wasserstrom, 1984; Roberts, 1984) little information concerning posttreatment follow-ups and success rates is publicly available. There have been virtually no studies on the relative effectiveness of couples versus individual therapy with spouse abusing couples (Neidig, 1985).[16] The few available assessments concerning treatment outcomes with spouse abusing couples have typically not employed control group comparisons. Although evaluations of couples therapy have yielded promising overall rates of subsequent nonviolence (e.g., Guerney, Waldo, & Firestone, 1987), one study that examined pre- versus posttreatment differences in measures of actual violence failed to show any significant changes (Deschner et al., 1986). Moreover, results of follow-up evaluations are invariably plagued by a serious attrition problem, which appears to be endemic to all longitudinal research on spouse abuse.

Police Interventions

Representative sample surveys of the general population provide various estimates of the extent to which police have been informed about the abuse: 17% of the severe abuse cases (Schulman, 1979); 30% of those abused in their lifetimes (Teske & Parker, 1983); and 55% of the spouse abuse victims in a national sample (Gaquin, 1977–78). With between one sixth and one half of the victims of serious abuse known to the police, the police constitute an important community contact for wife abuse cases.

At the same time, the traditional approaches to wife assault by law enforcement agents have been severely criticized as failing to protect the victim and to convey to the abuser that his behavior is unacceptable to the community (cf. Fields, 1978; Martin, 1976, 1985; Paterson, 1979; Taub, 1983). Police have typically preferred the simple approach of separating the parties, or (since the influential demonstration project by Bard, 1970) attempting to mediate the dispute, and have used arrest only as a last resort. These approaches sometimes incorporate actual counseling as well, with police–social worker

---

[16]A recent random-assignment experiment with nonviolent couples, however, failed to find any outcome differences between concurrent and conjoint methods of couples therapy (Hefner & Prochaska, 1984).

teams used in some communities (e.g., Carr, 1982; Holmes, 1981). Critics argue that these responses may do a serious disservice by leading abusive men to expect few negative consequences for their violence from the community. The responsibility for initiating legal sanctions has been placed on the victim, who remains vulnerable to additional assaults in the interim.

In addition to the legal system's pervasive pattern of discounting the seriousness of the offense, abused women who have sought legal redress have typically received unpredictable responses. For example, in Marion County, Indiana, 325 women who filed charges during 1978 were tracked for 6 months through the legal system (Ford, 1983). Ultimately, only 30 of the original complaints reached court to be adjudicated, and generally only after about 4 months and two continuances. Ford pointed out the fallacy in assuming that the criminal justice system would function on the victim's behalf if only she elected to use it:

> elements of chance were present at every juncture . . . chance arose due to variations in the ways officials performed their duties—police dispatchers did not apply uniform standards in dispatching cars; police officers sometimes gave erroneous information on the judicial process; deputy prosecutors did not have uniform standards for evaluating cases; different judges applied different standards when evaluating affidavits for approving warrants; and, police officers differed in their efforts to serve warrants. (p. 467)

In view of their experiences with the legal system, it is hardly surprising to find that (until recently) fewer than half of the battered women who called police viewed the officers' responses as helpful, and in fact, police were rated as the least helpful of all helper categories in two studies (Carlson, 1977; Fojtik, 1977–78; Roy, 1977; Saunders & Size, 1980).

Legal responses to wife abuse in many jurisdictions have changed in the last few years, partly as a result of landmark legal cases such as *Scott v. Hart* in Oakland, California, and *Bruno v. Codd* in New York City (Martin, 1985; Paterson, 1979; Roberts, 1984; Taub, 1983). Legislative changes in many jurisdictions have removed statutes that had barred officers from making arrests in misdemeanor cases unless they witnessed an assault, enlarging their discretionary power to make warrantless arrests in response to wife abuse. Other legislative changes have increased the sentencing flexibility of courts, providing alternatives to traditional criminal system punishments. Perhaps these changes explain why the recent study by Kennedy and Homant (1984) showed that 70% of the abused women in a shelter-based sample had found the police helpful to some degree—a pattern that contrasts sharply with the earlier studies of victims' reactions noted earlier.

A well-publicized study by Sherman and Berk (1984) has recently altered attitudes about policies governing the arrest of violent assailants in domestic disputes. Over an 18-month period, Minneapolis police responded to misdemeanor domestic assaults with one of three randomly-assigned treatments: arrest of the abuser, separation of the parties by ordering the abuser to leave the premises for 8 hours, or some type of advice that occasionally included informal mediation. Follow-up tracking of the couples continued for 6 months and included monitoring of any records concerning subsequent police contacts for wife abuse as well as interviews with the victims every 2 weeks. Arrest significantly reduced repeat offenses given in the police records below the level of recidivism associated with separation (13% vs. 26%) and the mediation recidivism rate did not differ from that of either of the other treatments. The victim self-report data also documented the deterrent effect of arrest (19% recidivism) but reordered the other two effects, with advice associated with the highest rate of repeat violence (37%).

Historically, the reluctance to make arrests in wife abuse situations was rationalized by the belief that without severe and speedy court sanctions, arrest was a waste of time. But Sherman and Berk (1984) found lower recidivism following arrest despite the fact that only 3 of the 136 arrested were formally sanctioned. The historical policy against arrest was also motivated, at least in part, by the fear that such action might actually worsen the violence. Increased violence was believed to be likely after arrest because of retributions against the victim for calling the police, or because having been labeled a wife abuser by the arrest might alter the abuser's self-concept and disinhibit future violence. The empirical evidence from this study does not support either of these fears. On the basis of these findings, Sherman and Berk argued that police should operate with the presumption of arrest in wife abuse incidents—arresting abusers unless exceptional circumstances mitigate against this approach in specific cases.

Although the study is notable for its use of random assignment, it is not without important methodological problems. Chief among these are the known failures of the random assignment design due to preplanned exceptions,[17] forgetfulness, or confusion (assignments were actually implemented in 99% of the arrest cases, 78% of the advice cases, and 73% of the separation cases), and an unknown incidence of design failures due to officers failing to comply with instructions in ways that differentially affected the three conditions (e.g., choosing to exclude certain types of situations from the random sequence of case assignments or allowing the next identified treatment to influence decisions about whether encountered cases should be considered to be misdemeanors and hence within the scope of the study).[18] Perhaps the most important reservation concerns the possibility that key features of the study may not be generalizable to other contexts. Minneapolis is not representative of urban areas in general, and the uniqueness of its police department as well as its specific policies and practices subsequent to arrest may have been critical to the effects of arrest found in this context. Similarly, the mediation effects here may be specific to the way this intervention was implemented, meaning that different forms of mediation may fare better relative to arrest.

Despite these limitations, the Sherman and Berk (1984) study began to affect police policy across the country soon after its findings were released to the public. To support the generalizability of the arrest effect in that study, Berk and Newton (1984) examined police records concerning wife battery incidents for a 28-month period in Santa Barbara County, California. Instead of using ordinary analyses of the correlation between arrest and subsequent wife abuse, Berk and Newton applied a recently developed technique that allowed them to approximate the internal validity of a randomized experiment (despite the fact that the arrests in the records had occurred entirely at the discretion of the police and not

---

[17]Officers were granted the discretionary power to upgrade separation or mediation assignments to arrest if a suspect attempted to assault them, a victim demanded arrest of the assailant, or both parties were injured. Empirical analyses of the randomization failures showed, however, that three additional variables, as reflected in police records, also led to an upgrading of the separation and advice treatments: whether the suspect was rude, whether weapons were involved, and whether a restraining order was being violated.

[18]Although there was considerable loss of couples during the follow-up period (only 62% of the victims completed the initial interviews and only 49% completed all 12 follow-up interviews over the 6 months) there did not appear to be differential loss across the three treatment conditions. In addition, whereas the police report follow-ups may have been distorted by the tendency for offenders who have experienced arrest to leave the scene after new assaults, the victim interviews were not subject to this bias yet revealed the same patterns of arrest effectiveness.

according to random assignment).[19] The results again confirmed the deterrence effect of arrest, showing that those offenders most likely to be arrested were also those most likely to commit wife battery again but that arrest deterred them from subsequent wife abuse.

The policy implications of these findings, however, are not clear. The effect of lowering recidivism was specific to those individuals whom police tended to arrest under the prevailing circumstances. There is no guarantee that the same pattern would hold if police arrest policies were to be changed. In addition, what exactly it was about the arrest of these individuals that reduced their subsequent wife abuse remains a puzzle. Thus, it may be misleading to promulgate general policies concerning arrest until the effective components of the arrest process are identified. Moreover, further analyses of the original data collected by Sherman and Berk have indicated that there is a rapid decay in the deterrent effect of arrest relative to the other police treatments over the course of the follow-up period (Tauchen, Tauchen, & Witte, 1986). By the end of this period there are no real differences across the three types of police interventions studied. This suggests that whereas police actions at the time of the violent incident may be more or less effective in interrupting the pattern of wife abuse, without other intervention methods, the violence quickly returns to its "steady state" level.

Community intervention programs (CIPs) are a relatively recent development in the area of legal response. Such systems systematically coordinate police, judicial, and social services responses at the community level. Police participation generally involves making probable cause arrests whenever possible in domestic violence situations. In some CIPs, the police will, at the time of such an arrest, notify local support or advocate groups (e.g., a battered women's shelter, a battering men's counseling program, a victim-witness support program, etc.), who will then contact the victim and/or abuser to provide support and discuss the alternatives and resources available to them. Some support or advocate programs follow-up on all calls to police involving domestic violence, regardless of whether any arrest was made. In the judicial system, prosecuting attorneys aggressively pursue these arrests in court, where judges may cooperate with the communitywide effort by sending the offenders to a diversion program in which they are mandated to complete successfully a counseling program for batterers in lieu of harsher legal sanctions, such as a jail sentence. As noted in the earlier section on men's programs, there is wide variation in the way courts mandate counseling and no information exists regarding the optimally effective method(s) of doing so.

Systematic evaluations of CIPs are in the formative stages and have thus far focused on measuring aspects of the newly implemented system itself, rather than on determining its effects on wife abuse. Gamache, Edleson, and Schock (1984) evaluated the implementation of CIPs in three suburban Minnesota communities using a quasi-experimental design. The design involved obtaining multiple baseline measures and multiple postintervention measures, and lagging the introduction of the intervention such that there was a 3-month interval between its introduction in the different communities. After beginning a CIP, all three communities showed shifts toward increased arrests, increased numbers of successful prosecutions, and increased use of mandated counseling by the courts. Clearly, the programs did effect a change in the communities' responses to wife abuse. Whether

---

[19]The technique requires one to model the mechanism by which cases are assigned to the different treatments and then test the impact of the treatments by calculating propensity scores, an approach that essentially partials out the effects in this assignment model (cf. Rosenbaum & Rubin, 1983, 1984, 1985).

and to what extent these responses in turn affect the actual occurrence of wife abuse remain unanswered questions.

Effectiveness of Interventions

The discussions in preceding sections indicate that there are relatively few publicly accessible evaluation studies of existing intervention programs. Moreover, the need for such studies is apparent across all categories of intervention, including intervention programs geared toward the women (and children), the men, or the couples experiencing husband-to-wife violence. This section will discuss some of the possibilities for future evaluations of spouse abuse programs.

Although the ultimate test of a program's effectiveness must be its impact on the violence itself, evaluations can provide information about underlying treatment processes by examining psychological effects or the acquisitions of specific skills. For example, studies of the effects of shelters on battered women have begun to go beyond measuring return rates and have assessed psychological changes in the women associated with their shelter stays (cf. Sedlak, 1983; Zuckerman & Piaget, 1982). Future studies might not only expand these efforts but might try to uncover exactly which aspects of shelter experiences are critical to which of the different psychological and behavioral effects observed. Similarly, recent evaluations of treatments for abusers have not only focused on follow-up assessments of abuse *per se,* but have also documented increased listening and anger management skills as well as reductions in marital disputes and improved marital relationships (cf. Deschner, 1984; Waldo, 1986). Future studies might focus on specifically linking reductions in abuse to changes such as these and on demonstrating which components of the treatment program are critical to these changes. Overall, evaluation studies would be of greater value if they were designed to assess the effects of different program components and to identify partial and localized successes.

Identifying why a program did not work, doing a "program autopsy," can be more useful to future interventions than being able to document a poorly understood success (cf. Garbarino, 1986). For example, in discussing the possible reasons why their group treatment program for batterers had so little impact, Grayson *et al.* (1984) suggested that 6 weeks was an insufficient treatment period and that the treatment might be more effective if the violence were sanctioned by more severe legal penalties. Such specific hypotheses suggest clear alterations in the program for future evaluation.

This last example also emphasizes another important consideration: whether and with whom a particular treatment is effective may depend importantly on exactly how it is implemented, and evaluation researchers could also contribute by exploring some of these possibilities. For example, court-mandated treatment of abusers may only be effective when offenders are given the choice between a treatment program and criminal justice procedures. Another possibility is that some types of offenders may be more likely to benefit from court-ordered counseling than others. The actual success of a program can be obscured if interactions such as these are not taken into account. Moreover, such interactions can be important guides to optimal allocations of scarce treatment resources. Future evaluations may be sufficiently fine-tuned not only to answer the primary question: "What works?" but to also address the more significant question: "What works with what type of client, under what conditions, with what type of provider?" (Saunders, 1984b, p. 2).

The reviews in previous sections indicate that extremely few evaluation studies have included some basis against which to compare posttreatment outcomes, such as with pretreatment baselines or with controls. Admittedly, meaningful evaluations can be performed without a comparison group if their focus is on identifying the factors associated with how well a program takes with different clients and in different circumstances (cf. Garbarino, 1986). It must be recognized, however, that such research is correlational only and more stringent tests involving random assignment to the treatment versus a control or comparison condition will eventually be needed for a rigorous demonstration that the observed outcomes were due to the program *per se*. At the same time, it is important that any control group be devised in an ethically responsible way (see the following), so that clients who are in need of treatment are not left untreated (cf. Saunders, 1984a, b). One strategy may be to provide the control group with a very different type of treatment. Researchers might also further develop the use of quasi-experimental designs (Campbell & Stanley, 1963; Cook & Campbell, 1979; Rosenbaum & Rubin, 1983, 1984, 1985), which have only recently been introduced in evaluations of wife abuse programs (Berk & Newton, 1985; Edelson *et al.*, 1985; Gamache *et al.*, 1984; Sedlak, 1983).

Another common obstacle to evaluation research in this arena is the serious attrition that plagues all spouse abuse programs. The loss of clients over the course of a program and during the follow-up period can seriously distort evaluation results, since those couples who are more difficult to locate are likely to be those who continue to be violent. This type of selective loss is so typical that Garbarino (1986) suggested that the very fact that a program maintains contact with participating families over a period of time may in itself be a reflection of the program's effectiveness. Although there is no simple solution to the distortions introduced by attrition, the conclusions drawn from any evaluation results will often need to be qualified on this basis.

A final factor to consider in gauging the impact of any intervention is its practical effectiveness. Evaluations must not only take into account the actual effect of the program on those who participate, but also the program's overall impact on the incidence and/or severity of the problem, that is, the program's reach (cf. Garbarino, 1986). Thus, a treatment program may have very substantial impact on those persons who participate, but if its format is so restrictive that it can serve only very few people in very special circumstances, then its practical effectiveness may be inadequate. For example, a residential treatment program that requires batterers to remain in the facility full-time for 6 weeks and that has space for only 10 residents will serve relatively few batterers over the course of a year and will only be able to serve those who can afford its time commitment (and expense). Alternatively, a program may be effective for its participants but may be so difficult to implement that it is unlikely to be offered by other service providers (or it may only prove effective when offered by a specific service provider). A program that can easily be exported to other service providers without any measurable loss of effectiveness will have a greater potential impact on the overall incidence of the problem of spouse abuse. Unfortunately, the issue of practical effectiveness has been virtually ignored in evaluation studies to date. However, if efforts to combat spouse abuse are to achieve a real reduction in the incidence of the problem, this issue warrants careful attention in future evaluation studies.

Ethical and Legal Issues

A highly sensitive problem with lethal potential, wife abuse presents a variety of ethical issues for service providers and researchers. Legal requirements, regulations, professional standards, and personal ethics represent four sources of prescriptions and prohibitions, each associated with specific types of sanctions and affording different degrees of discretionary latitude. Ethical issues in the area of spouse abuse revolve primarily around issues of confidentiality and the overriding responsibility to provide for the safety of all concerned.

The law can prescribe certain courses of action and impose criminal sanctions if the prescribed actions are disregarded. For example, certain professionals are mandated to report suspected child abuse or neglect. The courts for the most part, however, have ruled that people do not have a duty to warn or intervene in spouse abuse cases (Sonkin *et al.*, 1985). A notable exception to this pattern evolved in the past decade in California, where court rulings have reflected a clear philosophical shift on this point. California courts established a landmark case in 1976 (*Tarasoff v. The Regents of the University of California*, 17Cal.3d 425) when they ruled that psychotherapists have a responsibility to exercise "reasonable care" to protect a potential victim when a client makes a specific threat against a person. Two more recent rulings have further elaborated this requirement, dictating that it also applies when no specific threat has been made but the therapist has assessed a patient to be a danger to a specific person (*Jablonski v. Loma Linda Veterans Administration*, 712F2d. 391 9th Cir. 1983), and that such a therapist must not only warn the intended victim but also unintended victims in proximity to the victim, such as children, in-laws, roommates, etc. (*Hedlund v. Superior Court of Orange County*, 34Cal.3d 695 1983).

Governmental agencies may impose regulations that institutions must adhere to and that may be enforced by sanctions, such as rescinding funding for violations. The federal regulations governing research are relevant to spouse abuse studies. These require informed consent for any research participation. There is some question as to whether or not informed consent can be satisfied when men have been mandated for treatment by the criminal justice system. Some argue that, under these conditions, the inducement for the men to enter treatment is sufficiently coercive to consider that they cannot or have not provided informed consent for any participation in treatment-related research (cf. Saunders, 1984b). At present, this issue has been considered only on a case-by-case basis by local human subjects committees.

Professional standards comprise another source of ethical requirements or prohibitions. Professional licensing or ethical review boards may impose rules or standards of conduct that can be enforced by revocation of license, public censure, and possibly lawsuit. Issues of professional standards surrounding spouse abuse focus on difficulties associated with confidentiality and on insuring the safety of all concerned parties. The reactions of service providers to the recent California rulings reflect their concerns that these legal requirements may undermine existing standards of professional conduct. For example, some have voiced concerns regarding the therapist's risk of being sued for violating client confidentiality and about the impact of these requirements to breach confidentiality on clients' willingness to be honest. One resolution of this dilemma is that of Daniel Sonkin and his colleagues (Sonkin *et al.*, 1985) who deal with it by presenting the limits on confidentiality to the client at the outset. The client is informed that if he continues to have any contact with the partner, or if he gets involved in another relationship while in treatment, the therapists must have contact with that person. These contacts will be solely to discuss the client's progress in the program with regard to controlling the violence. Clients are also specifically warned that if they threaten to harm another in the therapists' presence, or are assessed to be a danger to another, the potential victim will be warned and the police will be notified. Finally, all clients are forewarned that the requirements of the child abuse reporting laws are respected. By making these provisions for mandated reporting requirements at the outset of treatment, Sonkin and his colleagues not only delineate the exact limits of client confidentiality, but also emphasize the seriousness and danger of the client's violence. Note, however, that the issue of confidentiality also intrudes on research activities where any follow-up evaluations mean that records must be kept not only of clients' names and addresses but also of their criminal (violent) behaviors. Such records may be subpoenaed at any time by a court if privileged communication or special federal research provisions are not available. Professional standards governing research dictate that this jeopardy to clients be minimized (Saunders, 1984b).

In view of the lethality potential of spouse abuse, it would be professionally unethical to use any method of treatment that could be dangerous for the woman or that would permit the violence to continue. Similarly, researchers must contend with the potential danger associated with traditional no-treatment or minimal-treatment control groups and provide some assurance against the recurrence of violence during any waiting period (Saunders, 1984b). In response to these concerns, many service providers have established specific policies or strategies for minimizing the danger surrounding reoffenses. For example, Sonkin's program goes beyond the requirements of the law in several respects: (a) all reoffenses are reported to the police (the client is encouraged to do so first), and (b) victims are contacted not simply for any necessary forewarning but as a regular course of action in order to determine the effectiveness of the treatment and whether any reoffenses have occurred.

Beyond legal, regulatory, and professional requirements, personal codes of ethics may also dictate particular cautions or duties based on beliefs about likely consequences and personal standards of acceptable practice. Personal codes of ethics are typically enforced by conscience, but may have the endorsement and support of peers as well. In the absence of clear-cut evidence concerning the effects of various treatment approaches, disagreements about the potential danger inherent in different approaches bring personal ethics into the discussions. Thus, debates about the advisability of different treatment approaches are often fueled by strong feelings about the ethics of the decision. Sonkin's approach to minimizing the likelihood of further violence, outlined earlier, is his personal resolution of a more general professional dilemma concerning how to minimize the recurrence of violence. Such procedures, dictated by a therapists' own ethical standards of conduct, serve to insure the safety of all potential victims.

As with most questions of ethics, those surrounding research and treatment in the area of spouse abuse have no simple and ready answers. Most professionals agree, however, that assuring the safety of all parties must be the paramount concern, outweighing any competing requirements that might apply.

FUTURE DIRECTIONS

Although it is neither possible nor advisable to forecast trends in research and treatment in a domain such as this one, the work reviewed in this chapter does point to several sorely needed developments in risk factor and program evaluation research.

First, general knowledge concerning the etiology of wife abuse would be substantially advanced by risk factor research that (a) controls for factors that may be confounded with the violence, such as marital distress; (b) clarifies the temporal relationship between risk factors and wife abuse, resolving whether a given correlate is a product or a precursor; and (c) attends to the possible interactive effects of risk factors for wife abuse.

Second, research directed toward identifying the unique risk factors for wife abuse in particular client populations would provide systematic bases for screening clients to identify cases of wife abuse. Also, given the relatively low frequency of wife abuse, screening and assessment would further benefit from more systematic development of sequential strategies that use preliminary screening mechanisms to focus more in-depth scrutiny on those couples more likely to experience wife abuse.

Third, there is a serious need for work that bridges the gap between risk factor research and treatment approaches. At present, little empirical evidence exists concerning risk factors related to the frequency and/or severity of wife abuse. Knowledge of these factors would have direct implications for secondary and tertiary prevention efforts, which comprise most existing interventions. At the same time, primary prevention has received relatively little attention to date. Further development of primary prevention efforts could capitalize on the considerable knowledge base concerning risk factors for occurrence. Advances on this point would benefit from studies of the impact of different primary prevention approaches.

Fourth, although great strides have been made in the devising a number of promising treatment approaches, these have been developed almost exclusively by clinicians ''flying by the seat of their pants'' (cf. Sonkin, 1984), with little systematic evaluation research to guide their revision or elaboration. Given the considerable diversity of treatment approaches that are now offered, it would appear feasible to begin the more systematic assessments of their relative effects which could indicate what treatment approach works with what type of client and under which conditions. More program evaluation studies, more carefully designed evaluation studies, and greater public access to the results of such studies would all contribute substantially to this goal.

As this chapter indicates, the past decade and a half has seen not only the birth, but also a tremendous growth in the knowledge base concerning wife abuse and in approaches to combat this serious problem. The future success of these efforts will depend on allocating limited resources wisely to provide those answers and offer those services that are most needed.

REFERENCES

Adams, D. C., & McCormick, A. J. (1982). Men unlearning violence: A group approach based on the collective model. In M. Roy (Ed.), *The abusive partner: An analysis of domestic battering* (pp. 170–197). New York: Van Nostrand Reinhold.

Adams, D., & Penn, I. (April, 1981). *Men in groups: The socialization and resocialization of men who batter.* Paper presented at the meeting of the American Orthopsychiatric Association.

Aguirre, B. E. (1985). Why do they return?: Abused wives in shelters. *Social Work, 30*(4), 350–354.

Ahlbom, A., & Norell, S. (1984). *Introduction to modern epidemiology.* Chestnut Hill, MA: Epidemiology Resources.

Alessi, J. J., & Hearn, K. (1984). Group treatment of children in shelters for battered women. In A. R. Roberts (Ed.), *Battered women and their families: Intervention strategies and treatment programs* (pp. 49–61). New York: Springer.

Bach, G. R., & Wyden, P. (1968). *The intimate enemy.* New York: Morrow.

Bagarozzi, D. A., & Giddings, C. W. (1983). Conjugal violence: A critical review of current research and clinical practices. *American Journal of Family Therapy, 11*(1), 3–15.

Bard, M. (1970). *Training police as specialists in family crisis intervention.* Washington, DC: U. S. Department of Justice.

Berk, R. A., & Newton, P. J. (1985). Does arrest really deter wife battery? An effort to replicate the findings of the Minneapolis spouse abuse experiment. *American Sociological Review, 50,* 253–262.

Berk, R. A., Berk, S. F., Loseke, D. R., & Rauma, D. (1983). Mutual combat and other family violence myths. In D. Finkelhor, R. J. Gelles, G. T. Hotaling, & M. A. Straus (Eds.), *The dark side of families: Current family violence research* (pp. 197–212). Beverly Hills, CA: Sage.

Bograd, M. (1984). Family systems approaches to wife battering: A feminist critique. *American Journal of Orthopsychiatry, 54*(4), 558–568.

Bowker, L. H. (August, 1984). *The effect of methodology on subjective estimates of the differential effectiveness of personal strategies and help-sources used by battered women.* Paper presented at the Second National Conference for Family Violence Researchers, Durham, NH.

Bowker, L. H., & MacCallum, K. (1981). *What works? A study of husbands' and partners' reactions to strategies and help-sources utilized by battered women.* Unpublished manuscript, University of Wisconsin, School of Social Welfare, Milwaukee, WI.

Brown, J. (1986). Predictors of husbands' and wives' rates of physical aggression. (Doctoral dissertation, The University of Utah, 1985). *Dissertation Abstracts International, 46,* 4053–B.

Bulcroft, R., & Straus, M. A. (1975). *Validity of husband, wife, and child reports of intrafamily violence and power.* Unpublished manuscript, University of New Hampshire, Durham, NH.

Campbell, D. T., & Stanley, J. C. (1963). *Experimental and quasi-experimental designs for research.* Chicago, IL: Rand McNally.

Carlson, B. E. (1977). Battered women and their assailants. *Social Work, 22,* 455–460.

Carr, J. J. (1982). Treating family abuse using a police crisis team approach. In M. Roy (Ed.), *The abusive partner: An analysis of domestic battering* (pp. 216–229). New York: Van Nostrand Reinhold.

Catalano, R., & Dooley, P. (1980). Economic change in primary prevention. In R. H. Price, R. F. Ketterer, B. C. Bader, & J. Monahan (Eds.), *Prevention in mental health: Research, policy and practice* (pp. 21–40). Beverly Hills, CA: Sage.

Colorado Association for Aid to Battered Women. (1979). *A monograph on services to battered women.* (DHHS Publication No. (OHDS) 79-05708). Washington, DC: U.S. Government Printing Office.

Cook, D., & Frantz-Cook, A. (1984). A systemic treatment approach to wife battering. *Journal of Marriage and Family Therapy, 10,* 83–93.

Cook, T. D., & Campbell, D. T. (1979). *Quasi-experimentation: Design and analysis issues for field settings.* Chicago, IL: Rand McNally.

Dalto, C. A. (1983). Battered women: Factors influencing whether or not former shelter residents return to the abusive situation. (Doctoral dissertation, University of Massachusetts, 1983). *Dissertation Abstracts International, 44,* 1277–B.

Daniel, J. H., Newberger, E. H., Reed, R. B., & Kotelchuck, M. (1978). Child abuse screening: Implications of the limited predictive power of discriminants from a controlled family study of pediatric social illness. *Child Abuse and Neglect, 2,* 247–259.

Davidson, T. (1978). *Conjugal crime: Understanding and changing the wifebeating pattern.* New York: Hawthorn.

Davis, L. V. (1984). Beliefs of service providers about abused women and abusing men. *Social Work, 29,* 249.

Deschner, J. P. (1984). *The hitting habit: Anger control for battering couples.* New York: The Free Press.

Deschner, J. P., McNeil, J. S., & Moore, M. G. (1986). A treatment model for batterers. *Social Casework: The Journal of Contemporary Social Work, 67*(1), 55–60.

Dobash, R. E., & Dobash, R. (1979). *Violence against wives: A case against the patriarchy.* New York: The Free Press.

Doherty, D. (1981). Salvation Army study of battered women clients. *Response to Violence in the Family, 4*(4), 5.

Edelson, J. L., Miller, D. M., Stone, G. W., & Chapman, D. G. (1985). Group treatment for men who batter. *Social Work Research and Abstracts, 21*(3), 18–21.

Elwood, R., & Jacobson, N. S. (1983). Spouses' agreement in reporting their behavioral interactions: A clinical replication. *Journal of Consulting and Clinical Psychology, 50,* 783–784.

Emery, R. E., Kraft, S. P., Joyce, S., & Shaw, D. (August, 1984). *Children of abused women: Adjustment at four months following shelter residence.* Paper presented at the meeting of the American Psychological Association, Toronto, Canada.

Fagan, J. A., Stewart, D. K., & Hansen, K. V. (1983). Violent men or violent husbands? Background factors and situational correlates. In D. Finkelhor, R. J. Gelles, G. T. Hotaling, & M. A. Straus (Eds.), *The dark side of families: Current family violence research* (pp. 49–67). Beverly Hills, CA: Sage.

Feazell, C. S., Mayers, R. S., & Deschner, J. (1984). Services for men who batter: Implications for programs and policies. *Family Relations, 33,* 217–223.

Ferraro, K. J. (1981). Processing battered women. *Journal of Family Issues, 2*(4), 415–438.

Fields, M. (1978). Wife beating: Government intervention policies and practices. In *Battered Women: Issues of public policy* (pp. 228–287). Washington, DC: U. S. Civil Rights Commission.

Finn, J. (1985). Men's domestic violence treatment groups: A statewide survey. *Social Work with Groups, 8*(3), 81.

Fleming, J. B. (1979). *Stopping wife abuse: A guide to the emotional, psychological and legal implications.* Garden City, NY: Anchor.

Fojtik, K. M. (1977–78). The NOW domestic violence project. *Victimology, 2,* 653–657.

Ford, D. A. (1983). Wife battery and criminal justice: A study of victim decision-making. *Family Relations, 32,* 463–475.

Gamache, D. J., Edelson, J. L., & Schock, M. D. (August, 1984). *Coordinated police, judicial and social service response to woman battering: A multiple-baseline evaluation across three communities.* Paper presented at the Second National Conference for Family Violence Researchers, Durham, NH.

Gaquin, D. A. (1977–78). Spouse abuse: Data from the National Crime Survey. *Victimology, 2,* 632–643.

Garbarino, J. (1980). Preventing child maltreatment. In R. Price, R. F. Ketterer, B. C. Bader, & J. Monahan (Eds.), *Prevention in Mental Health* (Vol. I, pp. 63–79). Beverly Hills, CA: Sage.

Garbarino, J. (October, 1986). *Prevention programs that work: Delivering services and measuring results.* Paper presented at the conference of the American Association for Protecting Children (American Humane), Denver, CO.

Geller, J. (1982). Conjoint therapy: Staff training and treatment of the abuser and the abused. In M. Roy (Ed.), *The abusive partner: An analysis of domestic battering* (pp. 198–215). New York: Van Nostrand Reinhold.

Geller, J. A., & Walsh, J. C. (1977–78). A treatment model for the abused apouse. *Victimology, 2,* 627–632.

Geller, J. A., & Wasserstrom, J. (1984). Conjoint therapy for the treatment of domestic violence. In A. R. Roberts (Ed.), *Battered women and their families: Intervention strategies and treatment programs* (pp. 33–48). New York: Springer.

Gelles, R. J. (1980). Violence in the family: A review of research in the seventies. *Journal of Marriage and the Family, 42,* 873–885.

Gelles, R. J. (August, 1984). *Applying our knowledge of family violence to prevention and treatment: What difference might it make?* Paper peresented at the Second National Conference for Family Violence Researchers, Durham, NH.

Gentry, C. E., & Eaddy, V. B. (1980). Treatment of children in spouse abusive families. *Victimology, 5,* 240–250.

Gilbert, N. (1982). Policy issues in primary prevention. *Social Work, 27*(4), 293–297.

Giovannoni, J. M. (1982). Prevention of child abuse and neglect: Research and policy issues. *Social Work Research and Abstracts, 18,* 23–31.

Goodstein, R., & Page, A. (1981). Battered wife syndrome: Overview of dynamics and treatment. *American Journal of Psychiatry, 138,* 1036–1044.

Grayson, J., Mathie, V. A., Wampler, D., Dennis, M., & Lynch, J. (August, 1984). *In response to spouse abuse: A men's group.* Paper presented at the meeting of the American Psychological Association, Toronto, Canada.

Gregory, M. (1976). Battered wives. In M. Borland (Ed.), *Violence in the family* (pp. 107–128). Atlantic Highlands, NJ: Humanities Press.

Guerney, B. G., Jr., Waldo, M., & Firestone, L. (1987). Wife-battering: A theoretical construct and case report. *American Journal of Family Therapy, 15*(1), 34–43.

Gully, K. J., Pepping, M., & Dengerink, H. A. (1982). Gender differences in third-party reports of violence. *Journal of Marriage and the Family, 44*(2), 497–498.

Hart, B. J. (1980, February). Testimony before the Subcommittee on Child and Human Development of the Committee on Labor and Human Resources. *Domestic Violence Prevention and Services Act, 1980.* United States Senate, Ninety-sixth Congress, Second Session on S. 1843.

Hefner, C. W., & Prochaska, J. O. (1984). Concurrent vs. conjoint marital therapy. *Social Work, 29,* 287–291.

Hofeller, K. H. (1980). Social, psychological, and situational factors in wife abuse. (Doctoral dissertation, Claremont Graduate School, 1980). *Dissertation Abstracts International, 41,* 408–B.

Holmes, S. A. (1981). A holistic approach to the treatment of violent families. *Social Casework: The Journal of Contemporary Social Work, 62,* 594–600.

Hudson, W. W., & McIntosh, S. R. (1981). The assessment of spouse abuse: Two quantifiable dimensions. *Journal of Marriage and the Family, 43*(4), 873–885.

Hughes, H. M. (1981). Advocacy for children of domestic violence: Helping the battered woman with non-sexist childrearing. *Victimology, 6,* 262–271.

Hughes, H. M. (1982). Brief interventions with children in a battered women's shelter: A model preventive program. *Family Relations, 31,* 495–502.

Hughes, H. M. (1986, August). *Child-focused intervention in shelters.* Paper presented at the meeting of the American Psychological Association, Washington, DC.

Hughes, H. M., & Barad, S. J. (1982). Changes in the psychological functioning of children in a battered women's shelter: A pilot study. *Victimology, 7,* 60–68.

Huston, K. (1986). A critical assessment of the efficacy of women's groups. *Psychotherapy, 23*(2), 283–290.

Jaffe, P., Wilson, S., & Wolfe, D. A. (1986, August). *Impact of group counseling for child witnesses to wife battering.* Paper presented at the meeting of the American Psychological Association, Washington, DC.

Jouriles, E., & O'Leary, K. D. (1984). *Interspousal reliability of reports of marital violence.* Unpublished paper.

Kalmuss, D. S., & Straus, M. A. (1982). Wife's marital dependency and wife abuse. *Journal of Marriage and the Family, 44*(2), 277–286.

Kalmuss, D. S., & Straus, M. A. (1983). Feminist, political, and economic determinants of wife abuse services. In D. Finkelhor, R. J. Gelles, G. T. Hotaling, and M. A. Straus (Eds.), *The dark side of families: Current family violence research* (pp. 363–376). Beverly Hills, CA: Sage.

Kennedy, D. B., & Homant, R. J. (1984). Battered women's evaluation of the police response. *Victimology, 9,* 174–179.

King, L. S. (1981). Responding to spouse abuse: The mental health profession. *Response to Violence in the Family, 4,* 6–9.

Kotelchuck, M. (1982). Child abuse and neglect: Prediction and misclassification. In R. H. Starr, Jr. (Ed.), *Child abuse prediction* (pp. 67–104). Cambridge, MA: Ballinger.

Langley, R., & Levy, R. C. (1977). *Wife beating: The silent crisis.* New York: E. P. Dutton.

Last, J. M. (1983). *A dictionary of epidemiology.* New York: Oxford University Press.

Lewis, B. Y. (1983). *The development and initial validation of the wife abuse inventory.* Unpublished doctoral dissertation, University of South Florida, 1983.

Lewis, B. Y. (1984, August). *Wife abuse and marital rape in a clinical sample.* Paper presented at the Second National Conference for Family Violence Researchers, Durham, NH.

Lewis, B. Y. (1985). The Wife Abuse Inventory: A screening device for the identification of abused women. *Social Work, 30*(1), 32–35.

Light, R. J. (1974). Abused and neglected children in America: A study of alternative policies. *Harvard Educational Review, 43,* 556–598.

Lindegren, T. M. (no date). *Survey of spouse abuse shelters: A family systems perspective.* Unpublished manuscript, University of New Hampshire, Durham, NH.

Lockhart, L. L. (1985). Methodological issues in comparative racial analysis: The case of wife abuse. *Social Work Research and Abstracts, 21*(2), 35–41.

Loseke, D. R., & Berk, S. F. (1981, August). *Defining "help": Initial encounters between battered women and shelter staff.* Paper presented at the First National Conference for Family Violence Researchers, Durham, NH.

Loseke, D. R., & Berk, S. F. (1982). The work of shelters: Battered women and initial calls for help. *Victimology, 7,* 35–48.

Lynch, C. G., & Norris, T. L. (1977–1978). Services for battered women: Looking for a perspective. *Victimology, 2,* 553–562.

Mace, D. R. (Ed.). (1983). *Prevention in Family Services.* Beverly Hills, CA: Sage.

Martin, D. (1976). *Battered wives.* San Francisco, CA: Glide.

Martin, D. (1985). Domestic violence: A sociological perspective. In D. J. Sonkin, D. Martin, & L. E. A. Walker (Eds.), *The male batterer: A treatment approach* (pp. 1–32). New York: Springer.

Mascia, C. A. (1983). A study of the treatment of battered women in emergency room settings. (Doctoral dissertation, Kent State University, 1983). *Dissertation Abstracts International, 44,* 1580–B.

Masumura, W. T. (1979). Wife abuse and other forms of aggression. *Victimology, 4*(1), 46–59.

McMurtry, S. L. (1985). Secondary prevention of child maltreatment: A review. *Social Work, 30*(1), 42–48.

Mettger, Z. (1982). Help for men who batter: An overview of issues and programs. *Response to Family Violence and Sexual Assault, 5*(6), 1–2, 7–8, 23.

Miller, D. (1980). Innovative program development for battered women and their families. *Victimology, 5*, 335–346.

Mott-McDonald Associates. (1979, May). *The report from the conference on intervention programs for men who batter.* Sponsored by Special Programs Division, Law Enforcement Assistance Administration. Washington, DC: U. S. Department of Justice.

Myers, C. W. (August, 1984). *The family violence project: Some preliminary data on a treatment program for spouse abuse.* Paper presented at the Second National Conference for Family Violence Researchers, Durham, NH.

Myers, T., & Gilbert, S. (1983). Wifebeaters' group through a women's center: Why and how. *Victimology, 8*(1–2), 238–248.

Neidig, P. H. (1985). Women's shelters, men's collectives, and other issues in the field of spouse abuse. *Victimology, 9*(3–4), 464–476.

O'Leary, K. D., & Arias, I. (August, 1984). *Assessing reliability of reports of spouse abuse.* Paper presented at the Second National Conference for Family Violence Researchers, Durham, NH.

Okun, L. E. (1983). A study of women abuse: 300 battered women taking shelter, 119 woman-batterers in counseling. (Doctoral dissertation, The University of Michigan). *Dissertation Abstracts International, 44*, 1972–B.

Pagelow, M. D. (August, 1977). *Battered women: A new perspective.* Paper presented at the International Sociological Association Seminar on Sex Roles, Deviance, and Agents of Social Control, Dublin, Ireland.

Pagelow, M. D. (February, 1978). Need assessment of victims of domestic violence. In *Research into violent behavior: Domestic violence.* [Hearings before the Subcommittee on Domestic and International Scientific Planning, Analysis and Cooperation, Committee on Science and Technology, U. S. House of Representatives, Ninety-fifth Congress, Second Session] (Appendix). (Publication No. 27-090-0). Washington, DC: U. S. Government Printing Office.

Pagelow, M. D. (1981). Factors affecting women's decisions to leave violent relationships. *Journal of Family Issues, 2*(4), 391–414.

Paterson, E. J. (1979). How the legal system responds to battered women. In D. M. Moore (Ed.), *Battered women* (pp. 79–99). Beverly Hills, CA: Sage.

Peltoniemi, T. (1981). The first 12 months of the Finnish shelters. *Victimology, 6*, 198–211.

Pizzey, E. (1974). *Scream quietly or the neighbours will hear.* Harmondsworth, Middlesex, England: Penguin.

Pleck, E., Pleck, J., Grossman, M., & Bart, P. (1978). The battered data syndrome: A reply to Steinmetz. *Victimology, 2*, 680–683.

Porter, C. A. (1983). Blame, depression and coping in battered women. (Doctoral dissertation. The University of British Columbia, 1983). *Dissertation Abstracts International, 44*, 1641–B.

Purdy, F., & Nickle, N. (1981). Practice principles for working with groups of men who batter. *Social Work with Groups, 4*, 111–122.

Rhodes, R. M., & Zelman, A. B. (1986). An ongoing multifamily group in a women's shelter. *American Journal of Orthopsychiatry, 56*(1), 120–130.

Ridington, J. (1977–78). The transition process: A feminist environment as reconstitutive milieu. *Victimology, 2*, 563–575.

Roberts, A. R. (1981). *Sheltering battered women: A national study and service guide.* New York: Springer.

Roberts, A. R. (1982). A national survey of services for batterers. In M. Roy (Ed.), *The abusive partner: An analysis of domestic battering* (pp. 230–243). New York: Van Nostrand Reinhold.

Roberts, A. R. (Ed.). (1984). *Battered women and their families: Intervention strategies and treatment programs.* New York: Springer.

Rosenbaum, P. R., & Rubin, D. B. (1983). The central role of propensity score in observational studies of causal effects. *Biometrica, 70*, 41–55.

Rosenbaum, P. R., & Rubin, D. B. (1984). Reducing bias in observational studies using sublcassification on the propensity score. *Journal of the American Statistical Association, 79*, 516–524.

Rosenbaum, P. R., & Rubin, D. B. (1985). Constructing a control group using multivariate matching sampling methods that incorporate the propensity score. *The American Statistican, 39*, 141–147.

Roy, M. (1977). A current survey of 150 cases. In M. Roy (Ed.), *Battered women: A psychosociological study of domestic violence* (pp. 25–44). New York, NY: Van Nostrand Reinhold.

Roy, M. (1982). The unmaking of the abusive partner. In M. Roy (Ed.), *The abusive partner: An analysis of domestic battering* (pp. 145–147). New York: Van Nostrand Reinhold.

Saunders, D. G. (1984a). Helping husbands who batter. *Social Casework: The Journal of Contemporary Social Work, 65,* 347–353.

Saunders, D. G. (August, 1984b). *Issues in conducting treatment research with men who batter.* Paper Presented at the Second National Conference for Family Violence Researchers, Durham, NH.

Saunders, D. G., & Size, P. B. (1980). *Marital violence and the police: A survey of police officers, victims and victim advocates.* Unpublished research report to the Wisconsin Council on Criminal Justice, Madison, WI.

Schlesinger, L. B., Benson, M., & Zornitzer, M. (1982). Classification of violent behavior for purposes of treatment planning: A three-pronged approach. In M. Roy (Ed.), *The abusive partner: An analysis of domestic battering* (pp. 148–169). New York: Van Nostrand Reinhold.

Schulman, M. (1979). *A survey of spousal violence against women in Kentucky.* Study No. 792701 conducted for Kentucky Commission on Women. Washington, DC: U. S. Department of Justice, Law Enforcement Assistance Administration.

Searle, M. (1985). Introduction. In D. J. Sonkin, D. Martin, & L. E. A. Walker (Eds.), *The male batterer: A treatment approach* (pp. xi–xiv). New York: Springer.

Sedlak, A. J. (August, 1983). *The use and psychosocial impact of a battered women's shelter.* Paper presented at the meeting of the American Psychological Association, Anaheim, CA.

Seward, R. (February, 1980). Shelters for battered women and their children. Testimony before the Subcommittee on Child and Human Development of the Committee on Labor and Human Resources. *Domestic Violence Prevention and Services Act, 1980.* United States Senate, Ninety-sixth Congress, Second Session on S. 1843.

Sherman, L. W., & Berk, R. A. (1984). The specific deterrent effects of arrest for domestic assault. *American Sociological Review, 49,* 261–272.

Snyder, D. K., & Scheer, N. S. (September, 1980). *Predicting adjustment following brief residence at a shelter for battered women.* Paper presented at the meeting of the American Psychological Association, Montreal, Canada.

Sonkin, D. J. (August, 1984). *Confronting the violence around us: Treatment of the male batterer.* Paper presented at the meeting of the American Psychological Association, Toronto, Canada.

Sonkin, D. J., Martin, D., & Walker, L. E. (1985). *The male batterer: A treatment approach.* New York: Springer.

Star, B. (1983). *Helping the abuser: Intervening effectively in family violence.* New York: Family Service Association of America.

Stark, E., & Flitcraft, A. (1981, August). *Therapeutic intervention as a situational determinant of the battering syndrome.* Paper presented at the First National Conference for Family Violence Researchers, Durham, NH.

Stark, E., Flitcraft, A., Zuckerman, D., Grey, A., Robison, J., Frazier, W. (1981). *Wife abuse in the medical setting: An introduction for health personnel.* Domestic Violence Monograph Series, No. 7, Rockville MD: National Clearinghouse on Domestic Violence.

Straus, M. A. (1977–1978). Wife beating: How common and why? *Victimology, 2*(3–4), 443–458.

Straus, M. A. (1979). Measuring intrafamily conflict and violence: The conflict tactics (CT) scales. *Journal of Marriage and the Family, 41,* 75–86.

Straus, M. A., Gelles, R. J., & Steinmetz, S. K. (1980). *Behind closed doors: Violence in the American family.* Garden City, NY: Doubleday.

Szinovacz, M. E. (1983). Using couple data as a methodological tool: The case of marital violence. *Journal of Marriage and the Family, 45,* 633–644.

Taub, N. (1983). Adult domestic violence: The law's response. *Victimology, 8,* 152–171.

Tauchen, G., Tauchen, H., & Witte, A. D. (1986). *The dynamics of domesitc violence: A reanalysis of the Minneapolis experiment.* (Working Paper #107). Wellesley, MA: Wellesley College, Department of Economics.

Tauchen, H. V., Witte, A. D., & Long, S. K. (1985, July). *Domestic violence: A non-random affair.* (Working Paper No. 1665). Cambridge, MA: National Bureau of Economic Research.

Teske, R. H. C., & Parker, M. L. (1983). *Spouse abuse in Texas: A study of women's attitudes and experiences.* (Publication No. 82-T-0003). Huntsville, TX: Sam Houston University, Criminal Justice Center.

Vaughan, S. R. (1979). The last refuge: Shelter for battered women. *Victimology, 4,* 113–150.

Waldo, M. (1987). Also victims: Understanding and treating men arrested for spouse abuse. *Journal of Counseling and Development, 65,* 385–388.

Waldo, M. (1986). Group counseling for military personnel who battered their wives. *Journal for Specialists in Group Work,* 132–138.

Waldo, M., Firestone, L., Anderson, C., & Guerney, B. G. (April, 1983). *Prevention of spouse abuse: Court referred group guidance.* Paper presented at the meeting of the American Personnel Guidance Association, Washington, DC.

Walker, L. E. (March, 1978a). *Feminist psychotherapy with victims of violence.* Paper presented at the mid-winter meeting of Division 29 Psychotherapy of the American Psychological Association, Scottsdale, AZ.

Walker, L. E. (February, 1978b). Psychotherapy and counseling with battered women. In *Research into violent behavior: Domestic violence.* [Hearings before the Subcommittee on Domestic and International Scientific Planning, Analysis and Cooperation, Committee on Science and Technology, U. S. House of Representatives, Ninety-fifth Congress, Second Session] (Appendix). (Publication No. 27-090-0). Washington, DC: U. S. Government Printing Office.

Walker, L. (1978c). Testimony in *Battered Women: Issues of Public Policy* (pp. 160–163). Washington, DC: U. S. Civil Rights Commission.

Walker, L. E. (1978d). Treatment alternatives for battered women. In J. R. Chapman & M. Gates (Eds.), *The victimization of women* (pp. 143–174). Beverly Hills, CA: Sage.

Walker, L. E. (1984). *The battered woman syndrome.* New York: Springer.

Weidman, A. (1986). Family therapy with violent couples. *Social Casework: The Journal of Contemporary Social Work, 67,* 211–218.

Yllo, K. (October, 1980). *The status of women and wife-beating in the U.S.: A multi-level analysis.* Paper presented to the National Council of Family Relations, Portland, OR.

Yllo, K. (1983). Using a feminist approach in quantitative research: A case study. In D. Finkelhor, R. J. Gelles, G. T. Hotaling, & M. A. Straus (Eds.), *The dark side of families: Current family violence research* (pp. 277–288). Beverly Hills, CA: Sage.

Yllo, K., & Straus, M. A. (1981). *Patriarchy and violence against wives: The impact of structural and normative factors.* Unpublished manuscript, University of New Hampshire, Family Research Laboratory, Durham, NH.

Zuckerman, D. M., & Piaget, A. E. (May, 1982). *The impact of shelters for battered women.* Paper presented at the First New England AWP (Association for Women in Psychology) Conference on the Psychology of Women, Boston, MA.

15

Neurological Factors

FRANK A. ELLIOTT

INTRODUCTION

The socioeconomic and cultural contributions to human destructiveness within the family circle are so many and so obvious that the roles of developmental and acquired neuro-psychological defects and metabolic disorders are often overlooked. In this chapter the emphasis given to biological factors in relation to pathologically aggressive behavior is not intended to derogate the importance of psychosocial forces, but rather is a reminder that to discuss aggression only in terms of such forces is somewhat like considering a car's performance without reference to the efficiency of its engine, steering, and brakes. It is obvious that severe damage in appropriate areas of the brain can impair cognition, perception, emotions, and behavior, but more subtle defects of the associational neocortex and limbic system can, and often do, escape detection unless special methods of investigation are used.

Organic defects have been found to be more common in children and adults with behavioral disorders than in the general population—in recidivist criminals (Monroe, 1970; Yeudall, 1979), violent juvenile delinquents (Lewis, Shamok, Pincus, & Glaser, 1979), the episodic dyscontrol syndrome (Bach-Y-Rita, Lion, Climent, & Ervin, 1971; Elliott, 1982; Hartocollis, 1968; Mark & Ervin, 1970; Monroe, 1970), borderline syndromes (Andrulonis & Glueck, 1980), atypical schizophrenias (Bellak, 1979), and antisocial personality disorders (Flor-Henry, 1983; Hare & Schalling, 1978; Mednick & Christiansen, 1977; Reid, 1978; Yeudall & Fromm-Auch, 1979). Similarly, many reports testify to a high prevalence of brain defects, often listed as minimal brain dysfunction, in children referred to child guidance clinics, whereas prospective and retrospective studies disclose that many of these children will become psychiatric or social casualties in adolescence or later (Anderson, 1972; Quitkin, Rifkin, & Klein, 1976; Robins, 1966; Rochford, Detre, Tucker, & Harrow, 1970; Satterfield, Hoppe, & Schell, 1982; Wender, 1971; Wood, Reimer, Wender, & Johnson, 1976).

On the other hand, Rutter and Giller (1984) concluded that "brain damage (however assessed) is present in only a tiny minority of delinquents," and Guze (1976) and

---

FRANK A. ELLIOTT • Department of Neurology, Pennsylvania Hospital, University of Pennsylvania, 3339 School House Lane, Philadelphia, PA 19144.

Schulsinger (1977) found that brain damage from birth complications did not contribute to psychopathic criminal behavior. However, Rutter and Giller do emphasize the link between delinquency and the hyperactive syndrome (which they do not regard as organic), and Guze's cases, though screened for gross organic disorders, were not examined for the sort of subtle defects found in minimal brain dysfunction and temporal lobe epilepsy.

Evidence of multiple defects was found by clinical examination, EEG, CAT scan, and neuropsychological tests in over 90% of 286 individuals with a history of repeated violence against family members and others (Elliott, 1982), suggesting a need for controlled studies on a more representative sample of domestic abusers.

Neurological Disorders Can Contribute to Family Violence

Overt neurological disabilities, such as mental retardation, cerebral palsy, and epilepsy can be a source of intrafamilial stress and are usually recognized and allowed for, but it is only too easy for the convoluted dynamics of family interactions to obscure the role of subtle, organically determined defects of cognition, perception, and emotional control in either aggressors or victims.

There are many symptoms and signs. Two of the most disruptive forms of antisocial behavior within the family (or out of it) are episodic dyscontrol in the form of unpredictable attacks of rage in response to minor provocation, and the recurrent callous brutality of aggressive psychopathy (the antisocial personality disorder of DSM-III). These will be discussed later.

Less dramatic symptoms can also contribute to conflict, notably in cases of minimal brain dysfunction. Slowness of thinking and a limited vocabulary hinder interpersonal communication and can lead to frustration and rage: for many, it is easier to hit than to talk. Some "organics" lack perception and miss the cues that are so essential to smooth social interactions—facial expression, tone of voice, and body language; consequently, they fail to perceive the anger or grief of others. Some do not recognize their own anger and tactlessness and fail to understand why they alienate people. Impulsiveness and lack of reflective delay are common in hyperactive children and in psychopathic adults. Thanks to a limited capacity for abstract thought, they fail to foresee the results of their ill-considered actions. Some lack a sense of fear and are therefore unduly combative and venturesome.

Others vexatious ingredients that are found in varying combinations are hyperactivity (or apathy), perseveration (e.g., persistence with a threadbare topic, as in fronto-temporal lesions), destructiveness, defective judgment, incapacity to fantasize, humorlessness, and emotional lability. Specific learning disabilities are common and even today are attributed too often to emotional problems.

The condition that casts the longest shadow in terms of future social deviance is the antisocial personality (Robins, 1966) with its impulsiveness, egocentricity, lack of empathy, unresponsiveness to discipline, and lack of guilt that so easily evoke antipathy and invite retaliation. "They tell me that I did not give him enough love, but believe me, doctor, he was a difficult child to love, right from the day he was born." Needless to say, the interactions between an antisocial child and a parent with emotional dyscontrol or psychopathy can be dire. A husband or wife who appears intelligent but cannot cope with practical matters because of the patchy cognitive defects of minimal brain dysfunction can incur the wrath of a spouse or adolescent children who do not understand the true state of affairs.

Gelles (1972) drew attention to another common situation—a violent attack by a husband who is enraged by sustained verbal abuse by an exasperated spouse who suffers from episodic dyscontrol.

Physiological Modulaters of Aggression

Genetics

The influence of genetics on behavior is avoided in much of the literature on family violence, but has to be faced because it plays a significant role in at least three syndromes that contribute to pathological aggression—episodic dyscontrol, minimal brain dysfunction (the attention deficit disorder of DSM-III), and the antisocial personality disorder. All three are more prevalent among aggressive criminals and delinquents than in the general population (Cantwell, 1975; Cloninger, Reich, & Guze, 1978; Lewis *et al.*, 1979; Mednick, 1977); and the same applies to episodic dyscontrol and minimal brain disfunction in batterers and abusers (Elliott, 1982).

Selective breeding for specific qualities was practiced in animal husbandry by the Greeks and has been used successfully for many generations in the production of highly aggressive bulls, dogs, and fighting cocks, and under laboratory conditions it has been possible to establish lines of abnormally aggressive dogs, Australian Dingoes, guinea pigs—and even rabbits (Ginsberg, 1979).

The XYY chromosomal anomaly was thought to predispose to violent criminal behavior and to be associated with high levels of plasma testosterone and testosterone synthesis, but the results are not consistent, and some geneticists consider that the issue is unsettled. On the other hand recent research has disclosed that a structural abnormality of the X chromosome is often associated with mental impairment varying from retardation to low-normal intelligence and learning difficulties, and sometimes with behavioral problems such as hyperactivity, violent outbursts, and autistic symptoms. Those bearing the fragile chromosome may exhibit large ears and enlarged testicles. Mental impairment has been found in about 80% of boys with this defect; girls are less often affected and about 1/3 of those with the abnormal chromosome are retarded or suffer a learning disability. Yet about 1/5 of the boys and 2/3 of the girls who inherit the chromosome appear entirely normal although they can act as carriers and may therefore have children or grandchildren with mental impairment. Recent estimates suggest that the abnormal chromosome, although not always the symptoms, may be found in about one in a thousand of the general population. If this figure is correct it means that this defect is second only to Down's Syndrome as a source of mental impairment and may also contribute to specific learning difficulties such as dyslexia and deviant behavior (Turner, Robinson, Lang, & Purvis-Smith, 1986).

In 1915, Davenport reported that an uncontrollable temper can run in families, involving several generations and affecting half the progeny in each generation. The writer has encountered several such pedigrees, involving two or three generations, sometimes in association with additional signs of minimal brain dysfunction. When violence "runs in the family," it is too often concluded that it is solely something that has been learned from parents, peers, and television. But this cannot be the whole explanation. Why is it that only some of the offspring of a violent household learn to be violent? And why are some individuals so extraordinarily resistant to powerful criminogenic forces such as criminal parents, poverty, broken homes, and racial discrimination (Mednick,

1977)? Conversely the generational transfer theory fails to explain the examples of habitual aggression that have no identifiable social origin.

The theory has been challenged by several observers, including Stacey and Shupe (1983) who found that in a sample of over 500 male spouse batterers 42% had *not* witnessed physical violence between their parents, 61% had *not* been physically abused in childhood, 59% had *not* been neglected by their parents, and 50% had *not* had an alcoholic father.

Eysenck & Eysenck (1978) vigorously criticized the emphasis placed by many sociologists on the environmental causes of antisocial behavior on the grounds that it is not sustained by modern biometric genetic analysis, and Reid's (1978) review of the literature on antisocial personalities supports the view that biological and social factors interact with each other to produce antisocial behavior—a conclusion also reached by Schulsinger (1977) and Mednick (1977).

Age and Aggression

The peak of physical violence in the home or in the street is in late adolescence and early adult life, after which it gradually declines in the sense that aggressive individuals usually become less so as they approach middle age. However, in the fifth decade or later pathological violence can occur for the first time in a formerly nonaggressive individual as a result of an organic brain insult, intoxication, or a functional psychosis. The link between youth and violence has been somewhat tenuously linked to testosterone levels in both males and females, but there are other factors to be considered. It is a matter of common observation that some people mature faster than others and that some individuals will not acquire the self-control, foresight, judgment, and social conscience that are commonly associated with the normal adult state until middle age. These functions are largely served by the frontal and temporal lobes, which are the last to mature in terms of myelination. Indeed, the process may not be complete until the third or fourth decade (Kaes, 1970; Yakovlev & Lecours, 1967); even the ascending reticular formation is not fully myelinated until the middle twenties. Thus far there is no information as to the rate of maturation in neurotransmitter systems, but there is evidence that the formation of new synaptic connections can continue in the human brain until advanced age. The persistence of the bilateral slow waves of childhood in the EEGs of adult aggressive psychopaths is consistent with the doctrine of physiological immaturity advanced by American and British authors 40 years ago.

Gender and Aggression

There are gender-determined differences between male and female brains in terms of speed of development, anatomy, cognitive skills, and behavior (Beach, 1976; Krieger & Hughes, 1980), and their effects on family violence are seen in several ways. Normal males, from cradle to grave, are more prone to physical violence than females. They are also more liable to physical conditions that often spell pathological aggression—the episodic dyscontrol syndrome, the attention deficit disorder, and the antisocial personality disorder.

The aggressiveness of the male is not solely a matter of learned behavior or cultural indoctrination, but is apparent from birth onward in goats, monkeys, dogs, and man, and seems to be the result of prenatal differentiation of the brain—the hypothalamic preoptic nucleus in particular—by androgens. If a pregnant monkey is given a large injection of testosterone a week before parturition, and the baby is female, the baby will have all the anatomical equipment of a female, but will usually behave like a male as regards aggressiveness and exploratory behavior, and later in life will be sexually unresponsive to males. This phenomenon is familiar to farmers: if a cow is carrying twins, one of each sex, the female offspring will look like a female but may behave like a male and will usually be sterile, thanks to the effects of testosterone from the male that reaches the female via the maternal circulation and puts the male imprint on her hypothalamus (Gorski, 1980). It seems that the brain is inherently female, its sexual differentiation depending on exposure to gonadal hormones at a critical period of prenatal development.

After birth, the hormonal endowment of both sexes plays a major role in their behavior (Beach, 1976; Moyer, 1976; Valzelli, 1981). The administration of testosterone increases aggression in both sexes, and castration reduces both sexual and irritable aggression in males. Higher levels of plasma testosterone have been found in violent women than in nonviolent women (Ehlers, Rickler, & Hovey, 1979). Androgen suppressors reduce sexual aggression in some males convicted of repeated offenses against children.

An important form of gender-related aggression is verbal abuse, which does much to fuel the fires of domestic strife (Gelles, 1972). In the writer's cases of domestic violence it was far more common in women than in men. Most women have a higher verbal IQ than most men, which may account for the fact that in English dictionaries there are ten terms for abusive women and none for men. People who have been exposed to it in childhood recall it with horror, and it often evokes physical retaliation, which sometimes results in homicide.

Another gender related contribution to domestic violence is the premenstrual tension syndrome characterized by depression, hostility, impatience and—especially in those with inadequate self-control—verbal and/or physical aggression. One study found that 62% of violent crimes committed by women occurred in the premenstrual week (Morton, Additon, Addison, Hunt, & Sullivan, 1953). This trend is confirmed by Dalton (1964). In France and Britain the syndrome has been accepted as an extenuation in violent crime. It is associated with a fall of progesterone level and a rise of prolactin (Valzelli, 1981). Many cases respond to the premenstrual administration of natural progesterone (Dalton, 1964). Unhappily, it was not available for Queen Victoria whose rages—which ceased during each of her nine pregnancies—terrified her Prime Minister and drove her husband into his study while royal fists pounded on the door (Duff. 1972).

THE ANATOMY OF AGGRESSION

Angry Aggression

Every human brain contains neurological and chemical systems for violent and destructive behavior, and for its control. We have inherited these systems, almost unchanged, from our reptilian and early mammalian ancestors, for which reason much of this equipment is situated in the phylogenetically ancient limbic system and brainstem (MacLean, 1973), which have extensive reciprocal connections with the prefrontal neocortex (Fuster, 1980; Nauta, 1972).

Aggression is not a unitary form of behavior, but appears in various forms depending on the objective: predatory, irritable, defensive, territorial, maternal-protective, inter-male, and instrumental (Moyer, 1976; Valselli, 1981). From clinical and neu-rophysiological points of view there are two main types in man: angry aggression and coldblooded violence. The latter is essentially predatory, in the etymological sense of the word. A subtype is compulsive violence.

The debate as to whether aggression is innate and instinctive, or a learned form of response is still unresolved (Wolfgang & Ferracuti, 1982). A formulation that best fits the facts is that the capacity for aggression is present in all of us, that most people learn to control it, and that this control can be reduced by biological factors that impair physiologi-cal inhibitory systems, and by psychosocial forces.

An early step toward understanding the physiology of rage was the demonstration by Goltz (1881) that in dogs decortication produced a restless animal which exhibited attacks of rage on minimal provocation. This was confirmed in other animals. Cannon (1926) and Bard (1928) showed that in cats this "sham rage" occurred when the posterior hypoth-alamus was separated from the forebrain. Much later it was found that in man, bilateral posterior hypothalmotomy prevented the rage attacks of the episodic dyscontrol syn-drome, and that relief could also be obtained by placing stereotaxic lesions bilaterally in other areas in the limbic system (Anterior cingulate gyrus and amygdala), and brainstem (thalamus and midbrain).

Additional light was thrown on the neural substrates of both predatory and angry aggression (which are not identical) and of related inhibitory systems by experimental procedures. For instance, in animals, attacks of rage can be terminated by electrical stimulation of points in the limbic system (e.g., septal region, amygdala, ventromedial hypothalamus), brainstem (head of caudate nucleus, thalamus), and midline cerebellar structures (Delgado, 1969; Moyer, 1976; Valzelli, 1981).

Clinical evidence helped to define the neurological substrate of aggression. It was noticed that episodic dyscontrol in formerly equable people sometimes followed head injury (Bowman, Blau, & Reich, 1974; Kaplan, 1899), and encephalitis (Wilson, 1940). It was also noticed as an early symptom of small localized tumors of the limbic system (Alpers, 1937; Bingley, 1958; Elliott, 1982; Luria, 1969; Malamud, 1967; Mark, Sweet, & Ervin, 1975; Smith, 1979), and of the brainstem (Barrett & Hyland, 1952; Cairns, 1950; Lassman & Arjona, 1967; Netzky & Strobos, 1952). Earlier reports of an associa-tion between deep midline lesions and aggressive behavior had prompted Papez (1937) to suggest that the limbic lobe is the neurological substrate of the emotions—a conclusion that outraged many who still believed the Cartesian doctrine that mind and brain are separate. However, it is now established that the brain contains identifiable interconnected assemblies of neurons, complete with specific neurotransmitters, which are the neu-rological substrate of angry aggression and are situated in phylogenetically ancient parts of the brain that are closely connected with the prefrontal neocortex.

Angry aggression does not occur without an exogenous or endogenous stimulus, and as we all know a given stimulus does not inevitably evoke rage. The response depends on the emotional or mental set and on many biological variables. Thus electrical stimulation of the hypothalamus or amygdala may cause rage in a caged monkey but not when the same animal receives the same stimulus (via radio signals) when running free out of doors (Delgado, 1969). It is difficult to produce anger by stimulation of the brain in man even in those who are liable to episodic rages, though it has been done (Delgado, 1967; Heath, Monroe, & Mickel, 1955; Mark & Ervin, 1970; Mark, Sweet, & Ervin, 1975; Smith,

1979). It is easier to evoke if the patient has been emotionally disturbed before the stimulation.

365

NEUROLOGICAL
FACTORS

The Anatomy of Predatory Aggression

In animals the form of violence we call predatory aggression can be triggered either by the presence of prey or by electrical stimulation of various points in the anterior and lateral hypothalamus, the preoptic nuclei, posterior thalamus, ventral midbrain tegmentum periaqueductal gray matter, and pons, and it can be suppressed by stimulation of the prefrontal cortex, ventromedial hypothalamus, and amygdala. In man the data are limited. Bilateral anterior cingulotomy has been effective in controlling persistent hostility and compulsive aggression, and stimulation of the antero-medial amygdala can elicit predatory assaultive behavior. Bilateral damage to the orbito-frontal area can produce features of psychopathic behavior—impulsiveness, lack of foresight, social irresponsibility, and either coldblooded aggression or explosive rage (Fuster, 1980; Luria, 1969).

The neurochemistry of all but the simplest forms of behavior is complicated, because so many neural circuits are involved. The pattern of neurotransmitters involved in irritable aggression differs from that in predatory attacks. The situation is further complicated by the activating effects of gonadal hormones on limbic circuits in the case of angry aggression and their reported lack of effect on predatory violence. At present too much remains unknown about the more than 40 neurotransmitters to permit a succinct or coherent account of this rapidly expanding field.

The Anatomy of Compulsive Violence

Charles Whitman of Austin, Texas, reported to a psychiatrist that he felt compelled to kill his wife, mother, and others. This he did in a carefully planned shooting spree. He was found to have a temporal lobe glioblastoma. He is not alone. Compulsive thoughts and aggressive behavior have been encountered in other cases of temporal tumor, as well as in temporal lobe epileptics and following head injury and encephalitis. They are not uncommon in minimal brain dysfunction. A severe obsessive-compulsive syndrome was a common sequel of encephalitis lethargica—apparently the result of brainstem damage; in one such case reported by Symonds (1975) the symptoms were abolished by bilateral frontal leucotomy. Lewin (1973) and others have also confirmed the therapeutic value of bilateral anterior cingulate ablation for severe obsessive-compulsive behavior. Flor-Henry (1983) accepted this as evidence that the frontal lobes are at fault, but on clinical grounds it appears that lesions in the temporal lobes and brainstem can also be responsible.

Compulsions to violence were described by 21 people examined by the writer on account of family aggression; there was evidence of neuropathology in 16: minimal brain dysfunction (7), head injury (3), encephalitis (1), multiple sclerosis (1), temporal lobe epilepsy (1), stroke (1), and bilateral fronto-temporal theta (2). In his classical description of primary obsessive-compulsive neurosis, Freud (1935) insisted that these individuals never carry out their violent impulses. Evidently this does not always apply to those whose inhibitory powers are impaired by organic brain defects, but it was noticed that they may attack surrogate victims instead of acting out their fantasies as in the example of an epileptic who felt driven to cut out his mother's eyes with a pair of scissors, but instead broke windows and beat up the family dog. A youth who had vivid "mind pictures" of killing his foster parents used to smash his glasses and break furniture; he had an unsuspected lucency in the left temporal lobe on CAT scan, and the left middle fossa was smaller than the right.

THE EPISODIC DYSCONTROL SYNDROME AND FAMILY VIOLENCE

Recurrent attacks of rage without adequate provocation and usually out of character are a common cause of physical and verbal abuse in the family. They were familiar to Benjamin Rush (1818) and to Falrêt (1960), and were admirably described by Kaplan (1899) in Germany as a sequel of head injury.

> Following the most trivial and impersonal causes, there is the effect of rage with its motor accompaniments. There may be the most grotesque gesticulation, excessive movement of the face and sharp explosiveness of speech. There may be cursing and outbreaks of violence which are often directed at things. There is an excessive reaction with inadequate adaptation to the situation that is so remote from a well considered and purposeful act that it approaches a pure psychic reflex. It may terminate in a convulsion.

Karl Meninger (Meninger & Maymen, 1956) drew attention to this form of dyscontrol in organic disorders, as did Hartocollis (1968), and the subject was further developed by Mark and Ervin (1970), Monroe (1970), Bach-Y-Rita, Lion, Climent, and Ervin (1971), Maletzky (1974), and Elliott (1976, 1982), who found that although somewhat similar episodes sometimes occur as an acting out of severe mental turmoil in both normal and mentally disturbed individuals, episodic dyscontrol is often associated with developmental or acquired biological defects. Frosch (1977) and Monroe (1970) have emphasized the differences between acting out and disorders of impulse control.

This account is based to a large extent on a study of 286 patients who were liable to recurrent attacks of rage. The following conditions were arbitrarily excluded from the study: overt and borderline psychotics, core psychopaths, the mentally retarded, individuals guilty of an isolated act of extreme violence, aggressive behavior solely triggered by the intake of drugs, and those who deliberately used aggressive behavior to manipulate situations.

The onset of dyscontrol attacks is often abrupt or may be preceded by a period of mounting dysphoria. Verbal abuse is marked by unwonted obscenity and profanity and accompanied by an apparent change of personality that greatly alarms children who are exposed to it. A cultivated Quaker lady of 60 interrupted a social occasion by starting to vilify her husband for no apparent reason. Her speech was garbled and her lips were flecked with foam as she glared at him. Finally, snarling with retracted lips, and growling like a dog, she left the room. Such attacks had occurred since a severe head injury at the age of 19, but they always happened at home and no doctor had ever witnessed one. Snarling, baring the teeth, and growling, often described by witnesses, also occurs in rabies (in which the main impact of the virus is on the hippocampus, cerebellum, and brain stem).

Physical violence often has a primitive quality—kicking, gouging, scratching, hitting, spitting, and biting. A wife is picked up bodily and thrown against the wall. Windows are broken, doors smashed, holes punched in walls. A young woman breaks her husband's arm. On the road a car is used as a weapon against pedestrians or other cars. The family cat is swung by its tail and its skull smashed against a wall. A man kills another by a single stab wound to the heart and then delivers 30 more stabs to the dead body. A young woman bites her 2-year-old daughter on the cheek, leaving a life-long scar. The attacks, whether verbal or physical, are usually followed by remorse, and suicide is not rare (Mark & Ervin, 1970).

Men who are violent at home are often guilty of violence elsewhere: fighting in bars, dangerously aggressive driving, and unnecessary altercations in public places (Bach-Y-Rita *et al.*, 1971; Mark & Ervin, 1970; Stacey & Shupe, 1983). In the writer's group, 40% of those who were violent at home were also pathologically aggressive in public.

The neurobiological correlates and causes of episodic dyscontrol can be divided into two groups: those that originate in early life and conditions arising in adolescence or later, causing rage attacks in a previously equable individual.

The first group consists of a heterogeneous collection of conditions: developmental and acquired, dating from infancy and mainly included under the rubric of minimal brain dysfunction (or the attention deficit disorder).

The most common neurological condition in the second group is severe head injury. Lagging far behind are encephalitis, postinfectious encephalopathy, stroke and subarachnoid hemorrhage, multiple sclerosis, Alzheimer's disease, tumor, Huntington's chorea, normal pressure hydrocephalus, and cerebral cysticercosis. Isolated incidents of rage can be caused by heat stroke and cerebral malaria. Metabolic conditions include Cushing's syndrome, hypoglycemia, and the common but controversial premenstrual tension syndrome.

The role of alcohol in intrafamilial psychodynamics is complex (Gelles, 1972; Steinmetz, 1978), but its pharmacological effects are established. It is a depressant, and Fenichel's description of it as a solvent of the ego is appropriate because its first action is to depress cortical inhibitory systems. This disinhibiting effect is particularly obvious in many of those with minimal brain dysfunction, antisocial personalities, and other organically determined disorders. However, its influence on behavior on any given occasion depends to some extent on the mental and emotional setting. People who are aggressive after drinking at home or in a bar may not be so affected when given the same dose in a laboratory experiment (Bach-Y-Rita, *et al.*, 1970; Maletsky, 1976; Marinacci, 1963). The same is true of hypoglycemia in man and electrical stimulation of limbic structures in monkeys (Delgado, 1969).

There can be no evasion of the issue; alcohol's dire contribution to family violence is evident in all social strata, whether in the form of Saturday night brawls in lower-class neighborhoods (Steinmetz, 1978), or the better camouflaged excesses of the privileged. Some drugs aggravate violence but they did not figure prominently in the writer's cases. Many subjects insisted that marijuana had a pacifying effect. One man attacked and killed a stranger 3 hours after taking PCP. Several stated, and relatives confirmed, that valium and phenothiazines aggravated the violence of organically determined dyscontrol.

MINIMAL BRAIN DYSFUNCTION (MBD) AND ATTENTION DEFICIT DISORDER

These names have been given to a hodgepodge of disorders that are heterogeneous as to symptomatology, suspected etiology, and neuropathology, and are found in children but can persist in modified form into adult life. The behavioral disorders that occur in many, but not all, hyperactive boys were first described in 1845 by Hoffmann, a German physician, in cautionary tales for children entitled "Der Struwelpeter" (Cantwell, 1975). The subject has been and still is controversial, but there is no doubt that the gallimaufry of symptoms so well described by Clements and Peters (1962), Anderson (1972), Wender (1971), Millichap (1975), and others are a common antecedent of psychopathology and social deviance in childhood, adolescence, and adult life. It is far more common in boys than in girls, and is characterized by attention deficits, hyperactivity (less often apathy), and impulsivity, associated in some cases with learning defects and "soft" neurological signs, which appear in a wide spectrum of combinations, short of mental retardation and cerebral palsy. Most of these people look and sound normal when casually encountered. MBD is estimated to involve about 3% of American children, according to DSM-III. Wender (1971) and others consider this figure to be too conservative.

The syndrome has been found to be unduly prevalent in patients with episodic dyscontrol (Bach-Y-Rita *et al.*, 1971; Elliott, 1982; Hartocollis, 1969; Mark & Ervin, 1970; Wood *et al.*, 1976), borderline syndromes (Andrulonis, 1980), atypical schizophrenia (Bellak, 1979), adult sociopathy, juvenile delinquency and adult criminality (Anderson, 1972; Berman, 1979; Cloninger *et al.*, 1978; Detre, Kupfer, & Taub, 1975; Guze, 1976; Lewis *et al.*, 1979; Milman, 1979; Monroe, 1970; Rockford *et al.*, 1970; Satterfield *et al.*, 1982). Residual MBD is also found in some adults who, despite average or even superior intelligence, somehow fail to live up to reasonable expectations and drift into idleness, frequent changes of job or spouse, dependence on family and Welfare, and substance abuse (Wood, Reimer, Wender, & Johnson, 1976). Some are parasitic and conspicuously defective in will power, and fall into Schneider's (1950) class of abulic psychopaths whose social importance lies in their capacity for petty larceny and fraud rather than criminal violence. They are thus a source of tension and frustration to other members of the family and can precipitate violent retaliation.

There is no information as to the prevalence of MBD among batterers and abusers in general. The writer identified it in 40% of 273 cases of episodic dyscontrol within the family. This figure, based on an expanded form of neurological examination (Critchley, 1969), reinforced by EEG, CAT scan, and neuropsychological tests, may be misleading because of referral bias and demographic factors. The majority were middle- or upper-class private patients, 95% were caucasian, males exceeded females by more than 3 to 1, and only 10 were prisoners. In addition, allowance must be made for the fact that specialized clinics attract many atypical cases.

Some of the many neurological manifestations of MBD in adults have been described elsewhere (Elliott, 1982). The symptoms, as described in DSM-III, apply primarily to children. Some outgrow them, and others manage to circumvent them as adults, though residua remain. These residua are often disregarded by physicians and patients alike. The former tend to discount the relevance of the signs to the behavioral disturbances, and the latter seldom volunteer information about their handicaps, which they have had all their lives and do not consider a matter for medical concern. Others suppress information about embarrassing defects (such as inability to knot a tie, catch a ball, ride a bicycle, spell, read with normal facility, distinguish right from left, dance or keep step to music, follow a map, jump rope, or do simple arithmetic). Many have a poor self-image, and some camouflage it with a macho veneer. Both patient and parents often fail to report antisocial behavior in childhood (Graham & Rutter, 1968), or use euphemisms to disguise it.

The cardinal symptoms are attention defects, impulsivity, and hyperactivity (less often, apathy), with or without additional neurological and neuropsychological signs—cognitive defects (notably specific learning problems such as dyslexia, dyscalculia, inability to spell, and a wide spectrum of dyspraxias), perceptual disorders, minor disturbances of speech and special senses, apraxias, clumsiness and other motor disorders short of cerebral palsy, and unreliability of sphincters.

Recent research, reviewed by Douglas (1983), shows that attentional difficulties represent only one of a group of related deficits that can have adverse effects on cognitive functions and behavior: including disinhibition of impulse response, ineffective modulation of arousal levels appropriate to the situation, excessive need for instant gratification, and absence of "reflective delay" (Monroe, 1970) before responding to external or internal stimuli. These symptoms, it will be noted, appear not only in hyperactive children but also in many adult psychopaths and in cases of bifrontal damage.

The apraxias and agnosias have been given scant notice in the literature on MBD, despite the pioneer work of Critchley (1964) and Gubbay (1975) and despite their diagnostic value in pointing to involvement of the associational neocortex (frontal, posterior parietal, and temporal). But like many other symptoms and signs, they will often escape notice unless the correct questions are asked because they are not identified by conventional neurological examination. Two examples follow.

Case 1. An Army Officer whose three wives had left because of his violence toward them during attacks of rage, and whose career was in jeopardy on account of explosive behavior, had failed to benefit from psychotherapy. Sketchy neuropsychiatric reports stated that he was neurologically normal, but closer examination revealed dyscalculia, left-right disorientation, difficulty in map reading, normal capacity for drawing in two dimensions but not in three, inability to use a golf club despite much practice, and failure to swing himself along the horizontal ladder in boot camp training exercises despite good athletic powers in other directions.

Case 2. A middle-aged women of superior intelligence who had been subject to episodic dyscontrol since childhood reported similar attacks in half the siblings in two generations and in one of her two sons. She was hyperactive, impulsive, impatient, socially imperceptive, and devoid of any sense of fear. Her verbal IQ was high, her mathematics below normal. She could not catch or hit a ball, yet her manual dexterity for mechanical work was exceptional. When dancing solo, her hands balled into fists with the thumbs flexed into the palm (a "frontal" sign). Sudden loud high-pitched sounds produced an exaggerated startle reaction, sometimes followed by rage.

Neuropathology

The scatter of neurological and neuropsychological defects implies multifocal pathology, but opportunities for histological studies in well-documented cases are rare indeed. Recent case reports (Galaburda & Kemper, 1979; Galaburda & Eidelberg, 1982) invalidate the common assumption that if the brain looks normal to the naked eye and under low power microscopic examination of random sections, it is normal. Far from it. A case of familial dyslexia, associated with clumsiness, difficulty in spelling, math, right-left discrimination, finger-agnosia, and occasional seizures revealed its secrets (patches of developmental dysplasia in the neocortex, limbic cortex, and thalami) only after stained whole brain slices (35μ) of the entire organ were examined under high power (Galaburda & Kemper, 1979). It is likely that new scanning methods will be able to identify multiple small lesions during life, but until then the neuropathology of individual cases will often remain conjectural.

Patches of developmental dysplasia and vascular anomolies have also been reported in epileptics (notably in temporal lobe cases) by Falconer, Serafetinides, and Corsellis (1969), Taylor, Falconer, Bruton, and Corsellis (1971), and Mathieson (1975). Multiple lesions are a feature of perinatal hypoxia (Millichap, 1975; Pasamanick & Knoblock, 1966; Towbin, 1971). The lesions of head trauma, encephalitis, and postfebrile encephalopathy are also multiple. But in many cases of MBD there is no conclusive evidence of structural brain damage other than the defects disclosed by neuropsychological tests.

Evidence has also been put forward that catecholaminergic mechanisms are involved in the hyperactivity syndrome (Rutter, 1983; Wender, 1971), and it appears likely that the syndrome may prove to have several causes.

TEMPORAL LOBE EPILEPSY AND AGGRESSION

The majority of epileptics do not develop significant personality disorders and are not especially prone to violent crime (Stevens, 1975). The prevalence of pathological aggressiveness in temporal lobe epileptics varies with the source of the material, being highest in those admitted to neurosurgical clinics that handle intractable cases. Rodin (1973) reported it in 6.8% of 700 cases from The Michigan Epilepsy Centre, and Curry, Heathfield, Henson, and Scott (1971) found it in 7% of 666 cases of temporal lobe epilepsy at a large London hospital. Elliott (1982) found a history of temporal lobe attacks in 30% of 286 cases of episodic dyscontrol, and Gastaut, Morin, and Leserve (1955) recorded paroxysmal violence in 50% of a large number of temporal lobe epileptics. Lewis, Pincus, Shamok, and Glaser (1982) reported psychomotor epilepsy in 18 out of 97 incarcerated boy delinquents.

When we look at people who are subject to episodic rage, the prevalence of temporal lobe epilepsy is greater than in the general population (Bach-Y-Rita *et al.*, 1971; Elliott, 1982; Lewis *et al.*, 1979; Mark & Ervin, 1970). Generally speaking, the seizures are infrequent, and are seldom convulsive. In addition, some patients report aggressive episodes with amnesia that cannot be proved epileptic on clinical grounds or the evidence of a scalp-EEG. Without depth electrodes it is unwise to be dogmatic about the nature of these ambiguous attacks, because abnormal behavior can be associated with seizure discharges from deep structures that are not recorded by scalp electrodes (Monroe, 1970; Wieser, Hailermariam, Regard, & Landis, 1985). Mark and Ervin (1970) reported the case of a 14-year-old girl who suffocated two of her small charges during attacks of rage, one of which was triggered by the baby's crying. Depth electrodes disclosed epileptic discharges in the temporal lobes that could be induced by the sound of a baby crying; the scalp EEG was normal.

Temporal lobe attacks can be so slight and so strange that they are not easily recognized as epileptic. This is especially likely if other mental symptoms are present. It is not enough to ask the patient about seizures or convulsions or attacks of unconsciousness because these symptoms are often absent, and the answer will often be in the negative. History taking demands a meticulous search for more subtle types of attack (Daly, 1975; Dreifuss, 1975), which may provide the only supplemental evidence of organic damage in cases of episodic dyscontrol and minimal brain dysfunction.

Episodic violence associated with epilepsy appears in four forms. The most common consists of interictal attacks of anything from irritability to destructive rages directed at people, animals, or things. Secondly, there are ictal rages that are probably rare; indeed, some epileptologists deny that they exist, but there are a few well-documented cases in which rage has coincided with a sudden seizure discharge recorded by deep electrodes (Mark & Ervin, 1970; Mark *et al.*, 1975; Smith, 1979). In such cases the violence is usually undirected and disorganized and is followed by complete amnesis. Thirdly, an attack of rage sometimes ends in a convulsion, as pointed out by Rush (1812) and Kaplan (1899). A 33-year-old woman who had occasional temporal lobe seizures preceded by chromatopsia, and frequent attacks of interictal rage over minor irritations in which she abused her children physically and verbally, was trying to open an aspirin bottle when the cap stuck. Instantly, the walls of the room "went red" and she heard herself screaming with rage. She then lost consciousness and was found having a convulsion. A seizure focus was found in the right temporal lobe. Both the rages and her occasional seizures were controlled by phenytoin. Fourth, violence can occur in postictal confusion if the patient is physically restrained.

Temporal lobe seizures come in many forms, and the form may change from time to time in the same patient, but they are usually characterized by a brief change in the quality and/or content of consciousness, sometimes accompanied by inappropriate behavior (Blumer, 1981; Daly, 1975). Disturbances of consciousness include moments of confusion, dreamy states, absence, double consciousness, or a sense of unreality, all of which can occur as split-second experiences in apparently normal people, unlike the ictal type that last at least several seconds. The patient may also experience forced thoughts or a persistent musical theme that cannot be remembered afterwards, or the attack may consist of visuo-auditory memories of something that has actually occurred in the past, or an olfactory experience. Perceptual aberrations include slowing or acceleration of ambient sounds such as the noise of traffic, and a sense of familiarity or unfamiliarity, a sense of floating or apparent alterations in the shape of objects, micropsia or macropsia, colored vision, and mistaken identification of faces.

Hallucinations are not infrequent. They may be formed or unformed and can be olfactory, gustatory, visual, auditory, or multimodal. The epileptic, unlike the psychotic, is usually able to describe his hallucinations with objectivity rather than with passion or fear (Rodin, 1973). ("I saw colored streamers coming down from the ceiling and I felt like I could reach out my hands and plait them together.") Disturbances of affect include a sudden sense of fear, or depression, or pleasure, or hatred, or anxiety, or occasionally anger. An exquisite sense of ecstasy was experienced by Dostoievski before his convulsions; onlookers commented that his face was transfigured with joy on these occasions (Blumer, 1981). Episodes of fear may occur by themselves or be accompanied by visual hallucinations, as in a young woman who saw a shadowy figure coming toward her holding a carving knife.

There are many forms of automatism including smacking of the lips, swallowing movements, repetitive water drinking, spitting, attacks of causeless laughter, or eating, cursive (running) attacks, disrobing in public, and gestures such as patting the top of the head, dusting off a sleeve, or repeatedly touching the face, which resemble mannerisms.

Interictal schizoid symptoms or antisocial behavior, including minor delinquency, may distract attention from occasional atypical temporal lobe seizures (Bear, Freeman, & Greenberg, 1981; Daly, 1975; Ferguson & Rayport, 1984; Glaser, 1964; Lewis *et al.*, 1979; Slater, Beard, & Glithero, 1963). But generally speaking these patients are not lacking in insight or affect and can often be made to laugh at themselves. Recurrent brief depressions may occur and there may be long-term intense introspection during which a patient is apt to write lengthy accounts of his feelings and religious experiences. Compulsions and phobias are encountered in temporal lobe epilepsy and progressive temporal lobe lesions. A case cited by Lishman (1978) is that of a temporal lobe epileptic who, following a nocturnal battering by her husband, became liable to intermittent phobias for men and for the dark which lasted about 10 days following each temporal seizure. A resting EEG showed rightsided fronto-temporal theta and delta waves as long as the phobias persisted.

Temporal lobe epilepsy and the behavioral disorders that spring from temporal pathology are great deceivers, mimicking a wide range of psychopathology and generating much controversy (Bear *et al.*, 1981; Ferguson & Rayport, 1984; Glaser, 1969; Heath *et al.*, 1955; Monroe, 1978; Slater *et al.*, 1963; Stevens, 1975; Williams, 1969). From the practical point of view, attention to the identification of temporal lobe pathology in violent people, including those who are responsible for intrafamily aggression, pays dividends because some respond favorably to adequate antiseizure medication even when the presence of epilepsy is suspected rather than proven.

HEAD INJURY

Over the past 40 years there has been a large increase not only in the incidence of head trauma but also in the number of severely injured people who survive because of improved methods of resuscitation. The latter applies also to neonates and children. The result is an increasing number of mentally and emotionally disabled people, many of whom are permanently crippled. They exhibit a wide spectrum of cognitive, perceptual, emotional, and behavioral symptoms, ranging from the irritability of the post concussional syndrome to the organic brain syndrome and antisocial behavior marked by either callous brutality or episodic rages (Bowman *et al.*, 1974; Roberts, 1979; Symonds, 1974). The change of personality that occurs in about 10% of serious injuries can have disastrous results (Roberts, 1979), and often does more to disrupt family peace than the cognitive defects that are also present in most cases. Posttraumatic episodic dyscontrol was responsible for violent attacks within the family in 17% of the writer's cases.

The physical sequelae of brain injury are often compounded by functional reactions, for as Symonds (1974) wrote, "Following a serious head injury the individual becomes less of a man and more of a child." The resulting neurotic patterns may obscure the underlying brain damage, and only too often family and friends feel that the victim could do better "if he wanted to." Needless to say, such attitudes do little to reduce domestic tension.

The more severe effects commonly follow injuries that have caused unconsciousness or amnesia for about a week, but repeated smaller head traumata—which are not rare in violent households—can also have serious cumulative effects. Even a single blow that stuns momentarily can cause multiple microscopic lesions in the brainstem, hypothalamus, and cerebral hemispheres. Whiplash injuries caused by the violent shaking of an infant by an angry parent or baby sitter can damage the brain without leaving external marks, a known cause of death and a possibility to be remembered in cases of unexplained unconsciousness followed by evidence of brain damage. It is prudent to appoint emotionally stable baby sitters. A case: following a modest head injury a young man developed episodic dyscontrol, especially after drinking, during which he battered his wife, who left him. While baby sitting for a girl aged 4, he started drinking. Hours later the child was found neatly tucked up in her cot. She had been sexually assaulted and fatally beaten. He had complete amnesia for the event.

The postconcussional syndrome—headaches, irritability, fatigability, dizziness, poor concentration, sensitivity to noise—can evoke anger if it is mistaken for moral turpitude, neurosis, or unwillingness to work. Another troublesome result of severe head trauma is posttraumatic epilepsy, which can appear as convulsions, focal seizures, or temporal lobe attacks, sometimes associated with interictal rages.

Among women the most common metabolic contributor to intrafamilial violence may be the premenstrual tension syndrome, if it is true that some 20% of women experience it in some degree during their reproductive years. However, hypoglycemia is the best documented. Wilder (1947) assembled an impressive bibliography on the subject. He stresses its importance as a cause of violent crime, including child abuse and other forms of family violence. In 1943 Hill and Sargant drove the point home with a widely publicized case of matricide triggered by hypoglycemia in an emotionally immature man who had suffered mild brain damage at birth. The authors were able to demonstrate a temporal relationship between a sharp fall of blood sugar, paroxysmal abnormalities in the EEG, and temporary mental disturbance. Green (1963) found that in nine individuals with focal cerebral lesions, a fall of blood sugar level induced by tolbutamide evoked focal slowing in the EEG.

A personal case: a respected citizen who was diabetic and had also developed occasional temporal lobe seizures in middle life took an evening dose of insulin but omitted to dine because he had an engagement. While parking his car he got into an altercation with a policeman, whom he assaulted. He then drove around the parking lot in a wild and pointless manner and attempted to run down another policeman, who promptly shot him in the arm and so brought the chase to an end. When apprehended he was belligerent and confused, and his blood sugar was found to be below 40 mgms.%. The confusion was abolished immediately by intravenous glucose; he had no recollection of anything he had done since leaving home.

Intermittent hypoglycemia is caused by a number of situations: prediabetes, diabetes, and hyperinsulinism in its various forms. Pancreatic insulinomas are notorious for producing intermittent psychiatric symptoms, especially attacks of rage with minimal provocation, for months or even years before they are recognized. The tumor is unsuspected in the early stages because usually there is no clearcut relationship between food intake, or the lack of it, and the hypoglycemic incident. The diagnosis therefore depends less on the history than on rigorous laboratory studies of the response of blood glucose to fasting and other provocations, and on blood insulin assays. It cannot be accurately diagnosed by a routine 3-hour glucose tolerance test (Lishman, 1978; Marks, 1974).

The extent to which hormones contribute to sexual dyscontrol is not fully established. Increases of testosterone levels influence aggression and sexual drives, and on the other hand, sexual difficulties resulting from impotence can prompt violent domestic outbursts (Straus, Gelles, & Steinmetz, 1980). Stacey and Shupe (1983) found that one in four battered women reported sexual abuse by husband or boy friend: the term included rape, perverse acts under the threat of physical punishment, and sexual mutilation. Walker (1979) described the diverse and perverse sexual practices of batterers, including bestiality—regression to primitive behavior that can also occur as a result of lesions in the brainstem, hypothalamus, and orbito-frontal areas. Damage to the temporal lobes usually decreases libido, as does temporal lobe epilepsy, but startling exceptions do occur, as in the case of a distinguished public figure whose unwonted sexual disinhibition was the first symptom of a mid-temporal glioma.

The Neurological Status of the Antisocial Personality Disorder

The antisocial personality disorder, as defined in DSM-III, has much in common with what the German literature calls the psychopathic personality (Schneider, 1950) and with Reich's impulsive character (Reich, 1925; Wishnie, 1977), and is consistent with

Harvey Cleckley's "mask of sanity" (1983) and Henderson's account of psychopathic behaviors (1939).

Considering its prevalence (3% of males, less than 1% of females) and its deserved noteriety as a troublemaker not only in the family but also in society at large, it is remarkable how seldom it is mentioned as a factor in domestic violence. This may be due in part to the fact that most individuals with this syndrome look and sound so normal that there is nothing to indicate what lies underneath the mask. Even colleagues and friends are misled. As Erich Fromm once remarked, they do not bear the mark of Cain on their foreheads. Only the family—and the police—know what they are really like.

Studies of behavioral changes following localized brain damage show that impulsiveness, and lack of a normal capacity for reflective delay (Monroe, 1970) are associated, as a rule, with prefrontal lesions. Indeed, a list of the behavioral results of bilateral prefrontal lesions in man strongly resembles the outstanding psychopathological features of the classical psychopath. These features include impulsivity, apathy or aggressiveness, egocentricity, incapacity for natural affection, absence of conscience, lack of insight, impaired foresight, inability to learn from experience, poor judgment, untruthfulness, absence of normal sense of fear, and a poor tolerance for alcohol.

For many years it has been taught that the core psychopath is usually somebody whose social and emotional development has been retarded because of extreme psychosocial adversity in infancy and childhood. This is consistent with the fact that aside from genetics and growth hormones, the postnatal development and maturation of the brain is largely dependent on appropriate external stimulation. As Longworthy pointed out in the 1930s, if one eye of a kitten is kept occluded for some weeks after birth, myelination ceases in the optic nerve and optic tract on that side, and sight does not develop. If an infant's leg is amputated, the pyramidal system destined for the limb does not mature. A large body of experimental work has confirmed that the full functional development of neural circuits depend on appropriate postnatal sensory, motor, and mental stimulation (Riesen, 1975). Also, Harlow and Mears (1979) demonstrated that if baby monkeys are separated from parents, surrogate mothers, and peers, their social and emotional development suffers, sometimes permanently. It has been found that in dogs, monkeys, and rats such isolation produces electrophysiological, histological, and biochemical alterations that are not present in control litter mates. Conversely, in rats, an enriched environment enhances histological and chemical development (Goldman & Lewis, 1978). These are instructive examples of the effects of environment on ontogeny.

The fact that many core psychopaths become significantly less antisocial in middle life supports the notion that emotional adversity in early life retards the maturation of the neurological substrate upon which social and emotional responses depend. The theory of a maturational lag is further supported by the fact that abnormalities in the EEG of the aggressive psychopath become progressively less common in middle life (Kiloh, McComas, & Osselton, 1972).

There are additional indications that physical disorders also contribute to the antisocial personality: (a) in a study of 280 criminals, Thompson (1953) found an excessive amount of specific learning defects associated with psychopathic personality traits and reported that only 6.4% of them were neurologically normal against 71.4% in a control series. One of his conclusions was that the psychopathic personality develops on a biosocial basis of psychological adversity working on a previously damaged brain. Persuasive evidence of the role of organicity in the antisocial behavior of criminal populations is also seen in (b) the results of neuropsychological tests (Monroe, 1978; Yeudall &

Fromm-Auch, 1979); (c) persistence into adult life of bilateral slow rhythms in the EEG, which are normal in children (Kiloh, McComas, & Ossleton, 1972); (d) the BEAM technique (brain electrical activity mapping) has disclosed abnormalities in the electrical activity of the frontal lobes of adolescent psychopaths; (e) psychopaths are resistant to the production of conditioned reflexes; in particular, they resist aversive conditioning, which helps to explain their failure to learn from painful experiences (Hare & Schalling, 1978); (f) their failure to respond to punishment, reward, rehabilitation, medication, and short-term psychotherapy is what is to be expected of an organic defect of the brain; (g) the improvement that many exhibit in middle life is consistent with the fact that some parts of the brain, notably the associational neocortex, continue to mature, as regards myelination, until middle age (Kaes, 1907; Yakovlev & Lecours, 1967); and finally, (h) evidence of genetic influence is provided by twin and adoption studies, the prevalence of psychopathy hysteria and psychosis in the family history of many psychopaths, and the prevalence of abnormal EEG's in their first-degree relatives (Cloninger *et al.*, 1978; Guze, 1976; Hare & Schalling, 1978; Mednick, 1977; Reid, 1978; Schulsinger, 1977).

It seems that both biological and environmental variables contribute to the antisocial personality, and that Benjamin Rush was right when, in an address to the American Philosophical Society (1786), he ventured to suggest that in these unfortunates, "there is probably an original defect of organization in those parts of the body which are occupied by the moral faculties of the mind."

BIOSOCIAL ROOTS OF DOMESTIC VIOLENCE

Although it is true that neurobiological disorders contribute to some episodes of family strife, it is obvious that they cannot be responsible for the current worldwide escalation of personal and collective violence, or for similar epidemics in the past that have occurred during times of great social, political, and philosophical change (Elliott, 1983; Kennan, 1954). As Tuchman (1978) has pointed out, in these periods increased aggressiveness has usually been accompanied by other evidence of regression—a growth of egocentricity at the expense of altruism, erosion of personal integrity at all levels of society, a drying-up of compassion, widespread dehumanization, unbridled material greed, a descent of sexual mores to animal levels, a lust for cruelty and sexual perversion in entertainment and art, recourse to superstition, and a revival of torture as an instrument of government policy and personal gratification.

Nor can neurobiological abnormalities by themselves fully explain the subculture of violence (Wolfgang & Ferracuti, 1982) that exists on a smaller scale in the lower social strata of many cities and is found in small pockets of population "characterized by residential propinquity and a shared commitment to the use of physical aggression as a mode of personal interaction and a device for settling problems." In these pockets there is much spouse battery and child abuse, many street gangs, and frequent brawls. Substance abuse is common, with alcohol in the lead as a promoter of violence. A member of a subculture in England is quoted by Parker and Allerton (1962) as saying:

> Violence is in a way like bad language, that a person like me has been brought up with, something I got used to very early in life as part of the daily scene of childhood as you might say. I don't at all recoil from the idea. . . . As long as I can remember I have seen violence in use all around me—my mother hitting the children, my brothers and sisters all whacking their mother or other children, the man downstairs beating his wife and so on.

A young woman from a New York slum said during a television interview, "And if I have kids I'll teach them to use a knife and a gun, and to be sure to hit first." Emil Durkheim (1897), who coined the word *anomie* for this state of lawlessness, attributed it to a sense of helplessness and inability to reach desired goals by legitimate means; under such conditions many feel lost, powerless, and frustrated and exhibit behavior that is deviant and out of character. George Kennan (1954) made similar observations:

> Whenever the autority of the past is too suddenly and too drastically undermined . . . Then the foundations of men's inner health and stability begin to crumble, insecurity and panic begin to take over, and behavior becomes erratic and aggressive.

This, too, is the message of Golding's *Lord of the Flies*.

The validity of Kennan's diagnosis is sustained by the relative immunity from violence in many small communities—secular and religious—that have maintained their rules of behavior; examples that spring to mind are the Society of Friends, Catholic Orders, Orthodox Jews, and Christian Fundamentalists such as the Plymouth Brethren. At a national level in recent years the Japanese have maintained extraordinarily low rates of domestic and street violence, thanks to child rearing practices and consistent opposition to the use of physical violence in the home, at school, and at work (Goldstein & Ibraki, 1983), and this despite their ferocity in war and their current devotion to violence in books, television, and movies (Halloran, Schodt, & Bailey, 1985). Similarly, physical (but not verbal) aggression is still taboo in most Chinese homes, thanks to the teachings of Confucius, which are reported to have survived as a constructive force in modern China (Bond & Wang Sung-Hsing, 1983) despite the excesses of the Cultural Revolution.

A neurophysiological basis for the value of consistency in training was supplied by Pavlov, who found that the behavior of dogs that have been conditioned by a system of rewards and penalties to respond to certain stimuli, such as a bell or an electric shock delivered at regular intervals, was grossly disturbed by any sudden change in the conditions of the experiment, as for instance by altering the intervals between signal and reward or by giving positive and negative signals in a confusing sequence or by sudden changes in the strength of the signal. The result was confusion, erratic behavior, irritability and eventually, apathy and indifference. Pavlov was confirming in the laboratory what animal trainers and children's nurses have known for a long time: the need for consistency and discipline in establishing acceptable and appropriate social responses. He and his colleagues also found that it was difficult and sometimes impossible to establish conditioned reflexes in dogs with unstable termperaments. In man the same is true of psychopaths, hysterics, and some brain-damaged individuals (Luria, 1969).

Many observers have emphasized the biosocial origins of antisocial behavior and of criminal violence in particular (Cloninger *et al.*, 1978; Detre *et al.*, 1975; Mednick, 1977), and the same type of interaction is seen in the batterers/abusers who have evaded legal notice. Some biological defects, whether developmental or acquired, increase vulnerability to antisocial influences (as in Schneider's abulics—psychopathic personalities whose inability to resist such influences leads them into criminal activities and substance abuse). It is possible that this vulnerability might be uncovered in many apparently normal people during times of anomie, when the rules of behavior are weakened.

PRESENT DUTIES AND FUTURE TASKS

Over the past 30 years evidence has accumulated that developmental and acquired neurological defects are far more common in violently aggressive individuals than in the population at large, but there has been no systematic examination of the neurological status of batterer/abusers *per se*. The need for such an investigation of a representative sample is suggested by the unexpected discovery of neurological and neuropsychological impairments, other than psychosis, in 94% of 286 cases of episodic dyscontrol, of whom 169 had confined their attacks to family members, and an additional 109 had been aggressive to family and others. The amount of neuropathology found was partly due to biased referrals—special clinics attract special cases—and partly to the use of the CAT scan and an expanded type of clinical examination designed to uncover subtle defects in cortical functions that tend to be missed by conventional examination; this applies especially to the signs of minimal brain dysfunction and the easily misunderstood symptoms of temporal lobe epilepsy. The clinical sieve must have a very fine mesh if it is to be effective in this context, as others have pointed out (Bach-Y-Rita, *et al.,* 1971; Mark & Ervin, 1970), and should be reinforced by an extended EEG examination, neuropsychological tests of the Halstead-Reitan genre, and metabolic studies when indicated. It is anticipated that the new metabolic scans will help to simplify what is now an expensive and time-consuming process, which many of these patients are reluctant to undergo.

There have been no rebuttals of the many reports of an undue prevalence of biological defects in habitually violent people, but doubts have been expressed as to their relevance to abnormal behavior except in those cases where violent aggression occurs for the first time in a previously equable person following a brain insult, as was the case in 102 of the writer's batterer/abusers. Reservations have also been voiced as to the practical usefulness of going to considerable trouble to establish the presence or absence of abnormalities that are usually ineradicable. The answer is that most of these patients are going to require pharmacological help, the nature of which will depend on a precise and comprehensive diagnosis. There is no universal pill for violence. Medications include those for episodic dyscontrol, hyperactivity, interictal rages, psychotic hostility, sexual dyscontrol, premenstrual aggression, the bipolar affective disorder, different forms of hypoglycemia, and compulsive violence (Carney, 1976; Elliott, 1984; Lion, 1972; Madden & Lion, 1976; Millichap, 1975; Monroe, 1970; Wender, 1971).

What is so discouraging about many batterers and abusers is that despite the availability of symptomatic therapies for some cases, at no time in their destructive careers have their neuropsychological handicaps been recognized. Nor, if recognized, have they been treated. The same point has been made by Mark and Ervin (1970), Berman (1979) and others.

Treatment almost always requires environmental/social interventions aimed at an avoidance of provocation and—so far as possible—modification of circumstances to fit the patients' temperamental and intellectual limitations (Chess & Thomas, 1984). This is central to effective management, and for this reason it is the psychiatrist and psychologist who must steer the ship. Few neurologists have the inclination or training to deal with behavioral deviance, but they can assist with the pharmacological conundrums that are apt to arise in these cases.

Selective psychosurgery is useful for incorrigibly violent patients who do not respond to medication. It has been used successfully in the United States and abroad. But, despite the conditional approval of a National Commission for the protection of human subjects of biomedical and behavioral research (1976), most neurosurgeons in this country see no option but to avoid the risks of catastrophic litigation in case of nonsuccess.

Prophylaxis

Once the habit of aggression is established, it is difficult to overcome, so there is a premium on prophylaxis in early life when the tantrums and other warning signs of developmental problems start to surface, whether they be due to environmental adversity, biological defects, or both. The 17th-century poet Alexander Pope wrote, "As the twig is bent, so the tree's inclined," and it is the task of developmental neuropsychiatry to evolve and apply timely interventions across a wide spectrum of neurological and psychosocial dilemmas (Rutter, 1980, 1983). There is ample evidence that antisocial behavior in children and adolescents can often be modified by appropriate treatment; examples are the improvements of social adjustment effected in ADD children by multimodal therapy programs such as that evolved by Satterfield, Satterfield, and Cantwell (1981), and the successes obtained by less formal efforts on the part of countless therapists, parents, and teachers to encourage the maturation and socialization of potential batterer/abusers.

REFERENCES

Alpers, B. J. (1937). Relation of the hypothalamus to disorders of personality. Report of a case. *Journal of Neurology and Psychiatry, 38,* 29–33.

Anderson, C. (1972). *Society pays: The high cost of minimal brain dysfunction in America.* New York: Walker.

Andrulonis, P. A. & Glueck, B. C. (1980). Organic dysfunction and the borderline syndrome. *Psychiatric Clinics of North America, 4,* 47–66.

Bach-Y-Rita, G., Lion, S., & Ervin, F. (1970). Pathological intoxication: Clinical and EEG studies. *American Journal of Psychiatry, 125,* 698–703.

Bach-Y-Rita, G., Lion, J. R., Climent, C. F., & Ervin, F. R. (1971). Episodic dyscontrol: A study of 130 violent patients. *American Journal of Psychiatry, 127,* 1473–1478.

Bard, P. (1928). Diencephalic mechanism for the expression of rage with special reference to the sympathetic nervous system. *American Journal of Physiology, 89,* 490–515.

Barrett, H. J., & Hyland, H. H. (1952). Tumors involving the brainstem. *Quarterly Journal of Medicine, 21,* 265–289.

Beach, F. A. (1976). *Human sexuality in four perspectives.* Baltimore, MD: Johns Hopkins University Press.

Bear, D., Freeman, R., & Greenberg, M. (1981). Behavioral alterations in patients with temporal lobe epilepsy. In D. Blumer (Ed.), *Psychiatric aspects of epilepsy* (pp. 197–228). Washington, DC: American Psychiatric Press.

Bellak, L. (1979). *Psychiatric aspects of minimal brain dysfunction in adults.* New York: Grune & Stratton.

Berman, A. (1979). *Minimal brain dysfunction: Factors leading to breakdown in adulthood. A developmental approach* (125–132). In E. Denhoff & L. Stern (Eds). New York: Masson.

Bingley, T. (1958). Mental symptoms in temporal lobe epilepsy and temporal lobe glioma. *Acta Psychiatrica Neurolica Scandinavia, 33,* 1–151.

Blumer, D. (1981). *Psychiatric aspects of epilepsy.* Washington, DC: American Psychiatric Press.

Bond, M. H., & Wang Sung-Hsing (1983). China: Aggressive behavior and the problem of maintaining order and harmony. In A. P. Goldstein & M. H. Segall (Eds.), *Aggression in global perspective* (pp. 58–74). New York: Pergamon Press.

Bowman, K. M., Blau, A., & Reich, R. D. (1974). Psychiatric states following head injury in adults and children. In E. H. Feiring (Ed.), *Brock's injuries of the brain and spinal cord* (pp. 570–613). New York: Springer.

Cairns, H. (1950). Mental disorders with tumour of the pons. *Folia Psychiatrica Neurologica,* (Netherlands) *53,* 193–203 .

Cannon, W. B. (1930). *Bodily changes in pain, hunger and rage* (2nd ed.). New York: Appleton Century.

Cantwell, D. P. (1975). *The hyperactive child.* New York: Spectrum.

Carney, F. P. (1976). Treatment of the aggressive patient. In D. J. Madden & J. R. Lion (Eds.), *Rage, hate, assault and other forms of violence* (pp. 223–248). New York: Spectrum.

Chess, S., & Thomas, A. (1984). *Origin and evolution of behavior disorders from infancy to early adult life.* New York: Brunner/Mazel.

Cleckley, H. (1982). *The mask of sanity.* St. Louis, MO: C. V. Mosby.

Clements, S. D., & Peters, J. E. (1962). Minimal brain dysfunction in the school age child. *Archives of General Psychiatry, 6,* 188–197.

Cloninger, C. R., Reich, T., & Guze, S. B. (1978). Genetic-environmental interactions and antisocial behavior. In R. D. Hare & D. Schalling (Eds.), *Psychopathic behavior: Approaches to research* (pp. 225–238). New York: Wiley.

Critchley, M. (1970). *The dyslexic child* (2nd ed.). London: Heinemann Medical Books.

Curry, S., Heathfield, K., Henson, R. A., & Scott, D. F. (1971). Clinical course and prognosis of temporal lobe epilepsy: A survey of 666 patients. *Brain, 94,* 173–190.

Dalton, K. (1964). *The premenstrual syndrome.* Springfield, IL: Charles C Thomas.

Daly, D. D. (1975). Ictal clinical manifestations of complex partial seizures. In J. K. Penry & D. D. Daly (Eds.), *Advances in Neurology* Vol. 11, pp. 57–84). New York: Raven Press.

Davenport, C. B. (1915). The feebly inhibited: Violent temper and its inheritance. *Journal of Nervous and Mental Disease, 42,* 493–628.

Delgado, J. M. R. (1969). *Physical control of the mind.* New York: Harper & Row.

Detre, T., Kupfer, D. J., & Taub, S. (1975). The nosology of violence. In W. S. Fields & W. H. Sweet (Eds.), *Neural bases of violence and aggression* (294–317). St. Louis, MO: W. H. Green.

Douglas, V. (1983). Attentional and cognitive problems. In M. Rutter (Ed.), *Developmental neuropsychiatry.* New York: Guilford Press.

Dreifuss, F. H. (1975). The differential diagnosis of partial seizures with complex symptomatology. In J. K. Penry & D. D. Daly (Eds.), *Advances in neurology* (Vol. 11, pp. 187–200). New York: Raven Press.

Duff, D. (1972). *Albert and Victoria.* London: Muller.

Durkheim, E. (1897). *Le suicide.* Paris: Ancienne Librairie Germer Bailliere.

Ehlers, C. L., Rickler, K. C., & Hovey, J. E. (1979). A possible relationship between plasma testosterone and aggressive behavior in a female outpatient population. In M. Girgis & L. Kiloh (Eds.), *Limbic epilepsy and the dyscontrol syndrome.* New York: Elsevier/North Holland.

Elliott, F. A. (1976). Neurological factors in violent behavior (The dyscontrol syndrome). *Bulletin of the American Academy of Psychiatry and Law, 4,* 297–315.

Elliott, F. A. (1982). Neurological findings in adult minimal brain dysfunction and the dyscontrol syndrome. *Journal of Nervous and Mental Disease, 170,* 680–687.

Elliott, F. A. (1983). Biological roots of violence. *Proceedings of the American Philosophical Society, 127,* 84–94.

Elliott, F. A. (1984). Episodic dyscontrol and aggression. In J. B. Green (Ed.), *Neurologic clinics* (Vol. 2, pp. 113–125). Philadelphia, PA: W. B. Saunders.

Eysenck, H. F., & Eysenck, S. B. (1978). Psychopathy, personality and genetics. In R. D. Hare & D. Schalling (Eds.), *Psychopathic behavior: Approaches to research.* New York: Wiley.

Falconer, M. S., Serafetinides, E. A., & Corsellis, J. A. N. (1969). Etiology and pathogenesis of temporal lobe epilepsy. *Archives of Neurology, 10,* 233–248.

Falrêt, J. (1860–1861). De L'état mental des épileptiques. *Archives of General Medicine, 16,* 666; *17,* 461; *18,* 423.

Ferguson, S. M., & Rayport, M. (1984). Psychosis in epilepsy. In D. Blumer (Ed.), *Psychiatric aspects of epilepsy.* Washington, DC: American Psychiatric Press.

Flor-Henry, P. (1983). *The cerebral basis of psychopathology.* Bristol: John Wright.

Freud, S. (1935). *A general introduction to psychoanalysis.* New York: Liveright.

Frosch, J. (1977). The relation between acting out and disorders of impulse control. *Psychiatry, 40,* 295–314.

Fuster, J. M. (1980). *The prefrontal cortex.* New York: Raven Press.

Galaburda, A. M., & Kemper, T. L. (1979). Cytoarchitectonic abnormalities in developmental dyslexia. *Annals of Neurology, 6,* 94–101.

Galaburda, A. M., & Eidelberg, D. (1982). Symmetry and asymmetry in the human posterior thalamus in a case of developmental dyslexia. *Archives of Neurology, 39,* 333–337.

Gastaut, H., Morin, C., & Leserve, N. (1955). Etude du comportement des epileptiques psychomoteurs de leurs crises. *Annals of Medical Psychology, 113,* 1–27.

Gelles, R. J. (1972). *The violent home.* Beverly Hills, CA: Sage.

Ginsberg, B. E. (1979). The violent brain. In C. R. Jeffery (Ed.), *Biology and crime.* Beverly Hills, CA: Sage.

Glaser, G. H. (1964). The problem of psychosis in temporal lobe epileptics. *Epilepsia, 5,* 271–278.

Goldman, P. S., & Lewis, M. E. (1978). Developmental biology of brain damage and experience. In C. W. Cotman (Ed.), *Neuronal plasticity.* New York: Raven Press.

Goldstein, S. B., & Ibaraki, T. (1983). Japan: Aggression and aggression control in Japanese society. In A. P. Goldstein & M. H. Segall (Eds.), *Aggression in global perspective* (pp. 313–324). New York: Pergamon Press.

Goltz, F. (1892). Der Hund ohne Grosshirn—siebente Abhandlung über die Verrichtungen des Grosshirn. *Pflugers Archives für die Gesampte Physiologie, 51,* 570–614.

Gorski, R. A. (1980). Sexual differentiation of the brain. In D. T. Krieger & J. C. Hughes (Eds.), *Neuroendocrinology* (pp. 215–222). Sundaland, MA: Sinauer Associates.

Graham, R., & Rutter, M. (1968). The reliability and validity of the assessment of the child: Interview with the parent. *Jouranl of Pediatrics, 114,* 581–592.

Green, J. B. (1963). The activation of EEG abnormalities by Tolbutaminde induced hypoglycemia. *Neurology, 12,* 192–200.

Greenfield, J. G. (1963). Infectious diseases of the nervous system. In J. G. Greenfield (Ed.), *Neuropathology.* London: Edward Arnold.

Gubbay, S. S. (1975). *The clumsy child.* Philadelphia: W. B. Saunders.

Guze, S. B. (1976). *Criminality and psychiatric disorders.* London: Oxford University Press.

Halloran, F. M., Schodt, F. C., & Bailey, J. (1985). Japan's new popular culture. *The Wilson Quarterly, 9,* 49–77.

Hare, R. D., & Schalling, D. (1978). *Psychopathic behavior.* New York: Wiley.

Harlow, H. F., & Mears, C. (1979). *The human model: Primate perspectives.* Washington, DC: Winston.

Hartocollis, P. (1968). The syndrome of minimal brain dysfunction in young adult patients. *Bulletin of the Meninger Clinic, 32,* 102–115.

Heath, R. G., Monroe, R. R., & Mickel, W. (1955). Stimulation of the amygdala in a schizophrenic patient. *American Journal of Psychiatry, 111,* 862–863.

Henderson, D. K. (1939). *Psychopathic states.* New York: W. W. Norton.

Hill, D., & Sargant, W. A. (1943). A case of matricide. *Lancet, 1,* 526–629.

Kaes, T. (1907). *Die grosshirnrinde des menschen in ihren wassen und in ihren fassengehalt: Ein gehirn anatomische atlas.* Jena: Fischer.

Kaplan, J. (1899). Kopftrauma und Psychosen. *Allgemeiner Zeitschrift für Psychiatrie, 56,* 292–297.

Kennan, G. (1954). *Realities of American foreign policy.* Princeton, NJ: Princeton University Press.

Kiloh, L. G., McComas, A. J., & Osselton, J. W. (1972). *Clinical electroencephalography.* London: Butterworth.

Kupfer, D. J., Detre, J. R., & Koral, J. (1975). Relationship of certain childhood traits to adult psychiatric disorders. *American Journal of Orthopsychiatry, 45,* 74–80.

Lassman, L. P., & Arjona, V. I. (1967). Pontine glioma in childhood. *Lancet, 1,* 913–915.

Lewin, W. (1973). Selective leucotomy: A review. In L. V. Laitenan & K. Livingstone (Eds.), *Surgical approaches to psychiatry* (pp. 69–73). Baltimore, MD: University Park Press.

Lewis, D. O., Shamok, S. S., Pincus, J. H., & Glaser, G. (1979). Violent juvenile delinquents. *Journal of the American Academy of Child Psychiatry, 18,* 307–319.

Lewis, D. O., Pincus, J. A., Shamok, S. S., & Glaser, G. H. (1982). Psychomotor epilepsy and violence in a group of incarcerated adolescent boys. *American Journal of Psychiatry, 139,* 882–887.

Lion, J. R. (1972). *Evaluation and management of the violent patient.* Springfield, ILL: Charles C Thomas.

Lishman, W. L. (1978). *Organic psychiatry.* Oxford: Blackwell Scientific Publications.

Luria, A. R. (1969). The frontal lobe. In P. J. Vinken & G. W. Bruym (Eds.), *Handbook of neurology* (Vol. 2, 735–757). New York: North Holland.

MacLean, R. (1973). A triune concept of the brain and behavior: Lectures 1, 2, 3. In T. J. Boag & D. Campbell (Eds.), *Clarence M. Hincks memorial lectures.* Toronto: University of Toronto Press.

Madden, D. J., & Lion, J. R. (Eds.). (1976). *Rage, hate, assault, and other forms of violence.* New York: Spectrum.

Malamud, N. (1967). Psychiatric disorders in intracranial tumors of the limbic system. *Archives of Neurology, 17,* 113–123.

Maletsky, B. M. (1974). The episodic dyscontrol syndrome. *Diseases of the Nervous System, 34,* 178–185.

Maletsky, B. M. (1976). The diagnosis of pathological intoxication. *Journal of Studies of Alcoholism, 37,* 1215–1228.

Marinacci, A. A. (1963). A special type of temporal (psychomotor) seizures following ingestion of alcohol. *Bulletin of the Los Angeles Neurological Society, 28,* 241–250.

Mark, V. H., Sweet, W., & Ervin, F. R. (1975). Deep temporal lobe stimulation and destructive lesions in episodically violent temporal lobe patients. In W. S. Fields & W. H. Sweet (Eds.), *Bases of violence and aggression.* St. Louis, MO: H. Green.

Mark. V. H., & Ervin, F. R. (1970). *Violence and the brain.* New York: Harper & Row.

Marks, V. (1974). Investigation of hypoglycemia. *British Journal of Hospital Medicine, 11,* 731–743.

Mathieson, G. (1975). Pathology of temporal lobe foci. In J. K. Penry & D. D. Daly (Eds.), *Advances in neurology* (Vol. 11, pp. 163–186). New York: Raven Press.

Mednick, S. & K. O. Christiansen (Eds.) (1977). *Biosocial bases of criminal behavior.* New York: Gardner.

Meninger, K., & Mayman, M. (1956). Episodic dyscontrol: A third order of stress adaptation. *Bulletin of the Meninger Clinic, 20,* 153–160.

Millichap, J. H. (1975). *The hyperactive child with minimal brain dysfunction*. Chicago, IL: Yearbook Medical Publishers.

Milman, D. (1979). Minimal brain dysfunction in childhood: Outcome in late adolescence and early adult years. *Journal of Clinical Psychiatry, 20*, 371–380.

Monroe, R. R. (1970). *Episodic hehavioral disorders*. Cambridge, MA: Harvard University Press.

Monroe, R. R. (1978). *Brain dysfunction in aggressive criminals*. Lexington, MA: Lexington Books.

Morton, J. H., Additon, H., Addison, R. G., Hunt, L., & Sullivan, H. (1953). A clinical study of premenstrual tension. *American Journal of Obstetrics and Gynecology, 65*, 1182–1191.

Moyer, K. E. (1976). *The psychobiology of aggression*. New York: Harper & Row.

Nauta, W. J. H. (1973). Connections of the limbic system with the frontal lobe. In L. V. Laitimen & K. Livingstone (Eds.), *Surgical approaches in psychiatry* (pp. 303–314). Baltimore University Park Press.

Netzky, M. G., & Strobos, R. R. (1952). Neoplasms within the midbrain. *Archives of Neurology and Psychiatry, 68*, 115–129.

Papez, J. W. (1937). A proposed mechanism of emotion. *Archives of Neurology and Psychiatry, 38*, 725–743.

Parker, T., & Allerton, R. (1962). *The courage of his convictions*. London: Hutchinson.

Pasamanick, B., & Knoblock, H. (1966). Retrospective studies in the epidemiology of reproductive casualty, old and new. *Merrill-Palmer Quarterly, 12*, 7–26.

Pincus, J. H., & Glaser, G. H. (1966). The syndrome of minimal brain damage in childhood. *New England Journal of Medicine, 275*, 27–30.

Plomin, R., DeFries, J. C., & McClearn, G. F. (1980). *Behavioral genetics*. San Francisco: W. A. Freeman.

Quitkin, F., Rifkin, A., & Klein, D. F. (1976). Neurological soft signs in schizophrenic and character disorders. *Archives of General Psychiatry, 33*, 841–853.

Reid, W. H. (1978). Genetic correlates of antisocial syndromes. In H. W. Reid (Ed.), *The psychopath: A comprehensive study of antisocial disorders and behaviors* (pp. 240–260). New York: Brunner/Mazel.

Reich, W. (1970). *The impulsive character* (English trans.). New York: New American Library. (Originally published 1925).

Riesen, A. H. (1975). *The developmental neuropsychology of sensory deprivation*. New York: Academic Press.

Roberts, A. (1979). *Severe accidental injury: An assessment of long term prognosis*. London: MacMillan Press.

Robins, L. (1966). *Deviant children grown up: Sociological and psychiatric study of the sociopathic personality*. Baltimore, MD: Williams & Wilkins.

Rochford, J. M., Detre, T., Tucker, F., & Harrow, M. (1970). Neuropsychological impairment in functional psychogenic diseases. *Archives of General Psychiatry, 22*, 114–119.

Rodin, E. A. (1973). Psychomotor epilepsy and aggressive behavior. *Archives of General Psychiatry, 38*, 210–213.

Rush, B. (1818). *Medical inquiries and observations on diseases of the mind*. Philadelphia, PA: John Richardson.

Rutter, M. (1980). *Changing youth in a changing society*. Cambridge, MA: Harvard University Press.

Rutter, M. (1983). *Developmental neuropsychiatry*. New York: Guilford Press.

Rutter, M., & Giller, H. (1983). *Juvenije delinquency*. New York: Guilford Press.

Satterfield, J. H., Satterfield, B. T., & Cantwell, D. P. (1981). Three-year multimodality treatment study of hyperactive boys. *Journal of Pediatrics, 98*, 650–655.

Schulsinger, F. (1977). Psychopathy: Heredity and environment. In S. Mednick & K. O. Christiansen (Eds.), *Biosocial bases of criminal behavior* (pp. 109–126). New York: Gardner Press.

Slater, E., Beard, A. W., & Glithero, E. (1963). The schizophrenia-like psychoses of epilepsy. *British Journal of Psychiatry, 109*, 95–150.

Smith, J. S. (1979). Episodic rage. In M. Girgis & L. S. Kiloh (Eds.), *Limbic epilepsy and the dyscontrol syndrome* (pp. 255–266). New York: Elsevier/North Holland.

Stacey, W. A., & Shupe, A. (1983). *The family secret: Domestic violence in America*. Boston, MA: Beacon.

Steinmetz, S. K. (1978). Wife beating: A critique and reformulation of existing theory. *Bulletin of the American Academy of Psychiatry and Law, 6*, 322–335.

Stevens, J. R. (1975). Interictal clinical complications of complex partial seizures. In J. K. Penry & D. D. Daly (Eds.), *Advances in neurology* (Vol. 2). New York: Raven Press.

Straus, M. A., Gelles, R. J., & Steinmetz, S. K. (1980). *Behind closed doors*. New York: Anchor Books.

Symonds, C. P. (1974). Concussion and contusion of the brain and their sequelae. In E. H. Feiring (Ed.), *Injuries of the brain and spinal cord* (pp. 100–161). New York: Springer.

Symonds, C. P. (1975). Reflections. In W. Penfield (Ed.), *The mystery of the mind* (pp. 91–101). Princeton, NJ: Princeton University Press.

Taylor, D. C., Falconer, M. R., Bruton, C. N., & Corsellis, J. A. (1971). Focal dysplasia of the cerebral cortex in epilepsy. *Journal of Neurology, Neurosurgery, and Psychiatry, 34,* 309–387.

Thompson, G. N. (1953). *The psychopathic delinquent and criminal.* Springfield, IL: Charles C Thomas.

Towbin, A. (1971). Organic causes of minimal brain dysfunction. *Journal of the American Medical Association, 217,* 1207–1214.

Tuchman, B. W. (1978). *A distant mirror: The calamitous 14th century.* New York: Ballatine.

Turner, G., Robinson, H., Lang, S., & Purvis-Smith, S. (1986). Preventive screening for the fragile X Syndrome. *The New England Journal of Medicine, 315,* 607–609.

Valzelli, L. (1981). *Psychobiology of aggression and violence.* New York: Raven Press.

Wender, P. A. (1971). *Minimal brain dysfunction in children.* New York: Wiley Interscience.

Wieser, H. G., Hailemariam, S., Regard, M., & Landis, T. (1985). Unilateral limbic epileptic status activity: Stereo EEG, behavioral and cognitive data. *Epilepsia, 1,* 19–29.

Wilder, J. (1947). Sugar metatolism in its relation to criminology. In R. W. Lindner & R. V. Seliger (Eds.), *Handbook of criminal psychology* (pp. 98–129). New York: New York Philosophical Library.

Williams, D. (1969). Neural factors related to habitual aggression. *Brain, 92,* 503–520.

Wilson, S. A. K. (1940). *Neurology* (Vol. 1). London: Edward Arnold.

Wishnie, H. A. (1977). *The impulsive personality.* New York: Plenum Press.

Wolfgang, M. E., & Ferracuti, F. (1982). *The subculture of violence.* Beverly Hills, CA: Sage.

Wood, D. R., Reimer, F., Wender, R., & Johnson, G. (1976). Diagnosis and treatment of minimal brain dysfunction in adults. *Archives of General Psychiatry, 33,* 1453–1600.

Yakovlev, R., & Lecours, R. (1967). In A. Minkowski (Ed.), *Regional development of the brain in early life.* Oxford: Blackwood.

Yeudall, L. F., & Fromm-Auch, A. (1979). Neuropsychological impairment in various psychopathological populations. In J. Gruzelier & P. Flor-Henry (Eds.), *Hemisphere asymmetries of function of psychopathology* (pp. 401–430). New York: Elsevier/North Holland.

16

Alcohol, Alcoholism, and Family Violence

KENNETH E. LEONARD and THEODORE JACOB

That excessive alcohol use may be related to family violence is by no means a new idea. William Hogarth's drawing of life in "Gin Alley" presents a striking visual image of the ills of alcohol: an intoxicated woman who neglectfully allows her small infant to fall from her arms. Temperance tracts in the 1830s and 1840s promulgated the view that alcohol, even in somewhat moderate doses, resulted in neglect of the basic needs of the family. Expenditures of family resources on alcohol rather than food and clothing and unusually cruel violence directed at children and spouse were repeatedly discussed. In 1832, for example, the Fifth Report of the American Temperance Society devoted several pages to instances where a father, while intoxicated, had murdered his wife or children:

> In the State of New York alone, in the course of a few weeks, not less than four men, under the influence of ardent spirits, murdered their wives, and with their own hands made their children orphans. . . . One of these men put to death not only his wife, but six of his children. (American Temperance Society Documents, 1972)

Despite this early view that excessive drinking was directly and causally related to family violence, specific research efforts directed at investigating this issue have been quite recent. In general, research in the area of alcohol and violence can be classified as either survey research or analog experiments. In the following sections, we will review the survey research concerning child abuse and marital violence, and then analog studies of alcohol and aggression that are relevant to the area of family violence.

CHILD ABUSE

A variety of different behaviors are often subsumed under the rubric of child abuse. The most commonly associated with this term is aggressive behavior toward the child beyond some arbitrary limit associated with the bounds of socially sanctioned physical punishment, and the terms *child abuse* and *physical abuse* toward the child are often seen

KENNETH E. LEONARD • Research Institute on Alcoholism, Buffalo, NY 14203. **THEODORE JACOB** • Division of Child Development and Family Relations, University of Arizona, Tucson, AZ 85721.

as synonymous. However, other conceptually distinct classes of behaviors are also commonly referred to as child abuse. These include sexual abuse, incest, neglect, abandonment, and emotional abuse.

The difficulty in defining and measuring such concepts has been addressed in the preceding chapters and will not be dealt with at length here. Suffice it to say that the judgments of these behavioral classes often require attributions of the intentionality of the parent and judgments as to the social appropriateness of the act, and necessarily involves beliefs concerning normal parent–child relationships. In cases of child abuse that are brought forward into the judicial/social work arena, these somewhat subjective decisions are made by a variety of different individuals with a variety of different standards. In the interests of justice and the child's welfare, this is perhaps as it should be. However, in terms of understanding these child abuse behaviors, it renders a difficult situation even more difficult. As has been noted with respect to other areas of research of socially deviant behavior that rely on the adjudication process to identify their samples, differences between groups that emerge may say as much about our norms and beliefs and about the adjudication process, as it says about the deviant behavior of interest. For example, similar behaviors are likely to be interpreted differently when exhibited by a relatively normal father as opposed to a father known to the social agencies for drinking problems. In fact, a drinking problem *per se* may be regarded as neglectful, regardless of whether, in fact, the child's emotional or physical needs were neglected. Thus, it is possible to find a spurious relationship between excessive drinking and child abuse because the two categories overlap, or because excessive drinking affects the probability that child abuse will be identified and labeled as such.

Definitional and measurement problems extend as well to the excessive alcohol consumption variables. Much of the alcohol and child abuse literature focuses on a single measure of excessive alcohol use, whether the abuser can be considered a problem drinker or an alcoholic. In many studies, it is not at all clear how the diagnosis of alcoholism was made and one suspects that the abuser, his (or her) spouse, or some social agency simply categorized the abuser with respect to his drinking habits. Similar to the problem noted earlier, it is plausible that a man who drinks heavily and neglects or abuses his children would be more likely to be labeled an alcoholic than another who drinks as much, but does not manifest this particular type of problem. In fact, even standard diagnostic practices that require social or familial impairment due to alcohol for an individual to receive the diagnosis of alcoholism, can produce a spurious association between alcoholsim and child abuse because the latter is one possible criteria of the former.

Another problem related to the measurement of excessive alcohol consumption is the failure of most studies to utilize more than one simple measure of alcohol use. A few studies have asked whether the perpetrator of the child abuse was drinking at the time of the abuse, but do not inquire as to the possible presence of alcohol problems. Thus, it is not possible to determine whether any obtained relationship is due to the acute effects of intoxication or to the socially debilitating effects of chronic excessive use, because these two variables are strongly related (people who use alcohol in a chronic, excessive fashion are more often experiencing the acute effects than those who do not use alcohol in this way). Beyond this consideration, however, it would be of interest to examine current and past alcohol use and alcohol problems in order to determine whether some specific pattern of alcohol use was related to some specific form of child abuse. However, to date, such research has been quite rare.

A final difficulty worth noting is simply the paucity of literature attempting to examine this issue. Few studies have been conducted and most of these have the methological problems mentioned earlier as well as others that will be mentioned in the following. Additionally, these few child abuse studies are frequently concerned with only one or two specific forms of child abuse, thus rendering comparisons between studies or conclusions regarding one specific form of abuse difficult to make. For this review, we shall not attempt to review the literature separately for each form of child abuse, but instead shall consider them together, drawing appropriate distinctions where necessary.

Much of our information concerning the role of alcoholism in child abuse is derived from studies that either did not use a control group, or compared several forms of child abuse with respect to the presence of alcoholism. Studies in the former category represent ''one-number estimates'' and do not provide persuasive evidence for an association between alcoholism and child abuse (Roizen, 1982). Nevertheless, such studies tend to suggest that a substantial number of child abusers are reported to be excessive drinkers. For example, Johnson and Morse (1968) reported on children known to the Department of Welfare to have been injured. After excluding those children who were victims of malnutrition or sexual abuse, one quarter of their fathers were believed to ''drink to excess.'' Kaplun and Reich (1976) studied murdered children, and identified 66 cases who were known to public assistance or child welfare of the 112 cases in which the child could be identified. Though the data are not analyzed separately for alcoholism, the authors indicate that 81% of the cases known to welfare were involved in some deviant behavior, with most being excessive drinkers. However, it should not surprise us that cases known to welfare should be deviant in some way. Model citizens are not known to welfare agencies. Browning and Boatman (1977) examined nine cases of father–daughter incest seen at a child psychiatry clinic and found alcoholism in five of the fathers, possible alcohol abuse in one father, and episodic drinking in one father.

There have been two studies that have started with a large, heterogeneous sample of families reported for child neglect or abuse, and have conducted creative internal analyses that shed some light on the role of alcohol in child abuse. MacMurray (1979) conducted an archival study of the Alberta Registry for Child Abuse and Neglect. Of the 1645 cases reported, 33% mentioned using alcohol. Importantly, when alcohol was mentioned, it was more likely that neglect or abuse was substantiated (84% of the cases) than when alcohol was not mentioned (65% of the cases). Further analyses suggested that this relationship was stronger for cases in which the suspected abuser was male than when the suspected abuser was female. Finally, when alcohol was mentioned in the case report, it was likely that the suspected abuser was described as either a problem drinker (44%) or an alcoholic (20%), and that the suspect was intoxicated at the time of the reported incident (83%). As in other archival studies, we can not know whether the absence of any mention of alcohol means that there was no alcohol involvement or whether there was alcohol involvement and the suspect successfully hid this or the caseworker felt it to be irrelevant. In the second study, Gil (1971) identified 13,000 cases of child abuse that were reported through legal channels for the year 1967–1968. Comprehensive cases studies were available for 1,400 of these. Using factor analysis to develop a typology, Gil was able to identify one type of child abuse to which alcohol intoxication at the time of the abuse was related. This type comprised approximately 13% of the sample and was related to the following factors: the perpetrator was male, mother was absent, abuse resulted from caretaker quarrel, and physical and sexual abuse coincide.

A variety of studies have examined alcoholism in one form of child abuse relative to other forms of child abuse. This is a step in the right direction; however, in the absence of a relatively normal control group, caution has to be exercised in interpretation. Julian and Mohr (1979) analyzed data from the National Study on Child Neglect and Abuse Reporting. Specifically, they compared validated father–daughter incest cases with sexual abuse cases, and found alcohol dependence to be twice as common in the incest group (32%) as in the sexual abuse group (14%). Martin and Walters (1982) examined 489 substantiated cases of abandonment, physical abuse, emotional abuse, neglect, and sexual abuse. Utilizing regression analyses, they found that the variable "mother promiscuous/alcoholic" correlated with abandonment whereas "father promiscuous/alcoholic" correlated with sexual abuse. The combination of promiscuity and alcoholism is unfortunate and does not allow a clean interpretation of the findings. Also, the absence of significant findings with respect to the other forms of child abuse cannot be interpreted as suggesting that alcoholism is not involved, only that alcoholism may be more involved with one form of child abuse than another.

Herman and Hirschman (1981) interviewed 40 women who reported a sexual relationship with their father during childhood and 20 women who reported "seductive" fathers but denied any incest. Women in both groups were recruited through an informal network of therapists, and were all, therefore, in therapy. Approximately 35% of both the incest and the control groups described their fathers as problem drinkers. There are a variety of issues that can be raised with respect to this study, from the potential bias of a sample collected in this fashion, to the unclear meaning of "seductive" fathers, to the absence of information concerning the reasons the control women were seeking treatment. Additionally, in the retrospective accounts, we do not know about the father's drinking status at the time at which he was involved with incest.

In one of the rare studies to use clear alcohol criteria and to examine alcoholism and drinking at the time of abuse, Rada, Kellner, and Winslow (1978) administered the Michigan Alcoholism Screening Test (MAST) to 382 imprisoned sex offenders. Of particular interest to the present review is one group of men convicted for incest. The proportion of individuals diagnosed as alcoholic (MAST score > 7) was approximately the same for those convicted of incest (48%) as for those convicted of child molesting (51%), exhibitionism (55%), or forcible rape (48%). When drinking in the event was examined the results were similar, with those convicted of incest slightly more likely to have been drinking (63%) than those in the other three groups (49% of the child molesters, 55% of the forcible rape cases, and 55% of the exhibitionists). Again, the possibility of alcoholism or intoxication being related to these latter crimes and the absence of a normal control group makes it difficult to know whether excessive alcohol use is related to incest or not. Perhaps the most interesting finding of this study was that for incest as well as for all of the other crimes, alcoholics were more likely to have been drinking during the event and nonalcoholics were more likely to have not been drinking. That is, alcoholism status and drinking at the time of the event were very highly related. Thus, it was not possible to actually examine the two drinking variables separately.

A few studies have examined alcohol and child abuse using relatively normal control groups. Elmer (1967) identified 31 families in which a child had been admitted to the children's hospital with an injury that was judged to be the result of abuse. In 12 instances the family was judged to be nonabusive on the basis of several possible criteria, but commonly because the injury was inflicted by a nonfamily member. Although specific data concerning alcohol were not reported, the author comments that "excessive drinking among the fathers" was characteristic of the abusive family group but not of the nonabusive family group. Among the many difficulties with interpreting this study, perhaps the most frustrating is that there is no way of knowing whether the mothers or the excessive drinking fathers were responsible for the abuse. Smith, Hanson, and Noble (1973) conducted a study in England using a normal control group and reported somewhat different results. These authors interviewed the parents of 134 battered infants and children under the age of five and parents of 53 control children matched for both age of child and mother. Again, specific figures are not provided and the identity of the batterer is not given. However, the authors failed to find substantial alcoholism in either group.

Whereas all of the above studies have examined alcohol use within samples of abusing parents, two studies have looked at the frequency of abuse and neglect in samples of alcoholic parents. Wilson and Orford (1978), in a small study of 11 families with an alcoholic parent, found violence toward children in four of these families. However, in one instance the perpetrator of the violence was the spouse of the alcoholic. In a more extensive study, Black and Mayer (1980) interviewed 92 alcoholic parents and 108 opiate addicted parents concerning child care. Some neglect was found in 100% of alcoholics and addicts. However, abuse was somewhat more common among alcoholics (27%) than among the addicts (19%). Additionally, alcohol or drug abuse in the spouse was related to abuse and neglect and other family violence. Although there were some group differences in the rate of abuse, the alcoholics and the addicts differed in several other regards that could have accounted for the results, including age, sex, race, education, current marital status, number of children, and number of arrests.

Summary

This is a difficult area of research to summarize. As noted earlier, the paucity of research and the ubiquity of major methodological and interpretive problems should make any conclusions drawn from this literature extremely tentative. The data do suggest that any relationship between alcohol use or alcoholism and child abuse will not account for major portions of variance in the child abuse variable. That is, if alcohol is involved in child abuse, its influence does not appear to be strong nor pervasive, but rather restricted to certain subgroups of abusers or types of abuse. Perhaps the most emphatic conclusion we can draw is that more and better research is desperately needed.

Wife Abuse

Many of the same problems described with respect to the child abuse literature also apply to the area of alcohol and wife abuse. However, more studies and more methodologically appropriate studies have been conducted in this area. Additionally, somewhat more diversified information has been collected with respect to the role of alcohol in wife abuse. This should not be taken to suggest that all is well with this literature. Methodological and conceptual problems abound. As in the child abuse literature, many studies lack control groups, use samples of convenience, and collect limited data on alcohol use. However, there are a few studies for which these problems are not the case.

A considerable body of research has developed in which abused women are asked to describe their husband's drinking patterns and this data uniformly supports the clinical literature in suggesting that many abusive husbands are considered by their wives to be alcoholic or problem drinkers. Roy (1982), for example, reported on 4,000 semistructured interviews with women calling a hotline for battered wives and found that 35% of the abusive partners were "problem alcoholics." Labell (1979) collected information from a predominantly white, working-class sample of women admitted to a women's shelter. Alcohol problems were reported for the husband by 72% of the sample, with 28% reporting that their husbands had drug problems. Fagan, Stewart, and Hansen (1983) reported on 270 interviews with victims of wife abuse and indicated that approximately one half of these women believed their husband to have a drinking problem. The highest level of alcohol problems was reported by Hilberman and Munson's (1978) study of women referred by a rural health clinic for a psychiatric evaluation because of the suspicion that they had been abused. Of the 40 black and 20 white women of very low socioeconomic status who were interviewed, 93% (56/60) indicated that alcoholism was a significant problem for their partner.

In the previously cited studies, and others addressing the same issue, considerable variability in both methods and results is evident. In most of these studies, women who were abused were identified when they presented for treatment of physical injuries (e.g., Hilberman & Munson, 1978; Rounsaville, 1978), sought aid from an abuse hotline (Roy, 1978, 1982), or admitted themselves to a women's shelter (Gayford, 1975; Labell, 1979). Additionally, some samples were drawn from rural communities (Hilberman & Munson, 1978), whereas others came from more urban areas (Rounsaville, 1978; Roy, 1977, 1980), and at least one sample came from England (Gayford, 1975). Other differences between the samples of abused women are also clearly evident with respect to race, socioeconomic status, and age. Also, the women were sometimes asked quite different questions from study to study regarding their husband's drinking patterns, with some answers being provided in terms of the husband being alcoholic, other answers in terms of having alcohol problems, and still other answers in terms of problem drinkers, probably alcoholics, or even frequently drunk. With such diverse samples and descriptions of spouses it is not particularly surprising that there is a considerable range of estimates of the proportion of abusing husbands who are alcoholic, and, in the absence of control samples, we cannot know whether these seemingly high levels of alcoholism in abusive husbands exceeds the levels in nonabusive husbands. Of equal importance, this variability in estimates should alert us to the possibility that there are other factors that may mediate or moderate any observed relationship between alcohol and wife abuse.

Only a few studies have utilized designs that allow for more definite conclusions. Hofeller (1982) compared abused women with control women matched with respect to education. The abused women were recruited from a local women's shelter where they had sought aid, whereas control subjects were rcruited from local women's organizations, church groups, or were personally referred. Husbands were rated as alcoholic by 38% of the abused women, but by only 4% of the control women. An additional 22% of the husbands of abused wives were rated as heavy drinkers, whereas none of the husbands of the control women received this rating. These two groups, though matched on education, probably differed in a number of important ways that could explain the results.

In an often cited study, Byles (1978) investigated family problems of 139 persons appearing in family court. Violence was reported as a problem by 52% of the sample and alcohol problems by 46%. More importantly, the presence of violence was related to alcohol problems, though we can only guess that it was the husband being violent and having alcohol problems. As with the previous study, other factors related to violence and alcohol problems could account for the relationship, though the author ruled out two such factors, incompatibility and indebtedness reported as problems.

A similar problem is evident in two other studies. Dvoskin (1981) interviewed 175 married women at a cervical cancer screening center, local beauty shops, and fabric stores, and identified 31 women who indicated that they had experienced a physical fight with their husband at least once and 144 who had never experienced such a fight. Of those who reported being in a physical fight, 42% indicated that their husband had a drinking problem, whereas only 12% of those who had not had a physical fight identified a drinking problem in their husband. However, the two groups also appear to differ in age, racial composition, and income level. Coleman and Straus (1979) interviewed a nationally representative sample of husbands and their wives with respect to violent behavior and frequencies of getting drunk. For men, 30% of those who acknowledged being "very often drunk" had engaged in severe violence, whereas only 5% or less of men who became drunk less frequently had engaged in severe violence. Approximately 15% of men who were drunk "almost always" were severely violent, suggesting a curvilinear relationship between frequency of being drunk and occurence of severe violence. A similar relationship was obtained for women. These studies (i.e., Byles, 1978; Coleman & Straus, 1979; Dvoskin, 1981; Hofeller, 1982) are significant advances over previous studies in a variety of ways. Most importantly, they do not rely on samples of women seeking assistance because of family violence, and, through comparisons with nonabused women, more strongly suggest that there is a relationship between alcohol problems and wife abuse. However, it is not possible on the basis of these studies to rule out conclusively other factors that may relate to alcohol and wife abuse, and thereby create a spurious relationship between the two.

One very recent study has attempted to examine the relationship between alcoholism and wife abuse while ruling out possible confounding factors. Leonard, Bromet, Parkinson, Day, and Ryan (1985) interviewed a rather homogeneous sample of male factory workers. In each interview, information was obtained regarding alcoholism status (the alcoholism section of the Diagnostic Interview Schedule; Robins, Helzer, Croughan, & Ratcliff, 1981), wife abuse (a modified version of the Straus Conflict Tactics Scale with the extremely violent items removed but physically aggressive items remaining), and level of marital satisfaction and dispositional hostility. Wife abuse was strongly related to a current diagnosis of alcohol dependence or alcohol abuse. Of those men who met criteria for such a diagnosis, 44% acknowledged physical conflict with their wife, but only 14% of those who did not meet criteria admitted to such abuse. Importantly, this relationship remained significant after controlling for marital satisfaction, hostility, and a variety of sociodemographic factors (e.g., religion, years married).

Thus, though much of the data bearing on the possible relationship between problem drinking or alcoholism and marital abuse is problematic, the findings are relatively consistent and do suggest an association between these variables. Of course, this is not to say that alcohol consumption *per se* is the culprit. As noted by Coleman and Strauss (1979) the relationship between habitual heavy alcohol consumption and violence does not by necessity indicate a relationship between acute consumption and episodes of violence.

Determining whether there is a relationship between acute alcohol consumption and family violence is perhaps one of the most difficult tasks in the family violence literature. The simplest approach to this problem has been to ask battered women whether their husband's violence has been connected to drinking or drunkenness. In Gayford's (1975) study, discussed earlier, the author reports that 44 of the 100 cases of wife abuse "occurred regularly" when the husband was drunk. In a similar vein, Walker states that "over half of the battered women in this sample indicated a relationship between alcohol use and battering" (p. 25). Approximately the same figures were obtained by Gelles (1972), who indicated that in 48% (21/44) of the violent families, drinking accompanied the abuse, and by Nisonoff and Bitman (1979), who indicated that of the women who had ever been hit by their spouse, 50% considered alcohol a factor.

Another simple approach is to ask the perpetrator of the violence about his drinking at the time. Three studies of marital violence have reported using this approach, though it has been commonly utilized in studies of alcohol and other forms of violence. Nisonoff and Bitman (1979), in the study described previously, also asked their random sample whether they had ever hit their spouse and if they had whether alcohol was a factor. For males who had hit their wives, 29% indicated that alcohol was a factor, whereas 21% of the females who had hit their husbands indicated this. In a large community survey, Pernanen (1979) asked respondents about the last episode of aggression with which they had been involved. Of those who reported that the last episode was marital violence, Pernanen observed that in 46% of the cases the respondent, the antagonist, or both had been drinking. That the level of alcohol involvement in nonmarital violence (violence between strangers) was higher does not indicate that alcohol consumption was unimportant in the marital violence, only that it was possibly of more importance in other instances of violence. Chimbos (1978) interviewed 34 men who were recently incarcerated for murdering their wives. Similar to results reported in other research concerning drinking and homicide (Mayfield, 1976; Shupe, 1954; Virkkunen, 1974; Wolfgang & Strohm, 1956), the offender and the victim were under the influence of alcohol in 53% of the cases, whereas the offender alone was under the influence in only 18% of the cases.

Instead of relying on the retrospective reports by those involved in the abuse, Bard and Zacker (1974) and Zacker and Bard (1977) trained police to observe the characteristics of domestic disputes. This procedure has its difficulties. As pointed out by Pagano and Taylor (1980), judgments of level of intoxication based on observation are of dubious reliability and validity. In the first study, Bard and Zacker (1974) trained biracial pairs of officers to observe, record, and intervene in cases of domestic dispute. On 1,388 occasions, these officers were involved in a domestic dispute. Either the complainant, the other person, or both were drinking in 56% of the incidents. However, drinking was as common in verbal disputes as in physical assaults, leading the authors to suggest that there was no relationship between drinking and physical assaults. In the second study, alcohol was present in 35% of the cases but again was unrelated to whether or not a physical assault had occurred.

Based on these findings, Bard and his associates concluded that alcohol is relatively unrelated to violence. However, they do not allow for the possibility that alcohol consumption was related to verbal disputes. By comparing physical assaults to verbal disputes, they may have simply been comparing two similar behaviors, verbal and physical aggression, both of which may be related to alcohol consumption. Furthermore, Bard did not recognize the possibility, as noted by Frieze and Schafer (1984), that the police intervention may have prevented the assaults, and thereby obscured any relationship between alcohol abuse and violence.

A few studies have provided more detailed information concerning the role of acute intoxication in wife abuse. Eisenberg and Micklow (cited in Langley & Levy, 1977) reported that 60% of the husbands were always drinking at the time of the attack, whereas 10% were occasionally drinking when the violence occurred. Similarly, Roy (1977) found that of those wife abusers described as occasional drinkers, 80% only assaulted their wives while drunk. According to the abused women in Hofeller's (1982) study, 20% of their husbands were always drunk when the violence occurred, 26% were usually drunk, 24% were sometimes drunk, 12% were rarely drunk, and 16% were never drunk.

Two studies present some data relating drinking pattern and acute intoxication to wife abuse. In Dvoskin's (1981) study, further analyses were conducted on the 31 women who acknowledged physical fights with their husbands. Of these violent men, alcoholics were more likely to have been drinking (77%) during the last violent episode than were nonalcoholics (44%). These data are reminiscent of findings reported by Rada, Kellner, and Winslow (1978) indicating that alcoholics who committed sex offenses with children were likely to have been drinking whereas nonalcoholics committing such crimes were not likely to have been drinking. It may be possible to ascribe drinking before violence in alcoholics to the fact that they are always drinking. However, the rate of drinking before violence in the nonalcoholics in Dvoskin's sample seems quite high, and may indicate a greater role for drinking in violent episodes among nonalcoholics than among alcoholics.

Corenblum (1983) provided information concerning alcoholism, drinking, and violence from a somewhat different perspective. Members of Alcoholics Anonymous were asked about hitting their spouses while sober and while drinking. Some subjects reported that they had never struck their spouses when they were sober. Of these, 44% had hit their spouses while they were intoxicated and 56% had not hit their spouses while intoxicated. Of those who admitted to hitting their spouses while sober, 84% also hit them while intoxicated. There are at least two possible explanations of these findings. First, there may be several subgroups among the alcoholics, those who never hit their spouses, those who hit their spouses whether they are sober or intoxicated, and those who hit their spouses only while intoxicated. Alcohol consumption may be importantly related to violence in the third group, whereas other factors may better predict violence in the second group. A second explanation is that these alcoholics are in different stages of spouse aggression; at the beginning, such aggression occurs only while drinking (for whatever reason) but then progresses to steady violent behavior regardless of whether alcohol is there as a precipitant, excuse, or cause. Unfortunately, data that might address this issue are not currently available.

Although these figures seem very impressive, their meaning is somewhat obscure. There are several reasons for this. Primarily, we have no null hypothesis value against which to judge these figures. That is, if there is no relationship between acute intoxication and wife abuse, what proportion of violence would be expected to have been committed by an intoxicated husband? Obviously, the co-occurence of intoxication and violence has more meaning when we are dealing with a nonalcoholic and rarely drunk sample. However, the data suggest that men who assault their wives are men who are frequently drunk (Coleman & Straus, 1979). As a result, violence and intoxication will co-occur by chance, and this rate of co-occurence will increase with increases in frequency of drunkenness, frequency of abuse, and amount of contact between the two spouses.

Considerations regarding base rate, therefore, should caution us against overinterpreting the reported links between episodes of violence and drinking. At the same time, the finding that many men who attack their wives when drunk also attack them when sober does not indicate that alcohol consumption is unrelated to wife abuse. As was argued earlier, this conclusion cannot be drawn in the absence of some expectation of the null hypothesis. For example, the man who is intoxicated 10% of the time that he is with his wife would be expected to be intoxicated in 10% of the violent episodes under the null hypothesis. The extent to which he deviates from this expectancy would indicate the influence of intoxication and intoxication-related factors. Secondly, the wife is not a static feature in this relationship. To the extent that she learns the antecedents of her husband's violence, she might find some means to minimize or escape from such episodes. Thus, if the wife discovers that her husband is more violent or more frequently violent when he has been drinking, she might behave in a passive and placating fashion, or she might avoid him altogether. When such a woman later becomes part of a research sample, she may indicate that drinking and violence were linked early in marriage. Because she developed ways to minimize the risk of violence when he is drinking, however, drinking and violence now seldom co-occur.

ANALOG STUDIES

Survey studies, such as the ones reviewed earlier, have provided valuable information concerning the relationship between alcoholism, alcohol consumption, and family violence. The value of such studies can be to indicate the likely extent of the problem, and to suggest possible high-risk groups for further study. Survey studies may also implicate other factors that might serve to moderate or mediate any observed relationship. Evidence suggestive of a causal relationship, however, will be rather indirect.

Unlike survey studies, analog studies begin with laboratory measures considered to be analogous to violent behavior and the construction of an experimental paradigm in which variation on these measures can be carefully related to planned variation in amount and context of alcohol consumption. The strengths of such an approach are many. First, this methodology allows us to examine the causal influence of alcohol by actually administering alcohol to subjects and comparing sober behavior with intoxicated behavior on measures of aggression and violence. Further refinement of any causal effect of alcohol can be accomplished through dose studies and through studies utilizing placebo or balanced placebo designs (Marlatt & Rohsenow, 1980). Second, elaboration of any causal effect with respect to moderator variables can be conducted. It is clear that neither alcoholism nor intoxication are necessary or sufficient causes of family violence. Many individuals drink to intoxication and do not manifest any aggressive behavior toward family members or strangers. Obviously, situational, personality, and interpersonal factors may modify the influence of alcohol or alcoholism on violence. Analog studies allow the investigator to manipulate many of these situational factors as well as to observe the influence of other factors in a more systematic and controlled fashion. Third, analog studies enable the investigator to examine the underlying interpersonal processes that are influenced by alcohol and that may lead to violence. Specifically, analog studies that allow for the observation and recording of actual, ongoing interactions may provide important information as to the processes and behavior patterns which characterize non-laboratory interactions. Changes in these patterns that occur when one or the other or both of the participants have been drinking may help to explain the way in which alcohol consumption influences an aggressive outcome. Finally, specific theoretical explanations of alcohol consumption and violence may be developed and tested within such analog studies.

Although there are many strengths to the analog study, one major issue may limit the usefulness of such an approach: the relationship between the analog measure of aggression and actual aggressive or violent behavior between family members in natural settings. There are two basic measures of aggression that have been used in laboratory studies of the alcohol/aggression relationship: the administration of different levels of a noxious stimulus, such as shock or noise, and the verbal expression of negative affect or cognitions within an interpersonal interaction. The implicit relationship between each of these analog measures and actual aggressive behavior is somewhat different.

The administration of shock is considered aggressive by virtue of its congruence with common definitions of aggression. The issue of importance, however, is whether the findings based on this procedure are generalizable to extra-laboratory aggression. Two considerations are of particular importance in this regard. First, there are unavoidable differences between the controlled and artificial laboratory setting and the naturalistic settings within which aggression commonly occurs. Second, most studies in this literature have utilized males as subjects and male strangers as targets, and as a result, associated findings may have little to say about marital or family violence. Obviously, caution must be exercised in attempts to use findings from such studies to explain family violence.

The issue is somewhat different when the analog measure is the expression of negative affect or cognitions: an index of verbal and not physical aggression. Whereas there are various measures of verbal aggression, the one most pertinent to this discussion involves the direct observation of a structured conflict situation with married couples and families. On the one hand, generalizability may be less of a concern because the conflict situation is selected for its relevance to the particular family. Furthermore, the responses exhibited by the family are not novel, but are part of their everyday repertoire of verbal behaviors. Finally, the family is observed in a naturalistic setting (e.g., the home) or a seminaturalistic setting (e.g., a living room set up within the interaction laboratory). The assumed link between verbal and physical aggression, however, is still a major issue. That is, if it cannot be demonstrated that verbal aggression leads to physical aggression, then any demonstration of a relationship between alcohol and verbal aggression involving family members may not be of great interest to the family violence issue. It has been argued by many, however, that there is an escalatory process in aggressive behavior in which the intensity of verbal aggression increases to a high level and results in physical aggression (Pernanen, 1976; Tinklenberg, 1973). Additionally, laboratory studies of aggression have frequently demonstrated that verbal provocation can serve to heighten physical aggression (e.g., Berkowitz & LePage, 1967; Rule & Percival, 1971). Straus (1974) also reported that there is a strong relationship between degree of reported verbal aggression and the degree of reported marital violence. Notwithstanding such arguments, however, it must be acknowledged that some cases of family violence probably do not arise from such an escalatory process, and that the verbal aggression analogs may not be applicable.

Alcohol and Laboratory Aggression

Studies of alcohol and aggression among college students commonly employ the adminstration of a noxious stimulus (shock, noise) as the laboratory analog of aggressive behavior. Three basic contexts have provided the rationale (to the subjects) for administering such stimuli: the teacher–learner paradigm (Buss, 1966), the perception-of-pain paradigm (Zeichner & Pihl, 1979, 1980), and the competitive-reaction-time paradigm (Taylor, 1967). In the teacher–learner paradigm, the subject is randomly selected to teach a confederate some task with shock or noise available to punish the learner for an incorrect response. The perception-of-pain paradigm allows the subject to administer shock to a target person who is presumably participating in a pain study. In turn, the target administers varying degrees of loud noise to the subject, obstensibly to inform the subject of the painfulness of the shock. The competitive-reaction-time paradigm pits the subject against an opponent in a reaction-time competition. The winner chooses the level of shock that is administered to the loser on the next trial, and the subject receives feedback concerning

KENNETH E.
LEONARD and
THEODORE JACOB

the level of shock the opponent selected for him. In fact, however, the opponent's shock settings and whether the subject wins and administers the shock or loses and receives the shock is predetermined by the experimenter. In general, the intensity of shock selected by the subject serves as the measure of aggression in all three paradigms.

Although these laboratory studies have generated considerable debate concerning different aspects of the alcohol-aggression relationship, several general conclusions do seem warranted. At the most basic level, it would appear that alcohol consumption does not uniformly induce aggressive behavior. Rather, several boundary conditions appear to be necessary in order for alcohol consumption to have an impact on aggressive behavior. First, the amount of alcohol consumed must be relatively high. Studies that utilize alcohol dosages resulting in blood alcohol concentrations well within the legal limits (.01 mg% to .05 mg%) do not typically find that alcohol increases aggression (Taylor & Gammon, 1975; Taylor, Vardaris, *et al.*, 1976). However, as blood alcohol content (BAC) attains the level of legal intoxication (.10mg%), one is considerably more likely to observe an increase in aggression. For example, Taylor and Gammon (1975) compared the behavior of subjects receiving no alcohol, low doses of alcohol, and high doses of alcohol. Subjects who consumed high doses of alcohol selected higher shocks for their opponents in the competition paradigm than did subjects who consumed no alcohol. Low doses of alcohol actually appeared to reduce shock settings relative to the no-alcohol control. These findings were replicated by Taylor, Vardaris *et al.* (1976).

A second boundry condition appears to be whether the context is generally threatening or instigative of aggressive behavior. Studies that utilize paradigms having minimal aggression-instigating cues tend not to report increased aggression due to alcohol consumption (Lang, Goeckner, Adesso, & Marlatt, 1975; Taylor, Gammon, & Capasso, 1976). In contrast, alcohol consumption in contexts that are generally aggression instigating seem to result in heightened aggressive behavior. For example, Taylor, Schmutte, Leonard, and Cranston (1979) examined the response of intoxicated and sober subjects to two intense provocations. Specifically, the opponent in the competitive paradigm attempted to administer shock purported to be twice the level of the subject's pain threshold. Intoxicated subjects reacted to these provocations in an exaggerated form relative to the sober subjects. Furthermore, Sears (1977) found that intoxicated subjects manifested a similarly exaggerated responsivity when the instigation to aggress was in the form of an observer urging the use of high shocks against a pacifistic opponent.

Beyond these two boundary conditions, some inhibitory cues reduce the aggressive behavior of intoxicated subjects, whereas other cues do not. In general, complex, subtle, or ambiguous cues do not seem to have this effect. For example, Zeichner and Pihl (1980) found that intoxicated subjects did not differentiate between a target who administered high-intensity noise with a malicious intent and a target who administered similar levels of noise with an ambiguous or neutral intent. Subjects who received placebos administered lower levels of shock to targets with a neutral intent than to targets with a malicious intent. In another study, Schmutte and Taylor (1980) found that intoxicated subjects with relatively high BACs did not decrease their shock settings in response to indications from the target that he was in considerable pain, whereas subjects with relatively lower BACs and subjects who received no alcohol did reduce their shock settings.

Several studies have found factors that serve to inhibit the aggressive responding of intoxicated subjects. Taylor, Gammon, and Capasso (1976) found that a clear statement of pacifistic intent reduced the level of aggression in intoxicated subjects. Taylor and Gammon (1976) found that an observer who urged the use of low shocks against a highly aggressive opponent was able to reduce substantially the aggression of intoxicated and sober subjects. Bailey, Leonard, Cranston and Taylor (1983) found that cues of a strongly self-relevant nature served to reduce the aggression of intoxicated and sober subjects in response to a nonaggressive, noninstigatory opponent. Thus, cues that lead to a redefinition of the situation may serve to reduce aggression in intoxicated subjects.

Although the studies reviewed earlier support the hypothesis that alcohol consumption increases aggressive behavior under certain conditions, there is considerable controversy regarding the mechanisms by which alcohol may come to exert such an effect. Traditionally, the aggression-inducing effects of alcohol consumption were viewed as a direct effect of the pharmacological impact of alcohol. It is clear, however, that this model cannot account for the many situations in which alcohol does not increase aggression, and there is an almost universal rejection of this direct disinhibition model, except perhaps in cases with temporal lobe dysfunctions (Mark & Ervin, 1970).

Although there are a number of alternative models (Graham, 1980), two perspectives have received special attention of late. The first approach, commonly referred to as the cognitive disruption model, argues that alcohol, through its pharmacological actions, impairs the individual's attentional and interpretive abilities; as a result, the probability of aggression is increased when the person is confronted with certain instigatory and inhibitory cues (Hull, 1981; Pernanen, 1976; Taylor & Leonard, 1983). The other approach, referred to as the learned disinhibition or expectancies approach, posits that alcohol enhances aggressive behavior because people have learned that they may behave in an uninhibited and aggressive fashion while drinking and get away with it; that is, the deviant behavior will be attributed to the effects of alcohol and the drinker can avoid responsibility for his actions. (Lang *et al.*, 1975; MacAndrew & Edgerton, 1969; Marlatt & Rohsenow, 1980).

Although it is beyond the scope of this chapter to evaluate these approaches in detail, several comments are necessary. First, administering subjects a placebo provides them the belief that they have consumed alcohol and, according to the expectancies model, enables them to behave aggressively while avoiding the responsibility for doing so. However, although increases in aggression in placebo subjects are sometimes reported (Lang *et al.*, 1975; Zeichner & Pihl, 1979), other studies have reported that placebos have no effect or may even reduce aggression (Rohsenow & Bachorowski, 1984; Shuntich & Taylor, 1972). Second, subjects with similar expectancies regarding the beverage they have ingested often behave quite differently as a function of the type of beverage (alcohol or placebo) or the amount of alcohol actually ingested. Thus, many studies have reported that subjects who actually consume alcohol behave more aggressively than subjects who believe they have consumed alcohol but, in fact, have not (Schmutte, Leonard, & Taylor, 1979; Shuntich & Taylor, 1972; Taylor & Gammon, 1976; Taylor, Schmutte, & Leonard, 1977; Zeichner & Pihl, 1979). Similarly, subjects who receive different doses of alcohol are provided with the same general belief that they have consumed alcohol, and yet they behave very differently. Thus, some of the evidence suggests that alcohol consumption may increase the probability of aggression through the responsibility-avoiding mechanism proposed by the expectancy theory, whereas other evidence suggests that the pharmacological factors resulting from the actual presence of alcohol also increase the probability of aggression.

Finally, whereas all of the previously cited studies were conducted using males as the targets of aggression, Richardson (1981) recently extended these findings to female targets. Relative to men who had been given a placebo, men who received a high dose of alcohol behaved in a highly aggressive manner against a female target, suggesting that the normative strictures against harming a female are to some extent overcome with alcohol.

In summary, there are several findings from laboratory studies of alcohol and aggression that may be relevant to the area of alcohol and marital violence. These studies indicate that alcohol consumption can cause an increase in aggressive behavior, suggesting that the observed relationship between alcohol and marital violence may be causal in nature. Further, these laboratory studies suggest that alcohol will have an effect on marital or family violence only when relatively large amounts of alcohol are consumed and when the situation is conducive to aggressive behavior. Obviously, these conditions are met quite frequently among families where one member is an alcoholic or a problem drinker, and may account for the high levels of marital violence seen in this population. However, these conditions are sometimes met even in families where no one is a heavy drinker, but where one or both individuals occasionally become intoxicated. Thus, alcohol consumption may lead to marital violence not only among alcoholics, but also among social drinkers. Laboratory studies also suggest that once aggression is instigated, subtle or ambiguous cues to behave nonaggressively have little impact, but cues that reinstate the norms of the situation (either through self-awareness, social pressure, or the explicit description of a nonaggressive norm) may reduce aggressive responding. However, in most instances of marital violence, the men involved probably do not hold norms for nonaggressive behavior with respect to their wives. Clinical reports certainly substantiate the view that many abusive men believe such aggression to be normative, and do not believe that they are acting in a deviant fashion. Thus, the reinstatement of the norms of the situation would be likely to have little influence on the ongoing abuse.

Finally, the theoretical models derived from this literature are particularly germane. The expectancies model has been used by Gelles (1977) and others to explain the association between alcohol use and marital violence. The cognitive disruption model, though not as consistently applied to wife abuse, is clearly relevant to this type of aggression.

Alcohol, Alcoholism, and Family Interactions

The second type of analog study relevant to the issue of alcohol and family violence is the interactional behavior of married couples and families. In these studies, actual interactions are observed, either naturally occurring interactions in the home or structured interactions in a quasi-naturalistic setting. As in laboratory studies of alcohol and aggression, this approach involves the manipulation and control of certain key variables, and thereby allows for causal statements linking alcohol and aggressive behavior. Further, as noted previously, it may be possible to identify the interactional processes that influence and perpetuate patterns of alcohol abuse through this method.

Over the past 15 years, there has been a growing interest in examining the marital and family interactions of alcoholics. Parallel with other family research, the purpose of these studies was to determine how family interactions influence the etiology and course of alcoholism, and the patient's response to treatment. Initial studies concerned with the interaction between alcoholics and their wives utilized interpersonal perception techniques or interactional games, rather than actual verbal interactions, and studied the alcoholic while sober, but not while drinking (Cobb & McCourt, 1979; Gorad, 1971; Kennedy, 1976; Mitchell, 1959). The results of these studies, though not uniformly positive, did suggest that the interactions of alcoholics and their wives differed from the interactions of social drinkers. In general, the interactions of alcoholics and their wives were characterized as negative and highly competitive, with the alcoholic behaving in such a way as to minimize or avoid personal responsibility for his behavior. Although these findings are interesting and potentially applicable to family violence, the most relevant studies are those in which actual interactions are observed and assessed while the alcoholic is sober and while he is drinking. At present, there are only a few such studies in the literature.

In the earliest of such studies, Billings, Kessler, Gomberg, and Weiner (1979) examined the marital interaction of alcoholic, distressed, and normal couples during sessions with and without the consumption of alcoholic beverages. Couples were involved in a standardized role play in which they were asked to imagine conflictual scenarios and to improvise these scenes, acting like they would if they were actually in the situation. The videotaped interactions were rated using the Interpersonal Behavior Rating System (Leary, 1957) and the Coding Scheme for Interpersonal Conflict (Raush, Barry, Hertel, & Swain, 1974). The results indicated that alcoholic couples engaged in more negative and hostile acts than did the normal couples. The maritally distressed group behaved in a fashion similar to the alcoholics. The availability of alcohol, however, had no impact on these negative behaviors. It should be noted that almost half of the subjects chose not to drink any alcoholic beverage when it was available, and among those who did drink, most drank one or two drinks. The alcoholic husbands achieved a blood alcohol concentration of only .026 mg%. Thus, the failure to find any effect of alcohol on marital interactions could be attributed to the relatively ineffective manipulation of alcohol consumption.

Jacob, Ritchey, Cvitkovic, and Blane (1981) studied eight families with alcoholic fathers/husbands and eight families with normal fathers/husbands. Two structured interaction tasks were employed. The first of these interaction tasks was the Revealed Difference Technique, which involved discussing and arriving at joint rankings of preferences for items in different content areas after each individual had already expressed his own preference in an earlier questionnaire. The second task involved discussions of personally relevant topics identified from the Areas of Change Questionnaire (Weiss, 1980). These tasks were completed by several different family combinations: mother-father, mother-children, and father-children. On one evening, these interaction tasks were completed with only nonalcoholic beverages available whereas on a second evening, the tasks were completed while the two parents were drinking alcoholic beverages. Unlike the Billings *et al.* study, all of the alcoholics in this study drank some amount of alcohol. On the average, the alcoholic husbands drank three drinks and attained a BAC of .08 mg% (.10% is considered legally intoxicated). The interactions were videotaped and rated with the Marital Interaction Coding System (MICS), yielding summary codes of positive affect, negative affect, agree/disagree, and problem solving.

Several findings are relevant to our discussion of family violence. First, on the relatively structured and somewhat impersonal RDT task, there were no differences as a function of group (alcoholic vs. normal), or drinking (drink night vs. no drink night) on the expression of negative or positive affect. However, when the more personally relevant ACQ task was examined, it was found that alcoholic couples (mother–father interactions) expressed significantly more negative affect than did normal couples. Importantly, alcoholic couples became distinctly more negative on drink night, whereas normal couples did not alter their affective expression as a function of alcohol. Consistent with this finding, wives of alcoholics disagreed more on drink night than on no-drink night whereas wives of normals disagreed less on drink night than on no-drink night. Finally, these differences

KENNETH E.
LEONARD and
THEODORE JACOB

in affect appeared primarily with the mother–father interactions, but not with the mother–children or the father–children interactions, possibly because of the variability of the age and sex of the children involved in the interaction.

Although these two studies suggest that alcoholics manifest high levels of negative affect and hostility, a recent study by Frankenstein, Hay, and Nathan (1984) reported somewhat different findings. Eight alcoholic couples were assessed while sober and after consuming a fixed dose of alcohol. Videotapes were made of the couples discussing marital problems and these tapes were coded with the MICS. The results indicated that alcohol led to increases in positive affect, and that this was primarily the result of increased positivity on the part of the wife.

Obviously, this study does not appear consistent with the hypothesis that alcohol consumption in alcoholics will lead to expressions of negative affect or verbal aggression. Indeed, it suggests quite the opposite — that drinking may have positive consequences for the alcoholic. Although this possibility is not commonly recognized by those in the family violence literature, several investigators from the fields of systems theory and marital/family studies have discussed such possibilities. In particular, Steinglass and Robertson (1981) and Steinglass (1983) suggested that drinking may have adaptive, and even positive consequences for an alcoholic family, and that these positive consequences can serve to reinforce and perpetuate excessive and abusive drinking. For Steinglass, abusive drinking continues because it is effective in providing a short-term solution to a familial problem. Of course, the adaptive consequence need not be positive in the sense that it is pleasurable; instead, alcohol-related interactions may allow for certain relationships that are important for individual and relationship stability yet difficult to achieve during periods of sobriety. Adaptive consequences can include a wide variety of response patterns, including ''increasing interactional distance (drinker goes off to drink in the basement), diminishing physical contact (no sex with someone who is drunk),'' or reducing ''interactional distance (making contact by fighting after the alcoholic spouse has been drinking).'' Increased expression of positive affect, as seen in the Frankenstein *et al.* study, could be viewed as an adaptive consequence of drinking, and as such, appear consistent with the model proposed by Steinglass.

Thus, these two literatures, family violence and family systems theory, suggest different roles for alcohol within the family. The family violence literature views alcohol as one of several factors that is associated with and may trigger aggressive behavior in the alcoholic, whereas the family systems literature argues that drinking may result in more positive outcomes that are adaptive — at least for certain types of alcoholics and their families. Though apparently contradictory, these positions are by no means mutually exclusive. For example, alcohol may, in a given person, result in positive effects under some circumstances and negative effects under other circumstances. Thus, the consideration of situational and contextual variables could lead to the development of conditional or interactional models that view the behavioral outcome as a joint function of alcohol consumption and contextual cues. This possibility is clearly suggested by the studies of laboratory aggression that indicate that alcohol does not facilitate aggression in the absence of aggression-provoking cues.

The differences between the two approaches can be reconciled in another manner. It is possible that for some types of subgroups of alcoholics, drinking leads to aversive interpersonal interactions, such as verbal attacks and violence, whereas for other alcoholics, drinking is associated with more positive interpersonal interactions. Some support for this hypothesis has been found in several recent studies of family interaction conducted in our laboratory.

In the first of these studies (Jacob, Dunn, & Leonard, 1983), alcoholic husbands and their nonalcoholic wives completed the MMPI, the Beck Depression Inventory, two measures of marital adjustment and satisfaction, and questions concerning drinking during the preceding month. Surprisingly, alcoholic husbands who had consumed relatively larger amounts of alcohol during the preceding month had lower scores on the MMPI, reported high levels of marital satisfaction, and had wives who also had low scores on the MMPI and the BDI and high levels of marital satisfaction. Of importance to the present discussion, only subjects who acknowledged a regular, steady pattern of drinking evidenced this pattern whereas the relationship was not significant for those alcoholics who described themselves as periodic or binge drinkers.

Preliminary analyses of recently collected family interaction data from our laboratory also support the possibility of differential effects of alcohol on different groups of alcoholics. In this study, families with an alcoholic, depressed, or normal father were studied using a similar methodology and coding system as reported earlier by Jacob *et al.* (1981). Based on the preliminary analyses, results replicated the earlier Jacob *et al.* (1981) study, indicating more negativity in alcoholic couples than in depressed or control couples, and an increase in negativity during drink night for alcoholic couples, but not for depressed or social couples. Subsequent post-hoc analyses, however, suggested that this increase in negativity occurred only with binge drinkers. In contrast, steady drinkers evidenced an increase in positive affect and problem solving on drink night. Although these results must be considered preliminary ones, they do suggest that alcohol may serve a positive, adaptive function for those alcoholics who manifest a relatively steady pattern of drinking, especially when drinking occurs primarily in the home. Binge alcoholics, who differ from steady alcoholics in ways other than drinking pattern, appear to respond in a relatively negative fashion when they have been drinking.

Summary

The analog studies reviewed earlier, including studies of laboratory aggression and family interactions, have demonstrated some important relationships. Unlike the interview studies, this literature indicates that alcohol consumption can lead to increases in aggressive behaviors that appear to be linked to violence. Among college students engaged in an aggressive encounter as well as married alcoholics discussing conflictual issues, the administration of alcohol increases the aggressive nature of their responses. This research also indicates that such increases are not uniform and that among certain persons or in particular situations increased aggressiveness is not observed. It is not possible at present to determine whether the increases, when they occur, are the result of cognitive impairment accompanying intoxication or of expectancies that antinormative behavior is permissable in intoxicated persons. However, it is likely that both processes may be at work, and that future analog studies have the potential of disentangling these effects.

Beyond the demonstration of the acute effects of alcohol on aggressive behaviors, the identification of mediating and moderating factors and the testing of theoretical conceptions of alcohol and aggression, analog studies have the potential to identify interpersonal processes underlying aggressive behavior. Of particular importance would be the comparison of those who report family violence with those who do not report any violence. Such studies are underway with respect to child abuse and neglect (Bousha & Twentyman, 1984; Twentyman & Martin, 1978), but not with respect to marital violence. More to the point would be an examination of the interactions of violent and nonviolent couples under the influence of alcohol and under the influence of a placebo.

DISCUSSION

The evidence reviewed in this chapter strongly suggests that alcoholism and acute alcohol consumption, particularly among certain alcoholics, is related to marital violence. The evidence with respect to child abuse is much weaker. Basically, the research indicates that a high percentage of those who engage in marital violence are alcoholics or at least very heavy drinkers, and that the marital violence is often associated with alcohol consumption. Laboratory studies of alcohol and aggression suggest that alcohol consumption can lead to increases in aggressive behavior in some people under certain circumstances. Further, studies of alcoholics interacting with their wives suggests that the consumption of alcohol results in increases in the expression of negative affect.

Despite the preponderance of evidence implicating alcohol use and alcoholism in much of marital violence, the precise role of these factors has not received systematic attention. Indeed, much of the relevant research did not explicitly focus on alcohol, but only included a few questions about alcohol (usually only a single question) that tended to be quite general. Contemporary reviews of much of the same literature discussed in this chapter often simply dismiss alcohol as not being the ''real cause'' of family violence (Martin, 1976). Others, with relatively little supportive evidence, relegate the role of alcohol to that of a post-hoc explanation and excuse that enables the violent husband and the abused spouse to deny any family deviance (Gelles, 1977). It is our position that alcohol use and alcoholism may influence family violence in a variety of direct and indirect ways, and that although suggestive evidence is available in some respects, we simply do not have enough data to confirm any hypotheses at this time. In the following section, we will discuss some of the ways in which alcohol and family violence could be linked, and suggest some approaches to assessing these links.

The first hypothesis that must be discussed is whether the findings considered may simply be spurious, the result of covariation between alcohol and marital violence and some other factor or combination of factors. That is, excessive drinking and violence may be produced by some other variable(s), whether individual characteristics, such as hostility or sociopathy, or family characteristics, such as marital satisfaction, family structure, or stress. Although this is certainly a possibility, the research on laboratory aggression and on marital interactions does not provide much support for this explanation. Additionally, at least one study (Leonard et al., 1985) found an association between excessive alcohol use and marital aggression after controlling for several potentially important extraneous variables. More research would be helpful, but it seems likely that the hypothesis that the relationship is completely spurious is not accurate.

Chronic excessive alcohol use can exert intense stresses on the family with or without resulting in family violence. These stresses may be economic in nature, resulting from the cost of alcohol and the loss of employment or employment at a level lower than the individual's abilities. Furthermore, there are significant costs that result from dealing with alcohol problems, such as traffic fines and higher insurance. Other family stresses may result when the alcoholic is not able or willing to fulfill his marital and parental roles and his spouse must take over. These features alone would be expected to increase overt family conflict, and in doing so would likely increase the probability of marital abuse. Additionally, there is evidence of a realignment of power structures in alcoholic families such that the hierarchy of father>mother>children is altered to mother>father>children (Jacob *et al.*, 1981). Indeed, in extreme cases, it might be expected that the alcoholic father may remove himself entirely from the hierarchy through his psychological or physical absence. Such family structures, where the mother is dominant, have been pinpointed by Straus (1973) as particularly prone to marital violence. The reason for this is unclear, although we might speculate that attempts by the father to exert dominance in the face of his wife's competence might lead to particularly harsh arguments and fights. Thus, the family stresses and the family structures that result from chronic excessive alcohol use may dispose a family toward violence.

Beyond the general impact of alcohol on family stress and structure, specific conflicts regarding drinking may erupt. Thus, excessive alcohol use may increase family violence by simple providing a highly charged personal topic of disagreement for husbands and wives. This would be particularly germane in cases where the alcoholic or heavy drinker returns home intoxicated and as a result, an argument ensues. This possibility has been suggested by Gelles (1972) and has received some preliminary support in that drunkenness is not an infrequent topic of arguments (Dvoskin, 1981).

Another way in which alcohol may relate to family violence is through its ability to serve as a "excuse" from both the abuser's and the victim's perspective (Coleman & Straus, 1979; Gelles, 1972). Thus, the abuser may vent his anger and frustrations, use drinking as an excuse, and be able to maintain a view of himself as nondeviant. His wife may believe this as well. This process was first discussed by MacAndrew and Edgerton (1969), who argued that disinhibited behavior is not a consistent feature of intoxication in all societies. Instead, such behavior appears in cultures which have adopted a "time-out" attitude toward alcohol whereby the normal social rules and sanctions are suspended during periods of intoxication. As applied currently, three different aspects of this hypothesis may be differentiated: (a) people hold expectations that alcohol consumption can result in aggression; (b) because alcohol is believed to cause the aggression, there is the expectation that an individual who behaves aggressively while intoxicated is held less responsible for his actions because there was an external cause; and (c) individuals who have been drinking feel less compelled to behave appropriately and feel free to act aggressively because they believe that they will be excused and their behavior blamed on the alcohol.

Several studies have suggested that people do, in fact, hold expectancies that alcohol will increase aggression (Brown, Goldman, Inn, & Anderson, 1980), though people hold these expectations more strongly with respect to other people's reactions to alcohol than to their own behavior (Rohsenow, 1983). A few studies have also found that alcohol in an aggressor can alter the assignment of causality for the aggressive behavior (Corenblum, 1983; Richardson & Campbell, 1980). However, the absolute decreases in blame attribution to the aggressor do not seem particularly impressive. For example, Richardson and Campbell (1980) indicated that when the male in a wife abuse scenario is depicted as sober, he was assigned 53% of the blame, with the victim, situation, and chance receiving the remainder. When he was depicted as drinking and intoxicated, he received 50% of the blame. Although these findings are consistent with an expectancies approach, they do not uniquely support the hypothesis that these expectancies lead to aggression, because it could be argued that a pharmacological effect of alcohol on aggression could have resulted in the expectancies.

Direct evidence that such expectations can lead to aggressive behavior was reviewed briefly when we considered theoretical accounts of the effects of alcohol on laboratory aggression. As we noted, the evidence suggests that such beliefs can, under certain circumstances, enhance aggressive behavior. For example, Lang *et al.* (1975) found that the expectation of receiving alcohol increased aggressive behavior among heavy social drinkers participating in a situation in which the target could not retaliate. However, such expectations do not uniformly enhance aggression (Rohsenow & Bachorowski, 1984; Shuntich & Taylor, 1972; Zeichner & Pihl, 1979). Beyond this, we can say very little. It is not known, for example, whether the role of alcohol as an excuse extends to marital interactions, or whether it is more applicable to other forms of aggressive interactions. Additionally, it is not known whether there are certain individuals, families, or situations for which this role of alcohol is particularly pertinent. Much more work is obviously necessary.

Alcohol, through its deleterious impact on attentional, interpretive, and decision-making processes, could lead more directly to instances of violence in a family. Although this approach to alcohol's impact argues for the importance of the pharmacological impact of alcohol, it also stresses the importance of the contextual setting, the characteristics of the individuals involved, and especially the interaction of the two (or more) individuals. Specifically, it is argued that alcohol alters the interaction of individuals in such a way that conflictual issues may be more likely to arise. Once generated, these issues are not likely to be dealt with satisfactorily, and are likely to escalate into a hostile and aggressive argument. In those people so disposed, the verbal assaults may escalate to physical violence. Alcohol affects these changes in several ways. First, by impairing the individual's ability to attend and interpret cues, the inebriated husband who is hostile to begin with and is in a stressful, conflictual marriage, would be likely to perceive cues from his wife in an aggressive light, whether this is accurate or not. For example, she may avoid him out of fear, but his perception could be that she is trying to punish him for his drinking. His reaction to this is likely to be hostile, and perhaps excessively so given his inability to process simultaneously cues that might mitigate his hostile response. Once this cognitive set is established, the cognitive disruptions reduce the likelihood that he will notice and correctly interpret subsequent contradictory cues as well. Further, his spouse, upon receiving an excessively hostile response, may counter with a defensive response of her own, thus establishing an escalatory cycle. If her response is not a hostile one, she may be unable for any number of reasons to formulate an unambiguously nonaggressive response that he can perceive as such, and escalation may occur anyway.

At present, most of the hypothesized links between alcoholism, acute alcohol use, and family violence have received scant research attention. Thus, these must be considered speculative. Future research is clearly necessary. However, certain pitfalls that have characterized previous work in this area need to be avoided. One major problem has been that much of the research linking alcohol and family violence has been atheoretical in nature. Although sophisticated systems approaches have developed with respect to family violence in general, there has been little speculation concerning how alcohol fits into such systems. As a consequence, the data concerning alcohol and family violence have been collected in an unsystematic fashion with many critical gaps.

A second issue is the multidimensional nature of family violence and alcoholism and alcohol use. There has been a tendency to treat family violence as a unitary concept, lumping such diverse phenomena as wife abuse, husband abuse, child neglect, child physical abuse, and sexual abuse. Although there are undoubtedly some common elements, it also seems clear that theoretically and/or empirically derived groupings would be preferable to indiscriminate combinations. Even within each of these somewhat specific categories (i.e., wife abuse, child abuse, etc.) it is likely that there are discrete subtypes that may have different chains of causality. The work by Frieze and Knoble (1980) is noteworthy in this regard. In a preliminary study, abused wives were interviewed with respect to a number of the details of their situation. These included whether alcohol or drugs were involved in the first, typical, and worst incidents of violence, whether drinking was an issue between her and her husband, whether her husband was a heavy drinker, and whether other forms of violence were present in the husband. On the basis of cluster analyses, five different groups were formed. Of importance, the role and importance of alcohol varied for each of these clusters, with one cluster where alcohol appeared to play a major role in the marital violence and a second where the marital violence was a part of a larger pattern of family violence with little contribution from alcohol.

In addition to different forms of abuse, there is the possibility that there are different stages to any given form of abuse. At the very least, it seems likely that the initial episodes of violence must differ from episodes after the violence has been firmly entrenched. Different factors may influence the initiation than influence the continuence or exacerbation of violence, and alcohol's impact may differ as well.

Finally, given the complexities and difficulties in conducting research on this issue, it is clear that there are many methodologies that can contribute to our understanding. These range from interviews with batterers and victims, to epidemiological investigations, to laboratory investigations of the effects of alcohol on aggression and communication, to structured observations of the interactions among abusive and nonabusive families. Currently, research is ongoing in all of these fields. What is needed, however, is an integrative focus among the different areas of research with more explicit ties between the diverse methodologies used to examine this issue.

REFERENCES

American Temperance Society (1972). *Permanent temperance documents of the American Temperance Society.* New York: Arno Press.

Bailey, D., Leonard, K. E., Cranston, J. W., & Taylor, S. P. (1983). Effects of alcohol and self awareness on human physical aggression. *Personality and Social Psychology Bulletin, 9,* 289–295.

Bard, M., & Zacker, J. (1974). Assaultiveness and alcohol use in family disputes. *Criminology, 12,* 281–292.

Berkowitz, L., & LePage, A. (1967). Weapons as aggression-eliciting stimuli. *Journal of Personality and Social Psychology, 7,* 202–207.

Billings, A., Kessler, M., Gomberg, C., & Weiner, S. (1979). Marital conflict-resolution of alcoholic and nonalcoholic couples during sobriety and experimental drinking. *Journal of Studies on Alcohol, 3,* 183–195.

Black, R., & Mayer, J. (1980). Parents with special problems: Alcoholism and opiate addiction. *Child Abuse and Neglect, 4,* 45–54.

Bousha, D. M., & Twentyman, C. T. (1984). Mother-child interactional style in abuse, neglect, and control groups: Naturalistic observations in the home. *Journal of Abnormal Psychology, 93,* 106–114.

Brown, S. A., Goldman, M. S., Inn, A., & Anderson, L. R. (1980). Expectations of reinforcement from alcohol: Their domain and relation to drinking patterns. *Journal of Consulting and Clinical Psychology, 48,* 419–426.

Browning, D. H., & Boatman, B. (1977). Incest: Children at risk. *American Journal of Psychiatry, 134,* 69–72.

Buss, A. (1961). *The psychology of aggression.* New York: Plenum Press.

Byles, J. A. (1978). Violence, alcohol problems and other problems in disintegrating families. *Journal of Studies on Alcohol, 39*, 551–553.

Chimbos, P. D. (1978). *Marital violence: A study of interspousal homicide.* San Francisco: R & E Research Associates.

Cobb, J. C., & McCourt, W. F. (1979, September). *Problem solving by alcoholics and their families: A laboratory study.* Paper presented at the Annual meeting of the American Psychological Association, New York.

Coleman, D. J., & Straus, M. A. (August, 1979). *Alcohol abuse and family violence.* Paper presented at the Annual meeting of the American Sociological Association. Boston, MA.

Corenblum, B. (1983). Reactions to alcohol-related marital violence: Effects of one's own abuse experience and alcohol problems on causal attributions. *Journal of Studies on Alcohol, 44*, 665–674.

Dvoskin, J. A. (1981). *Battered women: An epidemiological study of spousal violence.* Unpublished doctoral dissertation, University of Arizona.

Elmer, E. (1967). *Children in jeopardy: A study of abused minors and their families.* Pittsburgh, PA: University of Pittsburgh Press.

Fagan, J. A., Stewart, D. K., & Hansen, K. V. (1983). Violent men or violent husbands: Background factors and situational correlates. In D. Finkelhor, R. J. Gelles, G. T. Hotaling, & M. A. Straus (Eds.), *The dark side of families* (pp. 49–67). Beverly Hills, CA: Sage.

Frankenstein, W., Hay, W. M., & Nathan, P. E. (1985). Effects of intoxication on alcoholics' marital communication and problem solving. *Journal of Studies on Alcohol, 46*, 1–6.

Frieze, I. H., & Knoble, J. (1980, September). *The effects of alcohol on marital violence.* Paper presented at the Annual meeting of the American Psychological Association. Montreal, Canada.

Frieze, I. H., & Schafer, P. C. (1984). Alcohol use and marital violence: Female and male differences in reactions to alcohol. In S. C. Wilsnack & L. J. Beckman (Eds.), *Alcohol problems in women* (pp. 260–279). New York: Guilford Press.

Gaquin, D. A. (1977–78). Spouse abuse: Data from the National Crime Survey. *Victimology, 2*, 632–643.

Gayford, J. J. (1975). Wife battering: A preliminary survey of 100 cases. *British Medical Journal, 1*, 194–197.

Gelles, R. (1972). *The violent home.* Beverly Hills, CA: Sage.

Gelles, R. J. (1977). *Etiology of violence: Overcoming fallacious reasoning in understanding family violence and child abuse.* Child Protection Center of the Children's Hospital, National Medical Center, Washington, DC.

Gil, D. (1971). Violence against children. *Journal of Marriage and the Family, 33*, 637–698.

Gorad, S. L. (1971). Communicational styles and interaction of alcoholics and their wives. *Family Processes, 10*, 475–489.

Graham, K. (1980). Theories of intoxicated aggression. *Canadian Journal of Behavioral Science Review, 12*, 141–158.

Herman, J., & Hirschman, L. (1981). Families at risk for father–daughter incest. *American Journal of Psychiatry, 138*, 967–970.

Hilberman, E., & Munson, K. (1978). Sixty battered women. *Victimology, 2*, 460–471.

Hofeller, K. H. (1982). *Social, psychological, and situational factors in wife abuse.* Palo Alto, CA: R & E Research Associates.

Hull, J. G. (1981). A self awareness model of the causes and effects of alcohol consumption. *Journal of Abnormal Psychology, 90*, 586–600.

Jacob, T., Ritchey, D., Cvitkovic, J., & Blane, H. (1981). Communication styles of alcoholic and nonalcoholic families when drinking and not drinking. *Journal of Studies on Alcohol, 42*, 466–482.

Jacob, T., Dunn, N., & Leonard, K. (1983). Patterns of alcohol abuse and family stability. *Alcoholism: Clinical and Experimental Research, 7*, 382–385.

Jacob, T., Blane, H., & Dunn, N. (1986). Patterns of alcohol consumption and family adjustment. Manuscript in preparation.

Johnson, B., & Morse, H. A. (1968). Injured children and their parents. *Children, 15*, 147–152.

Julian, V., & Mohr, C. (1979). Father–daughter incest: Profile of the offender. *Victimology, 4*, 348–360.

Kaplun, D., & Reich, R. (1976). The murdered child and his killers. *American Journal of Psychiatry, 133*, 809–813.

Kennedy, D. L. (1976). Behavior of alcoholics and spouses in a simulation game situation. *Journal of Nervous and Mental Disease, 162*, 23–34.

Labell, L. S. (1979). Wife abuse: A sociological sudy of battered women and their mates. *Victimology, 4*, 258–267.

Lang, A. R., Goeckner, D. J., Adesso, V. J., & Marlatt, G. A. (1975). Effects of alcohol on aggression in male social drinkers. *Journal of Abnormal Psychology, 84,* 508–518.

Langley, R., & Levy, R. C. (1977). *Wife beating: The silent crisis.* New York: E. P. Dutton.

Leary, T. (1957). *Interpersonal diagnosis of personality.* New York: Ronald.

Leonard, K. E., Bromet, E. J., Parkinson, D. K., Day, N. L., & Ryan, C. M. (1985). Patterns of alcohol use and physically aggressive behavior. *Journal of Studies on Alcohol, 46,* 279–282.

MacAndrew, C., & Edgerton, R. B. (1969). *Drunken comportment: A social explanation.* Chicago, IL: Aldine.

MacMurray, V. D. (1979). The effect and nature of alcohol abuse in cases of child neglect. *Victimology, 4,* 29–45.

Mark, V. H., & Ervin, F. R. (1970). *Violence and the brain.* New York: Harper & Row.

Marlatt, G. A., & Rohsenow, D. J. (1980). Cognitive processes in alcohol use: Expectancy and the balanced placebo design. In N. K. Mello (Ed.), *Advances in substance abuse: Behaviorial and biological research.* Greenwich, CT: JAI Press.

Martin, D. (1976). *Battered wives.* San Francisco: Glide.

Martin, M. J., & Walters, J. (1982). Familial correlates of selected types of child abuse and neglect. *Journal of Marriage and the Family, 44,* 267–276.

Mayfield, D. (1976). Alcoholism, alcohol intoxication, and assaultive behavior. *Diseases of the Nervous System, 37,* 282–291.

Mitchell, H. E. (1959). Interpersonal perception theory as applied to conflicted marriages in which alcoholism is and is not a problem. *American Journal of Orthopsychiatry, 29,* 547–559.

Nisonoff, L., & Bitman, I. (1979). Spouse abuse. *Victimology, 4,* 131–140.

Pagano, M. R., & Taylor, S. P. (1979). Police perceptions of alcohol intoxication. *Journal of Applied Social Psychology, 10,* 166–174.

Pernanen, K. (1976). Alcohol and crimes of violence. In B. Kissin & H. Begleiter (Eds.), *The biology of alcoholism: Social aspects of alcoholism,* Vol. 4, (pp. 351–444). New York: Plenum Press.

Pernanen, K. (November, 1979). *Experiences of violence and their association with alcohol use in the general population of a community.* Paper presented at the Annual meeting of the American Society of Criminology. Philadelphia, PA.

Rada, R., Kellner, R., & Winslow, W. (1978). Drinking, alcoholism, and the mentally disordered sex offender. *Bulletin of the American Academy of Psychiatry and Law, 6,* 296–300.

Raush, H., Barry, W., Hertel, R., & Swain, M. (1974). *Communication, conflict and marriage.* San Francisco: Jossey-Bass.

Richardson, D. (1981). The effects of alcohol on male aggression toward female targets. *Motivation and Emotion, 5,* 333–344.

Richardson, D. C., & Campbell, J. L. (1980). Alcohol and wife abuse: The effect of alcohol on attributions of blame for wife abuse. *Personality and Social Psychology Bulletin, 6,* 51–56.

Robins, L., Helzer, J., Croughan, J., & Ratcliff, K. (1981). National Institute of Mental Health Diagnostic Interview Schedule: Its history, characteristics, and validity. *Archives of General Psychiatry, 38,* 381–389.

Rohsenow, D. J. (1983). Drinking habits and expectancies about alcohol's effects for self vs. others. *Journal of Consulting and Clinical Psychology, 51,* 752–756.

Rohsenow, D. J., & Bachorowski, J. (1984). Effects of alcohol and expectancies on verbal aggression in men and women. *Journal of Abnormal Psychology, 93,* 418–432.

Roizen, J. (1982). Estimating alcohol involvement in serious events. In *Alcohol and health monograph 1: Alcohol consumption and related problems,* Washington, DC: U. S. Government Printing Office.

Rounsaville, B. J. (1978). Theories in marital violence: Evidence from a study of battered women. *Victimology, 3,* 11–31.

Roy, M. (1977). A current survey of 150 cases. In M. Roy (Ed.), *Battered women: A psychosocial study of domestic violence* (pp. 25–44). New York: Van Nostrand Reinhold.

Roy, M. (1982). Four thousand partners in violence: A trend analysis. In M. Roy (Ed.), *The abusive partner: An analysis of domestic battering* (pp. 17–35). New York: Van Nostrand Reinhold.

Rule, B. G., & Percival, E. (1971). The effect of frustration and attack on physical aggression. *Journal of Experimental Research in Personality, 5,* 111–118.

Schmutte, G. T., & Taylor, S. P. (1980). Physical aggression as a function of alcohol and pain feedback. *Journal of Social Psychology, 110,* 235–244.

Schmutte, G. T., Leonard, K. E., & Taylor, S. P. (1979). Alcohol and expectations of attack. *Psychological Reports, 45,* 163–167.

Sears, J. (1977). *The effects of third-party instigation on the aggressive behavior of intoxicated and nonintoxicated subjects.* Unpublished master's thesis, Kent State University.

Shuntich, R. J., & Taylor, S. P. (1972). The effects of alcohol on human physical aggression. *Journal of Experimental Research in Personality, 6,* 34–38.

Shupe, L. M. (1954). Alcohol and crimes: A study of the urine alcohol concentration found in 882 persons arrested during or immediately after the commission of a felony. *Journal of Criminal Law and Criminology, 44,* 661–665.

Smith, S. M., Hanson, R., & Noble, S. (1973). Parents of battered babies: A controlled study. *British Medical Journal, 4,* 388–391.

Steinglass, P., & Robertson, A. (1981). The impact of alcoholism on the family. *Journal of Studies on Alcohol, 42,* 288–303.

Steinglass, P. (1983). The alcoholic family. In B. Kissin & H. Begleiter (Eds.), *The biology of alcoholism: The pathogenesis of alcoholism: Psychosocial factors Vol. 6* (pp. 243–306). New York: Plenum Press.

Straus, M. A. (1974). Leveling, civility, and violence in the family. *Journal of Marriage and the Family, 36,* 13–29.

Straus, M. A. (1973). A general systems theory approach to a theory of violence between family members. *Social Science Information, 12,* 105–125.

Taylor, S. P. (1967). Aggressive behavior and physiological arousal as a function of provocation and the tendency to inhibit aggression. *Journal of Personality, 35,* 297–310.

Taylor, S. P., & Gammon, C. B. (1975). Effects of type and dose of alcohol on human physical aggression. *Journal of Personality and Social Psychology, 32,* 169–175.

Taylor, S. P., & Gammon, C. B. (1976). Aggressive behavior of intoxicated subjects: The effect of third-party intervention. *Journal of Studies on Alcohol, 37,* 917–930.

Taylor, S. P., & Leonard, K. E. (1983). Alcohol and human physical aggression. In R. G. Geen & E. I. Donnerstein (Eds.), *Aggression: Theoretical and empirical reviews* (pp. 77–101). New York: Academic Press.

Taylor, S. P., Gammon, C. B., & Capasso, D. R. (1976). Aggression as a function of alcohol and threat. *Journal of Personality and Social Psychology, 34,* 938–941.

Taylor, S. P., Vardaris, R. M., Rawitch, A. B., Gammon, C. B., Cranston, J. W., & Lubetkin, A. I. (1976). The effects of alcohol and delta-9-tetrahydrocannabinol on human physical aggression. *Aggressive Behavior, 2,* 153–161.

Taylor, S. P., Schmutte, G. T., & Leonard, K. E. (1977). Physical aggression as a function of alcohol and frustration. *Bulletin of the Psychonomic Society, 9,* 217–218.

Taylor, S. P., Schmutte, G. T., Leonard, K. E., & Cranston, J. W. (1979). The effects of alcohol and extreme provocation on the use of a highly noxious shock. *Motivation and Emotion, 3,* 73–81.

Tinklenberg, J. (1973). Alcohol and violence. In P. Bourne & R. Fox (Eds.), *Alcoholism: Progress in research and treatment* (pp. 95–210). New York: Academic Press.

Twentyman, C. T., & Martin, B. (1978). Modification of problem interaction in mother-child dyads by modeling and behavioral rehearsal. *Journal of Clinical Psychology, 34,* 138–143.

Virkkunen, M. (1974). Alcohol as a factor precipitating aggression and conflict behavior leading to homicide. *British Journal of Addiction, 69,* 149–154.

Walker, L. (1979). *The battered woman.* New York: Harper & Row.

Weiss, R. (1980). *The area of change questionnaire.* University of Oregon: Marital Studies Program, Department of Psychology.

Wilson, C., & Orford, J. (1978). Children of alcoholics: Report of a preliminary study and comments on the literature. *Journal of Studies on Alcohol, 39,* 121–142.

Wolfgang, M. E., & Strohm, R. B. (1956). The relationship between alcohol and criminal homicide. *Quarterly Journal of Studies on Alcohol, 17,* 411–425.

Zacker, J., & Bard, M. (1977). Further findings on assaultiveness and alcohol use in interpersonal disputes. *American Journal of Community Psychology, 5,* 373–383.

Zeichner, A., & Pihl, R. O. (1979). Effects of alcohol and behavior contingencies on human aggression. *Journal of Abnormal Psychology, 88,* 153–160.

Zeichner, A., & Pihl, R. O. (1980). Effects of alcohol and instigator intent on human aggression. *Journal of Studies on Alcohol, 41,* 265–276.

17

Domestic Abuse

The Pariah of the Legal System

PATRICIA L. MICKLOW

Over the centuries, women and children have silently endured severe physical mistreatment at the hands of husbands, fathers, and other family members. Crimes of assault, rape, incest, and murder have been perpetrated against the weaker members of the family. Within a patriarchal legal system designed to adjudicate disputes between equals, the complaints of these disadvantaged members of society have often not been recognized. Traditionally regarded as property, they have been deprived of legal protection in the home and instead admonished to ''obey'' their husbands and fathers. It is illustrative of the powerlessness of their legal status that the first child protection requiring mandatory reporting of suspected child abuse and neglect was not adopted until 1963 and that no domestic abuse statutes were in effect in the United States prior to 1975.

These recent legislative reforms have begun to erode societal complacency and force a conservative legal system to acknowledge the serious and pervasive nature of the problem. Special pilot programs have been initiated in various cities to improve police and prosecutorial responses; trained victim/witness advocates are assisting traumatized victims through court proceedings. Legal scholars have proposed model legislation for remediating domestic violence and child sexual abuse. New theories of generational victimology have surfaced and the roots of crimes have been traced to the violent family.

Nevertheless, the legal system, and in particular the criminal justice system, have continued to avoid or trivialize the problem. This lack of effective response may be attributed to the callousness of the system, or the complexities of the issues, or perhaps the strength of society's need to deny the painful realities of such violent interaction between intimates. The legal system, in its most pristine state, is dependent upon a lack of familiarity between its contestants to achieve a measure of objectivity. The basic impulse of the system is to achieve anonymity so that decisions may be grounded on logic and facts and not on emotions. Domestic abuse cases require the adjudication of disputes between intimates where a prior history of emotional interdependence exists. Consequently, these cases do not easily adapt to the requirements of legal proceedings and are

PATRICIA L. MICKLOW • Judge, 96th District Court, Marquette County, MI 49855.

cast aside from traditional legal activities. Because of its objectionable nature, domestic abuse has become the pariah of the legal system.

This chapter focuses on the development of domestic abuse as a distinct and separate legal issue within our courts and legislatures. The first section reviews the legal traditions affecting court intervention into the family to regulate intrafamily violence. The second section presents an overview of the legislative reforms enacted within the past two decades in an effort to protect both adult and child victims of domestic abuse. In the third section, some major legal issues developing as a result of these reforms are examined, and the fourth section endeavors to identify the future directions of legal intervention and response.

THE LEGAL HERITAGE

Historically, the treatment of women and children under law has been extremely harsh (Brown, Emerson, Falk, & Freedman, 1971). Valued only as property or as a source of labor for the family economic unit, the law categorized married women and children with the mentally incompetent. In a nonegalitarian society, they ranked well below adult males in terms of personal autonomy. Even in early American life where equality was espoused as a principle of government, women and children continued to be denied personhood and bodily integrity. Certain unique legal policies were developed over the years to assure male dominance in the home (Cavanagh, 1971). These traditions, based on centuries of social conditioning and economic domination, have dramatically affected the position of women and children in society and have become formalized in our laws and legal institutions (Kanowitz, 1969).

Within this legacy of legal traditions, the medieval doctrine of *coverture*[1] profoundly influenced the status of married women and imposed onerous legal disabilities on most women. Under this rule, a woman lost her individual legal identity upon marriage (Blackstone, 1899). The husband and wife were deemed merged into one single legal entity identified only as the husband. Thus, a married woman became legally nonexistent. This ancient doctrine accounts for the fact that for several centuries married women were regarded as chattel of their husbands, legally incapable of owning or conveying property, of executing contracts, or of acting in any legal capacity. Although the Married Women's Property Acts, passed in the late 19th century, remedied some of these limitations, the ancient perception that women were to be treated differently than men and not accorded the full protection of the law has continued to be a persistent and reoccuring theme in American jurisprudence (Davidson, Ginsburg, & Kay, 1974).

Coverture produced several legal anomalies for women including the rule that the husband has a right of chastisement or corporal discipline over his wife. Because, under coverture, the husband became solely responsible for the acts and conduct of his wife, he was given the corresponding right to physically discipline her (Blackstone, 1899). Although it was cautioned that such discipline was to be moderate, legal authorities have claimed the colloquial phrase, "rule of thumb," is derived from the right of a husband to beat his wife with a stick "no thicker than his thumb" (Prosser, 1971, p. 136).

The first case decided in a U.S. court acknowledging the husband's right of physical

---

[1]The term *coverture* is derived from the phrases, *feme-covert*, or *foemina viro co-operta*. Because the wife is under the protection or *cover* of her husband, she is said to be *cover-baron*, and her condition during marriage is called her *coverture*. See Blackstone, 1899, *Commentaries*, pp. 442–445.

discipline over his wife occurred in 1824 (*Bradley v. State*). Stedman (1917), writing for the *Virginia Law Register,* stated that one of the reasons for this privilege of chastisement was that "a little wholesome chastising would make less noise and scandal than the publicity of a court trial." By 1864, a North Carolina court decided that the state should not interfere with domestic chastisement unless "some permanent injury be inflicted or there be an excess of violence" (p. 163). The right of chastisement was not expressly repudiated in the United States, however, until 1871 when an Alabama court (*Fulgham v. State,* p. 148) ruled in appalling explicit terms that

> the privilege, ancient though it be, to beat her with a stick, to pull her hair, choke her, spit in her face, or kick her about the floor, or to inflict upon her other like indignities is not now acknowledged by our law.

Similarly, the law has traditionally exempted husbands from the crime of marital rape. An 18th-century jurist, Sir Matthew Hale, has been credited as the author of this rule. (Hale, 1778). He decided that

> the husband cannot be guilty of a rape committed by himself upon his lawful wife, for by their mutual matrimonial consent and contract, the wife has given up herself in this kind unto her husband, which she cannot retract. (p. 629)

Hale cited no authority for this proposition but his theories have been mechanically applied in almost every jurisdiction until very recently (*State v. Smith,* 1981). The idea that the marriage contract implies consent to all sexual acts within the marriage, including those that are violent and physically forced, continues to be accepted today. Coverture also provides a rationale for assuming the wife's continuing assent to sexual acts, because upon marriage she would lack the ability to act independently of her husband. Historically, criminal liability was imposed only for those extreme situations where the husband forced his wife to have intercourse with another man.[2] Her consent to sexual intercourse with her husband could only be revoked by divorce.

Although major progress was achieved in 1920 when women were granted the right to vote after the passage of the 19th Amendment, substantial changes in the status of women did not occur. Women continued to occupy a separate and subordinate position as the common law heritage was continued in the form of discriminatory laws and institutions in every state (Davidson *et al.* 1974). The one reform that would guarantee equality for women under the law, the Equal Rights Amendment, has failed to pass congressional review or state ratification repeatedly. As a result, in sex discrimination cases a lesser legal standard is applied by courts than the strict scrutiny review required for certain suspect classifications, such as race (*Frontiero v. Richardson,* 1973; *Reed v. Reed,* 1971).

The fate of children under the law was even more dismal than that of women. Children of the poor were systematically put to work or apprenticed. According to a 1535 English statute, children between the ages of 5 and 14 "that live in idleness and be taken begging" could be "put to serve by the governors or cities, towns, etc., to husbandry or other crafts or labors," to minimize the costs of welfare (Areen, 1975, p. 894).

Under the feudal system, a minor's guardian could profit handsomely from marrying his ward to one of his own heirs or by selling the right to marry the child to a third party (Rossman, 1925). This practice was so lucrative that Henry VIII established the Court of

---

[2]As stated by Lord Hale, a wife may not be "prostituted to another" by her husband even though in marriage "she hath given up her body" to him. See 24 ALR 4th 105, Section 7, ftne. 22 quoting Hale (1736). *History of the pleas of the common crown,* p. 630.

Wards, which regulated guardianships of children by selling them to the highest bidder, accruing substantial revenues to the crown (Areen, 1975).

Although no reliable figures exist, thousands of children were separated from their families under the Elizabeth Poor law and shipped to the American colonies or impressed into the Merchant Marine (ten Brock, 1964). Later, workhouses were established to use this cheap source of labor more effectively. The early poor laws at least provided disadvantaged children with some skills in an age when no other public education or training was available. For all children, wealthy or indigent, the law provided little protection (Areen, 1975). No causes of action existed for children who were physically mistreated by their parents. Generally, any protection accorded children was motivated by their value as laborers or prospective marriage partners, rather than concern for their well-being.

The exploitation of children has not been confined to abuses of labor and discipline. The persistent use of children for the sexual gratification of adults was well established in Greek and Roman societies where child brothels, prostitution services, and marriages between boys and men were sanctioned (Algren, 1983–84; Thompson, 1984). The sexual abuse of slave children was commonplace. Over the centuries, the sexual victimization of children began to be perceived as immoral, although this new perception did not result in the development of significant protective measures for children from such abuse. The lowly status occupied by their mothers undoubtedly aggravated the problem and impeded effective protection actions (Algren, 1983–84).

Even though incest has been prohibited outwardly throughout history, that taboo has been consistently violated. Societal denial of incest has followed several courses from the widespread acceptance of Freud's theory of childhood incestuous fantasy to the family dysfunction theory proposed by Vincent DeFrancis in 1969 (Algren, 1983–84). Freud's theory not only shifted the blame for incest to the ''seductive'' child but provided a rationale for the notion that children lie or fantasize about incestuous experiences. Similarly, the family dysfunction analysis allocates partial culpability to both the child and to the mother/wife who is viewed as an inadequate sexual partner whose silence encouraged the role reversal to occur.

Related to the denial of incest is the requirement that a child's report of sexual abuse be independently corroborated as first established by an 18th-century legal commentator, John Henry Wigmore. Although modern critics have charged that his findings were distorted and prejudicial, some states still require such supporting evidence on the basis of his treatise (Algren, 1983–84; Skoler, 1984).

The first American case appealed to a higher court involving a conviction of parents for child abuse occurred in 1841 (*Johnson v. State*). The defendants were convicted of assault and battery for tying their child to a bed post, and whipping him. The case was remanded due to an improper jury instruction concerning the jury's duty to determine whether the punishment inflicted by the parents was excessive. It was not until 1874, however, that the first action by the state to intervene to protect a child from parental abuse occurred (Areen, 1975). The case received some notoriety since it involved an 8-year-old child who was reportedly rescued through the efforts of the newly formed New York Society for the Prevention of Cruelty to Animals. The court was implored to take action based on the argument that children were, after all, members of the animal kingdom. Subsequently, the first Society for the Prevention of Cruelty to Children was formed in New York City. However, it was poverty rather than cruelty that continued to be the major reason for intervention by the courts until the beginning of the 20th century.

A New York statute (N. Y. Laws) in 1922 became the first to exclude poverty from its definition of neglect as grounds for removal of a child from the home. Eventually, the *parens patriae* rule was expanded to permit the state to intervene to protect children from emotional, as well as physical harm (Areen, 1975). This crucial threshold in child protection was not crossed until 1963 when Idaho authorized intervention where a child was "emotionally maladjusted" or where a child who had been denied proper parental love or affection "behaves unnaturally and unrealistically in relation to normal situations, objects, and other persons" (Idaho Code, 1974). These reforms were given impetus by the growing body of child development literature that stressed the importance of meeting certain emotional needs of children. The experience of being raised within a family unit was regarded as particularly important.

Recognition of these theories led to new conflicts for the courts. The need to protect children from emotional and physical harm was weighed against the desire to avoid the separation of parents and children. Legitimate parental discipline had to be balanced against the need to protect children from unreasonable corporal punishment. By the turn of this century, there was also a definite movement away from institutional care for children, and today experts warn of the adverse effects of long-term or multiple foster care placements on children (Weisberg & Wald, 1984). The state, through the development of its social service intervention model, was to become the arbiter of acceptable parental behavior by midcentury. Recognition of the extent of child abuse, however, was minimal.

Two Decades of Reform

A flurry of legislative activity to respond to the plight of domestic abuse victims occurred in the two decades between 1960 and 1980. Special statutes defining child abuse and neglect and requiring mandatory reporting of suspected cases to authorities were enacted in all 50 states, the District of Columbia, and all territories of the United States (Alderman, 1979; Comment, Vanishing Exception, 1984; Thompson, 1984). Similarly, during the late 1970s new protective legislation was passed in every state and the District of Columbia to provide special remedies to adult and child victims of domestic violence (Lerman & Livingston, 1983).

The first concerns addressed were those involving the protection of children. Unlike adult victims, children who are victimized lack the knowledge, or, if very young, the ability to seek help themselves. The priority task was to develop an effective mechanism for the identification of child victims. Thus, mandatory reporting laws were created to alert authorities to suspected cases of abuse. These statutes were patterned after the required gunshot–knife wound reports existing in many states,[3] and initially required only physicians to report such cases. It quickly became evident that other medical professionals, such as nurses, medical examiners or coroners, psychiatrists, psychologists, and dentists were also in a position to identify the characteristics of abused children and should be required to report such suspicions as well.

The reporting responsibility was also imposed on other groups of professionals having regular contact with children (Thompson, 1984). All states, except New York, order teachers to make such reports. Forty-nine states and the District of Columbia require reporting from all social workers, and police officers must report in at least 45 states. A

---

[3]For example, Michigan Compiled Laws, Sec. 750.411 (1963) requires verbal and written reports to law enforcement agencies for nonaccidental injuries inflicted "by a gun, knife, or any other violence."

majority of jurisdictions have ordered that day care personnel or anyone entrusted with the care of children report suspected incidents of child abuse and neglect. Most of the jurisdictions impose only criminal liability on those professionals who are required to report but fail to do so. Only five states attach civil liability to such omissions.[4]

State statutes requiring mandatory reporting vary as to the responsibilities required in response to the reports filed. Most mandate that an investigation into the matter be initiated within a specific time after the report is received (usually 24 to 48 hours) to determine whether the information is verifiable. The responsibility for conducting the investigation is commonly assigned to a public social work agency. The agency personnel may then interview the parents and child and question any person having information about the matter including neighbors, relatives, or a professional who has treated the child. If the findings from the investigation warrant action to protect the child, the family may be offered services or treatment on a voluntary basis. If the family is unwilling to accept voluntary services (or such treatment proves to be unsatisfactory or ineffective), the agency may initiate civil proceedings in a juvenile or family court requesting court supervision on the grounds that the child has been abused or neglected as defined by the applicable statute.

The parents or guardians are generally provided all of the requisite legal formalities of due process: written notice of the allegations, legal representation, a hearing before an impartial fact finder, and the opportunity to present testimony and evidence (Landau, Salus, & Stiffarm, 1980). In most jurisdictions, a *guardian ad litem* or attorney is appointed to represent the child's interests. If the court determines that abuse or neglect has occurred, either after a hearing or through the admissions of the parent, a treatment or dispositional procedure follows in which the court decides whether the child should be removed from the home and placed in foster care or whether the family relationships may be maintained in the home under the supervision of the child protection agency. In arriving at its decision, the court commonly relies on studies and reports from professionals provided to the investigating agency (Weisberg & Wald, 1984).

If the child is removed from the home, the court is generally required to review the matter periodically, usually every 6 months, and determine whether or not any changes in the parents' behavior or the conditions of the home have occurred justifying the return of the child to the home. If the agency believes it is appropriate to remove the child permanently from parental custody, a separate hearing based on a higher standard of proof is required to terminate parental rights.

It should be noted that all states also have various criminal statutes in existence to use against the assailant in cases of physical abuse, such as assault and battery, assault with a weapon, and child cruelty. However, unless the injuries are particularly severe or life threatening or the cause of death, few agencies actively seek to impose these criminal sanctions in addition to the child protection proceedings (Note, The battering parent, 1984).

Beyond the child protection laws, certain statutory reforms to assist in the protection of child and adult victims of sexual abuse have been enacted in most states. Generally, each state relies on a combination of its child protection statues and various criminal

---

[4]See Arkansas Statutes Annotated Sec. 42.816(b) (1977); Colorado Revised Statutes Sec. 19.10-104(4)(b) (1978); Iowa Code Annotated Sec. 232 75(2) (West 1984–85); Michigan Compiled Laws Annotated Sec. 722.633(1) (West 1984–85); N. Y. Social Service Law Sec. 420(2) (McKinney 1976). Of these states, only Michigan has adopted a negligence standard as the basis for liability.

sexual conduct offenses to respond to cases of child sexual abuse by a parent, step-parent, or other adult within the home. In the late 1970s, legislatures began to overhaul their statutory schemes concerning sexual offenses (Algren, 1983–84) and deleted such unworkable and legally vague references as ''carnal knowledge,'' ''lewd and lascivious acts,'' and ''abominable crimes against nature'' that characterized most rape statutes (Bulkey, 1982). These reforms vastly improved the ability of law enforcement agencies to prosecute successfully various sexual crimes. The new laws explicitly defined a broader range of sexual offenses against adults and children, and generally provided a graduated system of sexual crimes based on severity with a corresponding tier of penalties. However, only half of the states now include sexual abuse within their child protection laws. Thus, the mandatory reporting provisions and the supervision and remedies available through juvenile court jurisdiction for intrafamilial child sexual abuse are not consistently triggered in child sexual abuse cases (Bulkey, 1982).

Another reform thrust is to provide civil protection orders for sexually abused children patterned after the domestic violence and battered women's remedies (Algren, 1983–84). These orders permit a civil court to order the offender out of the home rather than removing the child victim from his or her home, family, and school (Bulkey, 1983b). Civil protection orders may be drafted to include counseling and treatment orders, payment of support, restitution for medical expenses, or attorneys' fees (Bulkey, 1983b). Further, such orders are generally enforceable by criminal contempt proceedings. Protective orders are usually sought concurrently through juvenile court proceedings or civil protection orders to assure that the child will be in a safe environment and receive whatever services may be appropriate. Authorities may also charge an offender under criminal statutes to gain control over his conduct through incarceration or probation.

The most appropriate form of intervention in cases of child sexual abuse continues to be the subject of vigorous debate (Finkelhor, 1984). The more progressive programs disfavor punitive measures against the perpetrator, and encourage a family treatment mode to provide counseling and support to the victim and the entire family. Most experts agree, however, that certain coercive legal tools, such as the threat of prosecution, provide the incentive to effect these changes (Algren, 1983–84; Bulkey, 1983a). Alternatives to traditional prosecution include pretrial diversion and postconviction programs that focus on the rehabilitation of the offender with the threat that a penal sentence may be imposed if the defendant fails to cooperate.

The laws passed in the 1970s and early 1980s to provide protection to women victims physically assaulted by a husband or intimate also encompassed civil and criminal remedies (Lerman & Livingston, 1983). Advocates stressed the need for recognition of the criminal nature of these batterings to promote more effective responses from police, prosecutors, and judges (Eisenberg & Micklow, 1977). It was believed that if such incidents were acknowledged as crimes rather than trivialized as domestic disturbances, women victims would be assured of some relief. Of paramount concern was the interest in providing for the physical safety of domestic abuse victims through immediate arrest procedures, shelters, and hotlines. (Martin, 1976). Divorce proceedings and the injunctive protections usually available during such actions provided other entry points into the legal system for victims.

Even though prosecution was perceived to be the most appropriate remedy against abusers, the criminal justice system presented serious hurdles for women victims to overcome. Criminal laws were available in every jurisdiction to prosecute assailants for assaults; however, these laws were seldom enforced against domestic batterers (Comment, The battered wife's dilemma, 1981). Only in cases where the violence had escalated to a stage of severe injury or death were such incidents likely to be given priority by police or prosecutors.

Several justifications traditionally have been cited for this inaction. In general, prior relationship crimes are considered less serious than those involving strangers (Silberman, 1978), or at least, not as predictable. The criminal system differentiates between victims of assaults by strangers and victims of domestic assaults, creating a special category with a higher standard of intervention for the latter. The professionals in the system suffered from the same myths surrounding the nature and prevalence of the problem as that evidenced in society as a whole (Ellis, 1984; Lerman, 1981; Pastoor, 1984). The view that families could better survive by not permitting outside interference was, and still is, a strong justification for inaction. It was widely accepted that the home should be screened from the scrutiny of the state, and husbands and wives allowed to settle their "private" matters (Brodie, 1972). Outdated psychological theories about women, such as Freud's female masochism, were relied on to justify the reluctance of abuse victims to leave the home and the assailant (Langley & Levy, 1977; Martin, 1976; Stallone, 1984). Victims were thought to provoke, or even to enjoy, the violence. The violence was not seen as the responsibility of the batterer. Rather it was judged to be a product of the relationship or the result of the interaction of the individuals (Roy, 1977).

Understandably, the attrition rate of domestic assaults was high at every stage of the legal proceedings and usually did not survive the initial contact (Lerman, 1981; Pastoor, 1984). Victim noncooperation was probable. Police typically were discouraged after responding to multiple calls at a residence followed by victim withdrawal or recantation. Prosecutors were convinced on the basis of practical experience that they could not rely on domestic abuse victims and generally expected them to withdraw prior to any court appearance, an expectation that often generated that very result (Ellis, 1984; Lerman, 1984). Even if the victim's fear, or emotional or financial dependency on the assailant was recognized as a factor that contributed to her reluctance to testify, the practical difficulties of prosecuting all spouse abuse cases were sufficient to discourage already overloaded prosecutors. Many of them required the victim to appear physically to sign the complaint, or refused to authorize warrants until "a cooling off period" had expired in an effort to assure victim commitment to completion of the process (Ellis, 1984; Lerman, 1984).

From the point of view of the victim, however, many of these techniques had a chilling effect on her willingness to become involved in the criminal justice system (Eisenberg & Micklow, 1977). Many victims complained that police and prosecutors identified too closely with the assailant and failed to provide protection when contacted (Lerman, 1984; Woods, 1981). In some jurisdictions, police refused to respond to domestic disputes unless the use of a weapon was alleged. Even if the police did respond to a call for assistance and a criminal warrant was eventually authorized for the assailant's arrest, he would generally be able to post bond immediately and return home, often to inflict another assault. Criminal cases were fraught with delays and rescheduled hearings.

Similarly, if a wife attempted to terminate the relationship through civil divorce proceedings, the enforcement of any civil injunctive orders that may have been issued by the court in the interim could not occur until notice and a date for hearing were set by the court. This procedure often took several days and, of course, was ineffective in providing protection from multiple acts of violence (Lerman, 1984). Although violation of these protective orders invokes a criminal contempt citation, such transgressions did not automatically result in arrest without a written order from the court or a bench warrant.

Consequently, a pending divorce often caused more danger and less relief for abused wives than remaining in the marriage (Eisenberg & Micklow, 1977). Police could also ignore interspousal assaults during the pendancy of a divorce on the basis that "a civil action" was already initiated.

To address these issues, early efforts by feminists, legal services attorneys, and women's organizations led to the enactment of creative statutory schemes to enable women to gain equal access to the criminal justice agencies, the courts, and places of safety (Lerman & Livingston, 1983). First of all, warrantless arrest provisions were adopted to allow police to arrest immediately at the scene of a domestic dispute without the necessity of securing a criminal arrest warrant. Generally, most domestic assaults are misdemeanor crimes that require a warrant before an arrest is permitted, unless the offense occurs within the presence of the officer. As a result, officers rarely were allowed to arrest the assailant immediately. This specific reform now provides police agencies with the tool needed to defuse immediately a violent episode between intimates. In jurisdictions where it is utilized, it appears to be effective (Lerman, 1981; Sherman & Berk, 1984). It has the added benefit of emphasizing the message that society will not tolerate this type of violence in the home, a signal that domestic assailants traditionally have not received. Recently, some states have imposed additional responsibilities on police officers in these cases to provide specific services to victims if an arrest is not effected, such as requiring that the police officer stay until the victim is no longer in danger or mandating the police officer to use all means necessary to prevent further abuse. (Lerman, 1984; Lerman & Livingston, 1983).

The majority of the new laws, however, have concentrated on the expansion of injunctive-type orders to provide civil protections to victims (Lerman & Livingston, 1983). In most states, these protective orders have been made available regardless of whether the woman is married or has initiated divorce or separate maintenance proceedings. Although such statutes permit the court to order a potential assailant to desist from such abuse, many also insure that the abuser is denied access to the residence of the victim, prohibited from removing a minor child from the home without a court order, and in some cases, obligated to continue to provide financial support to the victim. Some of these orders may be initiated by the victim herself through the use of specially prepared forms available from the court. In almost every state, these injunctions are enforceable through a criminal contempt proceeding that essentially allows a civil court to impose a fine or incarceration in the county jail for violation of the orders. To assure prompt enforcement, some states have allowed a warrantless arrest immediately upon violation of such an order provided the defendant has received notice that such as order exists and proof of that notice is on file with a proper court or law enforcement agency.

The advantage of these protective orders are many. First, the victim herself may initiate the process for securing such an order and participate directly in its enforcement by reporting violations to the court. Second, the orders are flexible enough to provide for all of the forms of protection needed in most situations. Third, the court may impose punishment as soon as the assailant has received notice of the violation and appears at a hearing scheduled for that purpose. Because the assailant usually appears before the judge who originally signed the order, the court has a stake in guaranteeing enforcement of its own order.

Some difficulties with these orders, however, involve the crucial elements of cost and delay. If the victim is not allowed to prepare and file her own order, it is necessary for her to secure the services of an attorney and to compensate him or her for the preparation of the original motion and order as well as each subsequent violation of the order. Also, if no immediate arrest provision is available to enforce these orders, a significant delay may occur between the time of the violation and the ability of the victim to give notice to the defendant of the violation and secure a hearing date. The general tendency of the various jurisdictions, however, has been to continue to develop unique applications of the protective orders for domestic abuse victims and to expand, rather than limit, their use.

The most remarkable outcome of the battered women's movement has been the proliferation of shelters across the country. These shelters offer a variety of emergency services to abused women and their children and provide a structure for networking between communities and states. Services include emergency hotlines; individual and group counseling; advocacy services; emergency medical care, food, clothing and transportation; specialized services for children; and outreach services to inform the community of available resources. Foremost, however, these shelters and services provide the means to diffuse the violence immediately by providing the means for the victim leave the violent relationship. The support received from the staff and other residents at the shelters alleviates the sense of isolation most battered women experience. A significant number of states provide funding to support partially these grassroot organizations (Lerman & Livingstone, 1983), although inadequate, unstable funding still plagues almost every women's shelter and services project in the country. To address this issue, approximately half of the states have enacted a marriage license surcharge fee to fund domestic violence shelters and service programs (Lerman & Livingston, 1983). In addition to these fees, a few states impose a surcharge on divorce filing fees and others use fines imposed on abusers to provide shelter funds and services.

Reforms to criminalize violent marital rapes, however, have not been nearly as successful. By far the most brutal and insidious of all crimes between intimates, it has also been the least acknowledged. Until very recently, the courts were nearly unanimous in their view that a husband could not be convicted of rape against his wife under any circumstances, regardless of the force used (*State v. Smith,* 1981). This rule was codified in most states by language that specifically exempted husbands from the criminal rape statutes. Others have been implied in the laws of the state by reference to common law doctrine. Even the Model Penal Code (1962) retains the spousal exclusion by defining the act of rape as sexual intercourse between a male and "a female not his wife."

Despite extensive lobbying efforts, only a few states have totally abolished the exemption (Marital Rape Exemption, 1980). Many allow criminal prosecution only if the couple are living separately and/or have filed for divorce or separate maintenance actions. (Barry, 1980). Some states have deleted the exception for certain degrees of criminal sexual abuse only.

Even more distressing than the halting pace of the reforms is the decision in several jurisdictions to extend this "marital right" to unmarried persons (Barry, 1980; Marital Rape Exemption, 1980), despite the fact that the basis for such a rule was a valid marriage contract. Although many of these states require cohabitation as an element of the exemption, several provide partial immunity from prosecution for "date rape" in which the victim was the "voluntary social companion" of the defendant and had previously allowed him sexual contact.[5]

---

[5] It is noteworthy that courts have required an express or implied agreement between cohabiting unmarried partners before support ("palimony") or property division is ordered, whereas no such requirement has been present in the expansion of the marital rape exemption.

Consequently, the two decades of reform between 1960 and 1980 have generated some important changes in the laws to assist battered women and children. However, the reluctance of the legal system and state legislators to confront those situations where sexual assaults occur between intimates, and the uneven enforcement of the new laws, continues to plague the progress of providing needed protection to a distinct class of victims.

SPECIAL LEGAL ISSUES

Although many innovative steps have been undertaken to provide practical and effective responses to the problem, some new legal disputes, including constitutional conflicts, have surfaced in family violence cases. The development of the defense of self-defense to apply to battered women in homicide cases and the criminalization of marital rape are two examples of evolving legal questions directly resulting from the dramatic changes in the levels of awareness concerning intrafamily violence. Another complex issue precipitated by the recent legislative changes involves the need to reconcile privileged communications to professionals with mandatory reporting duties in child abuse cases. Finally, special procedures are being created for child sexual abuse cases, in response to the special difficulties posed by child witnesses giving in-court testimony. Although not exhaustive, these issues are illustrative of the extensive changes influencing our legal institutions.

Admissibility of Battered Woman's Syndrome in Homicide Cases

With certain reservations, a growing number of United States courts are admitting expert testimony concerning the battered woman's syndrome[6] in homicide cases to aid in establishing a claim of self-defense. Although this concept does not constitute a new defense for battered women who kill husbands or intimates (Recent Development; The Expert as Educator, 1982), the battered woman syndrome has a limited application in self-defense pleas. Generally, such evidence is only admissible to establish the complexities of the violent relationship and the effect violence has on the battered woman's perceptions of danger.

Traditionally, the law of self-defense exonerates a person who kills in the reasonable belief that such action was necessary to prevent death or serious injury, even if this belief is later proven to be mistaken. Thus, if a defendant reasonably believed that there was imminent danger to his or her life, the law may declare such aggressive actions justifiable.

In the case of a battered woman, where such a killing occurs during a violent episode, criminal charges usually are not brought against the woman if it is apparent she was acting in self-defense. However, in many of these cases, an interspousal homicide occurs hours or even days after the latest battering incident. If the batterer had no weapon or was not violently aggressive at the time of the fatal incident, the traditional application of the law of self-defense would lead to the conclusion that the battered woman could not have reasonably believed that she was in imminent danger at the time of the homicide.

---

[6]The *battered woman syndrome* refers to the unique psychological and behavioral reactions to common factors that are exhibited by a woman who is living in a violent relationship; the factors include fear, frustration, stress disorders, depression, economic and emotional dependence on the husband, hopes that the marital relationship will improve, poor self-image, isolation, and learned helplessness. See *State v. Kelly,* 35 CrL 2331 (Wash. Sup. Ct. 1984); *Ibn-Tamas v. U.S.,* 407 A2d 626 (D.C. 1979).

Commentators have observed that the traditional concept of self-defense has the element of a male contest, matching equal force with equal force, and therefore, is not technically applicable to the situation where a battered woman perceives her life to be in danger given a prior history of violent assaults (Comment, Self-defense, 1984). Previously, in cases where the actions of the battered woman did not conform to the traditional requirements of self-defense, a diminished capacity or insanity defense was often used to defend the woman's actions (Recent Development, The Expert as Educator, 1982). These defenses impose onerous consequences on a defendant because such an approach requires testimony of mental illness and may result in commitment to a mental institution. A successful defense of self-defense, however, results in acquittal.

The first successful use of expert testimony to establish the battered woman's syndrome in a self defense claim occurred in the landmark decision of *Ibn-Tamas v. United States* (1983). The defendant, who was 4 months pregnant at the time of the shooting, testified that on the day she shot her husband he had severely beaten her, threatened her with a gun, and told her that he would ''get her out of the house one way or another'' (p. 630). According to her testimony this was only one of many incidents of violence that had occurred during their marriage, and when she fired the gun at her husband she believed that he had a gun and was preparing to kill her (p. 631). The prosecution based its case of premediated murder on the fact that the deceased was not armed, had been ambushed on the stairs, and then shot at point-blank range as he lay wounded on the floor.

The trial court excluded the testimony on the battered woman's syndrome proposed by the defense and the defendant was convicted of second degree murder. On appeal, the District of Columbia Court of Appeals reversed the defendant's conviction on the basis that such expert testimony was admissible where it was offered to assist the jury in evaluating the woman's state of mind at the time the offense occurred. Ordinarily, experts are not permitted to testify about matters which are within the general knowledge or competency of the jurors. The appeals court, stating that the logical reaction of a woman in the defendant's position would have been to call the police from time to time or to have left her husband, concluded that expert testimony would have provided an interpretation of the facts that differed from the ordinary person's perception and was thus ''beyond the ken of the average layman'' (p. 635). The court observed that information to explain why the behavior of battered women is at variance with the ordinary lay perception could provide a basis from which a jury could understand why the defendant perceived herself in imminent danger at the time of the shooting.

Several other jurisdictions following the lead in *Ibn-Tamas* have admitted expert testimony on the battered woman's syndrome in support of self-defense claims. The Georgia Supreme Court (*Smith v. State,* 1981, p. 686), holding that the expert testimony should be admitted, stated that

> the expert's testimony explaining why a person suffering from battered woman's syndrome would
> not leave her mate, would not inform police or friends, and would fear increased aggression
> against herself, would be such conclusions that jurors could not ordinarily draw for themselves.

Other states where expert testimony concerning the syndrome has been admitted in reported cases include Maine (*State v. Anaya,* 1981); West Virginia (*State v. Dozier,* 1979), New Hampshire (*State v. Baker,* 1980); Florida (*Hawthorne v. State,* 1982); Kansas (*State v. Green,* 1982); New Jersey (*State v. Kelly,* 1984); and Washington (*State v. Allery,* 1984).

However, some jurisdictions have rejected such testimony in self-defense cases. The Ohio Supreme Court in *State v. Thomas* (1981) affirmed the defendant's conviction and upheld a trial court decision that had ruled expert testimony on the battered woman's syndrome inadmissible. In *Thomas,* the defendant testified that she feared for her life when she shot the deceased in self-defense. According to the testimony, she had suffered repeated abuse from her common law husband over a 3-year period and during a battering had picked up a gun lying on a nearby sofa. She testified that her husband then made a move toward her and she shot him because she knew the decedent would have taken the gun and killed her for having dared to pick up the weapon. The court ultimately ruled that the testimony on the battered wife syndrome was properly excluded by the trial court and that such testimony was irrelevant and immaterial to the issue of whether the defendant acted in self-defense at the time of the shooting. The court reasoned that the subject of the expert testimony was within the understanding of the jury, and that the battered wife syndrome was not sufficiently developed as a matter of commonly accepted scientific knowledge to warrant testimony under the guise of expertise (p. 140). Finally, the court contended that the prejudicial impact of such testimony outweighed its probative value. The court expressed the fear that the admission of such testimony "would tend to stereotype the defendant" causing the jury to "decide the facts based on typical, and not the actual, facts" (p. 140).

Earlier that same year, the Wyoming Supreme Court (*Buhrle v. State,* 1981) rejected the admission of such expert testimony although it did not bar all future use of evidence on the battered woman's syndrome. The court ruled that research relating to the syndrome was still in its infancy and that its recognition was limited to people actually engaged in the research. This case, however, is distinguishable on its facts from other similar homicide cases in that the wife went to the motel where her husband was staying carrying a rifle and rubber globes. After the shooting, which took place through the motel room door with the night chain still in place, the wife attempted to hide the gun and gloves and deny her role in the shooting. Similarly, a Missouri appellate court (*State v. Martin,* 1984) rejected the use of such testimony in a case where a wife had hired a "hit man" to kill her husband, claiming that she took such actions in self-defense.

Although some commentators (Acker & Toch, 1985) claim that the use of such expert testimony to buttress self-defense claims implies a hopeless problem that can only be remediated by violence, most of the courts that have considered the question have found the battered woman's syndrome admissible for the limited purpose of helping the jury to evaluate the claim of self-defense. Other experts (Comment, Self-defense, 1984; Recent Development. The Expert as Educator, 1982) suggest that the role of the expert as educator would dispel a jury's misconceptions about battered women and draw the focus of the testimony away from the implication that the battered woman's syndrome presents a new defense to murder.

The Criminalization of Spousal Rape

In those few states where the viability of the marital rape exemption has been questioned, the majority of courts have upheld the prohibition. Allowing a husband to be prosecuted for the rape of his wife, some have argued, violates the constitutional protections of due process and equal protection because the prevailing rule has always been to the contrary. Another legal attack on the rule has been based on the contention that the exemption was implicity incorporated into most states' statutory definition of that crime through the common law and thus does not require an express exemption to be legally in force. This argument, of course, would apply only in those jurisdictions where no explicit reference is made to a martial exemption in the rape statute. Very few legislatures or courts, however, have been persuaded that the exemption should be eliminated.

In a 1981 Massachusetts case, *Commonwealth v. Chretien,* a defendant charged with spousal rape asserted a constitutional due process defense on the basis that he had no fair notice that such conduct was now regarded as criminal under the laws of Massachusetts. Because the spousal exclusion had been in effect for so long, the defendant argued, the court should be precluded from applying a new interpretation of the law to his case. Although the court ultimately rejected this argument, it admitted that the due process claim might have been successful if the wife had not already obtained an interlocutory decree and lived separately from her husband even though the divorce was not yet final. The court reasoned that this decree was sufficient to put the husband on notice that his behavior was unlawful. The fact that the sexual assault had occurred in the presence of the couple's 9-year-old son also appeared to have had an impact on the court's decision.

The New Jersey Supreme Court in *State v. Smith,* in 1981 rejected similar claims by a defendant in a landmark opinion. New Jersey had recently enacted a new code of criminal justice that expressly excludes marriage to the victim as a defense against prosecution for sexual crimes. The incident with which the defendant was charged, however, had occurred prior to the effective date of the new code. At the time of the attack, the parties were living in separate cities and had been separated for over a year. The defendant was charged with breaking into his estranged wife's apartment and repeatedly beating and raping her over a period of several hours causing her severe injuries requiring hospitalization. The trial judge reluctantly granted the defendant's motion to dismiss the charge on the basis that the common law of the state implicitly incorporated a marital exemption from the crime of rape under the old statute. The appeals court affirmed the decision but on the basis that the due process clause of the 14th Amendment prohibited the retroactive application of new principles of law against the defendant. The New Jersey Supreme Court reversed both lower court rulings, refusing to apply Sir Matthew Hale's rationale that upon marriage an implied consent to intercourse became irrevocable. Observing that such reasoning may have been persuasive at a time "when marriages were effectively permanent," the Court stated that the rule should not prevail when those conditions have changed (p. 44). Similarly, the *Smith* court was not persuaded by the due process defense, stating that its holding was not an unforeseeable judicial enlargement of a criminal statute.

The strongest judicial rejection of the rule, however, has occurred recently in New York (*People v. Liberta,* 1984). In this case, the defendant, while living separately from his wife (as required by a Family Court protection order), forcibly raped and sodomized her in the presence of their 2½-year-old son. He was convicted of first-degree rape and first-degree sodomy at the trial court level and appealed the judgment. The New York rape statute in effect at the time contained a partial exemption that did not apply if the parties were living apart pursuant to a valid and effective court order. The New York Court of Appeals not only upheld the conviction, but struck the marital exemption from the first-degree rape and first-degree sodomy statutes so that any person who commits such acts "by forcible compulsion" (p. 579) is guilty regardless of marital relationship. Rejecting all of the traditional rationales advanced in support of the exemption, the court found no rational basis[7] for distinguishing between marital rape and nonmarital rape. Stating that "a married woman has the same right to control her body as does an unmarried woman," the opinion discarded the implied consent argument as "irrational and absurd" (p. 573). The court stressed that rape is not an erotic sexual act but a degrading, violent assault that violates the bodily integrity of the victim and frequently causes severe, long-lasting physical and psychic harm.

Although the New Jersey, Massachusetts, and New York courts may be illustrative of the direction of judicial opinions in the future, the overwhelming number of jurisdictions have clung to the rule or at least have seriously limited the remedies available. In both Missouri (*State v. Drope*, 1971) and North Carolina (*State v. Martin*, 1973), courts approved the principle that a husband may enforce his right to sexual intercourse with his wife without criminal responsibility. The New Mexico Supreme Court ruled in 1977 in *State v. Bell* that a wife is irrebuttably presumed to consent to sexual relations with her huband even if it is obtained through force and without consent. In *People v. Brown* (1981), the Colorado Supreme Court upheld the constitutionality of its marital rape exception for two reasons. First, the exemption allows the resumption of normal marital relations and encourages the state's interest in preserving the marriage. Second, the problems of proof inherent in such a case are avoided, and juries are not required to fathom the intimate sexual feelings and habits unique to the relationship. The court concluded that such a rule was neither arbitrary nor irrational. Other jurisdictions where the exemption has been upheld include Oregon (*State v. Aronhalt*, 1974; Texas (*Rozell v. State*, 1973); Pennsylvania (*Commonwealth v. Schilling*, 1981); Utah (*State v. Kennedy*, 1980); and Louisiana (*State v. Pratt*, 1970).

A more circuitous, and less justifiable approach, was presented in a recent Virginia case (*Kizer v. Commonwealth*, 1984). Construing a partial marital rape exemption that holds a husband criminally responsible if the wife conducts herself in a manner that established a *de facto* end to the marriage, the court held that the wife's vacillating conduct did not sufficiently manifest her intent to end the marriage to her husband. The couple no longer lived together, and had not had sexual intercourse for 6 months prior to the incident. The court found her actions "equivocal, ambivalent, and ambiguous" on the basis that she had returned to the husband once after the initial separation and had cancelled an appointment with a divorce lawyer. The court ignored the fact that at the time of the incident the wife was attempting to lock her apartment door when her husband kicked in the door to gain entry. The dissent also pointed out that the husband should have been aware of the termination of the relationship, because he had earlier filed suit to gain custody over the couple's son.

Policy reasons for continuing the marital rape exemption continue to be debated. Many within the criminal justice system believe that this type of situation should not have a criminal remedy but instead be resolved through a civil proceeding such as divorce or separation. Others fear that the dissolution of this rule would lead to frivolous complaints by wives against husbands to retaliate or gain a legal advantage against their husband in a divorce proceeding (Barry, 1980). The likelihood that married women will fabricate complaints is probably no greater than the possibility of unmarried women doing so and

---

[7]Where a statute draws a distinction based on marital status, the classification must be reasonable and must be based on "some ground of difference that rationally explains the different treatment" *Eisenstadt v. Baird*, 405 US 437, 447 (1972).

the criminal justice system is presumed to be capable of handling false complaints (*People v. Liberta,* 1984). Further, to allow a criminal remedy for a physical battering or assault but deny such a charge where the battering includes a sexual assault focuses on the sexual nature of the act or the relationship, ignores the actual criminal act that has occurred, and excuses the assailant from responsibility for his actions. To prohibit flatly criminal prosecution in all marital rape cases is too rigid a rule and allows the violent criminal a ready and defenseless victim. At a minimum, prosecution should be available in those cases where physical injury occurs or a weapon is used. These distinctions must be faced by the criminal justice system and state legislatures if women are to receive effective protection from sexual attack under law.

Privileged Communications and the Child Abuse Exception

The legal requirement that certain professionals have a duty to report suspected instances of child abuse and neglect to authorities often conflicts with their professional responsibility to respect the confidential communications disclosed by patients or clients. The law recognizes that certain relationships are worthy of protection for public policy reasons, and thus privileged (Note, Defendant v. Witness, 1978). Accordingly, the statements made to an attorney by a client or by a patient to a physician during the course of treatment are deemed relationships in which frankness is essential and privacy should be assured. The person who discloses private information to a professional is deemed the holder of the privilege, and such privileged communications cannot be revealed by the professional without the consent of the holder of the privilege. Although the laws of privilege vary from state to state, most jurisdictions have enacted statutes recognizing such privileges as physician-patient, psychotherapist-patient, psychologist-patient, and attorney-client.

These privileges reflect strong societal interests in encouraging persons to seek professional advice and treatment without fear of exposure; however, they are not absolute. Public policy arguments favoring disclosure must be weighed against the privacy issues involved. The state, for example, has a continuing interest in providing all evidence available for its legal proceedings. Each member of the community must sacrifice time, effort, and personal privacy to provide testimony necessary to learn the truth in legal proceedings (Comment, Vanishing Exception, 1984). With the passage of the mandatory reporting laws to detect child abuse and neglect, the states have articulated another compelling state interest favoring disclosure: the protection of minors from abuse and neglect. Although the purpose of these mandatory reporting laws is to identify child victims and provide appropriate state intervention to prevent further abuse, the abusers may be subject to criminal proceedings as a result of such reports. The initiation of criminal charges triggers the constitutional protections all defendants are entitled to, particularly the Fifth Amendment prohibition against self-incrimination (Note, The Psychotherapist–Patient Privilege, 1984). Disclosure of privileged communications in child abuse/neglect cases, therefore, may require the balancing of the need to protect children against the rights of the defendant to privacy and against self-incrimination.

As a result, many professionals (particularly mental health professionals) have found themselves in a conflicting and often confusing position. Because the new reforms generally abrogate all privileged relationships (some states except attorney/client privilege), professionals are often placed in the difficult position of being informed by a patient that he or she has abused a child. In some circumstances, the condition of the patient (i.e., severe alcohol or drug abuse, or certain forms of mental illness), may provide indirect evidence indicating the likelihood that child abuse or neglect may occur in that family in the future. The professional must determine not only the type of information to disclose but the extent of the information that must be revealed. For example, may the professional simply provide a statement to the authorities that an individual child is the victim of abuse or neglect, or must the professional provide all of the details disclosed by the patient? May more information be disclosed in court as opposed to out of court revelations? Is a professional required to report subsequent instances of abuse in the same family affecting the same child?

To complicate matters, the child abuse exemptions are not uniform between the states and are often vague and unclear. Some apply only to certain professionals; others only to particular proceedings, such as abuse or neglect hearings, but not termination of parental rights hearings. In approximately half of the states, professional privilege is abrogated only in a child abuse proceeding resulting from a required report (Weisberg & Wald, 1984). Thus, if no mandatory report initiated the proceeding, the privilege exemption is not applicable. Further, some pertinent information concerning suspected child abuse or neglect may be found in agency records rather than within confidential communications to a professional. Records are subject to other federal and state rules and regulations governing disclosure. Examples of these are records held by mental health agencies, schools, social welfare programs, and drug and alcohol abuse treatment programs.

In *People v. Stritzinger* (1983), the California Supreme Court grappled with many of the issues surrounding the privileged communications issue. In that case, the defendant allegedly sexually abused his 14-year-old stepdaughter over a 15-month period. When the victim's mother learned of these occurrences, she arranged appointment with a licensed psychotherapist for both the child and her stepfather. During her visit to the therapist, the child confirmed the sexual incidents with her stepfather, and the therapist reported the information to a child welfare agency as required by the California Child Abuse Reporting Act (1984). After the child welfare agency relayed this information to the police, a deputy sheriff telephoned the therapist to further investigate the report and learned that the therapist was scheduled to meet with the stepfather later that day. The investigating officer telephoned the doctor after the session and, although the therapist was reluctant to disclose the confidential communications made by his patient, the deputy sheriff cited the abrogation of privilege provision within the California Penal Code (1982). The doctor was persuaded to disclose that the stepfather had confirmed the child's earlier complaint. Later, the psychotherapist was allowed to testify at trial to the substance of these communications and the defendant was convicted of child molestation.

On appeal to the California Supreme Court, the issue presented was whether the trial court erroneously admitted the psychotherapist's testimony in violation of the psychotherapist–patient privilege or whether the California Child Abuse Reporting Act and the Penal Code provided an exception to the privilege that would allow the testimony. The court ruled that the privilege had been violated when the psychotherapist testified regarding his consultation with the defendant. Acknowledging that the child abuse exception imposes the affirmative duty to report all known and suspected instances of child abuse, the court found the time sequence of the counseling sessions significant. The court reasoned that by making his initial report, the doctor had satisfied his statutory reporting obligation and was not required to make subsequent reports of the same abuse. Thus, the psychotherapist–patient privilege was revived following the initial report and the psychotherapist could not be compelled to give testimony concerning the second counseling session with the stepfather.

The majority opinion in *Stritzinger* has been criticized as being too narrow an interpretation of the abrogation of privilege statute existing in California law at the time. (Comment, Vanishing Exception, 1984; Note, The Psychotherapist–Patient Privilege, 1984). By its action, the court effectively excluded those reports that may be permitted but are not mandated by the act from the exemption. The concurring opinion attempted to reconcile the statutory duty of the psychotherapist to report the child abuse with the patient's right to privacy under the Fifth Amendment.[8] Acknowledging that "there is obviously something revolting about the spectable of a psychotherapist testifying to a patient's confidences in which the patient is the defendant in a criminal action" (pp. 749–750), the concurrence held that the patient should be advised of the therapist's legal duty to testify against him concerning disclosures in advance of any counseling sessions. Then the patient may either choose to terminate the relationship or continue it, knowing the risk. The fear, of course, is that a child abuser will be discouraged from seeking psychological help for his problems if his therapist is allowed to testify as to his statements in a criminal proceeding. Should this concern be realized, the ultimate goal of preventing child abuse may be thwarted.

The legislatures of the various states will undoubtedly be required to address such conflicting public policies and to redefine the scope of the professional privileges. It may be desirable to strictly limit disclosure of confidential communications to the initial report in a child abuse case and exclude any subsequent admissions or indirect evidence within the knowledge of the therapist. Perhaps all patients should be warned of the risk in advance. Too narrow an interpretation of the abrogation of privilege statutes in various jurisdictions, however, could lead to situations where it is not possible to protect a child victim, particularly if the child is extremely young and unable to testify or provide any corroborating evidence. On the other hand, criminal defendants in child abuse cases cannot be denied the constitutional right to avoid self-incrimination, a right available to all other criminal defendants. The difficulty of framing an effective yet fair abrogation of privilege statute has not yet been accomplished. Until these conflicts are resolved, professionals will continue to face difficult choices between honoring their reporting duties as well as their confidentiality responsibilities. The most troubling aspect of this dichotomy is that children may suffer from abuse that could have been prevented.

Testimony, Hearsay, and the Child Sexual Abuse Victim

Many observers of the criminal justice system contend that a sexually abused child is victimized twice—first by the offender and secondly by the criminal justice system. Although it may be necessary for a child victim to provide testimony at a juvenile court hearing so appropriate protective measures and possibly counseling may be provided for the child and the family, the parent/offender in that type of proceeding is not entitled to the constitutional protections assured criminal defendants. If a crime is also charged, or even threatened, however, comprehensive constitutional rights accrue to the defendant

---

[8]The Fifth Amendment of the U.S. Constitution guarantees that no person shall be compelled in any criminal case to be a witness against himself. In *Griswald v. Connecticut*, 381 US 406 (1966), the U.S. Supreme Court declared that the Fifth Amendment in its Self-Incrimination Clause enables the citizen to create "a zone of privacy which the government may not force him to surrender to his detriment."

and the child victim may be subjected to the trauma of a public trial, multiple interviews, and cross-examination in the presence of the offender. Children, particularly those who are very young, may not be able to withstand such rigorous questioning. They may be incapable of recounting details or fixing the time and place of several incidents of sexual abuse. Adults, whether spectators, lawyers, or the offender himself, may easily confuse, frighten, or intimidate a child during such procedures. Consequently, some authorities have sought reform measures to exclude the public during the testimony of a child sexual abuse victim and to allow the child to testify outside the presence of the defendant without violating the constitutional rights of the accused.

The right of public access to criminal trials is guaranteed by the first Amendment to ensure that the individual citizen can effectively participate in or contribute to our republican system of self-government, according to the United States Supreme Court in the pivotal opinion, *Globe Newspaper Company v. Superior Court for the County of Norfolk* (1982). The court reasoned that "public scrutiny of a criminal trial enhances the quality and safeguards the integrity of the fact-finding process with benefits to both the defendant and to society as a whole" (p. 605). In this case, a Massachusetts trial court had excluded the press and public from a criminal rape trial involving three teenaged female victims on the strength of a Massachusetts statute that required that the press and the public be excluded from the courtroom during the testimony of a minor victim in a sex offense trial. The trial court ruling was challenged by the plaintiff on the basis that its First Amendment rights were violated.

Justice Brennan, writing for the majority, acknowledged that the right of access to criminal trials is not absolute but ruled that the compelling governmental interests advanced by Massachusetts were not sufficient to justify the mandatory closure rule. Thus, the statute was ruled unconstitutional. The interest in protecting minor victims of sex crimes from further trauma and embarrassment "could be served just as well" by requiring the trial court to determine whether the minor victim's well-being "necessitates closure" (p. 609) on a case-by-case basis. The other state interest of encouraging such victims to come forward and testify in a truthful and credible manner "is not only speculative in empirical terms but is also open to serious question as a matter of logic and common sense" (p. 610). The court observed that because the victim's identity and testimony are ultimately available to both the public and the press through transcripts, court personnel, or other sources, such privacy interests would not actually be furthered by the statute.

Chief Justice Berger, joined by Justice Rehnquist, dissented, pointing out the "disturbing paradox" of a ruling that allows states to mandate the closure of all proceedings to protect a 17-year-old charged with rape but with "callous indifference" does not permit the closing of part of a criminal proceeding to protect an innocent child who has been raped or otherwise sexually abused (p. 612). The dissent expressed the view that a law that excludes the press and public only during the actual testimony of the child victim rationally serves the state's overriding interest in protecting the child from "severe, possibly permanent, psychological damage" (p. 617). The dissenting Justices supported a mandatory rule on the basis that "victims and their families are entitled to assurance of such protection" and the closure determination should not be left to "the idiosyncrasies of individual judges" who may be subject to media pressures (p. 619).

Globe essentially forecloses any state or legislative efforts to require court protection of minor sex crime victims from public trial scrutiny. If *Globe* is not overruled by the court or modified in the future, sexually abused children will continue to be required to participate in public criminal trials unless a judge orders closure on a case-by-case basis pursuant to a constitutionally acceptable state statute.

Another difficulty encountered by child sexual abuse victims relates to the Sixth Amendment requirement that grants a criminal defendant the right "to be confronted with the witnesses against him." This rule guarantees that the complainant/witness, even a child, must testify in the presence of the offender, usually a painful, and often, intimidating experience for young victims of sexual crimes (Bulkey, 1982). The confrontation clause is most often encountered in child sexual abuse cases in those situations where the victim's condition should preclude the testimony in the presence of the offender, or when the prosecution desires to introduce out-of-court (hearsay) statements made by the child (Notes and Comments, The Sexually Abused Infant, 1984).

To mitigate the harm this requirement may cause victims, certain methods have been proposed to ease the burden upon the child victim as witness (Skoler, 1984). Some state statutes provide for videotaped depositions of the child victim's testimony to be used at trial in lieu of live testimony. Another proposal is to create a special child courtroom that would allow the prosecutor, defense counsel, and judge to be present during the child's testimony while the defendant observes the questioning by means of a one-way mirror. Presumably, the defendant would be able to communicate with his attorney through the use of a monitoring device. A third proposal recommends the use of a specially trained attorney to act as a child hearing officer (CHO) to protect the child during the proceedings. The CHO would participate as the child's advocate in usual court proceedings. The CHO would also conduct the questioning or interviewing of the child, and have the right to disallow or rephrase questions from others that may be too harsh or upsetting to the child.

One federal court has already ruled that the Sixth Amendment right to confrontation includes "a face-to-face meeting" during cross-examination (*United States v. Benfield*, 1979). In *Benfield*, an adult kidnap victim was prohibited from testifying in the presence of the defendant by her treating psychiatrist. A special deposition was ordered wherein the defendant was able to observe the proceedings on a monitor and halt the questioning by sounding a buzzer, but was excluded from the room in which the deposition took place. The victim/witness was unaware of the defendant's presence in the building. The United States Court of Appeals ruled that although a videotaped deposition supplies an environment substantially comparable to a trial, this procedural substitution was constitutionally infirm because the defendant was not permitted to be an "active participant" in the deposition (p. 821). Given this interpretation of the Sixth Amendment confrontation requirement, procedures that physically shield children from the presence of the defendant are not likely to withstand constitutional scrutiny.

Another testimonial problem surrounding the child sexual abuse victim involves the admissibility of out-of-court statements made by a child victim to third parties such as family member, physician, or social worker. Such statements are considered hearsay, and thus inadmissible, under the traditional rules of evidence. Generally, out-of-court statements are prohibited in court because the declarer is not present to be examined and tested by the opposing party for reliability and credibility during cross-examination. A child's statement to her mother about a sexual abuse incident is an example of a hearsay statement. The mother could not testify to this statement in lieu of the child's testimony unless the statement satisfies the requirements of a specific exception to the hearsay rule.

Several exceptions to the hearsay rule of inadmissibility have been developed over the centuries. The hearsay statement most often admitted in a child sexual abuse case is the "excited utterance" exception to the hearsay rule. This exception allows those spontaneous statements made while under the influence of a startling event to be admitted. These statements are regarded as inherently reliable because there is insufficient time for the declarer to fabricate or rehearse the statement. The critical test as to whether the statement satisfies the required spontaneity standard is usually measured by the time lapse between the event and the statement. In many jurisdictions, the spontaneity requirement has been relaxed for statements of child sexual abuse victims (Notes, A Tender Years Doctrine, 1984). Evidentiary statements have been admitted that were made days, weeks, and even months after the sexual assault (Skoler, 1984). Although such ploys have been used by courts to meet the special problems posed by child victims, they are not legally justifiable in cases where the time lapse is significantly long.

Other hearsay exceptions that may be used in child sexual abuse cases include the "complaint of rape" exception. This exception permits the admission of the rape complaint to overcome the idea that silence would be an indication that the act had not occurred. Another exception to the hearsay rule that may be useful is the declaration of present bodily feelings, symptoms, and conditions that usually would include statements made to a physician during treatment after such an assault.

However, all of the existing hearsay exceptions may not apply in certain cases of child sexual abuse, particularly where a significant time lapse has occurred or where the child only responds to questions and does not initiate discussion of the event spontaneously. If the age or condition of the victim precludes the viable possibility of future testimony, the admission of an out-of-court statement may be essential to successfully prosecute the case. Even if the child victim is available to testify, some commentators suggest that the child's out-of-court statements may be more inherently reliable and less subject to manipulation than future in-court testimony (Skoler, 1984). In cases where the child is subjected to intense pressure not to testify, such a conclusion is possible.

The federal rules of evidence, and in some cases, state evidentiary rules, contain a catch-all provision that allows the court to determine admissibility of certain out-of-court statements. In a recent South Dakota case, such a residual exception was successfully applied in a sexual abuse case (*State v. McCafferty,* 1984). However, the standards the court must apply to admit hearsay under the residual provision may be more strict than the confrontation clause requirements, and thus, not workable.

Several jurisdictions have opted to provide a new hearsay exception for child sexual abuse cases. Although the special hearsay statutes are substantially similar, there are some differences. Most require some degree of court evaluation through affirmative findings[9] in compliance with the reliability and unavailability tests set forth in *Ohio v. Roberts* (1980). In Washington, (Wash. Rev. Code, 1984), the statute provides that if the court finds at a hearing outside the jury's presence that the child's statement regarding sexual contact with another has sufficient "indicia of reliability" and the child testifies at trial, the statement is admissible provided the opponent has been given adequate notice. If the child is found

---

[9]The determination of reliability and trustworthiness must be met on a case-by-case basis. The court may consider such factors as the age of the child; his or her physical or mental condition; the circumstances of the alleged event; the language used by the child; the presence of corroborative physical evidence; the relationship of the accused to the child; the child's family, school, and peer relationships; any motive to falsify or distort the event; and the reliability of the testifying witness according to the Kansas Supreme Court in *State v. Myatt* (1985).

to be unavailable for testimony, corroborative evidence of the act is required. This statute was recently upheld as constitutional by the Washington Supreme Court (*State v. Ryan*, 1984).

The Kansas statute (Kan. State, Ann., 1983) is not limited to sexual abuse; it includes criminal proceedings as well as child deprivation and need of care proceedings. The court must find that the statement is "apparently reliable," that the child is unavailable as a witness, and that the child was not induced to make the statement. This statute has survived two recent appeals and found to be facially constitutional (*State v. Myatt*, 1985; *State v. Pendelton*, 1984).

The statute enacted in Colorado (Co. Rev. Stat., 1983) is substantially the same as the Washington statute except that the court is further required to instruct the jury as to how to determine the weight and credibility to be given the statement. Also, in Utah, the statute (Utah Code Ann. 1983) requires the court to determine whether "the interest of justice will be best served by admission" but does not specifically require an admissibility hearing. The determination must be based on a criteria of reliability.

Ironically, hearsay statements admitted under existing hearsay exceptions or under newly established hearsay exceptions for sexually abused child victims are more likely to satisfy the Sixth Amendment confrontation clause than special procedures for videotaped depositions and insulated courtroom testimony. Even though hearsay statements are not subject to cross-examination tests, they become superior vehicles for the admittance of evidentiary statements made by child victims in that they avoid Sixth Amendment constitutional challenges. Specially designed courtroom procedures that may provide complete cross-examination opportunities without direct face-to-face confrontation may be found to be constitutionally infirm.

FUTURE DIRECTIONS

Although the legal tools are now available in most jurisdictions to address the unique problems posed by prior relationship crimes, the incorporation of such changes into the legal system at a policy level has not yet occurred universally (Comment, The Battered Wife's Dilemma, 1981). Enforcement is uneven and sporadic.

Some police agencies still avoid arrests rather than implementing the new warrantless arrest procedures in violent domestic disputes (Pastoor, 1984; Woods, 1981). Prosecutors generally have not committed additional resources or personnel, or developed appropriate policy directives to handle violent and abusive families (Ellis, 1984). A majority of victims do not report the abuse to police agencies because they prefer to avoid involvement in the criminal justice system (Lerman, 1981). Professionals report a very small percentage of abused and neglected children to authorities (Thompson, 1984). Sexually abusive parents are not prosecuted in many cases because the child victim cannot withstand the trauma of a criminal trial that vigorously protects the rights of the offender over those of the victim (Algren, 1983–84; Bulkey, 1982, 1983a).

Yet no intervention model has been devised that can respond effectively to domestic abuse without using the threat of a legal sanction or remedy. Clearly, wrongs against the physical integrity of so many victims must be subject to some form of legal response if remediation of the problem is to occur. Assailants do not change willingly or seek counseling on a voluntary basis without some form of legal coercion. Acceptable methods for handling these cases must be found within the legal system.

Increased compliance with existing laws will undoubtedly occur through civil law suits against those individuals and agencies that have a duty to provide protection to victims under the law and fail to do so. Although personal injury law suits are too long and costly to provide a realistic option for most victims, certain highly publicized cases may successfully motivate better institutional responses. Such legal challenges are powerful vehicles for establishing accountability and compliance with domestic abuse laws. For example, a recent Connecticut case (*Thurman v. City of Torrington*, 1984) resulted in a judgment for a battered woman of $2.3 million after a United States District Court jury found that police officers had violated her constitutional rights by failing to protect her from a stabbing and beating by her estranged husband. Although this decision will undoubtedly be appealed, the *Thurman* case emphasizes to police agencies that domestic violence complaints can no longer be relegated to the bottom of the criminal justice barrel.

Similarly, in other jurisdictions, class action suits have been brought on behalf of battered women against police agencies, probation departments, and court personnel to guarantee access to the court system and prevent further discrimination in domestic violence complaints (Woods, 1981). Although several of these law suits have resulted in consent judgments and negotiated changes in police procedures in several cities, advocates of battered women report that police departments have not readily acceded to suggested changes in their policies and practices for handling complaints from battered women. It is possible that individual damage suits against agencies may provide a stronger financial incentive than class action suits requesting injunctive and declaratory relief.

Successful litigation strategies have also been developed in suits against mandatory reporters in certain jurisdictions for failure to report instances of child abuse that resulted in permanent injury or death to an abused victim. These actions have been brought primarily against physicians and hospitals but could also challenge the actions or omissions of other mandatory reporters depending on the circumstances. In one of the few reported cases, *Landeros v. Flood* (1975), the Supreme Court of California reversed the lower court decisions involving a child who suffered permanent injuries as a result of abuse by her mother and her mother's common law husband. The court held that the complaint did state a cause of action for malpractice, and that it was a question of fact for the jury as to whether the ability to recognize the battered child syndrome is within the skill of the ordinary prudent physician. In another California case, severe injuries sustained by a 5-month-old child that resulted in extensive and permanent brain damage led to a $5 million suit against four doctors for failing to report the attacks and against the city and police chief of the city for failing to investigate adequately when another doctor did file an abuse report. The suit was based on a theory of negligence *per se* in that the parties had a duty to the child under the California reporting statute. The suit was ultimately settled for $600,000 and a trust fund was set up to care for the child (Thompson, 1984). This type of action has the advantage of providing financial support for the treatment and care of an injured child as well as dramatically illustrating to other professionals that they have a duty to protect abused children.

The New York Court of Appeals (*Sorichetti v. City of New York*, 1985) recently approved a $2 million jury award to a 6-year-old child and $40,000 to her mother against a police agency for failing to prevent serious injuries to her child. During a court-ordered visitation period, the child was permanently disabled after her father repeatedly attacked her with a fork, a knife, a screwdriver, and then attempted to saw off her leg. The court held that the "special relationship" between the citizen and a police department necessary to hold the municipality liable was created by three factors in this case: the existence of a judicial order of protection ordering the father to avoid threatening or assaulting his wife, police knowledge of the man's violent history of assaulting his family, and police assurances to the wife that mislead her into believing that appropriate action would be taken to investigate the matter.

Other personal injury cases can be expected to be brought against public officials, including protective services agencies, courts, court personnel, and prosecutors. These suits may have mixed results depending on the level of sovereign immunity available in the jurisdiction for those officials who exercise discretionary decisions, particularly judges and prosecutors (Woods, 1981). Federal suits may also be pursued under Section 1983 of the Civil Rights Act (U.S. Code, 1968) provided a sufficient nexus is demonstrated between the municipality and the offending person or agency responsible for the inadequate protection (*Monell v. N.Y.*, 1978).

The criminal justice system must impact on the assailants in domestic abuse cases and not react solely to victims. Responsibility for their actions must be placed squarely on the offenders and institutional responses should be scrutinized to delete programs that provide excuses for violent conduct or allocate blame to innocent parties, such as the use of traditional mediation techniques (Stallone, 1984) to "settle" the terms of a violent relationship. Although the direction of such a focus on assailants should not necessarily be punitive, it must at the very least convey the clear message that the violent conduct is unacceptable.

This approach can be strengthened by the expansion of civil protection orders in adult and child abuse cases. Such orders should be used to provide flexible remedies for victims but at the expense of the assailants in terms of removal from the home, participation in counseling and treatment programs, and the victim's legal, medical, and shelter costs. Such protective orders should be refined and developed with the idea that victims retain as much control over their initiation where possible rather than abandoning such decisions to institutional initiatives and relegating adult victims to the status of children. Further, legislative reform efforts should focus on more specific definitions and careful drafting of the provisions to avoid the confusions inherent in the reporting system, for example, or the inequities in the area of marital rape. Increased preventative measures must also include the building of strong alliances between legal institutions and the many agencies involved in responding to these problems. Better communication, planning, and strategy development must be encouraged so that a rapprochement may be reached, and an integrated approach to all forms of family violence established.

CONCLUSION

Ultimately, the legal system must fully accept its role in the adjudication of domestic abuse cases, and accomplish the adjustments necessary to afford fair, perceptive, and consistent responses to victims and assailants. The compelling need to respond to violent actions in the family may no longer be sidestepped or avoided. The critical relationship between family violence and the generation of crime and other social problems must be recognized and understood in the legal profession and its institutions. More importantly, the professionals in the system must be willing to test nontraditional avenues of argument and procedure to provide innovative responses to the complicated and difficult demands of intrafamilial violence. Such demands may pose the greatest challenges the legal system, and in particular the criminal justice system, face in this century.

Acker, J. R., & Toch, H. (1985, March/April). Battered women, straw men, and expert testimony: A comment on State v Kelly. *Criminal Law Bulletin, 21,* 125.

Ahlgren, C. A. (1983–84). Maintaining incest victims' support relationships. *Journal of Family Law, 22,* 483.

Alderman, M. (1979). *Child abuse and neglect: State reporting laws* (DHHS Publication No. OHDS 80-30265). Washington, DC: U.S. Government Printing Office.

Areen, J. (1975). Intervention between parent and child: A reappraisal of the state's role in child neglect and abuse cases. *The Georgetown Law Journal, 63,* 887.

Barry, S. (1980, September). Spousal rape: The uncommon law. *American Bar Association Journal, 66,* 1088.

Blackstone, W. (1899). *Commentaries on the laws of England* (3rd ed.). Albany, NY: Banks.

Bradley v. State. 2 Miss. (Walker) 156 (1824).

Brodie, D. W. (1972). Privacy: The family and the state. *Law Forum, 4,* 743.

Brown, B. A., Emerson, T. I., Falk, G., and Freedman, A. E. (1971). The equal rights amendment. *Yale Law Journal, 5,* 871.

Buhrle v. State. 627 P.2d 1374 (Wy. 1981).

Bulkey, J. (Ed.). (1983a, January). *Innovations in the prosecution of child sexual abuse cases* (3rd ed.). Washington, DC: American Bar Association, National Legal Resource Center for Child Advocacy and Protection.

Bulkey, J. (Ed.). (1983b, April). *Child sexual abuse and the law* (4th ed.). Washington DC: American Bar Association, National Legal Resource Center for Child Advocacy and Protection.

Bulkey, J. (1982, October). *Recommendations for improving legal intervention in intra-family child sexual abuse cases.* Washington, DC: American Bar Association, National Legal Resource Center for Child Advocacy and Protection.

California Child Abuse Reporting Act, Cal. Penal Code, Sec. 11165-66 (West Supp. 1984); Sec.11167-74 (West 1982).

California Penal Code, Section 11171(b) (West 1982).

Cavanagh, B. K. (1971). ''A little dearer than his horse'': Legal stereotypes and the feminine personality. *Harvard Civil Rights-Civil Liberties Law Review, 6,* 260.

Colorado Revised Statues, Sec. 13-25-129 (1983).

Comment, The battered wife's dilemma: Kill or be killed. (1981). *Hastings Law Review, 32,* 895.

Comment, Self-defense: Battered woman syndrome on trial. (1984). *California Western Law Review, 20,* 485.

Comment, Vanishing exception to the psychotherapist-patient privilege: The child abuse reporting act. (1984). *Pacific Law Journal, 16,* 335.

Commonwealth v. Chretian, 417 N.E.2d 1203 (Ma. 1981).

Commonwealth v. Schilling, 431 A.2d 1088 (Pa. Super. 1981).

Davidson, K. M., Ginsburg, R. B., & Kay, H. H. (1974). *Text, cases and materials on sex-based discrimination.* St. Paul, MN: West.

Eisenberg, S. E., & Micklow, P. L. (1977, Spring/Summer). The assaulted wife: ''Catch 22'' revisited. *Women's Rights Law Reporter, 3,* 138.

Ellis, J. W. (1984, Spring). Prosecutorial discretion to charge in cases of spousal assault: A dialogue. *Journal of Criminal Law and Criminology, 75,* 56.

Finkelhor, D. (1984). *Child sexual abuse: New theory and research.* New York: The Free Press.

Frontiero v. Richardson, 411 U. S. 677 (1973).

Fulgham v. State, 46 Ala. 143 (1871).

Globe Newspaper Company v. Superior Court for the County of Norfolk, 457 U.S. 596, (1982).

Hale, Sir Matthew (1778). *History of the pleas of the common Crown* (Vols. 1 and 2). London: Sollom Emlyn of Lincoln's Inn, Esq.

Hawthorne v. State, 408 So2d 801 (F11. Dist. Ct. App. 1982).

Ibn-Tamas v. United States, 455 A2d 893 (DC, 1983).

Idaho Code, Sec. 16-1628(j) (Supp. 1974).

Johnson v. State, 21 Tenn. 183 (1841).

Kanowitz, L. (1969). *Women and the law: The unfinished revolution.* Albuquerque, NM: University of New Mexico Press.

Kansas Statutes Annotated, Sec. 60-640(dd) (1983).

Kizer v. Commonwealth, 321 S.E.2d 291 (VA. 1984).

Landau, H. R., Salus, M. K., and Stiffarm, T. (1980, May). *Child protection: The role of the courts* (DHHS Publication No. (OHDS) 80-30256). Washington, DC: U.S. Government Printing Office.

Landeros v. Flood, 50 Cal. App. 3d 189 (1975).

Langley, R., & Levy, R. C. (1977). *Wife beating: The silent crisis.* New York: E. P. Dutton.

Lerman, L. G. (1981, January/February). Criminal prosecution of wife beaters. *Response, 4*(3), 1–20.

Lerman, L. G. (1984). A model state act: Remedies for domestic abuse. *Harvard Journal on Legislation, 21,* 61.

Lerman, L. G., & Livingstone, F. (1983, September/October). State legislation on domestic violence. *Response, 6*(5), 1–28.

Marital rape exemption in the criminal law. (1980, October). *Clearinghouse Review, 538.*

Martin, D. (1976). *Battered wives.* San Francisco: Glide.

Model Penal Code (1962). Section 213.1(1). American Law Institute.

Monell v. New York City Department of Social Services, 436 U.S. 658 (1978).

New York Laws 1261, Ch. 547, Art. I, Sec. 2(4) (f) (McKinney, 1922).

New York Laws 3066, Ch. 686, Art. III, Sec. 312(a) (McKinney 1922).

Note, Defendant v. Witness: Measuring confrontation and compulsory process rights against statutory communications privileges (1978). *Stanford Law Review, 30,* 935.

Note, The battering parent syndrome: Inexpert testimony as character evidence. (1984), Spring). *University of Michigan Journal of Legal Reform, 17,* 653.

Note, The psychotherapist–patient privilege, the child abuse exception, and the protection of privacy through the Fifth Amendment. (1984). *Whittier Law Review, 6,* 1033.

Notes and Comments, The sexually abused infant hearsay exception: A constitutional analysis. (1984). *Journal of Juvenile Law, 8,* 59.

Notes, A tender years doctrine for the juvenile courts: An effective way to protect the sexually abused child. (1984). *Journal of Urban Law, 61,* 249.

Ohio v. Roberts, 448 U.S. 56 (1980).

Pastoor, M. K. (1984). Police training and the effectiveness of Minnesota ''domestic abuse'' laws. *Law and Inequality, 2,* 557.

People v. Brown, 632 P.2d 1025 (Colo. 1981).

People v. Liberta, 474 N.E.2d 567 (N. Y. 1984).

People v. Stritzinger, 668 P.2d 738 (CA. Sup. Ct. 1983).

Prosser, W. L. (1971). *Handbook of the law of torts* (4th ed.). St. Paul, MN: West.

Recent development, The expert as educator: A proposed approach to the use of battered woman syndrome expert testimony. (1982). *Vanderbilt Law Review, 35,* 741.

Reed v. Reed, 404 U.S. 71 (1971).

Rossman, G. (1925). Parens patriae. *Oregon Law Review, 4,* 233.

Roy, M. (1977). *Battered woman.* New York: Van Nostrand Reinhold.

Rozell v. State, 502 S.W.2d 16 (Tex. Crim., 1973).

Sherman, L. W., & Berk, R. A. (1984). The Specific effects arrest for domestic assault, *American Sociological Review, 49,* 261.

Skoler, G. (1984). New hearsay exceptions for a child's statement of sexual abuse. *The John Marshall Law Review, 18,* 1.

Silberman, C. E. (1978). *Criminal violence, criminal justice.* New York: Random House.

Smith v. State, 277 S.E.2d 678 (Ga. Sup. Ct. 1981).

Sorichetti v. New York, No. 304 (N. Y. Ct. App., July 9, 1985).

Stallone, D. R. (1984). Decriminalization of violence in the home: Mediation in wife battering cases. *Law and Inequality, 2,* 493.

State v. Allery, 682 P.2d 312 (Wash. en banc, 1984).

State v. Anaya, 438 A.2d 892 (Me. 1981).

State v. Aronhalt, 526 P.2d 463 (Or App, 1974).

State v. Baker, 424 A.2d 171 (NH, 1980).

State v. Drope, 462 S.W.2d 677 (Mo App, 1971).

State v. Green, 652 P.2d 697 (Ks. 1982).

State v. Kelly, 478 A.2d 364 (N. J. 1984).

State v. Kennedy, 616 P.2d 594 (Utah, 1980).

State v. Martin, 666 S.W.2d 895 (Mo. App. 1984).

State v. Martin, 194 S.E.2d 60, cert den 195 S.E.2d 691 (NC App, 1973).

State v. McCafferty, 356 N.W.2d 159 (S.E. 1984).

State v. Myatt, 697 P.2d 836 (Kan. 1985).

State v. Pendelton, 690 P.2d 959 (Kan. App. 1984).

State v. Pratt, 233 So.2d 883 (LA, 1970).

State v. Ryan, 691 P.2d 197 (WA. Sup. Ct., 1984).

State v. (J.) Smith, 227 S.E.2d 678 (Sup. Ct. GA, 1981).

State v. Smith, 426 A.2d 38 (N.J. Sup. Ct. 1981).

State v. Thomas, 423 N.E.2d 137 (OH, 1981).

Stedman, B. (1917). The right of husbands to chastise wife. *Virginia Law Register, 3,* 241.

ten Broek, J. (1964). California's dual system of family law: Its origin, development and present status (part I). *Stanford Law Review, 16,* 257.

Thompson, M. L. (1984). Civil suit: An abused child's only protection. *Probate Law Journal, 6,* 85.

Thurman v. City of Torrington, 595 F. Supp. 1521 (D. Conn. 1984).

United States v. Benfield, 593 F.2d 815 (8th Cri. 1979).

United States Code, Title 42, Sec. 1983 (1968).

Utah Code Annotated, Sec. 76-5-411 (1983).

Wash. Rev. Code Ann., Sec. 9A.44.120 (West Supp. 1984).

Weisberg, R., & Wald, M. (1984, Summer). Confidentiality laws and state efforts to protect abused or neglected children: The need for statutory reform. *Family Law Quarterly, 18*(2), 143.

Woods, L. (1981). Litigation on behalf of battered women. *Women's Rights Law Reporter, 7,* 39.

18

Family Violence in Cross-Cultural Perspective

DAVID LEVINSON

INTRODUCTION

The purpose of this chapter is to review and discuss the contributions cross-cultural studies have made or might make to our understanding of family violence. To cover as much territory as possible I have defined cross-cultural studies broadly to include any information collection and analysis approach that involves either the implicit or explicit comparison of two or more cultural groups. Cultural group is defined broadly as well, to include nations, political subdivisions within nations, ethnic groups, small-scale (primitive, nonliterate) societies, peasant societies, and so on. Following the work of Gelles and Straus (1979) family violence is defined as the action of a family member that will very likely cause physical pain to another family member. The term *beating,* such as wife beating or husband beating, is used throughout the chapter to refer to any violent act ranging from a slap to a beating with a stick to murder with a handgun.

The comparative approach implicit in most cross-cultural studies of family violence and explicit in only a few contributes to our understanding of family violence in a number of ways. First, cross-cultural studies expand our knowledge of the range of human actions that constitute family violence and factors relating to this violence, including types of families, types of family relationships, and methods of interpersonal conflict resolution. Second, cross-cultural studies enable us to analyze family violence in its cultural context, and thus come to grips with what family violence means to the participants and to the cultural group as a whole (Korbin 1977, 1981). Third, worldwide comparative studies, based on large samples of either nations or small-scale societies, are a powerful means of testing theories of family violence operationalized at the societal level (Lee, 1984; Straus 1985). Theories amenable to testing in this way include those that tie wife beating to sexual inequality, wife and child beating to a cultural acceptance of violence, and various forms of family violence to various forms of social organization. Fourth, cross-cultural studies, especially in developing regions of the world, enable us to study the effect of

DAVID LEVINSON • Vice President, Human Relations Area Files, Inc., 755 Prospect St., New Haven, CT 06520.

435

social change on family relationships, including violent ones. And, fifth, cross-cultural studies enable us to compare low-violence to high-violence cultures in order to identify factors or processes that may help control or prevent family violence.

Despite its potential contributions, cross-cultural family violence research as it is currently conducted is not without its limitations. Some of the limitations are indicated in Gelles and Cornell's (1983) suggestions for future research:

> What we need then is a knowledge of family violence built on cross-cultural research using precise and replicable definitions, measures, and research designs. Even more than this, we need cross-cultural research on family violence which empirically examines the factors that many investigators believe cause variation in the extent and patterns of family violence. Truly useful cross-cultural research on family violence should investigate social-structural variations, and variations in cultural meanings and norms concerning children and family life. (p. 162)

As Gelles and Cornell suggest, problems with current cross-cultural research include the lack of probability or representative samples and the failure to define and measure the cross-cultural variables that are often cited as the basic cause of cross-cultural variations in family violence. Beyond these methodological problems are some other more basic problems that currently limit the usefulness of cross-cultural studies. One, as noted by Korbin (1977) is the absence of a universal definition of family violence. This is something of a chicken-or-egg problem, as a broad definition can only be developed after cross-cultural studies have identified the full range of behaviors that can be categorized as family violence. A second problem is the failure to define the concept of culture and the related failure to establish criteria for delineating the boundaries of cultural groups (Naroll, 1973). Because anthropologists, the intellectual caretakers of the concept of the culture, have yet to develop a generally agreed-upon definition of the concept, it is hard to fault family violence researchers for failing to do so themselves. However, the question of where one culture ends and another begins is important in cross-cultural research designed to test casual theories. The issue is whether the behaviors or cultural factors under study developed independently in each group or diffused through cultural borrowing from one or two or three groups to the others. A third basic problem with cross-cultural studies is their failure to make explicit comparisons between two or more cultures. Part of the problem here rests with the methodological issues noted earlier. However, there is a more basic concern that many researchers and policy makers are content to assume that culture influences family violence without measuring and testing the actual influence of specific cultural factors.

This chapter is divided into nine sections. The following four sections provide descriptive details about various cross-cultural approaches used in family violence research, types of families found around the world, types of family violence, and the prevalence of selected types of family violence. Sections 5 through 7 contain summaries of cross-cultural research findings bearing on the sexual inequality, cultural patterning of violence, and social organization theories of family violence. Section 8 reviews research relevant to the effect of social change on family violence. In the final section, I discuss the role cross-cultural studies can play in helping us develop models and programs for the control and prevention of family violence.

CROSS-CULTURAL APPROACHES

At least six different cross-cultural research strategies have been or can be used by researchers interested in the comparative study of family violence. Although no single strategy can answer all relevant questions, in combination they can add substantially to our understanding of the nature, frequency, distribution, meaning, causes, prevention, and control of family violence. These six approaches are described in the following, with special attention given to the contribution each can make to our understanding of family violence.

Case studies of family violence in specific societies, nations, or subcultures have been appearing with increasing frequency in the family violence literature in recent years. We now have a long list of descriptive studies of family violence in North American, European, African, and Asian nations and ethnic groups. Most case studies provide descriptive information about the frequency and nature of family violence with additional demographic information about the individuals or families involved in the violent situations. Most of these studies are uncontrolled in the sense that no comparisons are made between the subjects and other individuals in the society. However, a few studies, such as White and Cornely's (1981) analysis of child abuse among the Navaho do compare abusive with nonabusive families on key demographic variables such as age, family size, family composition, socioeconomic status, and so forth. The major value of case studies is the descriptive information they provide about the nature and meaning of family violence in different cultural contexts. Unfortunately, the methodological weaknesses of many of these studies, such as biased sampling, undefined concepts, and untrustworthy data limit their usefulness for comparative and theory testing purposes.

Longitudinal comparisons involve the comparison of individuals or families or entire societies with themselves at two or more points in time. Longitudinal studies, although little used in cross-cultural family violence research, provide a potentially powerful tool for developing and testing theories of cause and prevention. Because temporal sequence is built into the research design, changes in the frequency or nature of family violence between two points in time can be related to economic, political, social, or environmental changes that occured between the original situation and the current one. For example, Erchak's (1984) analysis of wife beating among rural and urban Kpelle in Nigeria shows that wife beating only begins after couples move to the city, a shift he attributes to the absence of traditional patterns of social control in the city. The key difficulty with longitudinal studies is that there are many aspects of social change, such as urbanization, education, wage labor, a cash economy, influx of tourists, which may affect the family violence process. Controlling these factors can be a costly and time-consuming task.

Regional comparisons are used to identify similarities in family violence patterns among cultures in a particular geographical region. Unlike case and longitudinal studies the sample units are entire cultural groups rather than individuals or families. Regional comparisons operate on the belief that regional similarities can be attributed to historical contact between the neighboring cultures, which has led them to be similar on a number of basic cultural dimensions. Lozios' (1978) study of wife beating in rural Mediterranean cultures is a good example of this approach. He traces the high frequency of wife beating in Greece, Portugal, Sicily, and Cyprus to a basic value orientation that emphasizes male control and male honor. Regional comparisons are a valuable source of ideas about the case and prevention of family violence, not only in regard to specific regions but also for the world in general.

Intrasocietal comparisons involve the comparisons of family violence in subcultural groups in one society. As used so far, they come in two basic forms. First, there are cross-state comparisons, such as Yllo's (1983) study of wife beating and sexual inequality in the United States, where the sampling units are states, or political subdivisions of a nation. In these studies the emphasis is on economic and political rather than cultural variables, although there is often an assumption that cultural differences from one state to another may be important. Second, there are cross-ethnic comparisons, such as Erlich's (1966) study of family violence in which Bosians, Macedonians, Serbs, and other groups in Yugoslavia are compared. As with regional comparisons, intrasocietal comparisons provide ideas about the causes of family violence and a means of testing those ideas in a pluralistic societal context.

Small-scale comparisons involve the comparison of a small number of societies (usually two or three) for the purpose of relating differences in family violence to differences in legal, economic, or cultural factors from one society to the others. Less sophisticated studies of this type are often little more than two or three case studies discussed in a comparative framework. More sophisticated designs, which Straus (1985) refers to as cross-national replications, can be used as social quasi-experiments to measure the impact on family violence of cultural factors present in one society but absent in the others. Solheim's (1982) analyses of parental use of corporal punishment in Sweden and the United States and Tellis-Nayak and Donoghue's (1982) study of prescriptive norms in the United States, Ireland, and India are examples of this approach.

Hologeistic or *worldwide comparative studies* are used to test general theories of family violence with either worldwide samples of small-scale societies (*holocultural* studies) or worldwide samples of nations (*holonational* studies). These studies generally use samples ranging from 50 to over 100 societies or nations, with some attempt made to insure that the samples represent all major geographical and cultural regions of the world. Lee (1984) recently reviewed some of the methodological problems inherent in this approach, including nonprobability sampling, unreliable data, loss of cultural context, and the influence of cultural diffusion on statistical relationships. Despite these problems, there seems little doubt that if used carefully, hologeistic studies can make an important contribution to increasing our understanding of the relationships between societal level mechanisms, such as sexual inequality and family violence.

TYPES OF FAMILIES

The human family comes in five forms. The *matrifocal* family consists of a mother and her children. The *nuclear* family consists of wife/mother, husband/father, and their children. The *polygynous* family consists of a husband/father, two or more wives/mothers and their children. The *polyandrous* family consists of one wife/mother, her children, and two or more husband/fathers. And the *extended* family consists of individuals who are recognized as both husband/father and son/brother or wife/mother and sister/daughter at the same time. The nuclear family is by far the most common form. The polyandrous family is the rarest. The family members in each type of family occupy different kinship roles. Thus, each family type faces different interpersonal problems and has different organizational potentials. Table 1 lists the roles present in each type.

Obviously, the presence of different categories of kin and the different roles they fill creates the potential for different forms of family violence from one society to another. For example, in polygynous societies violence between co-wives is not uncommon (Burbank, in press).

The Matrifocal Family

Although not the dominant type of family in any society, the matrifocal family exists as an independent entity among certain groups in the Caribbean, Central America, South

America, and increasingly in North America (Adams, 1960; Kunstadter, 1963; Otterbein, 1965). The matrifocal family also existed as part of the matrifocal-matrilineal extended family system of the Nayar subcaste of south India (Gough, 1959).

When the matrifocal family does appear as a distinct family type, it evidently does so only in very specific circumstances. In the western hemisphere, it is mainly found in lower socioeconomic groups where the men must travel to find work or where the men have little status or economic security (Adams, 1960; Otterbein, 1965).

The Nuclear Family

A nuclear (conjugal, elementary) family is a small social group all of whose members, through birth, marriage, or adoption, stand in a relation of parent, child, spouse, or sibling to other members of the group (Bohannan, 1968; Murdock, 1949).

Adams (1960) sees the nuclear family as a collection of three dyadic relations: the conjugal or sexual; the maternal; and the paternal. The paternal relation is based on the

Table 1. Kin Roles by Family Type

Kin roles*	Matrifocal	Nuclear	Polygynous	Polyandrous	Stem	Lineal	Fully extended
M	+	+	+	+	+	+	+
F		+	+	+	+	+	+
W		+	+	+	+	+	+
H		+	+	+	+	+	+
D	+	+	+	+	+	+	+
S	+	+	+	+	+	+	+
Si	+	+	+	+	+	+	+
B	+	+	+	+	+	+	+
Co-W			+		+/−	+/−	+/−
Co-H				+	+/−	+/−	+/−
1/2 Sb			+	+	+/−	+/−	+/−
GM					+	+	+
GF					+	+	+
GC					+	+	+
A						+	+
U						+	+
Ni						+	+
Ne						+	+
C						+	+
PL						+	+
CL					+	+	+
SL					+	+	+

M—mother	Si—sister	GM—grandmother	Ni—niece
F—father	B—brother	GF—grandfather	Ne—nephew
W—wife	Co-W—co-wife	GC—grandchild	C—cousin
H—husband	Co-H—co-husband	A—aunt	PL—parent-in-law
D—daughter	1/2 Sb—half-sibling	U—uncle	CL—child-in-law
S—son			SL—sibling-in-law

Note. Whereas we recognize that the use of culture-bound kin terms such as aunt or uncle may be considered ethnocentric, for the summary purposes of this table, we feel that these general terms are sufficiently specific.
*A plus sign indicates that the kin role is present; a plus-minus sign indicates that the kin role may be present or absent.
(Reprinted from D. Levinson and M. J. Malone, 1981, *Toward Explaining Human Culture*. New Haven, CT: HRAF Press.)

other two. Whether or not a society recognizes a man's role in procreation, his role and status as father are almost always a function of his role as mother's husband. Adams thinks that the sexual and maternal dyad are especially important:

> The conjugal or sexual dyad is particularly significant because it is the reproductive unit of society, the maternal dyad is the temporal link between successive generations of adult dyads . . . since the mother is the only adult in the maternal dyad, and the wife is the only female in the sexual dyad, they can be joined most readily by identifying the wife with the mother. (1960, pp. 40–41)

Although some would argue that Murdock (1949) overstates the case, there is considerable cross-cultural support for his conclusion that

> The nuclear family is a universal human social grouping. Either as the sole prevailing form of the family or as the basic unit from which more complex familial forms are compounded, it exists as a distinct and strongly functional group in every known society. (p. 2)

The Polygynous Family

There is some disagreement over whether to classify the polygynous family as a form of the nuclear family. Murdock (1949) views the polygynous family as a group of nuclear families with a common husband/father. This view conflicts with the position that the polygynous family is a group of matrifocal families sharing one husband/father.

There are three sets of relations in polygynous families that are not present in nuclear ones: (a) the relationship between co-wives referred to by Bohannan as shared sexuality (all of the wives share sexual relations with the same husband); (b) the relationship between siblings, or limited shared descent; and (c) the relationship between children and the wives who are not their mothers. Each type of relationship may lead to feelings of rivalry, jealousy, hostility, and antagonism that each polygynous family must control in order to function and survive. Among these factors that may help maintain social order within the polygynous family are clearly defined roles, equitable distribution of tasks, sororal polygyny (co-wives are sisters), and equitable treatment of co-wives by the husband.

Although polygynous families are always in the minority even in societies where they are favored, they tend to be the goal of all men in those societies. They are highly desirable because more wives mean more prestige and more material wealth. Wives also often desire additional wives for their husbands—additional wives lighten their workloads and increase the prestige and wealth of the family. In most polygynous families, wives are an economic asset. Whether they cultivate, or make craft products to sell, their work increases the wealth of the family.

The Polyandrous Family

As with polygyny, polyandrous marriage must be based on a relationship that the society recognizes as marriage; for this reason, wife sharing is not considered polyandry. For a family to be classified as polyandrous, each of the husbands must be eligible to be considered the legal father of at least one of the woman's children.

Polyandry is very rare and why it exists is not clear. A number of suggestions have been proposed. Leach (1961, p. 110) suggested that polyandry is closely tied to a need to keep real property together. Prince Peter (1965, p. 206) saw polyandry as an adaptation to "a difficult and insecure natural environment." Others have linked it to female infanticide.

The Extended Family

Extended families contain a number of relationships not found in other families. Affinal relationships exist between parents-in-law, children-in-law, and siblings-in-law. Relations between in-laws are often difficult and disruptive, and it is not surprising that they are often handled through institutionalized rules of behavior, such as avoidance and joking relationships. The unique lineal relationship in extended families is that between grandparents and grandchildren. Apple (1956) reported that the grandparent–grandchild relationship seems to be freest and easiest in societies where the grandparents have little authority over their own children. And, there may be relationships involving cousins, aunts, uncles, nieces, and nephews in more than one generation. Rules of residence and descent largely determine which relationships will be emphasized and which will be ignored. Rules regarding cousin marriage also effect the relationships.

There are a number of kinds of extended families and there are a number of ways to classify them. Nimkoff (1965, p. 19) classifies four types based on structure:

1. Stem family—two nuclear families in adjacent generations with one son/husband or daughter/wife who is a member of both families
2. Lineal family—one nuclear family in the senior generation and two or more nuclear families in the junior generation
3. Fully extended family—the families of at least two siblings or cousins in each of at least two adjacent generations
4. Joint family—two or more nuclear families who form a corporate economic unit

Although extended families are sometimes seen as relatively free of family violence (Whitehurst 1974), it should be noted that life in extended families can be and often is quite stressful. As Pasternak, Ember, and Ember (1976, p. 14) pointed out,

> In addition to the ordinary problems of living in a one-family household, the members of an extended family household might be faced with conflicts of authority between senior and junior individuals or between siblings, conflicts of loyalty because of competing interests of spouses and kinsmen, and other conflicts which may arise merely from the larger number of possible dyads, triads, and so forth.

Using a cross-cultural sample of 60 societies, Pasternak and his associates go on to suggest that extended family households occur primarily in situations where both the husband and wife work outside the home and where replacement help for domestic chores is unobtainable.

TYPES OF FAMILY VIOLENCE

Table 2 lists different types of family violence classified by the life stage of the victim. The list includes events where both the aggressor and the victim are family members, and events (initiation rites, child marriage) where one family member allows another to be placed in a situation where the latter will very likely be harmed. This list was compiled through a search of ethnographic reports in the Human Relations Area Files data archive, a review of the articles in Korbin's (1981) reader on child abuse and neglect, and cross-cultural reports published in *Child Abuse and Neglect*.

Table 2 indicates that, when viewed cross-culturally, family violence covers a wide range of human behaviors. However, before assuming that there is no limit to the types of injury family members will inflict on one another, it is important to remember that most of these types of violence occur in only a few societies around the world. For example, sale of infants for sacrifice, child marriage, forced homosexual relationships for adolescents, and forced suicide by wives are quite rare. And, other practices, such as scarification at puberty, are rapidly disappearing. It is also important to keep in mind that just because a practice occurs in a society does not mean that it occurs with any degree of frequency. Infanticide, for example, is reported as occuring in a majority of the world's societies, but

Table 2. Forms of Family Violence by Stage of Life

Infancy
    Infanticide
    Sale of infants for sacrifice
    Binding body parts for shaping (head, feet, etc.)
    Force feeding
    Harsh disciplinary techniques, such as cold baths
Childhood
    Organized fighting promoted by adults
    Ritual defloration
    Harsh socialization techniques (beating, kicking, slapping, burning, twisting ears, etc.)
    Child marriage
    Child slavery
    Child prostitution
    Drugging with hallucinogens
    Parent–child homicide/suicide
    Child labor
    Sibling fighting
    Nutritional deprivation
    Corporal punishment in schools
    Mutilation for begging
Adolescence (puberty)
    Painful initiation rites (circumcision, supercision, clitoridectomy, sacrification, cold baths, piercings, sleep deprivation, whippings, bloodletting, forced vomiting)
    Forced homosexual relations
    Harsh socialization techniques
    Gang rape of girls
Adulthood
    Killing young brides
    Forced suicides by young brides
    Wife beating
    Husband beating
    Husband–wife brawling
    Matricide
    Patricide
    Forced suicide of wives
    Wife raiding
    Marital rape
    Parent beating
Old Age
    Foresaking the aged
    Abandonement of the aged
    Beating the aged
    Killing the aged
    Forcing the aged to commit suicide

in no society does it occur frequently, and in most it occurs rarely. Although the data to measure the relative frequency or these types of family violence is not yet available, my review of the literature suggests the wife beating, physical punishment of children, sibling violence, infanticide, and harsh initiation rites at puberty are the ones that occur in the greatest number of societies.

The Prevalence of Family Violence

As part of our NIMH-supported holocultural study of family violence in 90 small-scale and peasant societies, we have obtained data about the frequency and severity of various forms of family violence in non-Western societies. Although not a probability sample, the 90 societies form a representative sample of societies from major cultural and geographical regions of the world.

The information about family violence in these 90 societies was gleaned from ethnographic reports on these societies included in the Human Relations Area Files data archive. The archive contains some 6,000 reports on the ways of life of 330 different cultural groups around the world. The reports are cross-referenced and indexed for easy and rapid retrieval. Most of the reports are ethnographies written by cultural anthropologists who lived with and observed the ways of life of these societies. Included are 14 societies from sub-Saharan Africa including the Zulu and Kung Bushmen, 10 from the Middle East including the Kurd of Iran and the Somali, seven European peasant groups including the Rural Irish and Serbs, 17 North American and 16 South American tribal societies and ethnic groups, 13 Oceanic societies including the Javanese and Lau Fijians, and 13 Asian societies including the Central Thai and the Santal of India.

Wife beating is the most common form of family violence, occuring in 84.5% of the 90 societies. Wife beating occurs at least occasionally in all or nearly all households in 18.8% of societies surveyed, in a majority but not all households in 29.9% of societies surveyed, in a minority of households in 37.8% of societies surveyed, and rarely or never in 15.5% of societies in the sample. Our data are comparable with that of other cross-cultural studies, based on different worldwide samples and different definitions of wife beating, which indicate that wife beating is present in from 71% to 92% of societies (Broude, 1983; Justinger, 1975; Masamura, 1979; Naroll, 1969; Schlegel, 1972; Whyte, 1978; Zelman, 1974).

In 8.9% of the societies in our sample, wife beating occurs only when the husband is intoxicated. In another 5.6% of the societies, beatings occur when the husband is sober or intoxicated. In the remaining 70% of societies wife beating usually occurs when the husband is sober.

Wife beating incidents resulting in death or permanent injury occur in 46.6% of societies. In 45.5% of societies, sexual jealousy, suspicion of adultery, or actual adultery motivates wife beating. In 25.5% of societies wife beating is provoked by insubordination or disobedience by the wife. In 23.3% the wife's failure to meet household responsibilities provokes abuse.

Husband beating occurs in a majority of households in 6.7% of societies and in a minority of household in 20.2%. In the other 73.1% of societies it is either rare or unheard of. Husband beating occurs only in societies where wife beating also occurs, although the two do not always occur simultaneously. In four societies husband–wife brawling is the common pattern, as opposed to either husband or wife beating alone. Burbank (1986) recently provided cross-cultural data suggesting that adultery or sexual jealousy is a major

Table 3. Relationships among Types of Family Violence

	(1)	(2)	(3)	(4)
(1) Wife beating		.38 (*n*=90)	.29 (*n*=48)	.41 (*n*=90)
(2) Child punishment			.64 (*n*=48)	−.03 (*n*=90)
(3) Sibling beating				.39 (*n*=48)
(4) Husband beating				

reason women beat their husbands as well as a major reason why women assault other women.

Physical punishment of children including spanking, slapping, beating, scalding, burning, pushing, pinching, and the like, occurs in 74.4% of societies. Physical punishment is regularly used in 13.3% of societies, is frequently used in 21.1%, is infrequently used in 40%, and is rarely or never used in 26.5% of societies.

Physical violence between nonadult siblings occurs in 43.7% of societies, being routine in 22.9%, infrequent to frequent 20.8% and rare or absent in 56.2%.

Intervention by outsiders in wife beating situations occurs in 91.2% of societies. Immediate intervention by kin or neighbors occurs in 17.6% of societies, the wife is provided temporary shelter in another household in 14.7%, the wife can obtain a judicial hearing or invoke supernatural sanctions in 17.6%, the wife can obtain a divorce in 11.8%, any of the above are available only when the beating exceeds norms governing severity or the reason for the beating in 29.4%, and intervention is unavailable in 8.8%.

As shown in Table 3, the frequency of one type of family violence is generally related to the frequency of other types (all coefficients are *gammas*). Additionally, infanticide, which occurs in 78.5% of societies, although rarely in most, is also related to family violence (*gamma*=.60, *n*=67, with wife beating; .11, *n*=67, with physical punishment; .44, *n*=36, with sibling beating, and .84, *n*=67 with husband beating).

The information summarized indicates that most people in the world are no strangers to family violence. It seems reasonable to conclude that most people in the world have either been the victims or the perpetrators of family violence at some point in their life. At the same time, we must recognize that few societies allow family violence to go unnoticed, with some form of intervention meant to protect the victim available in nearly all societies. Determining what types of intervention are effective in preventing family violence and what types of intervention are effective in preventing family violence and what societal conditions encourage the use of those interventions is an important next step for cross-cultural research on family violence.

SEXUAL INEQUALITY AND WIFE BEATING

Perhaps no idea so dominates current thinking about the causes of wife beating as the notion that wife beating results from or is a reflection of cultural values, rules, and practices that afford men more status and power than women. Analysis based on a feminist perspective (Martin, 1976), a review of the development of Western legal systems (Davidson, 1977), a regional comparison of Mediterranean cultures (Lozios, 1976), a study of social change in Yugoslavia (Erlich, 1966), and a study of wife beating victims (Ferraro, 1983), among others, all suggest that culturally sanctioned male dominance over females is a basic cause of wife beating. Unfortunately, none of these or any other studies to date actually establish a link between wife beating and sexual inequality. What is missing from the research program is a broad, systematic comparative study that allows comparison of the frequency of wife beating in cultures where female status is low with the frequency of wife beating in cultures where female status is relatively high. (Because in virtually all societies female status is never higher than that of men, high status for women means status equal to that of men.) If sexual inequality theory is valid, we would expect to find more wife beating in societies where women have relatively low status.

Although testing sexual inequality theory seems like a relatively straightforward task, it is anything but. Cross-cultural studies on female status have pointed to a number of conceptual and theoretical problems that must be addressed before any cross-cultural study of female status can produce meaningful results. One key problem is raised by Whyte (1978a,b) in his holocultural study of 56 indicators of female status in 93 small-scale societies. Whyte's (1978b, p. 214) statistical analysis leads him to conclude that:

> This finding calls into question much existing thought about women's roles. Cross-culturally, there appears to be no such thing as the status of women. It is perfectly possible for women in one society to have important property rights while being excluded from key religious posts and ceremonies; they may also do most of the productive work or have an important role in political life while suffering under a severe sexual double standard.

Whyte goes on to identify nine independent dimensions of female status: property control, kin power, value of life, value of labor, domestic authority, ritualized female solidarity, control of sex, ritualized fear of women, and joint male–female participation.

Although female status or lack of status seems less diffuse at the national level, Mascia-Lees' (1984) study of 98 nations suggests separate economic and family-educational-political dimensions to female status. These two broad studies suggest that in any study of sexual inequality and wife beating, status must be measured with a variety of independent indicators.

A related distinction was raised by Sanday (1981a) in her study of female power and male aggression toward women in 93 small-scale societies. Sanday pointed out a distinction between mythical male dominance and real male dominance. Real male dominance is present when men are violent toward women (they abduct them for marriage, beat their wives, live apart from them, etc.) and when women have little or no economic or political power in the community. Mythical male dominance is present when the violence is present but when women do have real power in the community. This pattern suggests that researchers need to measure female status in the private and public domains of culture.

A third conceptual distinction is noted by Schlegel (1977), who suggests that any study of status needs to focus on the three components of status—power, prestige, and rewards.

A final concern that investigators need to keep in mind is that any link they establish between wife beating and sexual inequality begs the broader question of why sexual inequality exists at all. Discussion of this question is beyond the bounds of this chapter, but the interested reader can find summaries of major theories of sexual inequality in Mascia-Lees (1984).

Three holocultural studies provide information about the relationship between sexual inequality and wife beating. Masamura (1979) suggested that sexual inequality is unrelated to wife beating because his data for 86 societies show no relationship between the frequency of wife beating and either patrilocal postmarital residence or patrilineal descent. Unfortunately, postmarital residence and descent are, at best, imprecise measures of sexual inequality. Schlegel's (1972) data indicate that wife beating is allowed in 77% of matrilineal societies. Schlegel's data further suggests that descent is less a determinant of frequency of wife beating than of who may beat the wife. In some matrilineal societies both the woman's husband and her brother may beat her. Who may beat her seems dependent in large part on whether it is the husband or the brother who is dominant in the household. Lester (1980) used a sample of 71 small-scale societies and claims to support sexual inequality theory, although he provides no indication of how female status is actually measured.

Our on-going holocultural study of family violence provides some preliminary information about sexual inequality theory. Gamma coefficients between wife beating frequency and 13 indicators of inequality are presented in Table 4. The inequality variables are scaled so that a positive relationship suggests a relationship between frequent wife beating and inequality. The coefficients in the Table suggest that in most areas of cultural activity inequality is unrelated to wife beating. However, the findings also suggest that in the economic and family domains wife beating is related to sexual inequality. Where female work groups are absent, where men control the distribution of the fruits of family labor, where women cannot acquire independent wealth, where men own the dwelling, and where men have the real power in the household, women are more likely to be beaten by their husbands.

Because the household tends to be the basic economic unit in small-scale societies and because these five factors are intercorrelated with one another, it seems reasonable to argue that these findings support an economic interpretation of the sexual inequality theory of wife beating. It seems that wife beating occurs most frequently in societies where men control the wealth and make most decisions in the household, regardless of a woman's status outside the home. However, it is worth noting that an examination of the distribution of the data indicates that relatively equal status between the sexes in household control and economic matters is a predictor of infrequent wife beating. Wife beating is absent altogether mainly in societies where women are dominant in the home and in economic matters and where they can amass personal wealth.

These cross-cultural findings mesh well with Kalmuss and Straus' (1982) finding that in United States families, economic dependence on the husband is a major predictor of severe wife beating. Economic dependence is reflected in the wife being unemployed, the

Table 4. Wife Beating Frequency and Female Status

Factor	Gamma	N
Domestic authority	.65	80
Female work groups	.53	77
Control of fruits of labor	.40	80
Acquisition of wealth	.34	76
Dwelling ownership	.33	75
Widow remarriage freedom	.26	87
Infanticide sex preference	.21	54
Menstrual taboo restrictions	.19	78
Property inheritance	.15	81
Divorce freedom	.13	64
Female initiation ceremonies	.12	78
Postmarital residence	.11	88
Premarital sex restrictions	.06	86

presence of children under the age of 5 years in the home, and the husband earning 75% or more of the family income. However, these findings are not in total agreement with Yllo's conclusions (1983, 1984) concerning sexual inequality and wife beating in the United States. Yllo reports a curvilinear pattern, with wife beating less frequent in states where women's status approaches that of men and more frequent in states where women's status is either lowest or highest. At the interactional level, she reports a similar pattern, with wife beating lowest where decision making is shared and highest where either the husband or wife dominates the process. As Yllo and others suggest, the United States pattern may reflect a transitional state where family norms and societal norms governing status are somewhat incongruent. This interpretation is supported by Erlich's (1966) study of social change in Yugoslavia, which suggests that the shift from a male-dominant to an egalitarian social order is a multigenerational process, with the frequency of family violence likely to rise first and then drop during the process.

The cross-cultural and intracultural research discussed provides support for a multidimensional conceptualization of female status and power and for the economic inequality theory of wife beating. At the same time, these findings suggest that broad statements linking sexual inequality in all its forms to wife beating are counterproductive as they mask the real linkages that provide us with some hints on how to control and prevent wife beating. Knowing that it is economic clout in the home that is strongly related to wife beating rather than the value placed on women's lives or a double standard in premarital sex is an important first step in identifying societal rules and practices that must be changed to reduce the frequency of wife beating.

CULTURAL PATTERNING OF AGGRESSION

In its broadest form, the cultural pattern model of human aggression suggests that cultures may be characterized by a basic, underlying set of values and beliefs that emphasize aggression and violence. Thus, in these cultures aggression is likely to be present in most spheres of activity including interpersonal relationships, child-rearing practices, religious beliefs and ceremonies, warfare practices, games and sports, etc. The culture pattern model is often viewed as an alternative to the drive discharge or catharsis model of aggression, which rests on the premise that all individuals and groups have an innate level of aggression that must be periodically discharged (Sipes, 1973). In contrast to the culture pattern model, the drive discharge model predicts that if aggression is present in one sphere of activity it will likely be absent in others.

As applied to family violence, the cultural patterning of aggression can be interpreted in four ways. First, the *subculture of violence* hypothesis suggests that violence is a learned behavior shared by members of groups whose value systems encourage the use of violence (Wolfgang & Ferracuti 1967). Although not yet employed empirically in family violence research, the subculture of violence hypothesis could serve as a framework for explaining high levels of family violence in subcultural groups in societies where the level of family violence is low in general. The *cultural consistency* hypothesis suggests that family violence is a reflection of basic values that shape the norms governing family life, conflict resolution, child-rearing practices, and so forth. Carroll (1980) used the idea of cultural consistency to develop models that explain the high level of parental violence toward children among Mexican-Americans and the low level among Jewish-Americans. *Family socialization into violence* theory suggests that violence is transferred from one generation to the next by individuals who witness or are victims of family violence in their childhood homes. Although there is still much controversey about women learning to be victims, most researchers would be comfortable with Straus' (1983) limited conclusions that: "The idea that child-abusing parents were themselves victims of abuse, and that wife beating husbands come from violent families, is now widely accepted" (p. 217). The fourth approach to the cultural patterning of family violence, the *cultural spillover* hypothesis (Baron & Straus 1985) suggests that:

> the more a society tends to endorse the use of physical force to attain socially approved ends (such as order in the schools, crime control, and international dominance), the greater the likelihood that this legitimation of force will be generalized to other spheres of life where force is less socially approved, such as the family and relations between the sexes. (p. 13)

Both Masamura (1979) and Lester (1980) have provided holocultural tests of the hypothesized link between wife beating and other forms of aggression in society. Although both claim to support the hypothesis, their findings are actually somewhat contradictory. Masamura finds wife beating associated with high rates of theft, personal crime, aggression, suicide, homicide, feuding, and warfare. Lester finds wife beating associated with cruel treatment of war captives, drunken aggressiveness, and mutilation of children but unrelated to homicide, suicide, and warfare frequency. A third study, by Levinson (1981), suggested that rare or infrequent wife beating is associated with rare or infrequent physical punishment of children, but that frequent wife beating does not consistently predict frequent use of physical punishment.

From a cross-cultural viewpoint, the only statement we can make with any degree of certainty about the cultural patterning of family violence is that children are more likely to be punished physically in societies where people believe that supernatural spirits are malevolent and punishing (Lambert, Triandis, and Wolf 1959; Prescott 1975; Rohner 1975; Spiro & D'Andrade, 1958; Whiting 1967). Not only is this proposition supported by these five independent holocultural studies but also by Otterbein and Otterbein's (1973) study of caretakers in the Bahamas.

Although cross-cultural studies have yet to make a major contribution to testing the cultural pattern model of family violence in its various forms, two groups of holocultural studies suggest that cross-cultural research can make a major contribution in this area. One group of studies suggests that there is a link between violence directed at women and other forms of aggression. Minturn, Grosse, and Haider (1969) found rape associated with male genital mutilations at puberty; Sanday (1981b) found rape associated with raiding for wives, and interpersonal violence; Baron and Straus (1985), in a comparison of United States states, observed that rape is associated with legitimate violence.

A second group of studies suggest that aggressive child rearing practices are linked to various adult behaviors, beliefs, and cultural norms and practices. Pain infliction in child rearing has been related to polygynous marriage, inferior status for women, aggressive deities, and tobacco use by both sexes (Blum, 1969; Prescott, 1975); physical punishment to a long menstrual taboo (Stephens, 1962); and severe socialization to complex and representative art design (Barry, 1957). Additionally, an emphasis on aggression in child-rearing has been associated with warfare, displaced aggression, fear of others, and aggression explanations and therapies for illness (Kiev, 1960; Prothro, 1960; Russell, 1972; Whiting & Child, 1953).

One of the major problems facing researchers attempting to study violence and aggression cross-culturally is the complexity of these two concepts and the wide range of behaviors that can be classified as aggression. In our study of family violence we have tried to control this complexity problem by placing aggressive behaviors in three categories: (a) aggression between household residents; (b) aggression between acquaintances (relatives, neighbors, co-workers, etc.), and (c) aggression between strangers (people from other communities, animals, inanimate objects). When the relationship between wife beating and other forms of aggression are analyzed in this framework, we find that wife beating is part of a pattern involving aggression between household members and aggression between acquaintance to resolve disputes. Similarly, physical punishment of children seems to be part of a pattern characterized by the use of violence to punish and reinforce societal norms, as evidenced by violent punishments for crimes and the use of pain in initiation ceremonies.

SOCIAL ORGANIZATION

Social organizational theories of family violence rest on the premise that the basic causes of family violence can be found in the structural features of a society that order the relationships among family members. As with the sexual inequality and cultural patterning of aggression theories, social organization theories require testing at the societal level through systematic comparisons of societies that vary on the key organizational features.

The type of family characteristic of a society and the composition of the family are the two major social organizational features that are seen as directly related to family violence. Holocultural studies consistently demonstrate that the best assurance that an infant or child will be treated warmly and affectionately in nuclear and extended families, and have his or her needs met, is the availability of alternative caretakers in the household (Levinson, 1979; Minturn & Lambert 1964; Rohner 1975; Whiting, 1960). The presence of multiple caretakers in the home almost guarantees that an infant or child will be indulged and accepted, although who the caretakers are makes a difference. Siblings, for example, are not especially warm and loving, but fathers and grandparents in the home on a day-to-day basis help ensure that a child will be held and treated warmly. On the other hand, an infant or child is more likely to be rejected or neglected when raised by his or her mother alone. A woman in continual contact with her child is more likely to abuse that child emotionally than a woman who has other adults in the home or nearby to help her. Mothers who are often away from the home do not tolerate insubordination from their children, but are not much concerned about irresponsible behavior.

These studies also suggest that household type seems to affect child rearing practices. In extended family households where multiple caretakers are readily available, infants are frequently indulged. In nuclear family household where only two caretakers are generally available, infants may or may not be indulged. And, in mother–child households where the mother is the only caretaker, children run a fair risk of being neglected and sometimes rejected in the form of physical and verbal abuse.

Unfortunately there is little systematic cross-cultural research bearing on the related question of whether societies with nuclear family households have higher rates of wife beating than societies with extended family households. The possible link between nuclear families (especially the social isolation and potential for hostility in nuclear families) and wife beating has been emphasized for some years by Straus and his associates (Straus, Gelles, & Steinmetz, 1980) and others (Mahmood, 1977; Whitehurst, 1974); and requires careful cross-cultural study. The only formal cross-cultural test is Whiting and Whiting's (1976) study of 39 societies, which supports the hypothesis that wife beating is more frequent in societies with independent as opposed to extended family households.

On a broader scale, a number of researchers report that the level of societal scale or complexity may also influence child-rearing practices. Rohner finds that people in complex societies—those with high levels of political integration and social stratification and a fixed settlement pattern—tend to reject their children to a somewhat greater extent than people in less complex societies. This pattern is supported by Pryor (1977) who finds a positive relationship between the level of economic development of a society and the frequency of use of nonpermissive and punitive disciplinary techniques in child rearing. Similarly, Petersen, Lee, and Ellis' (1982) study of 122 societies suggests a link between societal complexity and the use of physical punishment in child rearing. However, Petersen and his associates go a step further and suggest a broader causal sequence involving a societal emphasis on adult supervision of other adults, which leads to conformity as a child rearing goal and that, in turn, leads to the use of physical force to shape children's behavior.

Obviously, there is a great deal of room and a pressing need for more cross-cultural research on the links between social organization and wife beating and husband beating. The research on child rearing and especially the use of physical punishment in child rearing has produced a number of stimulating conclusions. Because ample data on violence between adult family members is available, we should begin to see equally useful research conclusions about these types of family violence appearing in the near future. One clear need is for a test of the nuclear/extended family hypothesis of wife beating. Again, this is an area where cross-cultural analysis can make a major contribution to our understanding of family violence as study of family structure requires the use of a cross-cultural sample that includes the full range of family types that occur in societies throughout the world.

SOCIAL CHANGE AND FAMILY VIOLENCE

Much of the recent interest in cross-cultural studies of family violence has focused on the possible effects of social change on family relationships in developing nations. Of 14 studies bearing directly on this issue, 10 suggest that Westernization, urbanization, industrialization, colonization, and the like, encourage a breakdown of traditional forms of family organization and a disintegration of informal social controls. This breakdown leads in turn to increased levels of stress and violence among family members. Social change is linked to the use of children as beggars, pimps, and domestic laborers in Sri Lanka (deSilva, 1981); to child neglect and abandonment by the Zulu of South Africa (Loening 1981); to patricide, infanticide, and extortion of money from parents in Nigeria (Nkpa, 1981); to filial violence, usually directed at the mother, in Japan (Kumagai, 1983); to wife beating among the Hare in Canada (Savishinsky, 1970), the Kpelle in Liberia (Erchak, 1984; Gibbs, 1984), and peasants in Yugoslavia (Erlich, 1966); and to increased violence by youths in Tahiti (Spiegel, 1981). On the other hand, a decrease in wife beating frequency has been attributed to the awarding of legal rights to women in rural Greece (Sanders, 1962) and to Azande women in central Africa (Evans-Pritchard, 1937), to the direct intervention of British colonial officials in Uganda (Mair, 1940), and to the influence of Protestant missionaries on the Highland Quechua of Ecuador (Muratoria, 1981).

Although these studies suggest that social change influences the nature and frequency of family violence in developing regions, it should be noted that this finding is anything but conclusive. For the most part, these and other studies of social change and family violence are uncontrolled case studies conducted with a limited amount of data pertaining to small samples of individuals at one point in time. The major exception is Erlich's (1966) analysis of changes in structure and relationships in Yugoslav families from the turn of the century until 1941. Because family researchers seem unaware of this early study, its approach and conclusions warrant some space here. From 1936 to 1941 Erlich and her associates gathered historical and contemporary data from over 300 villages in the Macedonia (Albanian and Christian), Bosnia (Moslem and Christian), Serbia, Croatia, and Littoral regions of Yugoslavia. By comparing regional patterns at different points in time over a 50-year period and by comparing the regional and village patterns to one another, Erlich effectively utilized longitudinal and intersocietal comparisons to gauge the effect of social change on Yugoslav family life.

Until about the turn of the century in some regions and until later in others, Yugoslav peasant families were organized into large, patriarchial, patrilocal households called *zadrugas*. Each *zadruga*, numbering up to 40 members, was ruled by the oldest male, although his sons could influence his decisions, and his wife had authority over other women (usually daughters-in-law and granddaughters) in the zadruga. Sons spent their whole lives in the zadruga of their birth, whereas daughters married out into other zadrugas in the village. Except for personal items, all property including land and live-stock was owned by the zadruga. A shift to a money economy beginning around 1900, political disruptions caused by World War I, and the economic depression of the 1930s led to a gradual break-up of the zadrugas, first into smaller extended families and ultimately into nuclear families.

Erlich's tracing of the disintegration of the zadrugas and rise of nuclear family suggests a clear relationship among family type, wife beating frequency, and female authority in the home. In the traditional zadruga, men held all authority and women were never beaten. In transitional extended family households, women's authority increased, but so too did the frequency of wife beating. Finally, in villages where small extended families or nuclear families became the rule, wife beating was rare and female authority in the household about equal that of men. In the Littoral region, which is farthest along in the transition to nuclear family households, (a process that has taken some 80 years) wife beating is nonexistent and women share equally in decision-making in 85% of the villages.

Erlich's approach and findings contain some important lessons for students of social change and family violence. First, it is important to view social change as an ongoing, open-ended process rather than as a narrow cause and effect sequence. Second, social change involves both external and internal pressures, although in the modern world external forces seem to be more important. Third, data concerning the social change process under study must be collected for the entire time period during which change takes place. And, fourth, although social change seems in the short run to lead to an increase in family violence, in the long run a new social order may be established and the level of violence decreases.

IMPLICATIONS FOR CONTROL AND PREVENTION

As with all approaches to family violence, cross-cultural studies are conducted with the hope that they will contribute to controlling and preventing family violence. The assumption is that what we learn about family violence and related matters in one society can be put to use in other societies. Although cross-cultural studies have some way to go before they maximize their potential contribution to our understanding of family violence, they do provide some information relevant to the control of family violence. First, it seems fairly clear that the presence of kin or neighbors who will intervene in violent or potentially violent situations is a characteristic of societies with low rates of wife beating and the regular use of nonviolent child rearing practices. This finding strongly suggests that, in the absence of intervening neighbors, shelters for battered women, and swift criminal justice and social welfare intervention must play a prominent role in any effort to control family violence. Second, it seems that social change involving industrialization, urbanization, and other major forces, is often followed by an increased rate of family violence. However, there is also some evidence suggesting that once the new social order is stabilized, the rate of family violence decreases. Third, it is important to remember that there is a long list of human behaviors that can be classified as types of family violence, with virtually each type considered abuse in some societies but legitimate behavior in others.

In the sample of 90 small-scale societies currently being used in our holocultural study of family violence, 16 societies can be described as essentially free or untroubled by family violence. In these societies spouses rarely or never beat each other, parents never or rarely physically punish their children, and siblings rarely fight with one another. In short, any physical violence between family members is considered to be abusive and a violation of societal norms. These 16 societies cover a broad range of cultural types, ranging from the hunting and gathering Bushmen of the Kalahari Desert to the Kurdish villages of Iran to Lapp herders of Scandinavia to the Papago Indians of the American Southwest. What do these societies have in common that distinguishes them from other societies with either moderate or high rates of family violence? Our preliminary analysis suggests that four factors are especially important. First, spouses enjoy sexual equality with joint decision making in household and financial matters, equal freedom to divorce for both men and women, and no double standard governing premarital sex. Second, marriage is monogamous and the divorce rate relatively low, suggesting marital stability and emotional and economic dependence between spouses. Third, disagreements between adults in the society are resolved peacefully through avoidance of conflict situations, mediation, or disengagement, rather than violently or through threats of violence. Fourth, immediate outside help by neighbors who intervene or provide shelter is provided to family members who are victims or are threatened with physical harm by other family members. Although these findings are tentative, pending further theoretical and methodological analysis, they do suggest that we can learn something about controlling family violence by studying other cultures.

REFERENCES

Adams, R. N. (1960). An inquiry into the nature of the family. In R. L. Carneiro & S. E. Dole (Eds), *Essays in the science of culture* (pp. 30–49). New York: Thomas Crowell.

Apple, D. (1956). The social structure of grandparenthood. *American Anthropology, 58,* 656–663.

Baron, L., & Straus, M. A. (1985). *Legitimate violence and rape: A test of the cultural spillover theory.* Unpublished paper, Family Research Laboratory, University of New Hampshire.

Barry, H. III. (1957). Relationship between child training and the pictorial arts. *Journal of Abnormal and Social Psychology, 54,* 380–383.

Blum, R. H. (1969). *Society and drugs.* San Francisco: Jossey-Bass.

Bohannan, P. (1968). An alternative residence classification. In P. Bohannan & J. Middleton (Eds), *Marriage, family, and residence* (pp. 317–323). Garden City, NY: Natural History Press.

Broude, G. J., & Greene, S. J. (1983). Cross-cultural codes on husband–wife relationships. *Ethnology, 22,* 263–280.

Burbank, V. K. (in press). Female aggression in cross-cultural perspective. *Behavior Science Research.*

Carroll, J. C. (1980). A cultural-consistency theory of family violence in Mexican-American and Jewish-ethnic groups. In M. A. Straus & G. T. Hotaling (Eds.), *The social causes of husband–wife violence* (pp. 68–85). Minneapolis, MN: University of Minnesota Press.

Davidson, T. (1977). Wife beating: A recurring phenomenon throughout history. In M. Roy (Ed.), *Battered women* (pp. 2–34). New York: Van Nostrand Reinhold.

deSilva, W. (1981). Some cultural and economic factors leading to neglect, abuse and violence in respect to children within the family in Sri Lanka. *Child Abuse and Neglect, 5,* 391–405.

Dobash, R. E., & Dobash, R. P. (1979). *Violence against wives.* New York: The Free Press.

Erchak, G. M. (1984). Cultural anthropology and spouse abuse. *Current Anthropology, 25,* 331–332.

Erlich, V. S. (1966). *Family in transition: A study of 300 Yugoslav villages.* Princeton, NJ: Princeton University Press.

Evans-Pritchard, E. E. (1937). *Witchcraft, oracles and magic among the Azande.* Oxford: Claredon Press.

Ferraro, K. J. (1983). Rationalizing violence: How battered women stay. *Victimology: An International Journal, 8,* 203–214.

Gelles, R. J., & Cornell, C. P. (1983). *International perspectives on family violence.* Lexington, MA: D. C. Heath.

Gelles, R. J., & Straus, M. A. (1979). Determinants of violence in the family: Toward a theoretical integration. In W. R. Burr, R. Hill, I. Nye, & I. Reiss, (Eds.), *Contemporary theories about the family (Vol 1,* pp. 549–581). New York: The Free Press.

Gibbs, J. L. Jr. (1984). On cultural anthropology and spouse abuse. *Current Anthropology, 25,* 533.

Justinger, J. M. (1978). *Reaction to change: A holocultural test of some theories of religious movements* (Doctoral dissertation, State University of New York at Buffalo, 1978). Ann Arbor: University Microfilms International.

Kalmuss, D. S., & Straus, M. A. (1982). Wife's marital dependency and wife abuse. *Journal of Marriage and the Family, 44,* 277–286.

Kiev, A. (1960). Primitive therapy: A cross-cultural study of the relationship between child training and therapeutic practices related to illness. *Psychoanalytic study of society, 1,* 185–217.

Korbin, J. (1977). Anthropological contributions to the study of child abuse. *Child Abuse and Neglect, 1,* 7–24.

Korbin, J. E. (1981). *Child abuse and neglect: Cross-cultural perspectives.* Berkeley, CA: University of California Press.

Kumagai, F. (1983). Filial violence in Japan. *Victimology: An International Journal, 8,* 173–194.

Kunstadter, P. (1963). A survey of the consanguine or matrifocal family. *American Anthropologist, 65,* 56–66.

Lambert, W. W., Triandis, L. M., & Wolf, M. (1959). Some correlates of beliefs in the malevolence and benevolence of supernatural beings: A cross-societal study. *Journal of Abnormal and Social Psychology, 58,* 162–169.

Leach, E. R. (1961). *Rethinking anthropology.* London: Athlone Press.

Lee, G. R. (1984). The utility of cross-cultural data. *Journal of Family Issues, 5,* 519–541.

Lester, D. (1980). A cross-culture study of wife abuse. *Aggressive Behavior, 6,* 361–364.

Levinson, D. (1979). Population density in cross-cultural perspective. *American Ethnologist, 6,* 742–751.

Levinson, D. (1981). Physical punishment of children and wife beating in cross-cultural perspective. *Child abuse and neglect, 5,* 193–195.

Loening, W. (1981). Child abuse among the Zulus: A people in transition. *Child Abuse and Neglect, 5,* 3–7.

Lozios, P. (1978). Violence and the family: Some Mediterranean examples. In J. P. Martin (Ed.), *Violence and the family* (pp. 183–196). Chichester: Wiley.

Mahmood, T. (1977). Child abuse in Arabia, India and the West—Comparative legal aspects. In J. M. Eekelaar & S. N. Katz (Eds.), *Family violence: An international and interdisciplinary study* (pp. 281–289). Toronto: Butlerworths.

Mair, L. P. (1940). *Native marriage in Buganda.* London: Oxford University Press.

Martin, D. (1976). *Battered wives.* San Francisco: Glide Publications.

Masamura, W. T. (1979). Wife abuse and other forms of aggression. *Victimology: An International Journal, 4,* 46–59.

Mascia-Lees, F. E. (1984). *Toward a model of women's status.* New York: Peter Long.

Minturn, L., & Lambert, W. (1964). The antecedents of child training: A cross-cultural test of some hypotheses. In L. Minturn & W. Lambert (Eds.), *Mothers of six cultures* (pp. 343–346). New York: Wiley.

Minturn, L., Grosse, M., & Haider, S. (1969). Cultural patterning of sexual beliefs and behaviors. *Ethnology, 8,* 301–318.

Muratorio, B. (1981). Protestantism, ethnicity, and class in Chimborazo. In N. E. Whitten (Ed.), *Cultural transformations and ethnicity in modern Ecuador* (pp. 506–534). Urbana, IL: University of Illinois Press.

Murdock, G. P. (1949). *Social structure*. New York: Macmillan.

Naroll, R. (1969). Cultural determinants and the concept of the sick society. In S. C. Plog & R. G. Edgerton (Eds.), *Changing perspectives in mental illness* (pp. 128–155). New York: Holt, Rinehart & Winston.

Naroll, R. (1973). The culture-bearing unit in cross-cultural surveys. In R. Naroll & R. Cohen (Eds.), *A handbook of method in cultural anthropology* (pp. 721–765). New York: Columbia University Press.

Nimkoff, M. F. (1965). Types of family: The social system and the family. In M. F. Nimkoff (Ed.), *Comparative family systems* (pp. 12–60). Boston, MA: Houghton-Mifflin.

Nkpa, M. K. V. (1981). Social change and the problems of parent abuse in a developing country. *Victimology: An international journal, 6,* 167–174.

Otterbein, C. S., & Otterbein, K. (1973). Believers and beaters: A case study of supernatural beliefs and child rearing in the Bahama Islands. *American Anthropologist, 75,* 1670–1681.

Otterbein, K. F. (1965). Caribbean family organization: A comparative analysis. *American Anthropologist, 67,* 66–79.

Pasternak, B., Ember, C. R., & Ember, M. (1976). On the conditions favoring extended family households. *Journal of Anthropological Research, 32,* 109–123.

Petersen, L. R., Lee, G. R., & Ellis, G. J. (1982). Social structure, socialization values, and disciplinary techniques: A cross-cultural analysis. *Journal of Marriage and the Family, 44,* 131–142.

Prescott, J. W. (1975). Body pleasure and the origins of violence. *Bulletin of the Atomic Scientists, 31,* 10–20.

Prince Peter of Greece and Denmark. (1965). The Tibetan family system. In M. F. Nimkoff (Ed.), *Comparative family systems* (pp. 192–208). Boston, MA: Houghton Mifflin.

Prothro, E. T. (1960). Patterns of permissiveness among preliterate peoples. *Journal of Abnormal and Social Psychology, 61,* 151–154.

Pryor, F. L. (1977). *The origins of economy*. New York: Academic Press.

Rohner, R. P. (1975). *They love me, they love me not: A worldwide study of the effects of parental acceptance and rejection*. New Haven, CT: HRAF Press.

Russell, E. W. (1972). Factors of human aggression: A cross-cultural factor analysis of characteristics related to warfare and crime. *Behavior Science Notes, 8,* 275–312.

Sanday, P. R. (1981a). *Female power and male dominance*. New York: Cambridge University Press.

Sanday, P. R. (1981b). The socio-cultural context of rape: A cross-cultural study. *Journal of Social Issues, 37,* 5–27.

Sanders, I. T. (1962). *Rainbow in the rock: The people of rural Greece*. Cambridge: Harvard University Press.

Savishinsky, J. S. (1970). *Stress and nobility in an Artic community: The Hare Indians of Colville Lake, Northwest Territories* (Doctoral Dissertation, Cornell University, 1970). Ann Arbor: University Microfilms.

Schlegel, A. (1972). *Male dominance and female autonomy*. New Haven, CT: HRAF Press.

Schlegel, A. (1977). Toward a theory of sexual stratification. In A. Schlegel (Ed.), *Sexual stratification* (pp. 1–40). New York: Columbia University Press.

Sipes, R. G. (1973). War, sports, and aggression: An empirical test of two rival theories. *American Anthropologist, 57,* 64–86.

Solheim, J. (1982). A cross-cultural examination of use of corporal punishment on children: A focus on Sweden and the United States. *Child Abuse and Neglect, 6,* 147–154.

Spiegal, J. P. (1981). Ethnopsychiatric dimensions in family violence. In M. R. Green (Ed.), *Violence and the family* (pp. 79–89). Boulder, CO: Westview Press.

Spiro, M. E., & D'Andrade, R. G. (1958). A cross-cultural study of some supernatural beliefs. *American Anthropologist, 60,* 456–466.

Stephens, W. N. (1962). *The Oedipus complex: Cross-cultural evidence*. New York: Free Press.

Straus, M. A. (1983). Ordinary violence, child abuse, and wife-beating: What do they have in common? In D. Finkelhor, R. J. Gelles, G. T. Hotaling, & M. A. Straus (Eds.), *The dark side of families* (pp. 213–234). Beverly Hills, CA: Sage.

Straus, M. A. (June, 1985). Methodology of collaborative cross-national research on child abuse. Paper presented at the U.S.-Sweden Joint Seminar on Physical and Sexual Abuse of Children, Satra Burk, Sweden.

Straus, M. A., Gelles, R. J., & Steinmetz, S. K. (1980). *Behind closed doors; violence in the American family*. New York: Anchor Press.

Tellis-Nayak, V., & Donoghue, G. O. (1982). Conjugal egalitarianism and violence across cultures. *Journal of Comparative Family Studies, 8,* 277–290.

White, R. B., & Cornely, D. A. (1981). Navajo child abuse and neglect study: A comparative examination of abuse and neglect of Navajo children. *Child Abuse and Neglect, 5,* 9–17.

Whitehurst, R. N. (1974). Alternative family struciures and violence-reduction. In S. K. Steinmetz & M. A. Straus (Eds.), *Violence in the family* (pp. 315–320). New York: Harper & Row.

Whiting, J. W. M. (1960). Resource mediation and learning by identification. In I. Iscoe & H. Stevenson (Eds.), *Personality development in children* (pp. 112–126). Austin, TX: University of Texas Press.

Whiting, J. W. M. (1967). Sorcery, sin, and the superego: A cross-cultural study of some mechanisms of social control. In C. Ford (Ed.), *Cross-cultural approaches* (pp. 147–168). New Haven, CT: HRAF Press.

Whiting, J. W. M., & Child, I. L. (1953). *Child training and personality: A cross-cultural study.* New Haven, CT: Yale University Press.

Whiting, J. W. M., & Whiting, B. B. (1976). Aloofness and intimacy of husbands and wives: A cross-cultural study. In T. Schwartz (Ed.), *Socialization as communication* (pp. 91–115). Berkeley, CA: University of California Press.

Whyte, M. K. (1978a). *The status of women in preindustrial societies.* Princeton, NJ: Princeton University Press.

Whyte, M. K. (1978b). Cross-cultural codes dealing with the relative status of women. *Ethnology, 17,* 211–237.

Wolfgang, M. E., & Ferracuti, F. (1967). *The subculture of violence: Towards an integrated theory of criminology.* London: Tavistock.

Wright, G. C. (1970). Projection and displacement: A cross-cultural study of folktale aggression. In D. R. Price-Williams (Ed.), *Cross-cultural studies* (pp. 348–360). Baltimore, MD: Penguin.

Yllo, K. (1983). Sexual equality and violence against wives in American states. *Journal of Comparative Family Studies, 14,* 67–86.

Yllo, K. (1984). The status of women, marital equality and violence against wives. *Journal of Family Issues, 5,* 307–320.

Zelman, E. A. (1974). *Women's rights and women's rites: A cross-cultural study of woman power and reproductive ritual* (Doctoral dissertation, the University of Michigan, 1974). Ann Arbor: University Microfilms International.

19

Research Issues Concerning Family Violence

ROBERT GEFFNER, ALAN ROSENBAUM, and HONORE HUGHES

INTRODUCTION

After decades of professional inattention and neglect, the area of family violence has received substantial publicity in recent years, and more research is being conducted now than ever before. Several factors have contributed both to the inattention and to the burgeoning interest. Researchers in this area come from a variety of disciplines, including psychology, sociology, criminology, medicine, law, and others. Communication between these fields has been inadequate, conceptual schemata and research strategies are often divergent, and there is sometimes competition between the professions. As a consequence, numerous inconsistencies in methodology, results, and interpretation have emerged, and these contribute to the confusion regarding the etiology and demography of family violence.

Difficulties inherent in studying violent families have discouraged many potential investigators from pursuing research in these areas. In addition, discrepancies between the popular conceptions of the family and the realities of family violence, the shame and stigma often associated with such problems, and public policies protecting the sanctity of the home have tended to obscure the very serious magnitude of domestic violence. As a result of these and other issues, the development of family violence research has been impeded.

However, there has been a gradual improvement in the last two decades. Laws that mandate the reporting of child maltreatment to agencies specializing in working with families have been implemented in every state. Shelters for abused wives and their children have proliferated, and with them have come the development of programs for abused women, abusive men, and their children. National coalitions for child abuse, sexual assault, and domestic violence have sprung into existence. A national clearinghouse for domestic violence research has been established at the University of Texas at

ROBERT GEFFNER • Department of Psychology, University of Texas at Tyler, Tyler, TX 75701. ALAN ROSENBAUM • Department of Psychiatry, University of Massachusetts Medical School, Worcester, MA 01605. HONORE HUGHES • Department of Psychology, University of Arkansas, Fayetteville, AR 72701.

Tyler, and research programs focusing on family violence are being added at many universities.

Researchers and practitioners also have more sources for publication of research and sources for interventions concerning this type of violence because there are four new journals in the field (*Journal of Family Violence, Journal of Interpersonal Violence, Sexual Coercion and Assault,* and *Violence and Victims*). It is anticipated that an increase in the number of conferences and journals will enhance the quality and quantity of research being conducted. The national clearinghouse for spouse abuse research already reports such an increase in research; they catalogued 450 references for the 13-year period from 1972 to 1985, but over 100 additional references in just the last 8 months of 1985.

Because more studies are being reported concerning family violence, the purpose of this chapter is to focus on the issues involved in conducting research in this area. There are several concerns that will be addressed, including conceptual issues, methods and design, intervention and/or treatment evaluation, ethical issues, and future directions. A methodological critique of previous research and suggestions for improvement are presented. There are several general issues that encompass varied aspects of family violence research, and these are discussed first. Examples of research in child physical abuse, child sexual abuse, and marital violence are discussed throughout this chapter, as well as a very recent area (children who witness family violence).

CONCEPTUAL ISSUES

The degree of research sophistication for the various areas of family violence appears to be directly related to the amount of attention that the area has received. For example, child physical abuse came to the forefront in the 1960s, and the methodological rigor in this area is more advanced in comparison to marital violence and child sexual abuse. The initial studies in the various areas of family violence were generally anecdotal, and tended to focus more on clinical issues and demographic characteristics. However, contemporary researchers are now looking more carefully at conceptual issues and reevaluating their research strategies accordingly. Some of the major issues being discussed are definitions, assessment, and epidemiology.

The operational definition of abuse has important ramifications for all aspects of research. For example, researchers have identified the lack of generally accepted definitions of physical abuse, neglect, and sexual abuse as a major difficulty in each of these areas (Besharov, 1981; Finkelhor & Hotaling, 1984; Gelles, 1982; Mrazek & Mrazek, 1981). In epidemiological research, the lack of accepted definitions has produced a wide variety of estimates of incidence and prevalence rates, depending on how broadly or narrowly the particular form of maltreatment is defined. Problems with nonuniform definitions occur in nonepidemiological studies as well. The use of idiosyncratic definitions by individual researchers leads to results that cannot be compared across studies because the subject populations are very likely to be different.

The usual approach in physical abuse of children regarding the issue of definition is to employ the criteria used by the local social service workers (i.e., a documented case of physical abuse or neglect), which is a practical, though inadequate, solution because substantiation judgments differ by state, by county, and even by worker. In the last 5 years, a major step toward the alleviation of many of the problems associated with definitions has been taken with the completion of the National Study of the Incidence of

Severity of Child Abuse and Neglect (1981). One of the purposes of this study was to develop systematic definitions of child abuse and child neglect that took into account the details of the suspected event or neglectful behavior and the evidence on which the reporters' suspicions were based. The development of these criteria for abuse and neglect led to more systematic data gathering and more complete reporting of information, which has improved the quality and comparability of the research published in the last several years.

At the present time, issues regarding definitions of sexual abuse are very salient. In most studies the definitions employed have been broad and the victims included in the studies have experienced diverse types of sexually abusive acts (Mrazek & Mrazek, 1981; Sablatura, 1985). Whereas earlier investigators have included adult exhibitionism in the definition, recent researchers, with the exception of Finkelhor (1985; Finkelhor & Hotaling, 1984), have more restrictively defined child sexual abuse as involving physical contact.

In contrast to the previous two areas of child maltreatment, the study of children who witness parental violence has only recently become a recognized research area, and its development is still in the very basic stages. Whereas in the previous two areas many of the researchers are cognizant of the importance of a standardized definition, most authors in child witness research assume that children are exposed to violence if it is present in the children's home, and they make ambiguous statements, such as that the children "frequently observed" or "were aware" of the violence (e.g., Elbow, 1982; Hilberman & Munson, 1978). This assumption is made even in studies in which the Conflict Tactics Scale (Straus, 1979) was administered to obtain information about the amount and type of violence (Brown, Pelcovitz & Kaplan, 1983; Wolfe, Zak, Wilson, & Jaffe, 1986). However, a few researchers did ask the battered women in their samples whether their children had witnessed marital violence. Hershey (1982) inquired of the women in her sample whether their children had witnessed episodes of violence (91% were reported to have done so), though she provides no definition of the term *violence* as she used it, nor an estimate of frequency, intensity, or duration.

The problem of definition has also been important in marital violence research. An informal survey conducted for this chapter of over 30 marital violence investigations published since 1980 indicated that only five investigators described the criteria used to define the abused sample. Further, the nature of the criteria was inconsistent across studies. Goldberg and Tomlanovich (1984) distinguished victims of domestic violence from nonvictims on the basis of a yes or no response to the statement: "at some time my boyfriend/husband or girlfriend/wife has pushed me around, hit me, kicked me or hurt me" (p. 3260). It should be noted that at least two or these items (pushed me around and hurt me) could be interpreted in nonphysical ways. Dalton and Kantner (1983) asked the question "have you yourself been battered or abused?" in order to classify subjects. Even though they went on to define abuse as "the physical and emotional maltreatment of a woman by her husband or ex-husband or even male companion or boyfriend" (p. 706), there is clearly much room for variability. Most typically, subjects are included in the abused sample if they described themselves as abused, attended a shelter for abused women, or met some nonoperationalized criteria.

Thus, definitions used to include particular people in family violence samples have not yet been widely agreed on by researchers. Operational definitions of violent acts that would be accepted by researchers and consistently used may resolve many of the discrepancies across studies.

ROBERT GEFFNER
ET AL.

The methods and design in family violence research have become the focal point for those who are attempting to improve the rigor of the studies. Several concerns have been raised, including issues relating to sampling, epidemiology, measurement techniques, experimental design, and data analysis.

A general problem with many studies in family violence arises from an author's failure to provide adequate detail in the research report when describing the subjects, methods of assessment, procedures involved, etc. Careful description of important parameters of the investigation is essential for understanding the results and for replicating the study. Specificity is also crucial for treatment outcome studies as regards the descriptions of the intervention procedures and the delineation of the outcome criteria.

Sampling

Bias due to sampling methods and reporting is a frequent problem, especially with regard to generalizability. Results obtained from samples that are unrepresentative of the larger population (e.g., prisoners, college students, shelter residents) are likely to be misleading or inaccurate if the interpretations of those findings are not appropriately circumspect. A reporting bias may also be an important source of confusion and distortion in studies in this area. Jason (1984) pointed out that a reporting bias exists when some characteristic of a person or family leads them to have more contact with sources of child abuse reports than another family might. That particular characteristic may then become associated with an increased risk of abuse when in fact it may be related to increased risk of being suspected of abuse.

Although improvements have been noted in sample selection for child physical abuse, a number of problems still remain. Many of the families included in investigations were quite heterogeneous and frequently the number of subjects was quite small. Other difficulties included lumping together children of a wide age range (e.g., 4 to 14 years) as well as different types of abuse. In some studies, the question as to whether children were subject to multiple forms of abuse was not specified, and in several instances children were identified as abused and neglected, but were put into the abuse group because that form of abuse was considered to be more serious.

Most of the investigators conducting research in the sexual abuse of children have also used small samples, including case studies, as well as subjects who are generally unrepresentative of the population as a whole. According to Sablatura (1985), four types of samples have typically been utilized. These are (a) children and families who are studied soon after the sexual abuse was disclosed or reported; (b) women who had been sexually abused as children and are currently receiving mental health services; (c) deviant, or what Tierney and Corwin (1983) call prescreened populations of adults or adolescents (e.g., prisoners, prostitutes, runaways); and (d) college students.

Much of the empirical information we have about marital violence has been obtained from samples recruited at centers providing services to battered wives. These centers include agencies and clinics providing outpatient services, as well as residential facilities (shelters and safe homes). Some researchers (Goldberg & Tomlanovich, 1984; Rounsaville, 1978) have relied on hospital emergency room samples. Clearly, the samples obtained from each of these facilities might be expected to differ. Women seeking outpatient services are most likely to be living with their spouses. Women recruited at emergency rooms are more likely to have been physically injured at that time. Women recruited at shelters have separated from their spouses, possibly reflecting more marital dissatisfaction, a longer duration of abuse, and/or more personal and psychological resources on the part of the wife.

A review of the marital violence literature reveals that *marital violence* is probably a misnomer. In fact, few, if any, studies require a legal marital relationship. In reality, *spouse, wife,* and *husband* are typically used generically to refer to a man or woman involved in an intimate marriage-like relationship. Our informal survey, albeit incomplete, did not identify any studies that specifically excluded unmarried "spouses." Although Straus suggests empirical criteria based upon his Conflict Tactics Scales (Straus, 1979), they are seldom employed in assigning subjects to groups. The use of quantified criteria in defining the abused sample seems a worthwhile methodological consideration.

Thus, there has not been a consensus among researchers concerning the appropriate subjects to include in their samples. In addition, the method used to obtain samples has often been based more on practical matters (i.e., availability) rather than on empirically sound operational definitions. Furthermore, subjects seeking any form of service should be distinguished from undiscovered cases who have not presented at any agency or otherwise identified themselves. In fact, there is some evidence of differences between discovered and undiscovered cases. Gelles (1976) reported that abused wives were more likely to have come from families of origin in which they either witnessed parental violence or were abused themselves. Rosenbaum and O'Leary (1981), on the other hand, failed to find differences between abused wives and their nonabused counterparts on this variable. This apparent discrepancy may be due to Gelles' sample consisting largely of undiscovered cases, whereas Rosenbaum and O'Leary studied women who had presented at an agency serving abused wives. Systematic study of potential differences between samples appears warranted. It is important that investigators adequately describe their samples so that such comparisons can be facilitated.

There is some evidence that the quality of the family relationship may affect the data obtained concerning the abuse. For example, Rosenbaum and O'Leary (1981) differentiated between those abused wives who were able to involve their husbands in counseling and those who were not. On almost every variable, abused wives who were seen without their husbands could be differentiated from those seen with their husbands in the way they described their spouses and themselves. It could, therefore, be reasonably expected that differences would be obtained between shelter samples and agency samples. Similarly, it has been reported (Rosenbaum & O'Leary, 1981; Telch & Lindquist, 1984) that the level of marital discord is an important factor accounting for differences between violent and nonviolent couples. This suggests that even within agency samples, and certainly across different types of samples (clinics, emergency rooms, family and criminal courts, shelters, undiscovered, etc.), differing levels of marital satisfaction might produce differential findings.

Although initial research in family violence focused upon the victims, no doubt due to their availability as subjects, more recently the proliferation of programs for perpetrators (Frank & Houghton, 1982; Rosenbaum & O'Leary, 1986) and couples (Geffner, Franks, Patrick, & Mantooth, 1986; Geller & Wasserstrom, 1984) has provided samples of abusers for research purposes. Some of these perpetrators have been court-referred or even mandated into treatment as a condition of probation or order of protection. Differences between court mandated and self-referred subjects and potential differences between self-referred subjects and those refusing to participate in treatment need to be examined further. Frank and Houghton provide an excellent description of their program for batterers, most of whom are court-mandated into treatment. They report that their workshop participants express a great deal of anger and resentment. Rosenbaum and O'Leary (1986) and Geffner, Jordan, Hicks, and Cook (1985) operate similar programs for batterers and couples, respectively; most of their participants are self-referred, voluntary participants, and they did not find such dynamics, despite attempts to facilitate expression of these feelings. It is likely that these differences are due to whether or not the samples are court mandated.

Many of the recent studies surveyed in the preparation of this chapter utilized randomized sample selection procedures. Szinovacz (1983), for example, reported that over 80% of the couples in her sample were randomly selected from telephone directories. She further reported that relatively high refusal rates did occur, and that her sample was largely college educated, predominantly caucasian and of middle to high socioeconomic status. Such biases precipitate speculation that actual violence rates may be substantially higher than those derived from her data. They also provoke criticism regarding the external validity of many family violence investigations.

Another problem related to sampling involves deciding who the respondent should be, and dealing with contradictory data provided by spouses within a couple, by parents, by children, etc. Frequently, the nature of the respondent is determined adventitiously. For example, Straus, Gelles, and Steinmetz (1980) obtained information from whichever spouse was home and willing to provide it. Thus, if the wife was the respondent, she provided information about herself and her husband. Data provided by husbands were then combined with those provided by wives. Rosenbaum and O'Leary (1981) obtained the bulk of their data about both spouses from the wives. Although some data were available from the husbands, they were not combined with the wife data. In order to assess whether the data provided by the wives about the husbands was accurate, reliability between husbands and wives was calculated for those variables on which data from husbands and wives were available. The results indicated only moderate levels of agreement (just under 50%) between spouses. Similar findings concerning respondent reliability are likely to exist in other areas of family violence as well.

Epidemiology

The issues of sampling and definition have had the most influence on studies of epidemiology in family violence. The definition used determines the sample selected, and this then influences the reported incidence rates. For example, in marital violence research the Conflict Tactics Scale (Straus, 1979) has been used to select subjects. The CT Scale inquires as to whether specified behaviors have occurred during the past 12 months and also whether they have ever happened. Walker (1983), however, considered a woman battered if "she reported that she had been battered at least two times by a man with whom she had an intimate or marital relationship" (p. 84). Rounsaville (1978), on the other hand, required the violence to have occurred during the previous month. The time frame that one adopts has been demonstrated to influence the data obtained. Straus *et al.* (1980), for example, reported an incidence of 16% when the time frame is the previous year, but an incidence figure of 25% if the time frame is the entire relationship. We might also expect differential short- and long-term effects of violence, as well as differential recall, depending on the recency of the violence. It might be suggested, therefore, that the criteria for inclusion in the abuse group and the time frame be specified in the methods section of reports of family violence research.

Other suggestions relevant for epidemiological research include carefully selecting samples in order to obtain the most representative group possible, and assessing accurately the most important etiologic characteristics. An explanation of social epidemiology and strategies for its implementation in child abuse research are discussed in McClelland and Battle (1984).

Careful assessment of the suspected risk factors in an epidemiological study is also important. As much as possible, nondemographic variables need to be measured with standardized instruments which are reliable and valid for the particular population, supplemented with a comprehensive interview. An example of an especially well-conducted epidemiological study, one concerning the ''psychological ecology'' of the neglectful mother, is provided by Polansky, Gaudin, Ammons, and Davis (1985).

Methodological improvements in the investigation of the incidence and prevalence of child sexual abuse, of the characteristics of families, and of the treatment of family members have been occurring slowly, but steadily. Continued study of the prevalence and incidence rates of child sexual abuse is essential in order for investigators to make more precise estimates of the need for services and to gain increased understanding of the etiology of the phenomenon. Two of the best epidemiological studies of the prevalence of child sexual abuse conducted recently are by Kercher and McShane (1984) and Russell (1983, 1984). These investigations were carefully conducted, with definitions of sexual abuse specifically delineated and the samples randomly selected, though some methodological differences between the investigations make comparison difficult.

Research Design

Two important concerns relating to the design of the investigation are the use of control groups and whether the data are gathered prospectively or retrospectively. Without a matched control group, it is impossible to ascertain whether one's findings are associated with the occurrence of maltreatment, or with other subject variables, such as socioeconomic status, level of education, personality functioning, level of stress, and so on. A major requirement for retrospective designs is for the control group to have an equal probability that an abusive event would be detected. For example, the potential for bias exists when there are unequal chances for abuse to be identified in target and control children (Leventhal, 1982).

Many of the early research initiatives in family violence were uncontrolled or poorly controlled surveys. Nonparametric or descriptive statistics were the rule and dramatic or shock value took the place of inferential statistics and experimental rigor. Rosewater (1984), for example, reported the MMPI patterns of abused wives in the absence of any control sample. Parenthetically, because these investigations have not actually been experimental, the term *comparison* group would probably be more correct than control group.

The usual design selected for research in child physical abuse is what Leventhal (1982) calls the case-control study, in which the investigation is conducted retrospectively, resulting in numerous problems unless the groups are very carefully matched on a number of relevant dimensions. In the past 5 years, greater numbers of investigations have been conducted employing the prospective design that Leventhal labels the observational cohort study. In this type of study, two groups of subjects are followed for a specified time period; one group is identified as high risk for the abuse and the other as low risk. Leventhal clearly specifies the abuse factors, presents techniques to minimize bias, and matches groups on demographic variables.

Although this type of design minimizes some of the sources of distortion, some problems related to sample selection and evaluation remain. One positive feature of this prospective-type design is that certain criteria thought to be risk factors for maltreatment can be tentatively identified. Two recent observational cohort studies produced structured interviews and criteria that can now be evaluated for usefulness in screening for high-risk families (Altemeier, O'Connor, Vietze, Sandler, & Sherrod, 1984; Murphy, Orkow, & Nicola, 1985).

In the decade between 1970 and 1980, there was a fairly dramatic increase in the number of controlled studies published in child physical abuse (e.g., Plotkin, Azar, Twentyman, & Perri, 1981). In the past 5 years that trend has continued. Currently, the issue seems to be whether the control subjects have been adequately matched on the relevant variables. A concern for physical abuse and neglect researchers is that in the vast majority of the cases, the controls were selected on the basis of lack of reports of maltreatment. Unless some check is made on the presence of maltreatment in control families, even if only by asking the parents to fill out the Conflict Tactics Scale, no one can be certain that the control families are maltreatment free.

Most of the early investigations concerning sexual abuse did not gather information from comparison or control groups; even among studies conducted in the last 5 years, only a small minority of investigators included control groups (Sablatura, 1985). In addition, there are no prospective follow-up studies; all are retrospective. The studies of Herman and Hirschman (1981), Meiselman (1980), and Tasi, Feldman-Summers, and Edgar (1979) are good models for obtaining reasonable comparison groups. For adults who were victimized as children, an appropriate comparison might consist of four groups, including differing combinations of adults who were abused as a child or not, and are in psychotherapy or not. For families for whom the disclosure has been recent, long-term follow-up investigations need to be conducted. Ideally, two matched nonabusive comparison groups would also be followed, one in which the adult partners were not happily married and the other in which the couples reported a satisfactory marriage.

Marital violence research has not yet attained a level of methodological sophistication commensurate with that of more established topics. There persists a generalized failure to employ appropriate control or comparison groups. When comparison groups are used, they are often defined as a generic nondomestic violence sample (e.g., Gellen, Hoffman, Jones, & Stone, 1984). In addition, most studies have conceptualized marital violence as a unitary phenomenon, though there are some notable exceptions. Snyder and Fruchtman (1981), for example, attempted to identify subgroups of abusive relationships, based primarily on husband–wife configurations. Straus *et al.* (1980) reported percentages for three relationship subtypes; these were (a) husband abusive, wife not abusive, (b) wife abusive, husband not abusive, and (c) husband and wife mutually abusive. Although there is, to date, little evidence for systematic differences between these subgroups, it is also true that potential differences have not been empirically assessed. It makes intuitive sense that these groups be differentiated and potential differences examined.

Several recent research efforts have demonstrated the importance of including a comparison group of nonabused/nonabusive, maritally discordant wives/husbands, in order to ascertain that any differences obtained between satisfactorily married couples and abusive couples are not artifactual. In the absence of the availability of adequate comparison groups, marital satisfaction should be evaluated statistically. It is suggested that marital violence research employ a three-group design with samples of (a) maritally violent, (b) nonviolent, maritally discordant, and (c) satisfactorily married. Again, our informal survey of the recent literature indicated that only a few studies have employed this type of design (Rosenbaum & O'Leary, 1981; Telch & Lindquist, 1984).

Selection of an appropriate comparison sample may also be problematic. Despite the best efforts of researchers to select nonabusive comparison groups, family violence is so prevalent that even families who have not admitted abuse to their therapists may be somewhat abusive. Even satisfactorily married couples may have experienced some violence at some point in their relationship. It seems prudent to suggest that comparison samples be screened utilizing a measure of abuse, and that every effort be made to eliminate those reporting abuse from the control groups.

Measurement Procedures

Many different types of assessment procedures have been utilized to obtain information in various investigations of family violence. In epidemiological studies, mailed questionnaires or structured interviews are usually employed. Reviewing hospital charts and case histories is also a common method for gathering information. However, standardized measures of functioning are rarely administered and specific criteria for clinical judgments of depression or good adjustment are often omitted.

The measures selected are extremely important because that choice influences the results of descriptive investigations and treatment outcome studies. If the assessment procedures are different, even if the criteria are labeled similarly, results cannot be compared across investigations. Different methods employed to gather data (e.g., clinical impression, unstructured interviews, standardized measure of personality functioning, clinical material obtained from reviews of case histories, or reports from social service agencies or courts) yield diverse types of information. Biases may also result from the use of measurement instruments that are not reliable and valid for the sample under study, or whose psychometric properties are generally inadequate.

In addition to the problems associated with the actual measures, distortions in information may occur from the procedures utilized. Biases may be exacerbated if the individuals evaluating the family members are not blind to the hypothesis of the study or the status (research or control) of the subjects. Biased information may be obtained if the data come from only one source, especially one of the family members. A very common difficulty that leads to inaccurate and misleading conclusions is the assumption on the investigator's part that the current assessment of the family members' functioning represents the same level of adjustment seen prior to as well as at the time of the report or disclosure of the abuse. Information that is gathered retrospectively is likely to be somewhat distorted, because one's memory, especially regarding emotionally charged situations, tends to be selective.

Although the use of standardized instruments and structured interviews improves the descriptive process somewhat, arriving at composite descriptions is still fraught with difficulty. The particular definitions of behavior or diagnostic labels are inextricably tied to the methods used to assess the behavior. Discrepancies exist between the findings of researchers who rely on informal observations or interviews, and those who utilize structured instruments, with the former more likely to report difficulties in the subject's adjustment. However, the investigators who employ standardized scales have reported measurement problems, with the primary difficulties encountered being those that are inherent in the use of self-report procedures. Whereas the informal assessments are subject to investigator bias, self-report measures are vulnerable to the effects of subject distortion, including responses made in a guarded fashion, in an exaggerated ''cry for help'' manner, or in a socially desirable way. This latter tendency has been reported to be especially problematic in the assessment of self-esteem (Emery, Kraft, Joyce, & Shaw, 1984; Hughes & Hampton, 1984).

Many of the early reports of the functioning of children living in violent homes consisted of impressions and descriptions based on informal observation or unstructured interviews with battered women (Elbow, 1982; Hershey, 1982; Hilberman & Munson, 1978; LaBell, 1979). More recently, a number of investigators have begun employing standardized measures of psychological functioning and/or structured diagnostic interviews with the child witnesses and their mothers (Brown *et al.,* 1983; Hughes & Barad, 1983; Hughes & Hampton, 1984; Wolfe *et al.,* 1986).

Rosenberg (1984) modified the Conflict Tactics Scale to include the question ''How often has this occurred in front of your child'' after each strategy listed on the instrument, with the result that both frequency and intensity information are available. Emery *et al.* (1984) and Kraft, Sullivan-Hanson, Christopoulos, Cohn, and Emery (1984) have also employed this modification of the CTS. A similar approach to specifying the parameters of marital hostility was used by Hershorn and Rosenbaum (1985). They assessed parental violence by employing a version of the O'Leary Porter Scale (OPS), a 10-item instrument on which mothers report how often various forms of hostility (e.g., sarcasm, physical violence) were witnessed by their children (Emery & O'Leary, 1984; Porter & O'Leary, 1980). This measure also provides frequency and intensity information, though neither the modified CTS nor the OPS yields an estimate of duration. It should be noted that the CTS is still the most frequently employed measure of spousal violence despite questions regarding its validity and reliability (Jouriles & O'Leary, 1985; Szinovacz, 1983).

The literature on marital violence commonly includes such terms as jealousy, masochism, assertion, and defective home environment as important etiological factors, yet the majority of the published studies fail to operationalize adequately these constructs. Most studies either did not utilize standardized measures, or combined standardized measures of some constructs (most commonly violence and marital satisfaction) with nonstandardized measures and interview data. Only about 30% of the studies surveyed for this chapter utilized standardized dependent measures. Although the structured interview can provide important information that may be lost when more objective measures are employed, interviewer bias and vague definitions of constructs can seriously distort interview data. Walker (1979), for example, relied primarily on data collected by interviewers who shared her feminist viewpoint. Inclusion of standardized, empirical measures represents a way of minimizing the effects of experimenter bias.

Two promising avenues for more accurate behavior description and data collection are a structured, diagnostic interview (e.g., Brown *et al.,* 1983) and direct behavioral observations (e.g., Margolin, John, Gleberman, Miller, & Reynold 1985). Though both types of assessment are very time consuming, these methods of data collection would be extremely useful supplements to the self-report instruments in family violence research.

Concerns about measures are not restricted to reliability and validity issues. The CTS, for example, elicits information regarding the frequency of occurrence of each of the violent behaviors assessed without regard to the impact of that behavior on the victim in terms of the physical and psychological damage inflicted. Furthermore, the scales fail to reflect whether a violent behavior was retaliatory or initiative. Thus it cannot be determined whether violence by either partner was in response to violence by the other. The development of measures that could be subjected to a sequential analysis would enhance our knowledge of the nature of family violence.

It should also be noted that because many of the violent behaviors occurring between spouses or within families are relatively infrequent, reports of reliability based on occurrence and nonoccurrence are significantly inflated; this suggests that reliability based only on occurrence should be reported. A further question concerns discrepancies between family members. Because social desirability would suggest that subjects would be more predisposed to deny violence that had occurred than they would to admit violence that had not occurred, it seems prudent to accept the veracity of a report of violence by any family member (either as perpetrator or victim) for purposes of classification. Caution, however, is advised regarding the use of one person to provide information about the other.

Assessment procedures used in common by several investigators would greatly enhance opportunities for comparison of results, and to that end Tierney and Corwin (1983) suggested employing multiple measures that assess constructs from several different theoretical levels. Based on their review of the assessment literature in sexual abuse and their theoretical framework, they provided a list of suggested measures that could be adopted by workers in the field, regardless of the specific area of research interest in family violence.

Data Analysis

The level of sophistication and appropriateness of statistical analyses employed by researchers is another area of methodological concern. Once appropriate statistical techniques for data analysis have been selected, interpretation of the results become important. Problems are frequently encountered when investigators attempt to separate out the antecedent conditions, correlates, and effects of the maltreatment (Tierney & Corwin, 1983). Researchers seem to imply that the associations established between the abuse and identified factors lead to knowledge of the ''causes'' (for example, Mrazek & Mrazek, 1981, list ''effects of child abuse''). In actuality, no causes have yet been identified, only features or variables that are related in an as yet unknown way to the abuse the child has suffered.

Paralleling the increase in the use of control groups in family violence research has been a rise in the utilization of inferential statistics and more sophisticated analyses. However, these techniques are still the exception rather than the rule. Many researchers continue to employ only descriptive statistics. Hershorn and Rosenbaum (1985), Hughes, Rau, Hampton, and Sablatura (1985), Rosenberg (1984), and Wolfe, Jaffe, Wilson, and Zak (1984) all provide good examples of typical analyses conducted when control groups are utilized. There are even suggestions for multivariate analyses as the field progresses.

Another issue concerns the use of aggregate data versus within-couple or within-family data for analysis. For example, there is ample evidence that spouses differ substantially in their answers to seemingly objective questions (Szinovacz, 1983), complicating interpretation of couple data. This significant problem is often obscured by the use of aggregate data (i.e., data from husbands and wives in general), because within couples the responses are somewhat more discrepant and inter-rater reliability is actually much lower. Unfortunately, the use of aggregate data is more common than the use of couple data (Klein, 1982).

ROBERT GEFFNER
ET AL.

Methodological difficulties abound in treatment research, and intervention in family violence is no exception. According to Smith, Rachman, and Yule (1984), the two major sources of methodological problems in this area are the high degree of suspiciousness and noncooperation among the families, and the ethical considerations encountered when working with families in which there is life-threatening behavior. Several researchers have stated that the few families who are most likely to profit from interventions need to be identified (Gabinet, 1983; Green, Power, Steinbok, & Gaines, 1981; Rivara, 1985). Wodarski (1981) conceptualized abuse as multidetermined and recommended a comprehensive treatment approach, which he described, as well as procedures for assessment of initial functioning and outcomes.

A series of articles by Smith and her colleagues (Smith, 1984; Smith & Rachman, 1984; Smith et al., 1984) provides a most useful discussion of behavioral interventions for child abuse (including their model treatment evaluation study) and of methodological issues. They discuss the problems of sample attrition and appropriate control groups; for ethical reasons, they recommend the use of treated control groups (i.e., by the protective service workers) whereas the experimental group receives the additional interventions. Smith et al. suggested that the usual criteria for treatment effectiveness are too global and they recommend multiple outcome measures assessing the quality of life for the child. They also discuss the need for long-term follow-up and suggest using behavioral treatment in a diagnostic fashion (i.e., identifying the distinguishing features of families which do not profit from treatment). This approach in general seems applicable to other areas of family violence as well.

Recommendations regarding the methodology employed in the treatment literature for sexual abuse are not difficult to make because there are so few investigators who have attempted to evaluate their treatment programs. Probably the best known and most extensively evaluated program is the California Sexual Abuse Treatment Program conducted by Giaretto (1981) and evaluated by Kroth (1979). One of the most positive features of Kroth's research includes the detail and specificity of the information provided, which greatly facilitates a replication of the evaluation procedure. In addition to the three groups of variables he used as outcome criteria, he also assessed the parents' perceptions of the treatment. Another noteworthy aspect of Kroth's report is that he discusses negative findings. This study would be a good model for other family violence researchers to follow in evaluating interventions.

However, the level of sophistication of research methodology is not at the point where questions of "what therapy provided by what therapist for what clients, for what problems, produces what kinds of effects" are able to be addressed (Kendall & Norton-Ford, 1982, p. 434). Rather, preliminary evaluations of treatment problems on a number of dimensions are being conducted to assess the success of the treatment.

As one might surmise, based on how recently children who are exposed to violence between their parents have become the subject of any research, no evaluation of the effectiveness of treatment with child witnesses has been conducted to date. The information that is available regarding intervention with children consists mostly of anecdotal accounts and descriptions of children's programs in shelters for battered women. Carefully collected outcome data and the use of control groups are definitely needed in this area. Some general descriptions of intervention programs in shelters exist (Carlson, 1984; Hughes, 1982), with a more detailed description of a group approach to treatment provided by Alessi and Hearn (1984). Although this latter approach is based on a sound theoretical foundation, it has not been evaluated empirically. The only comprehensive, family-oriented approach to intervention reported in the literature is described by Gentry and Eaddy (1980). They coordinated family-systems-based, educationally focused group interventions for parents and children with the treatment individual family members might be receiving from health care professionals, though the results of their pre- and postintervention assessments were not reported.

The selection of appropriate outcome indexes and issues related to follow-up are two significant problems with all forms of outcome research, family violence included. Some investigators have accepted violence reduction as an acceptable (i.e., successful) outcome, whereas others require cessation of violence in order for therapy to be considered successful. However, there are several problems with this practice. First, it suggests that violence can be objectively scaled. Is being pushed better than being punched? Not if the push results in a concussion. Is being beaten once better than being beaten three times? Only if the beatings are of equal severity. Determining whether abuse has diminished is much more complex and unreliable than determining whether or not violence has occurred at all. Second, there is little reason to believe that some reduction in violence would automatically improve the family relationship. The occurrence of any violence serves as a threat that constrains the behavior of the victim and produces psychological stress. Accepting reduction of violence as a successful outcome indicator communicates the message that some violence is permissable in the relationship.

Selection of an adequate follow-up interval is also an important methodological concern for treatment outcome research with abusive populations. It is often observed that violence rarely occurs once counseling (family, couple, or individual) commences. It is also characteristic of many abusive couples, for example, that violence is an infrequent event (Rosenbaum & O'Leary, 1986). This suggests that posttherapy evaluations that show a cessation of violence may actually be capitalizing on a naturally occurring nonviolent interval, rather than reflecting a successful therapeutic intervention. Walker (1979) reflected this phenomenon in her depiction of the cycle of violence. The cycle includes three phases: the build-up, the violence, and the honeymoon, only one of which involves physical violence. Although Walker made no claims regarding the length of the various phases, she did imply that the actual period of violence may be sandwiched between much longer periods of nonviolence. In order to minimize the possibility of taking advantage of the low base rate of occurrence of violence, Rosenbaum and O'Leary (1986) recommend that nonviolent follow-ups of at least 6 months post treatment be required before judging an intervention successful.

Another issue concerns who should be contacted to provide outcome information. If a couple is being seen conjointly, it makes sense to solicit outcome data from both spouses; however, in situations where only the husband is being treated, as in men's groups, the question arises as to whether the husband's self-report should be accepted or whether the wife should be contacted for corroboration. Although it might be suggested that the wife would be a more reliable source of such information, it could also be argued that because acceptance of responsibility for one's own behavior is a major goal of most men's groups, it would be counterproductive to that goal to suggest that the husband cannot be trusted to provide accurate information (Rosenbaum & O'Leary, 1986). In the absence of an empirical demonstration of the accuracy of abusive husband's self-report of nonviolence, it might be useful to obtain some corroborating evidence of treatment success for male-directed treatment strategies. In general, the report of the victim or the person reporting the violence should be accepted in determining outcome because it would be the less socially desirable response.

ETHICAL ISSUES

An area that has not been discussed adequately by researchers in family violence is ethical concerns. The subjects in these studies may be in physical or psychological danger, and there are often clinical as well as legal ramifications. Confidentiality, privacy, informed consent, nontreatment groups, and legal reporting of abusive relationships carry much more weight than in other types of research, and often create ethical dilemmas for the researcher.

In conducting research with families in which children have been maltreated, an important ethical issue that must be addressed is the handling of informed consent. Due to the nature of these investigations and the potential for subtle (and not so subtle) coercion, this issue is especially salient. When subjects do refuse to participate, this potential source of bias must be addressed. There is some evidence that children who are not given parental permission to take part in research studies may differ along some important dimensions from those who do participate (Beck, Collins, Overholser, & Terry, 1984). Some useful guidelines regarding ethical issues in research with abused children have been recently proposed by Kinard (1985). Although the focus of the article is children who are physically abused, the points made are relevant for cases of sexual abuse and spousal violence as well.

Two major issues must be addressed in informed consent procedures: who can give consent for children to be research participants and how informed must this consent be. Kinard pointed out that the consent issue is made more complex in abuse situations because of the potential adversarial relationship between children and parents. This is one of the reasons that a waiver of the requirement for parental consent in the cases of child abuse can be obtained (Department of Health and Human Services, 1983). Kinard discussed advantages and disadvantages of different plans for provision of consent, including designated professionals, review boards, and advocates for children. Kinard also reminded researchers that regardless of the source of the consent for the participation of children in studies, agreement from the children themselves should also be obtained.

The second issue of how informed must consent be is especially important, because child abuse is an instance in which full disclosure of the purpose of the research is very likely to result in distorted findings. Parents may refuse to participate and not allow their child to participate, or may avoid revealing behavior that others might consider undesirable. Kinard suggested that with child abuse, the deception involved in stating in an initial description that the purpose of a study is to focus on child development may be justified.

After consent is obtained, special provisions must be made to prevent potential problems when a child becomes distressed by the testing or interviewing, when a child's answers indicate emotional problems, or when a child reveals either directly or indirectly that he or she might be experiencing abuse. Kinard recommended that the researcher prepare a debriefing process for all participants, and be especially sensitive to cues from the children that indicate they are upset. Researchers need to probe gently for the source of the distress, and attempt to calm the child and clarify misperceptions, if they are present. Another dilemma arises when a child's answers indicate emotional problems. Kinard suggested that the need for intervention for the child warrants a breach of the child's confidentiality. Nonclinically trained investigators might consider selecting a clinical psychologist to act as a consultant in order to deal with these difficult determinations. If a decision to inform the child's parents is made, the reasons for the choice should be discussed with the child.

Issues of informed consent and refusals to participate are important for generalizability and for the ethical pursuit of knowledge. Exemplary models for handling informed consent and for discussing people who refused to participate are provided by Lahey, Conger, Atkeson, and Treiber (1984), and Bauer and Twentyman (1985), respectively. Additional discussion of these topics by family violence researchers is still needed, however.

Another ethical issue is applicable to certain types of marital violence research. It must be kept in mind that in cases where the husband is not a participant, some research strategies, such as calling the wife on the phone or mailing questionnaires to her home, might place her in some jeopardy vis-à-vis her husband. Even when the husband is a participant, he may put pressure on her to disclose her answers to him or to withhold certain information from the researchers. Consideration should be given to having the husband and wife complete questionnaires in different rooms and extra care should be taken to assure privacy and confidentiality. Close supervision of the couple by an agent of the investigator may help to reduce coercion and increase the wife's sense of security, thus maximizing the chances of obtaining accurate information. These suggestions would apply to other areas of family violence research as well.

Perhaps the most difficult dilemma occurs when the investigator suspects that a child is being abused or discovers potential abuse in the course of conducting the research. All states currently have laws that mandate the reporting of child maltreatment by persons in specified occupations, which include psychologists, physicians, educators, sociologists, nurses, and so forth. The states vary with regard to the agency to which the report is to be made, the nature of the offense, and the penalty for nonreporting. In addition, it is widely recognized that therapists have a ''duty to take proper care'' that obligates therapists to protect potential victims of their clients if they have knowledge that the client intends to do harm. This too has legal implications and therapists have been held liable for damages in several states. Although these mandates are intended for practitioners, the question arises as to how researchers who become aware of ongoing or potential abuse in the course of data collection are expected to respond.

Let us take a hypothetical example. Researcher X. is studying marriages. The subject couples have volunteered and have been promised anonymity and confidentiality. One of the wives reports, in response to a written questionnaire item, that her husband is abusing their daughter. Although the couple is only identified by a number, the researcher becomes aware of the response while checking the data for completeness before the couple leaves, and thus is aware of the information and the couple's identity. What are the legal and ethical obligations for dealing with this discovered abuse?

As often occurs, the legal and ethical obligations may be inconsistent. Legally, the researcher may protect anonymity and confidentiality of research data by obtaining a Certificate of Confidentiality. Section 303 (a) of the Public Health Service Act states in part that:

> the Secretary [of H.E.W.] may authorize persons engaged in (bona fide) research on mental health . . . to protect the privacy of individuals who are the subject of such research by withholding from all persons not connected with the conduct of such research the names or other identify-

ing characteristics of such individuals. Persons so authorized to protect the privacy of such individuals may not be compelled in any Federal, State, or local civil, criminal, administrative, legislative, or other proceedings to identify such individuals.

It should be noted, however, that there is some question as to how this impacts on "duty to take proper care."

Persons obtaining these certificates should protect themselves by carefully reading the provisions and consulting with legal counsel at the research site. With respect to child abuse reporting, if such a certificate has been obtained, the data are protected from judicial scrutiny, thus precluding enforcement of any reporting mandates. However, the ethics of hiding behind such an umbrella can certainly be questioned. In our example, the researcher who fails to make a report is sanctioning the continued abuse of the child. On the other hand, if couples have been promised anonymity and confidentiality, then reporting could legitimately lead to charges of misrepresentation, which could easily introduce a self-selection bias into future samples and damage the reputation of the researcher. Similarly, informing couples at the outset that certain information will be reported to the authorities might introduce a serious confound into the data set, especially if abuse is one of the variables under investigation.

Filing abuse reports, similar to making referrals, not only violates the confidentiality of the parent and child, but may sometimes increase the risk of harm to the child. However, Kinard (1985) strongly suggested that the investigator is morally and ethically bound to report the abuse. Any failure to report suspected abuse actually increases the risks to the child because the potential for harm in that instance is much greater than when a report is made. Kinard stated that when in doubt, it is essential to err on the side of the child's safety. The same would be true in other abusive circumstances. Although sexual and spouse abuse situations may differ on the specifics, the general ethical and moral issues are quite similar.

What do we do? Unfortunately it is easier to identify a problem such as this than it is to solve it. We can only outline the issues and possible methods of dealing with this dilemma and then leave it to the individual researchers to follow their own consciences. The following are possible methods for dealing with this situation:

1. A Certificate of Confidentiality can be obtained that will protect the researcher from legal liability. More information regarding this can be obtained from Judith T. Galloway, Legal Assistant, Office of the Administrator, Alcohol, Drug Abuse, and Mental Health Administration, Parklawn Building, Room 13C-06, 5600 Fishers Lane, Rockville, MD 20857.

2. Do not look at the data when there is any way for you to identify the subjects. Have the data coded by persons without access to the subject's identity. If you are going to follow this procedure, it would probably be useful to have a Certificate of Confidentiality as well.

3. Do not ask any questions that might elicit information concerning current abuse. Walker (1984) reworded her questionnaires to focus on past abuse and perceptions of abuse so that the chances of obtaining information about actual current maltreatment were greatly minimized This satisfied the ethical obligations as well as confidentiality, but it can alter the focus of the research as well.

4. Notify subjects during the "informed consent" aspect of the study that you may have to report information related to child maltreatment or intent to harm another to the authorities. Make the necessary reports if such information is divulged, but be cautious in any generalizations concerning your data.

This chapter has presented a methodological critique of family violence research. The areas that we have focused on as relevant examples in this field include child abuse (physical and sexual), child witnesses of violence, and marital violence. Suggestions for improvement in the research in these areas have been discussed more often in recent years, and changes have been occurring. Thus, it seems appropriate at this point to present recommendations for future research in each of these areas, with the hope that these suggestions can be applied by researchers to the other areas of family violence.

Child Physical Abuse

Identifying families included in investigations based on a uniform definition of child physical abuse and neglect would greatly enhance comparability across these types of studies. One would then have a certain amount of confidence that the abusive events were all of a similar nature, according to a clearly articulated criteria. Especially noteworthy in this regard are the recent studies conducted by Twentyman and his colleagues at the University of Rochester (Bauer & Twentyman, 1985; Bousha & Twentyman, 1984; Hoffman-Plotkin & Twentyman, 1984; Smetana, Kelly, & Twentyman, 1984), in which the protective services workers use carefully defined standardized criteria for physical abuse that are based on the results of the National Incidence Study.

Once uniform definitions of maltreatment are obtained, then samples may be separated according to the abusive event or characteristics of the participants. Sorting subjects into more homogeneous groups is important because evidence has been accumulating that shows that physical abuse and neglect have quite different consequences for the child (Egeland, Stroufe, & Erickson, 1983). Better specification of characteristics of the abuser and the family structure are also important in sample description. For example, to date, few studies have specifically differentiated mothers from fathers as the offending parent (Martin, 1983).

Regarding issues of assessment and design, Leventhal (1982) and Plotkin *et al.* (1981) are good resources. Plotkin addressed assessment and hypothesis testing and emphasized that data must be obtained in ways that are reliable and valid for the population that is being measured, and that multiple sources of information need to be utilized. Leventhal (1982) provided an excellent description and explanation of three commonly used research strategies and identifies similarities and differences among them. He delineated which methodological issues are the most important to consider within each research strategy.

Appropriately matched comparison groups are also necessary in order to separate the factors that are related to the abuse from other variables. Especially good examples of this type of matching and the use of multiple strategies for assessment are the studies by Egeland *et al.* (1983), Hoffman-Plotkin and Twentyman (1984), and Lahey *et al.* (1984). However, one difficulty with comparison groups in this area is that virtually every investigator uses the lack of official reports of abuse as the criterion for "nonabusive." Thus, there is no certainty that the control children are not currently physically abused or neglected. A possible solution to this dilemma would be to administer the Conflict Tactics Scale to the nonabusive families as a measure of physical punishment, though these results would still be dependent on behaviors the parents are willing to admit.

Sufficient empirical research has been conducted in this area of family violence for the development of coherent theories of physical child abuse (e.g., Belsky, 1980; Keller & Erne, 1983) by which researchers explain their findings and formulate new questions to be investigated. Each of the four or sometimes five factors that are hypothesized to contribute to the etiology of maltreatment (e.g., individual child characteristics, parent–child interactions, sociocultural variables) provides different areas upon which investigators from various areas or disciplines can focus. One researcher in this area (Krugman, 1985) listed four areas as challenges for the future: (a) evaluation of treatment programs; (b) continued long-term investigation of survivors of physical child abuse and neglect; (c) focus on the child; and (d) focus on prevention. Integrated, coordinated efforts related to these four areas of challenge and to the different levels of analysis as suggested by theories will ultimately be the most efficacious approach.

Future research especially needs to be focused on continuing the prospective, longitudinal studies in order to identify more definitively families that are at high risk for physical abuse and neglect. The prospective studies conducted have already resulted in the development of promising and much needed screening instruments and provide excellent examples of follow-up studies (Altemeier *et al.*, 1984; Milner, Gold, Ayoub, & Jacewitz, 1984; Murphy *et al.*, 1985). Only through epidemiological studies are the causes of child maltreatment going to be identified (McClelland & Battle, 1984). Once the etiological factors have been delineated, then the focus of efforts in the area can turn to prevention.

Child Sexual Abuse

A number of suggestions made in the previous section are also relevant here, with a special emphasis on more specific definitions of sexual abuse, better sample description, use of multiple measures for assessment, and inclusion of appropriate control groups. As was mentioned previously, a uniform definition of sexual abuse needs to be adopted, possibly following the lines suggested by Finkelhor and Hotaling (1984). Mrazek and Mrazek (1981) and Finkelhor and Hotaling provide recommendations for additional demographic characteristics of the family and details regarding the sexual abuse that they feel must be gathered and reported at some length. In addition, informed consent procedures need to be addressed and refusal-to-participate rates reported.

One of the phenomena associated with a newly developing field is that its body of research often develops haphazardly and in a piecemeal fashion, with no clearly articulated theory or set of theories to guide the investigations. Research in the area of child sexual abuse has evolved to the point where some comprehensive macroscopic hypotheses are being formulated (Finkelhor, 1985; Tierney & Corwin, 1983). However, with investigators from a number of different professional fields interested in child sexual abuse, diverse theories from disparate viewpoints abound. Additional research remains to be conduced before answers to some of the more complex questions can be obtained. However, a truly prospective study would be very difficult to conduct for many reasons (e.g., average age of victim is 8 years, most incidents of sexual abuse go unreported); therefore, it would be beneficial at this point to concentrate on carefully conducted follow-up studies. Again, prevention would be the ultimate goal.

At the present time, Tierney and Corwin (1973) provide the best discussion and integration of theoretical issues available. They pull together various viewpoints and propose some testable hypotheses, complete with recommendations for outcome criteria and assessment procedures; they also include a comprehensive listing of suggested scales and instruments. Their systems model involves assessment of the family member's functioning along with two matched comparison groups, one in treatment for other types of problems and one group of normal families. These recommendations should be extremely helpful to researchers in providing a framework in which programmatic studies could be conducted.

Child Witnesses of Family Violence

At this point, very few conclusions can be drawn regarding child witnesses of parental violence. The most fruitful avenues to pursue are those that will help investigators understand the incidence and prevalence of exposure to parental violence, and identify the effects of such exposure. A large-scale national probability sample survey similar to the one conducted by Straus *et al.* (1980) would be very beneficial.

Accepted definitions of exposure to violence and methods of assessing that exposure are crucial. Scales that provide measures of the parameters of violence and exposure to it, such as intensity, frequency, and duration are necessary. The modified CTS and the OPS provide researchers with assessments of intensity and frequency and may be useful in this regard. Careful sample delineation is essential to these basic descriptive investigations. Information about whether a child has been physically or sexually abused, marital status of the mother, whether the male in the household is the biological father, duration of the relationship and of the abuse from the parent, and whether the family lives in a rural or urban area are important for an accurate understanding of the children's background and current living situation. Demographic characteristics of the parents, including types of abuse in their early history are essential details to obtain.

Central to issues of sample description is the likelihood that researchers are only coming into contact with a select group of child witnesses: those whose mother sought assistance either from a shelter or a mental health agency. However, the relative homogeneity of these families provides researchers with a place to begin, especially given the wide variety of methods for assessment of psychological functioning. Perhaps carefully describing these child witnesses and even identifying subgroups within this select sample will be a first step in understanding their adjustment. Some progress in identifying subgroups of child witnesses has been made (e.g., Hughes & Hampton, 1984; Webster-Stratton, 1985); when delineating small groups of subjects, it is important to differentiate among (a) children whose parents are violent with each other but not with the children, (b) children who are exposed and subject to parental violence, and (c) children who are victims of maltreatment though no spouse abuse occurs.

Whereas the majority of the research conducted in this area has been purely descriptive, recently a number of researchers have utilized a variety of control groups, although all such groups have fairly small numbers of subjects. In one study, all of the children were from a clinical population, with the groups differentiated on the basis of whether or not violence occurred between the parents (Brown *et al.*, 1983). Other investigators have included two comparison groups. Rosenbaum (Hershorn & Rosenbaum, 1984; Rosenbaum & O'Leary, 1981) used the male children of three groups of women; these groups consisted of (a) women who were victims of physical spouse abuse, (b) women who were in a discordant, though nonviolent, marital relationship, and (c) women who were happily married. Wolfe *et al.* (1984) focused their efforts on three groups of families; one group of women and children were current residents of a shelter for battered women, another group consisted of former residents who had not been exposed to violence for approximately 6 months, and a control group recruited from the local communities and matched on family income and child's age and gender. The use of various types of comparison groups is needed in future research, and more emphasis on such methodological designs is recommended.

In designing treatment outcome studies in this area, much could be gained from following Barrett, Hampe, and Miller's (1978) recommendations related to the evaluation of child psychotherapy. Investigators of child witnesses to parental violence are probably decades away from being able to specify what type of treatment, under what circumstances, for which types of clients, is most effective, though that certainly is an admirable goal. Researchers in this area must also begin utilizing theories of family violence to guide their investigations. Some combination of theoretical formulations from child physical abuse, along with theories from child sexual abuse and spouse abuse, would be heuristic. Five factors seem to be necessary for an integrated, interactive model; these include (a) characteristics of the individual child, (b) characteristics of the individual parent, (c) family interaction patterns (e.g., parent-parent, parent-child, sibling-child), (d) family climate (e.g., economic level, other stresses, situational factors), and (e) social/community/cultural context. Longitudinal investigations need to be conducted so that better understanding of the generational cycle of violence can be obtained.

Marital Violence

In order to instigate a process of upgrading the standards for research in marital violence, many of the recommendations made concerning the previous areas are applicable. Suggestions for marital violence research include (a) the specification of criteria for defining the abused/abusive group; (b) the inclusion of a comparison sample of nonviolent, maritally discordant spouses; (c) the use of couple rather than aggregate data when appropriate (self-report data rather than the use of one spouse as an informant on the other should be accepted, except in determining whether violence has occurred; in this case the spouse reporting violence should be used); (d) the use of standardized measures in defining the sample as well as in operationalizing the constructs under investigation; (e) the use of inferential in addition to descriptive statistics; and (f) providing adequate criteria (nonoccurrence rather than diminution of violence) and follow-up intervals (6 months or more) in outcome research with maritally violent populations.

Methodologically, the field would also benefit from the development of better measures of violence. This might involve incorporating several aspects of violence: the actual behavior (slapping, punching, kicking, etc.), the frequency of occurrence, the consequences (bruising, bleeding, pain, medical intervention, etc.), the sequence of events (who hit first, initiative vs. retaliatory violence, etc.), and the intent. Once new measures are developed it might be useful to utilize them to establish norms for the various behaviors. The determination of norms might help refine the definitions of abuse used in designating group composition in marital violence research.

Perhaps it is premature at present, but marital violence researchers should gradually be moving toward more sophisticated designs that identify subgroups within the violent population. Current designs that either combine abused or abusive spouses from different sources (agencies, shelters, emergency rooms, police records, etc.) or focus on only one source and generalize results to the population at large are probably obscuring important differences between subgroups.

Family violence research has evolved over the past 20 years into a legitimate field of study. Improvements in methodology are quite apparent in the child physical abuse area, with the other areas lagging somewhat behind. At this point two changes seem to be needed: an integration of the various areas of abuse under the rubric of family violence, and the development of coherent theories that could assist with this synthesis, explain past and current findings, and help guide research in these areas. Violence, whether as physical abuse, neglect, sexual abuse, or exposure to violence, must be conceptualized in a synergistic fashion in order to provide the proper context for understanding the phenomenon.

The current emphasis on family violence provides the field with an ideal structure for conceptualization and investigation of the etiologies of all types of violence in the family. Large prospective studies need to be conducted in order to identify more definitively the aspects of family life, for individuals and on a collective basis, which contribute to high risks of maltreatment. The intergenerational transmission of violence is one commonly held belief that needs investigation and can be most effectively studied by longitudinally following each family member.

One subgroup of the family system that has received little attention are the siblings of the maltreated child who may or may not be exposed or subject to the same type of violence as the target child. Siblings are frequently overlooked, and that subsystem seems to be the last piece of the puzzle to be included in investigations. Recent research has provided some initial evidence for the importance of including sibling violence within the purview of the field (e.g., Crittenden, 1984; Post, Willett, Franks, House, & Back, 1982).

In terms of a contextual understanding, several comprehensive theories have been proposed that describe child abuse as being multiply determined, with a number of factors that interact to produce an abusive event. The total person–situation context must be considered, with factors from the sociocultural, family climate, interpersonal, and intrapersonal levels included. Although such a large perspective may lead one to feel overwhelmed at the enormity of the task, it also makes clear that there are a number of fronts upon which researchers can focus, and each one is important to study. Investigators in various areas of family violence can benefit from the model provided by the researchers in the child abuse area. There is much to be learned from their struggles with definitions, sample selection, assessment procedures, designs, outcome criteria, and statistical analyses. A substantial amount of the necessary technology is ready to be implemented, including the separation of groups of families on relevant variables, using multiple measures, and confronting issues regarding informed consent.

Researchers can also benefit from the knowledge, concepts, and techniques of other areas of psychology, including social psychology (especially the current research on aggression) and developmental psychology (particularly the broad area of parent–child and peer interactions). Because family violence is so widespread and touches diverse people and many aspects of society, a multifaceted approach with many people working on a number of different fronts in a coordinated effort to integrate the accumulated knowledge is the only approach that ultimately will be effective. Otherwise researchers could continue, as we have done for too long, in the isolated manner of the proverbial blind men who evaluated the elephant.

Finally, it would be unfair to close without a disclaimer of sorts. The present chapter may leave the reader with the somewhat jaundiced view that family violence researchers are not competent researchers. However, this is not the case. More realistically, the current status of research in this area reflects a number of problems. Marriage and family dynamics involve complex phenomena; two or more individuals, each of whom carries their own unique psychological baggage, are interacting on a continuous, intimate basis with each other, with in-laws, friends, etc., and are affected by a host of environmental stressors (finances, jobs, health issues, etc.). It would be naive to suggest that the factors that evolve into family violence have simple, main-effect type of explanations.

In addition, subjects in violent families have not been readily accessible. The proliferation of shelters, agencies specializing in working with abusive families, and programs for perpetrators are all recent developments. Further, perpetrators are often unwilling to participate in research or therapy. Abusers and their victims who do not attend agencies or come to the attention of police, emergency rooms, and the like are not typically represented in research data. Lastly, the status of research in this area reflects the fact that this is a topic that has only recently received research attention and, with all due respect to Piaget, is only in its sensorimotor stage of development. However, improvement has been occurring, and it is hoped that we will enter the next stage of development in the near future.

REFERENCES

Alessi, J. J., & Hearn, K. (1984). Group treatment of children in shelters for battered women. In A. R. Roberts (Ed.), *Battered women and their families: Intervention strategies and treatment programs* (pp. 49–62). New York: Springer.

Altemeier, W. A., O'Connor, S., Vietze, P., Sandler, H., & Sherrod, K. (1984). Prediction of child abuse: A prospective study of feasibility. *Child Abuse and Neglect, 8,* 393–400.

Barrett, C. L., Hampe, I. E., & Miller, L. (1978). Research on psychotherapy with children. In S. L. Garfield & A. E. Bergin (Eds.), *Handbook of psychotherapy and behavior change: An empirical analysis* (2nd ed., pp. 411–436). New York: Wiley.

Bauer, D. M., & Twentyman, C. T. (1984). Abusing, neglectful, and comparison mothers' responses to child-related and non-child-related stressors. *Journal of Consulting and Clinical Psychology, 53,* 335–343.

Beck, S., Collins, L., Overholser, J., & Terry, K. (1984). A comparison of children who receive and who do not receive permission to participate in research. *Journal of Abnormal Child Psychology, 12,* 473–580.

Belsky, J. (1980). Child maltreatment; An ecological integration. *American Psychologist, 35,* 320–335.

Besharov, D. J. (1981). Toward better research on child abuse and neglect: Making definitional issues an explicit methodological concern. *Child Abuse and Neglect, 5,* 383–390.

Bousha, D. M., & Twentyman, C. T. (1984). Mother–child interactional style in abuse, neglect, and control groups: Naturalistic observations in the home. *Journal of Abnormal Psychology, 93,* 106–114.

Brown, A. J., Pelcovitz, D., & Kaplan, S. (August, 1983). *Child witnesses of family violence: A study of psychological correlates.* Paper presented at the annual meeting of the American Psychological Association, Anaheim, CA.

Carlson, B. E. (1984). Children's observations of interparental violence. In A. R. Roberts (Ed.), *Battered women and their families: Intervention strategies and treatment programs* (pp. 147–167). New York: Springer.

Crittenden, P. M. (1984). Sibling interaction: Evidence of a generational effect in maltreating infants. *Child Abuse and Neglect, 8,* 433–438.

Dalton, D. A., & Kantner, J. E. (1983). Aggression in battered and non-battered women as reflected in the hand test. *Psychological Reports, 53,* 703–709.

Department of Health and Human Services. (1983). Additional Protection for children involved as subjects in research. *Federal Register, 48,* 9814–9820.

Egeland, B., Sroufe, L. A., & Erickson, M. (1983). The developmental consequence of different patterns of maltreatment. *Child Abuse and Neglect, 7,* 459–469.

Elbow, M. (1982). Children of violent marriages: The forgotten victims. *Social Casework, 63,* 465–471.

Emery, R. E., Kraft, S. P., Joyce, S., & Shaw, D. (August, 1984). Children of abused women: Adjustment at three months follow-up. In H. M. Hughes (Chair), *Impact of marital and family violence on children in shelters*. Symposium conducted at the annual meeting of the American Psychological Association, Toronto.

Emery, R. E., & O'Leary, K. D. (1984). Marital discord and child behavior problems in a nonclinic sample. *Journal of Abnormal Child Psychology, 12*, 411–420.

Finkelhor, D. (1985). *Child sexual abuse*. New York: The Free Press/Macmillan.

Finkelhor, D., & Hotaling, G. T. (1984). Sexual abuse in the National Incidence Study of Child Abuse and Neglect: An appraisal. *Child Abuse and Neglect, 8*, 23–33.

Frank, P. B., & Houghton, B. D. (1982). *Confronting the batterer: A guide to creating the spouse abuse workshop*. New York: Volunteer Counseling Services of Rockland County.

Gabinet, L. (1983). Child abuse treatment failures reveal need for redefinition of the problem. *Child Abuse and Neglect, 7*, 395–402.

Geffner, R., Franks, D., Patrick, J. R., & Mantooth, C. (August, 1986). Reducing marital violence: A family therapy approach. In R. A. Geffner (Chair), *New approaches for reducing family violence*. Symposium conducted at the annual meeting of the American Psychological Association, Washington, DC.

Geffner, R. A., Jordan, K., Hicks, D., & Cook, S. K. (August, 1985). Psychological characteristics of violent couples. In R. A. Geffner (Chair), *Violent couples: Current research and new directions for family psychologists*. Symposium conducted at the annual meeting of the American Psychological Association, Los Angeles, CA.

Gellen, M. L., Hoffman, R. A., Jones, M., & Stone, M. (1984). Abused and nonabused women: MMPI profile differences. *Personnel & Guidance Journal, 62*, 601–604.

Geller, J., & Wasserstrom, J. (1984). Conjoint therapy for the treatment of domestic violence. In A. R. Roberts (Ed.), *Battered women and their families: Intervention strategies and treatment programs* (pp. 33–48). New York: Springer.

Gelles, R. J. (1976). Abused wives: Why do they stay. *Journal of Marriage & the Family, 38*, 659–668.

Gelles, R. J. (1982). Toward better research on child abuse and neglect: A response to Besharov. *Child Abuse and Neglect, 6*, 495–496.

Gentry, C. E., & Eaddy, V. B. (1980). Treatment of children in spouse abusive families. *Victimology: An International Journal, 5*, 240–250.

Giaretto, H. (1981). A comprehensive child sexual abuse treatment program. *Child Abuse and Neglect, 5*, 263–278.

Goldberg, W. G., & Tomlanovich, M. C. (1984). Domestic violence in the Emergency Department: New findings. *Journal of the American Medical Association, 251*, 3259–3264.

Green, A. H., Power, E., Steinbook, B., & Gaines, R. (1981). Factors associated with successful and unsuccessful intervention with child abusive families. *Child Abuse and Neglect, 5*, 45–52.

Herman, J., & Hirschman, L. (1981). *Father–daughter incest*. Cambridge, MA: Harvard University Press.

Hershey, D. (April, 1982). *Domestic violence: Children reared in explosive homes*. Paper presented at the annual meeting of the Eastern Psychological Association, Baltimore, MD.

Hershorn, M., & Rosenbaum, A. (1985). Children of marital violence: A closer look at the unintended victims. *American Journal of Orthopsychiatry, 55*, 260–266.

Hilberman, E., & Munson, K. (1978). Sixty battered women. *Victimology: An International Journal, 3*, 460–471.

Hoffman-Plotkin, D., & Twentyman, C. J. (1984). A multimodal assessment of behavioral and cognitive deficits in abused and neglected preschoolers. *Child Development, 55*, 794–802.

Hughes, H. M. (1982). Brief interventions with children in a battered women's shelter: A model preventive program. *Family Relations, 31*, 495–502.

Hughes, H. M., & Barad, S. J. (1983). Psychological functioning of children in shelters for battered women: A preliminary investigation. *American Journal of Orthopsychiatry, 53*, 525–531.

Hughes, H. M., & Hampton, K. L. (August, 1984). Relationships between the affective functioning of mothers and their children. In H. M. Hughes (Chair), *Impact of marital and family violence on children in shelters*. Symposium conducted at the annual meeting of the American Psychological Association, Toronto.

Hughes, H. M., Rau, T. J., Hampton, K. L., & Sablatura, B. (August, 1985). Effects of family violence on child victims and witnesses. In M. Rosenberg (Chair). *Mediating factors in adjustment of child witnesses to family violence*. Symposium presented at the annual meeting of the American Psychological Association, Los Angeles, CA.

Jason, J. (1984). Centers for Disease Control and the epidemiology of violence. *Child Abuse and Neglect, 8*, 279–382.

Jouriles, E. N., & O'Leary, K. D. (1985). Interspousal reliability of reports of marital violence. *Journal of Consulting and Clinical Psychology, 53,* 419–421.

Keller, H. R., & Erne, D. (1983). Child abuse: Toward a comprehensive model. In A. P. Goldstein (Ed.), *Prevention and control of aggression* (pp. 1–36). New York: Pergamon Press.

Kendall, P. C., & Norton-Ford, J. D. (1982). Therapy outcome research methods. In P. C. Kendall & J. N. Butcher (Eds.), *Handbook of research methods in clinical psychology* (pp. 429–460). New York: Wiley-Interscience.

Kercher, G. A., & McShane, M. (1984). The prevalence of child sexual abuse victimization in an adult sample of Texas residents. *Child Abuse and Neglect, 8,* 495–501.

Kinard, E. M. (1985). Ethical issues in research with abused children. *Child Abuse and Neglect, 9,* 301–311.

Klein, D. (1982) *The problem of multiple perception in families.* Unpublished manuscript, University of Notre Dame.

Kraft, S. P., Sullivan-Hanson, J., Christopoulos, C., Cohn, D. A., & Emery, R. A. (August, 1984). *Spouse abuse: Its impact on children's psychological adjustment.* Paper presented at the annual meeting of the American Psychological Association, Toronto.

Kroth, J. E. (1979). *Child sexual abuse: Analysis of a family therapy approach.* Springfield, IL: Charles C Thomas.

Krugman, R. D. (1985). The coming decade: Unfinished tasks and new frontiers. *Child Abuse and Neglect, 9,* 119–121.

LaBell, L. S. (1979). Wife abuse: A sociological study of battered women and their mates. *Victimology: An International Journal, 4,* 258–267.

Lahey, B. B., Conger, R. D., Atkeson, B. M., & Treiber, F. A. (1984). Parenting behavior and emotional status of physically abusive mothers. *Journal of Consulting and Clinical Psychology, 52,* 1062–1071.

Leventhal, J. M. (1982). Research strategies and methodologic standards in studies of risk factors for child abuse. *Child Abuse and Neglect, 6,* 113–123.

Margolin, G., John, R., Gleferman, L., Miller, C., & Reynold, N. (August, 1985). Abusive and nonabusive couples' affective responses to conflictual discussions. In R. A. Geffner (Chair), *Violent couples; Current research and new directions for family psychologists.* Symposium presented at the annual meeting of the American Psychological Association, Los Angeles, CA.

Martin, J. (1983). Maternal and paternal abuse of children: Theoretical and research perspectives. In D. Finkelhor, R. J. Gelles, G. T. Hotaling, & M. A. Straus, (Eds.), *The dark side of families: Current family violence research* (pp. 293–304). Beverly Hills, CA: Sage.

McClelland, R. W., & Battle, S. F. (1984). Applying social epidemiology to child abuse. *Social Casework, 65,* 212–218.

Meiselman, K. C. (1980). Personality characteristics of incest history psychotherapy patients: A research note. *Archives of Social Behavior, 9,* 195–197.

Milner, J. S., Gold, R. G., Ayoub, C., & Jacewitz, M. M. (1984). Predictive validity of the Child Abuse Potential Inventory. *Journal of Consulting and Clinical Psychology, 52,* 879–884.

Mrazek, P. B., & Mrazek, D. A. (1981). The effects of child sexual abuse: Methodological considerations. In P. B. Mrazek, & C. H. Kempe (Eds.), *Sexually abused children and their families* (pp. 235–245). New York: Pergamon Press.

Murphy, S., Orkow, B., & Nicola, R. M. (1985). Prenatal prediction of child abuse and neglect: A prospective study. *Child Abuse and Neglect, 9,* 225–235.

National Center on Child Abuse and Neglect. (1981). *Study Findings: National Study of the Incidence and Severity of Child Abuse and Neglect.* DHHS Pub. #(OHDS) 81-30325, Washington, DC.

Plotkin, R. C., Azar, S., Twentyman, C. T., & Perri, M. G. (1981). A critical evaluation of the research methodology employed in the investigation of causative factors of child abuse and neglect. *Child Abuse and Neglect, 5,* 449–455.

Polansky, N. A., Gaudin, J. M., Ammons, P. W., & Davis, K. B. (1985). The psychological ecology of the neglectful mother. *Child Abuse and Neglect, 9,* 265–274.

Porter, B., & O'Leary, K. D. (1980). Marital discord and childhood behavior problems. *Journal of Abnormal Child Psychology, 8,* 287–295.

Post, R. D., Willett, A. B., Franks, R. D., House, R. M., & Back, S. M. (1982). Childhood exposure to violence among victims and perpetrators of spouse battering. *Victimology: An International Journal, 6,* 156–166.

Rivara, F. P. (1985). Physical abuse in children under two: A study of therapeutic outcomes. *Child Abuse and Neglect, 9,* 81–87.

Rosenbaum, A., & O'Leary, K. D. (1981). Children: The unintended victims of marital violence. *American Journal of Orthopsychiatry, 51,* 692–699.

Rosenbaum, A., & O'Leary, K. D. (1986). Treatment of marital violence. In N. Jacobson, & A. Gurman (Eds.), *Clinical handbook of marital therapy* (385–405). New York: Guilford Press.

Rosenberg, M. S. (August, 1984). Intergenerational family violence: A critique and implications for witnessing children. In H. M. Hughes (Chair), *Impact of marital and family violence on children in shelters.* Symposium conducted at the annual meeting of the American Psychological Association, Toronto.

Rosewater, L. (August, 1984). *MMPI patterns of abused wives.* Paper presented at the Second Family Violence Research Conference, Durham, NH.

Rounsaville, B. J. (1978). Battered wives—Barriers to identification and treatment. *American Journal of Orthopsychiatry, 48,* 487–494.

Russell, D. E. H. (1983). The incidence and prevalence of intrafamilial and extrafamilial sexual abuse of female children. *Child Abuse and Neglect, 7,* 133–146.

Russell, D. E. H. (1984). The prevalence and seriousness of incestuous abuse: Stepfathers vs. biological fathers. *Child Abuse and Neglect, 8,* 15–22.

Sablatura, B. (1985). *Mediating variables in the short- and long-term effects of child sexual abuse.* Unpublished master's thesis. University of Arkansas.

Smetana, J. G., Kelly, M., & Twentyman, C. J. (1984). Abused, neglected, and nonmaltreated children's conceptions of moral and social-conventional transgressions. *Child Development, 55,* 277–287.

Smith, J. E. (1984). Non-accidental injury to children—I: A review of behavioral interventions. *Behavioral Research and Therapy, 22,* 331–347.

Smith, J. E., & Rachman, S. J. (1984). Non-accidental injury to children—II: A controlled evaluation of a behavioral management programme. *Behavioral Research and Therapy, 22,* 349–366.

Smith, J. E., Rachman, S. J., & Yule, B. (1984). Non-accidental injury to children—III: Methodological problems of evaluative treatment research. *Behavioral Research and Therapy, 22,* 367–383.

Smith, S. L. (1984). Significant research findings in the etiology of child abuse. *Social Casework, 65,* 337–346.

Snyder, D. K., & Fruchtman, L. A. (1981). Differential patterns of wife abuse: A data-based typology. *Journal of Consulting & Clinical Psychology, 49,* 878–885.

Straus, M. A. (1979). Measuring intrafamily conflict and violence: The Conflict Tactics Scales. *Journal of Marriage & the Family, 41,* 75–88.

Straus, M. A., Gelles, R. J., & Steinmetz, S. K. (1980). *Behind closed doors: Violence in the American family.* New York: Anchor Press/Doubleday.

Szinovacz, M. E. (1983). Using couple data as a methodological tool: The case of marital violence. *Journal of Marriage & the Family, 45,* 633–644.

Tasi, M., Feldman-Summers, S., & Edgar, M. (1979). Child molestation: Variables related to differential impacts on psychosexual functioning in adult women. *Journal of Abnormal Psychology, 88,* 407–417.

Telch, C. F., & Lindquist, C. U. (1984). Violent versus nonviolent couples: A comparison of patterns. *Psychotherapy, 21,* 242–248.

Tierney, K. J., & Corwin, D. L. (1983). Exploring intrafamilial child sexual abuse: A systems approach. In D. Finkelhor, R. J. Gelles, G. T. Hotaling, & M. A. Straus (Eds.), *The dark side of families: Current family violence research* (pp. 102–116). Beverly Hills, CA: Sage.

Walker, L. E. (1979). *The battered woman.* New York: Harper & Row.

Walker, L. E. (1983). Victimology and the psychological perspectives of battered women. *Victimology: An International Journal, 8,* 82–104.

Walker, L. E. (1984). *The battered woman syndrome.* New York: Springer.

Webster-Stratton, C. (1985). Comparison of abusive and nonabusive families with conduct-disordered children. *American Journal of Orthopsychiatry, 55,* 59–69.

Wodarski, J. S. (1981). Treatment of parents who abuse their children: A literature review and implications for professionals. *Child Abuse and Neglect, 5,* 351–360.

Wolfe, D. A., Jaffe, P. J., Wilson, S., & Zak, L. (August, 1984). Impact of family violence upon children's adjustment. In H. M. Hughes (Chair), *Impact of marital and family violence upon children in shelters.* Symposium conducted at the annual meeting of the American Psychological Association, Toronto.

Wolfe, D. A., Zak, L., Wilson, S., & Jaffe, P. (1986). Child witnesses to violence between parents: Critical issues in behavioral and social adjustment. *Journal of Abnormal Child Psychology, 14,* 95–104.

Author Index

483

Subject Index

DATE DUE

APR 1 0 '02			
APR 1 5 '02			
1 20 '02			
JUN 2 0 '02			
JUN 2 5 '02			
NOV 0 3 2003			

HIGHSMITH #45115